Ophthalmology
Clinical and
Surgical Principles

Ophthalmology
Clinical and Surgical Principles

Louis E. Probst, MD
National Medical Director and Surgeon
TLC The Laser Eye Centers
Chicago, Illinois

Volunteer Clinical Assistant Professor
Department of Ophthalmology
University of Wisconsin School of Medicine and Public Health
Madison, Wisconsin

Julie H. Tsai, MD
Clinical Assistant Professor
Albany Medical College
Albany, New York

George Goodman, OD
Senior Manager of Clinical Affairs
Refocus Group, Inc
Dallas, Texas

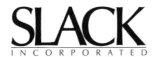

SLACK
INCORPORATED

WW
39
061
2012

Published by: SLACK Incorporated
                  6900 Grove Road
                  Thorofare, NJ 08086 USA
                  Telephone: 856-848-1000
                  Fax: 856-848-6091
                  www.slackbooks.com

Contact SLACK Incorporated for more information about other books in this field or about the availability of our books from distributors outside the United States.

Library of Congress Cataloging-in-Publication Data

Ophthalmology : clinical and surgical principles / [editedy by] Louis E. Probst, Julie H. Tsai, George Goodman.
     p. ; cm.
  Includes bibliographical references and index.
  ISBN 978-1-55642-735-0 (pbk.)
  I. Probst, Louis E. II. Tsai, Julie H. III. Goodman, George, OD.
  [DNLM: 1. Eye Diseases--diagnosis--Handbooks. 2. Eye Diseases--therapy--Handbooks. 3. Ophthalmologic Surgical Procedures--Handbooks. WW 39]

  617.7--dc23
                         2011037584

Dedication

To my wife, Kate, and three children, Louis, Coleson, and Parker. You are my greatest challenge and inspiration.

Louis E. Probst, MD

To my daughter, Sofia, who has opened my eyes to new possibilities; my husband, Tom, who consistently inspires me and always supports me 100% in all aspects of my life; and to my students, who continue to teach me as much as I strive to teach them.

Julie H. Tsai, MD

To my children, Aaron, Hannah, Ethan, and Ryan. Never quit striving to be the best you can be. You are my inspiration and my joy. I am so incredibly proud of each of you.

George Goodman, OD

Contents

Acknowledgments

All books of this depth and scope become collaborative efforts. This book would not have been completed without the assistance of George Goodman, OD, who managed to resurrect this project with his significant tenacity and editorial prowess. Julie H. Tsai, MD also stepped in to assist in the middle of the process and provided 2 excellent chapters. I must also thank the staff of SLACK Incorporated, particularly John Bond, Jennifer Briggs, and Amy McShane for their unrelenting support and confidence during the long and challenging editorial process that seemed insurmountable on several occasions. Finally, I thank all of the authors who have shown incredible patience with this project after so many questions, e-mails, and revisions. Without this incredible collection of talented and industrious individuals, this book would not have come to fruition.

Louis E. Probst, MD

I thank my coeditors for their tenacity and perseverance: Dr. Probst for his faith and patience when it seemed that the vision for this book would not come to pass; and Dr. Goodman for his endless efforts in making that vision a reality. I also thank the staff at SLACK Incorporated for their support and assistance through the entire process.

Julie H. Tsai, MD

I would like to thank Dr. Lou Probst for being a great mentor and for giving me the opportunity to contribute to this book project. I would also like to thank my wife for being incredibly supportive and patient during the countless hours of working on this manuscript.

George Goodman, OD

About the Editors

As National Medical Director of TLC The Laser Eye Centers, the largest laser vision provider in North America, *Louis E. Probst, MD* has performed over 100,000 LASIK procedures over 16 years; has written 5 reference textbooks on refractive surgery and LASIK, over 80 book chapters on ophthalmology and LASIK, and over 50 articles in peer-reviewed publications; and has designed 10 instruments for LASIK. Dr. Probst has given hundreds of lectures at national and international level meetings on his various innovations and insights into improving patient outcomes in ophthalmology and refractive surgery.

Dr. Probst has been an innovator in many refractive surgery techniques that include the treatment of LASIK flap striae, cross cylinder ablation techniques for the treatment of high mixed astigmatism, bioptics for the correction of high hyperopic astigmatism, single-use instrumentation for LASIK, flap/zap femtosecond LASIK, custom zone CustomVue LASIK, and customized oval flap LASIK techniques.

Dr. Probst serves as the chief surgeon at several TLC laser center locations in Illinois, Wisconsin, South Carolina, and Florida and is a member of the Clinical Advisory Group of TLC to which provides guidance and recommendation for over 500 ophthalmologists and 5000 optometrists who work within the TLC system. Dr. Probst also serves as a trainer and educator at TLC for surgeons interested in learning about the latest techniques and technology. Dr. Probst also trains residents and fellows in ophthalmology as a volunteer assistant professor at the University of Wisconsin.

Julie H. Tsai, MD is an Assistant Professor of Ophthalmology and is heavily involved in resident training. She has served as the Residency Program Director for 2 training programs and continues to promote ophthalmic education and mentorship through her work in various committees and organizations on both local and national levels. She has written several chapters and peer-reviewed publications and has been an invited lecturer on topics involving anterior segment reconstruction, cornea, and uveitis.

George Goodman, OD currently serves as the Senior Manager of Clinical Affairs for Refocus Group, Inc, in Dallas, Texas. Prior to working for a medical device company, Dr. Goodman served as the Clinical Director at TLC The Laser Eye Centers in Chicago where he worked for the National Medical Director, Dr. Louis E. Probst. Before relocating to Chicago, Dr. Goodman was the Co-Founder and Clinical Director of Advanced Laser Center of Oklahoma in his hometown of Oklahoma City, Oklahoma. He began his career by working with his father and grandfather in private practice.

Dr. Goodman has the following associations: Board Member of the Optometric Council on Refractive Technology (OCRT); Co-Founder of the Optometric Education Council of America (OEC); Speaker—Inspire, Allergan, Alcon, Zeiss; Adjunct Faculty—Northeastern State University Oklahoma College of Optometry; Member—American Optometric Association (AOA), Oklahoma Association of Optometric Physicians (OAOP), and Illinois Optometric Association (IOA). Dr. Goodman previously served on the Board of Directors and the Medical Advisory Board for the Oklahoma Lupus Association. Dr. Goodman has written and published 3 books. He also served as the author and executive editor of "Focus on Co-Management," TLC The Laser Eye Center's monthly affiliate newsletter.

Contributing Authors

Peter Bergenske, OD (Chapters 2 and 3)
Director of Professional and Clinical Support
Alcon Laboratories, Inc.
Fort Worth, Texas

Catherine M. Birt, MA, MD, FRCS(C) (Chapter 8)
Associate Professor
Department of Ophthalmology and Vision Sciences
University of Toronto
Toronto, Ontario, Canada

Louis C. Blumenfeld, MD (Chapter 10)
Clinical Instructor
University of Central Florida School of Medicine
Orlando, Florida

Paul Ernest, MD (Chapter 9)
Associate Clinical Professor
Kresge Eye Institute
Wayne State Univeristy
Detroit, Michigan

Founder
TLC Eyecare of Michigan
Jackson, Michigan

Thomas J. Federici, MD (Chapter 12)
RETINAcare Consultants
Albany, New York

Robert S. Gold, MD (Chapter 10)
Pediatric Ophthalmology and Adult Eye Muscle Disorders
Eye Physicians of Central Florida, A Division of Florida Pediatric Associates, LLC
Maitland and Orlando, Florida

Khalid Hasanee, MD, FRCS(C) (Chapter 8)
Assistant Clinical Professor,
Division of Ophthalmology, Department of Surgery
Michael G. DeGroote School of Medicine, McMaster University
Hamilton, Ontario, Canada

Edward J. Holland, MD (Chapter 6)
Director, Cornea Service
Cincinnati Eye Institute
Professor of Ophthalmology
University of Cincinnati
Cincinnati, Ohio

T. Mark Johnson, MD, FRCS(C) (Chapter 13)
Attending Surgeon
Retina Group of Washington
Chevy Chase, Maryland

Clinical Assistant Professor
Georgetown University
Washington, D.C.

Jemshed A. Khan, MD (Chapter 5)
Clinical Professor of Ophthalmology
Kansas University School of Medicine
Kansas City, Kansas

Khan Eyelid and Facial Plastic Surgery
Overland Park, Kansas

Andrew G. Lee, MD (Chapter 11)
Chair, Department of Ophthalmology
The Methodist Hospital
Houston, Texas

Professor of Ophthalmology, Neurology, and Neurosurgery
Weill Cornell Medical College

Adjunct Professor of Ophthalmology
The University of Iowa and Baylor College of Medicine

Clinical Professor of Ophthalmology
The University of Texas Medical Branch
Galveston, Texas

Irmingard Neuhann, MD (Chapter 9)
Private Practice
Munich, Germany

Thomas Neuhann, MD (Chapter 9)
Director
Eye Center
Prof. Neuhann & Colleagues
Munich, Germany

Director
Eye Department
Red Cross Hospital
Munich, Germany

Paul Rafuse, PhD, MD, FRCS(C) (Chapter 4)
Associate Professor
Dalhousie University
Department of Ophthalmology and Visual Sciences
Halifax, Nova Scotia, Canada

Naval Sondhi, MD (Chapter 10)
Consultant
Pediatric Ophthalmologist
Midwest Eye Institute
Indianapolis, Indiana

Jeff Steeves, MD, CCFP, FRCS(C) (Chapter 1)
Lecturer
Faculty of Medicine
Dalhousie University
Halifax, Nova Scotia, Canada

Preface

Why write another ophthalmology book when there are already several quality books available? After careful review and analysis, we believed that it was possible to create a better one—a book that was comprehensive enough to be useful for an ophthalmology resident but practical enough to be a resource for the family doctor or the ophthalmic technician and a book that was easy to read so the information could be rapidly assimilated. In other words, our goal was to create a book that we would enjoy using ourselves.

A great book requires great authors. We were fortunate to be able to benefit from the expertise of world experts in each of the subspecialties of ophthalmology. Each of these authors is a recognized leader in his or her field and has written papers and books on the subject of his or her chapter. Our job as editors was simply to ensure the consistency between each of these excellent contributions.

As with our experience with previous publications that we have authored and edited, this project required more than 100-fold the effort than was originally anticipated with the genesis of the original concept. The fruits of this effort can be seen by the quality of the final product, with well-organized, consistent structure and hundreds of beautiful illustrations. We hope that the reader finds this a valuable resource.

Foreword

Although Darwin was able to persuade much of the world that a modern eye could be produced gradually from a much simpler structure, he did not even attempt to explain how the simple light sensitive spot that was his starting point actually worked.
Michael Behe

As an editor, Dr. Louis Probst has previously orchestrated several books in his area of special expertise, refractive surgery, which now serve as the foundations for the knowledge of that specialty. Now, demonstrating amazing energy and a career-long commitment to education, he delivers a superb work covering a broader range of topics. *Ophthalmology: Clinical and Surgical Principles* again demonstrates his ability to create a book focused on the needs of the practicing ophthalmologist or eye care professional.

This book is appropriately arranged into 2 sections: Basic Sciences and Clinical Sciences. Within the Basic Sciences section, the anatomy chapter is unusually interesting due to the numerous beautiful illustrations, detailed information, and occasional injection of a clinical pearl that keeps the material relevant. The chapters on pharmacology, optics, and the ocular exam are appropriate, relevant, and concise. These chapters will likely serve as reference material for the reader of the more clinical chapters that follow. The Clinical Sciences section is composed of chapters that represent each of the subspecialties of ophthalmology. While each chapter is authored by different experts in each field, there is an impressive level of consistency in the format of each chapter, which all contain an impressive collection of illustrations and the generous use of tables to allow easy assimilation of comparison of information. There is clearly an effort to be comprehensive; however, there is also particular attention paid to the more common ocular diseases. The most modern concepts, medications, technology, and techniques are all addressed within each subspecialty chapter.

In summary, this is a book that is current, concise yet comprehensive, and targeted to provide information that will improve clinical and surgical care to the benefit of patients. The selected authors are all experts with wide experience in their field. The writing and format is consistent and easy to read. The illustrations are numerous and of excellent quality. I found within each chapter several clinical pearls and nuggets of wisdom to apply in my own practice. While there are many textbooks in this arena, the clinical ophthalmologist who invests in this book will be rewarded. Dr. Probst and colleagues, thank you for sharing your experience and knowledge.

Richard L. Lindstrom, MD
Founder and Attending Surgeon, Minnesota Eye Consultants
Adjunct Professor Emeritus, University of Minnesota, Department of Ophthalmology
Associate Director, Minnesota Lions Eye Bank

Introduction

There are 10 keys concepts and unique features that have been applied in this book with the goal of making it comprehensive, practical, and readable.

1. **Subspecialty organization:** Many general ophthalmology books are organized anatomically, which does not reflect the way modern-day ophthalmology is practiced. If a student is on a retina rotation, he or she should be able to study and think about the retina and vitreous like a retinal specialist. Therefore, each subspecialty of ophthalmology is represented by a specific chapter.

2. **Consistent point form layout:** Long paragraphs can be difficult to assimilate when the reader is looking for the salient information quickly in the clinical setting. We have used the standard subject headings of definition, etiology, symptoms, signs, differential diagnosis, evaluation, management, and prognosis whenever appropriate.

3. **Practical emphasis:** While each chapter is comprehensive and concise, there is clear emphasis on the common disease presentations for each area so that the information learned can be applied to the real world.

4. **Succinct synopsis of the fundamentals:** While the clinical aspects of ophthalmology are of the most practical value, the fundamentals of anatomy, pharmacology, optics, and the ocular exam are key components to understanding the full spectrum of ocular disease.

5. **Intelligent presentation:** While this book will appeal to a broad audience, it aims for the educational level of an ophthalmology resident.

6. **Surgical descriptions:** This area is often omitted from general ophthalmology texts; however, ophthalmology is a surgical specialty. Readers will be interested and inspired to learn about the surgical options for the disorders.

7. **Pictures:** Ophthalmology is a visual specialty so high-quality pictures are essential. This book has an incredible collection of more than 400 color figures.

8. **Tables:** Summary tables are excellent learning aids. This book attempts to make use of tables whenever appropriate.

9. **Suggested readings:** Suggested readings for the key papers or studies provide a starting point for those readers interested in the source or authors for further information.

10. **Study questions:** The study questions at the end of each chapter allow readers to test their knowledge and prepare for examinations.

SECTION I

BASIC SCIENCES

Anatomy of the Eye and Orbit

Jeff Steeves, MD, CCFP, FRCS(C)

Outline

Probst LE, Tsai JH.
Ophthalmology: Clinical and Surgical Principles (pp. 3–52).
© 2012 SLACK Incorporated

Introduction

A solid knowledge of the anatomy of the eye and orbit is important for a full understanding of the functioning of the normal ocular system and is crucial for the diagnostic interpretation of the signs and symptoms of a diseased state. This overview will approach the eye from the surface. The structures will be explored anterior to posterior, similar to how patients are examined.

Eyelids

Eyelid Margin
- 2-mm thick and 30-mm long

Anterior Lamellae
- Composed of skin and orbicularis muscle

Posterior Lamellae
- Composed of the tarsal plate and conjunctiva

Palpebral Fissure
- The space, or opening, between the lids
- Maximum width is at junction of the nasal and middle third in Caucasians and African Americans, and at the midpoint in Asians.
- Temporal flare is the lateral shift of this maximum width in patients with thyroid eye disease.

Upper Eyelid
- Larger and more mobile than the lower eyelid
- When open, the lid margin crosses the corneal limbus around 10 and 2 o'clock.
- When closed, it covers the entire cornea and ocular surface.

Lower Eyelid

- Sits at the lower limbus, with the lid margin crossing the corneal limbus at 4 and 8 o'clock positions
- Rises only slightly with lid closure

Lateral Canthus

- The eyelids meet at the lateral canthus and form a 60-degree angle.
- The lateral canthus lies 2 mm higher than the medial canthus in Caucasians and African Americans and 5 mm higher in Asians.

Medial Canthus

- The upper and lower lids meet at the medial canthus, which sits 6-mm nasal to the eye.
- The medial 5 mm of eyelid is slightly elevated with the punctum lacrimale at the summit. The opening is 0.4 to 0.6 mm in diameter. The punctum extends into the tear lake sitting over the caruncle.

Eyelashes

- Short, thick, curved hairs
- Typically darker than scalp hair
- Do not gray with age
- Replaced every 100 to 150 days
- Upper eyelid has approximately 150 eyelashes
- Lower eyelid has approximately 75 eyelashes
- Aligned in 2 to 3 rows
- Emerge from the anterior border of the eyelids

Glands

- Sebaceous glands of Zeis open into each follicle.
- Ciliary glands of Moll produce sweat exit within or between each follicle.
- Meibomian gland
  - Orifices exit the posterior aspect of the lid margin and mark the junction between eyelid skin and conjunctiva.

Gray Line

- Can sometimes be seen running along the lid margin between lashes and meibomian gland orifices
- Delineates a vestigial structure called Riolan's muscle and represents the division of anterior and posterior lamellae of the lid
- This plane can be surgically split with minimal scarring.

Layers of the Eyelid

Skin

- Thinnest in body, 0.5-mm keratinized stratified squamous epithelium

Subcutaneous Tissue

- Loose, elastic fibers, almost devoid of fat

Orbicularis Oculi

- Striated muscle, closer to skin than any other muscle (Figure 1-1)
  - Palpebral portion
    - Arises from anterior and posterior lacrimal crests and contributes to medial canthal tendon
    - Sweeps elliptically around eye joining the lateral palpebral raphe
    - Small bundle of muscles at lid margin becomes Riolan's muscle

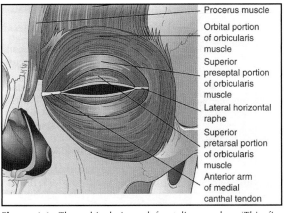

Figure 1-1. The orbicularis and frontalis muscles. (This figure was published in *Atlas of Clinical and Surgical Orbital Anatomy.* Dutton JJ., Copyright Elsevier [1994].)

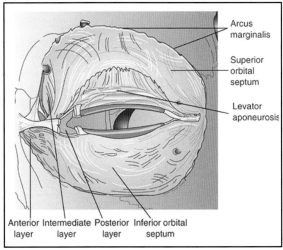

Figure 1-2. The orbital septum. (This figure was published in *Atlas of Clinical and Surgical Orbital Anatomy.* Dutton JJ., Copyright Elsevier [1994].)

- o Pretarsal section over tarsus
  - ▪ Overlies orbital septum and is responsible for blinking reflex and nasolacrimal duct pumping
- o Orbital portion
  - ▪ Extends concentrically from the lid to the orbital rim and onto the cheek and temple
  - ▪ Responsible for voluntary eye closure

Orbital Septum

- Dense fibrous sheath separates eyelids from orbital fat (Figure 1-2)
- Acts as a barrier against trauma and limits diffusion
- Fibrous layer originating at the orbital rim where it is continuous with periosteum
- Perforated by all nerves and vessels that leave the orbit
- Acts as a retaining wall for orbital fat. It is weakest in the inferior medial lid.
- With age, fat can prolapse from the orbital space into the lid.
- The septum acts as a barrier for infection (preseptal versus orbital cellulitis) and can restrict the migration of blood (ie, black eye). It also lies anterior to the following structures:
  - o Lacrimal gland (palpebral and orbital potion)
  - o Trochlea of superior oblique (SO)
  - o Lateral canthal tendon
  - o Orbital fat

Tarsal Plates

- Dense fibrous tissue (not cartilage) that give eyelids firmness and shape (Figure 1-3)
- 25-mm long, 1-mm thick
- Upper lid tarsus is 10-mm wide, and lower lid tarsus is 5-mm wide.
- Attachments of upper tarsus include the orbital septum and levator.
- The septum and lower lid retractors (capsule-palpebral fascia) attach to the lower tarsal plate
- Müller's muscle (superior tarsal muscle) is a sympathetically driven muscle originating on the undersurface (deep) of levator and attaching to the upper surface of upper tarsus. It assists in eyelid elevation. There is a similar muscle in the lower eyelid.
- Embedded within the tarsal plates are 25 modified sebaceous glands (meibomian glands) consisting of a central canal connecting 10 to 15 acini. The oily secretion helps retard tear evaporation.

Tendons and Ligaments

- Canthal tendons (Figure 1-4)
  - o Extensions of the orbicularis muscle that attach to the periorbital (periosteum) of the bones

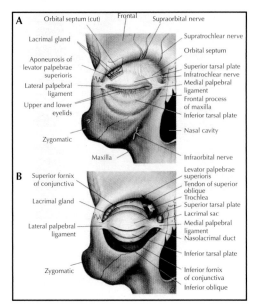

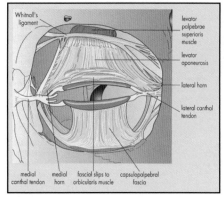

Figure 1-4. The levator aponeurosis and the medial and lateral canthal tendons. (This figure was published in *Atlas of Clinical and Surgical Orbital Anatomy.* Dutton JJ., Copyright Elsevier [1994].)

Figure 1-3. Right eye. (A) The superior and inferior tarsal plates, orbital septum, and lacrimal gland. (B) The superior and inferior tarsal plates, conjunctiva, and lacrimal gland, sac, and duct. (*Clinical Anatomy of the Eye.* Snell RS, Lemp MA. Copyright © 1989. Reproduced with permission of Blackwell Scientific Publications.)

Medial Canthal Tendon

- More complex than the lateral
- Holds the tarsal plate and lid medially
- Divides in 2
    - Anterior limb attaches to the frontal process of the maxilla of the anterior lacrimal crest.
    - Posterior limb attaches to posterior lacrimal crest. The 2 limbs surround the nasolacrimal sac.
- The lower border of the ligament is distinct with an indefinite upper border.

Lateral Canthal Tendon

- Poorly developed and attaches to a lateral tubercle of the zygomatic bone
- Posterior to the lateral raphe of the orbicularis

Nerve Supply of Eyelids

Sensory

- Upper lid (cranial nerve branch V1)
    - Branches include the following:
        - Infratrochlear
        - Supratrochlear
        - Supraorbital
        - Lacrimal
- Lower lid (cranial nerve branch V2)
    - The infraorbital nerve of V2 (the terminal portion of the maxillary). The infratrochlear contributes to the medial aspect.

Motor

- CN VII
    - Temporal and zygomatic branches to orbicularis muscle

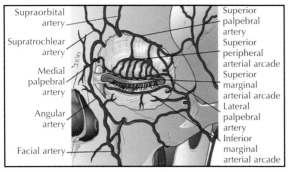

Figure 1-5. Arterial supply of the eyelids. (This figure was published in *Atlas of Clinical and Surgical Orbital Anatomy*. Dutton JJ., Copyright Elsevier [1994].)

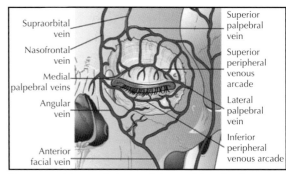

Figure 1-6. Venous drainage of the eyelids. (This figure was published in *Atlas of Clinical and Surgical Orbital Anatomy*. Dutton JJ., Copyright Elsevier [1994].)

- CN III
  - ○ Levator and extraocular muscle (EOM)
- Sympathetic nervous system (SNS)
  - ○ Müller's and inferior tarsus muscles

Arterial Supply of Eyelids

Lateral Lid

- Internal carotid artery (ICA) → ophthalmic artery → lacrimal artery → superior and inferior lateral palpebral arteries → peripheral and marginal arterial arcade (Figure 1-5)

Medial Lid

- External carotid artery → facial artery → angular artery → inferior and superior palpebral arteries → peripheral and marginal arterial arcades

Marginal Arcade

- 3 mm from lid margin between orbicularis and tarsus

Peripheral Arcade

- Near lid crease between orbicularis and septum
- Arcades anastomose with themselves and receive blood supply from surrounding vessels and posterior route (ICA → ophthalmic artery → muscular branches → anterior ciliary artery → posterior conjunctival artery → anastomose to arterial arcades).
- The peripheral and margin arcades allow anastomoses of ICA and external carotid artery circulation.

Venous Drainage of Eyelids

- Numerous small veins drain the lids (Figure 1-6).
  - ○ Superior drainage goes into the supraorbital and then the superior orbital vein in the orbit.
  - ○ Lateral drainage involves the superficial temporal to internal jugular vein.
  - ○ Medial drainage includes the angular vein to the internal jugular vein.
  - ○ Deeper lid structures are drained by the orbital veins.

Lymphatic Drainage

Submandibular

- Drain the medial one-third of the upper lid and the medial two-thirds of the lower lid

Preauricular

- Drain the lateral two-thirds of the upper lid and the lateral one-third of the lower lid

Retractors of the Eyelids

- Serve to open the eyes

Upper Eyelid

Levator Palpebrae Superioris Muscle

- Strong striated muscle that elevates the upper lid
- Muscular portion is 40 mm in length
- Aponeurotic portion is 14- to 20-mm long
- Originates at the lesser wing of the sphenoid above the annulus of Zinn (above optic canal)
- Aponeurosis descends posterior to the orbital septum to insert on the upper anterior surface of the tarsal plate.
- Tendinous fibers pierce orbital septum and orbicularis to attach anteriorly to skin, creating the upper lid crease.
- Aponeurosis is wider than the levator muscle belly.
- Lateral expansion, called horn, attaches to the zygomatic tubercle along with the lateral canthal tendon.
- Medial expansion fuses with the orbital septum and medial canthal tendon.
- Nerve supply
  - Superior branch of the oculomotor nerve (CN III) that passes through or, less commonly, around the superior rectus (SR) muscle to enter the inferior surface of levator
- Clinically, stretching or dehiscence of the levator aponeurosis with age results in ptosis, lid thinning, and upward migration or loss of the lid crease. Lid excursion may remain normal.

Müller's Muscle

- Thin sheet of smooth muscle arises from the inner surface of the aponeurosis starting at about Whitnall's ligament and inserting onto the upper edge of the tarsal plate.
- 12- to 15-mm long, thin
- Raises eyelid about 2 mm
- Nerve supply
  - Sympathetic fibers from ICA
- Blood supply
  - Peripheral arterial arcade (between aponeurosis and Müller's muscle)
- Clinically, fear, excitement, or hyperthyroidism that activates the sympathetically driven Müller's muscle can enhance upper (and lower) lid retraction. Damage to the sympathetic chain (Horner's syndrome) can cause mild lid ptosis.

Whitnall's Ligament

- Condensation of levator muscle sheath attaching medial to trochlea and laterally to orbital wall 10 mm above tubercle
- Laterally splits lacrimal gland into palpebral and orbital lobes
- The levator changes direction at Whitnall's, heading down to tarsus.
- Prevents excessive lid elevation

Lower Lid

Capsulopalpebral Fascia

- Analogous to levator aponeurosis
- Originates from inferior rectus (IR) sheath, divides to encircle inferior oblique (IO), reunites to form Lockwood's ligament, then fuses with orbital septum and attaches to inferior edge of tarsal plate

Lockwood's Suspensory Ligament

- Analogous to Whitnall's ligament
- Arises from capsulopalpebral fascia with horns spreading out diffusely medially and laterally
- Supports the globe from below

Inferior Tarsus Muscle

- Analogous to Müller's muscle
- Arising from and internal to capsulopalpebral fascia
- Sympathetic innervation

Conjunctiva

- Thin mucous membrane continuous from corneal epithelium to eyelid skin
- Histologically composed of nonkeratinized stratified columnar (2 to 5 layers) cells
- Transitions to nonkeratinized squamous epithelium near the limbus and near meibomian orifices of the eyelid
- Contains goblet cells that produce mucin
- Loose substantia propria provides the connective tissue base.
- Accessory lacrimal gland ducts (up to 50) open to the free surface of conjunctiva.

Palpebral Conjunctiva

- Thin mucous membrane adherent to tarsal plates (often called tarsal conjunctiva) and lining sulcus
- Difficult to grasp tarsal conjunctiva as it is tightly adherent to tarsus

Bulbar Conjunctiva

- Overlying globe, thin, translucent, and loosely attached to episcleral tissue
- Fusion at cornea is called conjunctival limbus
- Bulbar conjunctiva is only loosely adherent to underlying substantia propria in fornices, but becomes firmly attached to sclera at the limbus. This becomes a useful place to grasp with forceps when performing forced duction testing.

Conjunctival Fornices

- The potential spaces under the lids. Conjunctiva is loosely attached to fascial sheaths of the extraocular muscles and levator so will move with contraction.
- Superior fornix is 10 mm above limbus.
- Inferior fornix is 8 mm.
- Laterally, it increases to 14 mm.

Plica Semilunaris

- Narrow fold of bulbar conjunctiva near caruncle
- Vestigial nictitating membrane

Caruncle

- Tissue containing accessory dermal appendages (hair and glands) located in medial canthal area

Blood Supply

- Tarsal conjunctiva
  - o Marginal and peripheral arcades send deep branches.
- Fornices
  - o Peripheral arcade
- Bulbar conjunctiva
  - o Anterior ciliary arteries

Veins

- Numerous, draining to palpebral veins, or directly to superior or inferior ophthalmic veins

Nerves (Sensory)

- Bulbar conjunctiva receives innervations from anterior ciliary nerves (of nasociliary from V1).
- Superior fornix innervated by frontal and lacrimal branches of V1.
- Inferior fornix receives branches from infraorbital (of V2) medially and lacrimal (of V1) laterally.

Lacrimal Apparatus

- Includes
  - Lacrimal gland
  - Punctum
  - Lacrimal canaliculi
  - Lacrimal sac
  - Nasolacrimal duct
  - Nasal cavity

Lacrimal Gland

- Located in superior temporal anterior orbit
- Divided into 2 portions on the medial side by levator aponeurosis
  - Orbital (larger, superior)
    - Found in fossa of superolateral orbital rim (frontal bone) behind orbital septum
  - Palpebral (smaller, inferior)
    - One-third the size of orbital portion located beneath the levator and into upper lid
  - Twelve ducts pass from the orbital lobe through the palpebral lobe to enter the superior conjunctival fornix
- Histology
  - Arranged in a tubuloacinar structure consisting of columnar cells with central lumens
- Blood supply
  - Lacrimal artery
    - Supplied by the ophthalmic artery branch of the internal carotid
    - Also possibly supplied by the infraorbital artery with branches from the maxillary artery
- Nerve supply
  - Receives parasympathetic innervations from the lacrimal nerve
  - Pathway involves the secretory motor lacrimatory nucleus of facial nerve → sphenopalatine (pterygopalatine ganglion) → postganglionic fibers to maxillary nerve → zygomatic branch → zygomaticotemporal nerve → lacrimal nerve
  - Also receives sympathetic innervations via the following pathway:
    - Postganglionic fibers from superior cervical ganglion → internal carotid plexus → deep petrosal nerve → maxillary → zygomatic → zygomaticotemporal nerve → lacrimal nerve
  - Sensory innervations from CN V1 → lacrimal nerve

Punctum

- Opening in lid on slight elevation called the papilla lacrimalis
- Projects backward 2 degrees to tone of orbicularis into the tear lake
- Must be everted to visualize
- Superior is more medial than the inferior.

Lacrimal Canaliculi

- Histologically composed of thin elastic stratified squamous epithelium
- Vertical component, 2 mm; horizontal component, 8 mm
- Both run medially and at the junction with the lacrimal sac, they may (80% to 90%) or may not join to form common canaliculus.
- Enter lacrimal sac 2.5-mm below the apex
- Lie behind medial palpebral ligament and are surrounded by fibers of the orbicularis muscle
- During blink, canaliculi are shortened, pulled medially, and compressed to cause pumping action.

Lacrimal Sac

- Located in the lacrimal fossa of the lacrimal bone and frontal process of the maxilla
- 10-mm long
- Superior section of this blind sac is covered by periosteum and surrounded by medial canthal tendon
- Histologically composed of fibroelastic tissue lined by 2 layers of columnar cells
- Surrounded by lacrimal fascia. This is attached to the anterior and posterior lacrimal crests.
- Valve of Rosenmüller prevents reflex of fluid into the canaliculi.

Nasolacrimal Duct

- Connects lower end of the lacrimal sac with the inferior meatus of nose
- 18-mm long
- Proceeds inferiorly, angled in a posterolateral direction
- When passing a probe down the nasolacrimal duct, remember direction is down, back, and lateral
- Thinner in middle section
- Lies in nasolacrimal canal (formed by maxillary and lacrimal bone)
- Enters inferior meatus under inferior turbinate 2.5-mm posterior to nares
- Nasal opening partially covered by mucosal flap (Hasner's valve)
- Attached to the periosteum of canal
- Histologically consists of 2 layers of columnar epithelium, some ciliated, which line the duct

Nasal Cavity

- The nasal cavity (or nasal fossa) is a large air filled space above and behind the nose in the middle of the face.
- Function
  - The nasal cavity conditions the air to be received by the other areas of the respiratory tract. Owing to the large surface area provided by the nasal conchae, the air passing through the nasal cavity is warmed or cooled to within 1 degree of body temperature. In addition, the air is humidified, and dust and other particulate matter is removed by vibrissae, short, thick hairs present in the vestibule. The cilia of the respiratory epithelium move the particulate matter toward the pharynx where it passes into the esophagus and is digested in the stomach.
- Walls
  - The lateral wall of the nasal cavity is mainly made up by the maxilla; however, there is a deficiency that is compensated by the perpendicular plate of the palatine bone, the medial pterygoid plate, the labyrinth of the ethmoid and the inferior concha.
  - The nasal cavity is enclosed by the nasal bone above.
  - The floor of the nasal cavity, which forms the roof of the mouth, is made up by the bones of the hard palate: the horizontal plate of the palatine bone posteriorly and the palatine process of the maxilla anteriorly. To the front of the nasal cavity is the nose, while the back blends, via the choanae, into the nasopharynx. The paranasal sinuses are connected to the nasal cavity through small orifices called ostia.
  - The nasal cavity is divided in 2 by a vertical fin called the nasal septum. On the sides of the nasal cavity are 3 horizontal outgrowths called nasal conchae (singular "concha") or turbinates. These turbinates disrupt the airflow, directing air toward the olfactory epithelium on the surface of the turbinates and the septum. The vomeronasal organ is located at the back of the septum and has a role in pheromone detection.
- Cilia and mucus
  - Cilia and mucus along the inside wall of the nasal cavity trap and remove dust and pathogens from the air as it flows through the nasal cavity. The cilia move the mucus down the nasal cavity to the pharynx where it can be swallowed.
- Segments
  - Respiratory segment
    - Lined with ciliated pseudostratified columnar epithelium (also called respiratory epithelium). The conchae are located in this region. The respiratory segment has a very vascularized lamina propria allowing the venous plexuses of the conchal mucosa to engorge with blood,

restricting airflow and causing air to be directed to the other side of the nose. This cycle occurs approximately every 20 to 30 minutes. Nose bleeds (epitaxis) in the inferior concha are common in this region.

- o Olfactory segment
  - ▪ Lined with a specialized type of pseudostratified columnar epithelium known as *olfactory epithelium*, which contains receptors for the sense of the smell. This segment is located along the dorsal roof of the nasal cavity. Histological sections appear yellowish-brown due to the presence of lipofuscin pigments. Olfactory mucosal cell types include bipolar neurons, supporting (sustentacular) cells, basal cells, and Bowman's glands. The axons of the bipolar neurons form the olfactory nerve (cranial nerve I) which enters the brain through the cribiform plate. Bowman's glands are serous glands in the lamina propria, whose secretions trap and dissolve odoriferous substances.

- Blood supply
  - o There is a rich blood supply to the nasal cavity. In some animals such as dogs, the capillary beds flowing through the nasal cavity help cool the blood flow to the brain.
  - o Blood supply comes from branches of both the internal and external carotid artery, including branches of the facial artery and maxillary artery. The named arteries of the nose are:
    - ▪ Sphenopalatine and greater palatine arteries, branches of the maxillary artery.
    - ▪ Anterior ethmoidal artery, a branch of the ophthalmic artery
    - ▪ Branches of facial artery supplying the vestibule of the nasal cavity.

- Nerve supply
  - o Innervation of the nasal cavity responsible for the sense of smell is via the olfactory nerve, which sends microscopic fibers from the olfactory bulb through the cribiform plate to reach the top of the nasal cavity.
  - o General sensory innervation is by branches of the trigeminal nerve (V1 and V2):
    - ▪ Nasociliary nerve (V1)
    - ▪ Nasopalatine nerve (V2)
    - ▪ Posterior nasal branches of maxillary nerve (V2)
  - o There are 2 passages in the nasal cavity (not to be confused with nostrils).
  - o The entire nasal cavity is innervated by autonomic fibers.
  - o Sympathetic innervation to the blood vessels of the mucosa causes them to constrict, while the control of secretion by the mucous glands is carried on postganglionic parasympathetic nerve fibers originating from the facial nerve.

Tenon's Fascia

- Thin membrane surrounding eyeball
- Inner surface of smooth, delicate bands of connective tissue attach Tenon's to sclera. The potential space is called the episcleral space.
- Outer surface has coarse trabeculations running through orbital fat
- Anteriorly attached firmly to sclera, 1.5-mm posterior to limbus
- Posteriorly fused to sclera around optic nerve merging with meninges of optic nerve
- Inferiorly thickens and extends medially and laterally to form Lockwood's suspensory ligament
- Pierced posteriorly by
  - o Ciliary nerves and vessels, vortex veins
  - o Six muscles with fascial sheath reflected onto muscles (Figure 1-7)
    - ▪ Expansion on lateral rectus (LR) and medial rectus (MR) extends laterally and medial to orbit, forming check ligaments.
    - ▪ Extensions from inferior rectus and IO extend to lower tarsus.
    - ▪ Extensions from SR to levator
- Provides support and maintains position of eye
- Functionally acts as "pulleys" for the extraocular muscles
  - o Enucleation removes the globe and leaves Tenon's and muscle. They can support the prosthesis.
- Operation on the IR or IO must consider the effect of lower lid retractors and eyelid position due to the extensions to the lower tarsus.

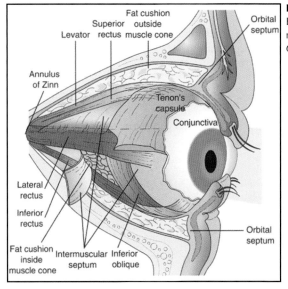

Figure 1-7. Muscle cone. (This figure was published in Campolattaro BN, Wang FM. Anatomy and physiology of the extraocular muscles and surrounding tissues. In: Yanoff M, Duker JS, eds. *Ophthalmology*. 2nd ed. Copyright Elsevier [2004].)

Eyeball (Globe)

- Size
  - ○ Anteroposterior (AP) diameter is 24 mm.
  - ○ Vertical diameter is 23 mm; horizontal is 23.5 mm
- Location
  - ○ In anterior orbit, closer to orbital roof and lateral wall
  - ○ Lateral canthus is posterior to eye, most exposed

Sclera

- Thickness 1 mm (thinner in children)
- Thinnest under muscle insertions (0.3 mm)
  - ○ The sclera is thinnest behind the rectus muscles, complicating recession of muscles in strabismus surgery. Eye trauma can result in blow out under muscle.
  - ○ 0.6-mm thick at limbus

Openings in Sclera

Optic Nerve

- 3-mm medial and 1-mm superior to posterior pole, bridged by lamina cribrosa
- Lamina cribrosa is an area of weakness (ie, cupping of optic nerve as it stretches outward with intraocular pressure [IOP] elevation).
- Small opening around optic nerve for long and short ciliary nerves
- Four to 5 openings for vortex veins, approximately 4-mm posterior to equator
  - ○ Intraocular tumors can migrate through the passages to exit the eye (optic nerve, vortex vein canals)
- Opening for anterior ciliary arteries (2 per muscle except LR with 1), found anterior to muscle insertions

Layers of Sclera

Episclera

- Composed of loose connective tissue connecting to Tenon's fascia, becomes thinner more posteriorly

Stroma

- Dense fibrous tissue.; collagen bundles in mat-like pattern resulting in white color
- Older people develop yellowish hue of sclera from fatty infiltration.

Lamina Fusca Sclera

- Thin irregular layer of melanocytes and collagen fibers allowing a weak attachment to choroid; forms a potential space (suprachoroidal space)
- Collagen diseases (eg, Ehlers-Danlos syndrome, Stickler's syndrome) can allow sclera to stretch and thin, resulting in axial myopia.

Blood Supply of Sclera

- Anteriorly from external episcleral plexus
- Posteriorly from branches of long and short ciliary arteries

Cornea

- Diameter
  - Vertical
    - Averages 11.5 mm
  - Horizontal
    - Averages 12.5 mm
- Thickness
  - 550 μm in center, thicker (700 μm to 1 mm) at limbus
- Radius of curvature
  - Anterior surface
    - 7.8 mm
  - Posterior surface
    - 6.2 to 6.8 mm
- Refractive index
  - 1.36
- Refractive power
  - 43 diopters (D) (anterior +49 D, posterior −6 D)

Layers of Cornea

- See Figure 1-8

Epithelium

- 50- to 60-μm thick
- Five layers of stratified nonkeratinized epithelium
  - Deep single layer basal cells, columnar
  - Desmosomes connect adjacent cells
  - Secrete basement membrane (BM) type IV collagen
  - Hemidesmosomes anchor BM to Bowman's
  - Folds of columnar cells near limbus (called Palisades of Vogt) increase surface area of basal cells for new cell production
    - Turnover 3 to 6 days
  - Middle layer
    - Polyhedral "wing"-shaped cells linked by desmosomes, protective layer
  - Outer layer
    - Two or 3 cell layers of flattened squamous cells held by desmosomes
- Trauma to epithelium is quickly repaired by migration of epithelial cells and maturation and migration (centripetal) of basal cell layer

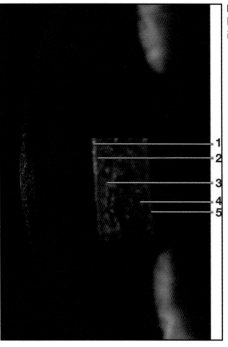

Figure 1-8. Histological layers of the cornea. (1) Epithelium. (2) Bowman's layer. (3) Stroma. (4) Descemet's. (5) Endothelium. (This figure was published in *Corneal Atlas*. 2nd ed. Krachmer JH, Palay DA. Copyright Elsevier [2006].)

Bowman's Layer

- 10 µm below the epithelial BM
- Fine interwoven collagen fibrils (type I)
- Secreted from basal epithelial cells and stromal keratocytes
- Ends at limbus, deep surface merges with stroma
- Not a true BM
  - ○ Does not regenerate and is replaced by fibrous tissue
- Thickens with age

Stroma (Substantia Propria)

- Makes up at least 90% of corneal thickness (480 to 900 µm)
- Collagen fibrils (mostly type 1) run parallel to each other in 2-µm layers
- 300 lamellae each run parallel to the surface of the cornea from limbus to limbus
- Tightly organized orientation allows cornea to be transparent
- Glycosaminoglycans containing water can alter lamellar spacing and result in corneal opacity (ie, corneal edema).
- Accumulation of fluid in the cornea disturbs the regular spacing of collagen fibrils causing corneal cloudiness and reduction of vision.
- Upon injury, tissue is repaired via fibrosis.
- Condensation in the stroma occurs with age.
  - ○ Extracellular accumulation of lipid is called arcus senilis

Descemet's Membrane

- 10-µm thick, strong, type IV collagen (secreted from endothelial cells)
- Banded layer (fetal) 3 µm, does not thicken with age, has striations
- Nonbanded layer (adult) thickens with age, 2 to 10 µm, not organized
- Anchors endothelium. Terminates abruptly at limbus, becoming continuous with trabecular tissue of sinus canal. This ring is known as Schwalbe's line.
- Is elastic, can curl up when disrupted, and is repaired by the endothelial cells
- Thickens with age
- Protrusions of Descemet's membrane in periphery are called Hassall-Henle bodies

Endothelium

- 5-μm single layer of polygonal-shaped, flattened cells
- Tight junctions allow cells to act as a barrier, while mitochondria, endoplasmic reticulum, and Golgi bodies service the pumping mechanism.
- Elevations in IOP (ie, acute glaucoma) can open gap junctions between endothelial cells and allow passage of aqueous humor into the stroma

Corneal Blood Supply

- None → avascular
- Anterior ciliary vessels at limbus allow for diffusion.
- Tear film and aqueous humor provide nutrients via diffusion.
- Due to its avascularity and absence of Langerhans cells in epithelium, the cornea is considered an immunologically privileged site.
- Vascular migration from infection or inflammation can occur.
- Upon resolution, corneal vascularization can reverse, leaving "ghost vessels."

Nerve Supply to Cornea

- Cranial nerve V → cranial nerve V1 (ophthalmic division) → long posterior ciliary nerves
- Annular plexus formed in sclera near limbus.
- Seventy to 80 nerves lose myelin sheath and enter stroma in radial fashion.
- Axons divide and create anterior epithelial plexus. Small branches pierce Bowman's and form intraepithelial plexus.

Limbus

- 1.5 to 2.0 mm wide
- Anatomic limbus
  - Schwalbe's line (termination of Descemet's)
- Surgical limbus
  - Blue area where clear cornea merges with sclera
  - An incision through the surgical limbus will enter the eye anterior to the trabecular meshwork
- Posterior limbus
  - Under conjunctiva, where blue merges with opaque sclera
- Outer groove called "external scleral sulcus" at the junction of the steeper corneal radius of curvature and the flatter sclera
- Internal scleral sulcus contains the trabecular meshwork and Schlemm's canal. Posterior rim of this sulcus is the scleral spur. This is where the largest resistance to outflow is found—the endothelial linings that form vacuoles that connect the basal to apical layers of the cells of the trabecular meshwork transiently creating a channel for aqueous fluid to exit into the canal (Table 1-1).

Schlemm's Canal

- Channel located in the corneoscleral junction, lying in the internal scleral sulcus
- Sclera posteriorly, trabecular meshwork internally
- Lined with endothelium, canal is not a continuous channel, but breaks up in areas and then reforms.
- Drained by approximately 25 small collecting channels that empty into deep scleral venous plexus. Larger aqueous veins pass through sclera and drain clear aqueous humor directly to conjunctival veins at the limbus.

Uveal Tract

- Layers
  - Iris
  - Ciliary body
  - Choroid

TABLE 1-1. STRUCTURAL CHANGES AT THE LIMBUS

Corneal epithelium	Becomes conjunctival (bulbar) epithelium
Bowman's layer	Continuous with substantia propria of conjunctiva and Tenon's
Stroma	Gradually becomes sclera
Descemet's membrane	Terminates at Schwalbe's line, trabecular meshwork then begins
Endothelium	Continues as endothelium lining trabecular meshwork and covering anterior iris

Iris

- Thin pigmented, contractile structure acting as diaphragm to create the pupil
- Separates anterior from posterior chamber
- Lightly touches the lens centrally
- Pupil diameter can vary from 1 to 8 mm, and 25% of the population has a slight difference in size (anisocoria).
- The iris is 12 mm in diameter and is thickest 2 mm from the pupillary margin. Thinnest at base where it attaches to the anterior ciliary body, called the ciliary margin or root of the iris.
- Color
  - Variation from light blue to dark brown
  - Blue color results from absorption of longer wavelengths (red) and reflection of shorter wavelengths (blue).
  - More pigment in melanocytes results in a brown iris.
  - The irides of infants born with blue eyes may become progressively darker as pigment accumulates.
- The 2 structures of the iris
  - Anterior stroma (from mesenchyme)
  - Posterior pigmented epithelium (from neural crest)

Iris Stroma

- The stroma of iris contains the following:
  - Highly vascular connective tissue (collagen, fibroblasts, melanocytes, matrix)
  - Nerve fibers
  - Smooth muscle of sphincter papillae
  - Myoepithelial cells of dilator papillae
  - Anterior surface
    - Devoid of epithelium
    - Velvety appearance with bands of connective tissue forming a radiating meshwork
    - Oval openings, called Fuchs' crypts, allow aqueous humor deeper into stroma.
    - Collarette lies 2 mm from the pupillary margin. Bands extend radially from the collarette, and the iris is thickest here. The collarette divides the pupil into the pupillary zone and the peripheral ciliary zone.
    - Radial ridges indicate the presence of vessels from the major arterial circle of the ciliary body. The branches form an incomplete minor vascular circle near the papillary margin.
    - The pupillary zone is a 1-mm wide ring of smooth muscle around the pupil.
    - Parasympathetic nerve fibers from short ciliary nerves contract muscle, constricting the pupil.
    - The ciliary zone contains the dilator papillae muscle.
      - These cells arise from pigmented epithelial cells in the posterior iris.
      - The apical portion remains in the epithelial layer while a basal process projects into the stroma to join other processes to become the dilator muscle.
      - They are thus called myoepithelial cells.
      - Sympathetic nerve fibers from the superior cervical ganglion cause iris dilation.

Epithelial Layer of Iris (Posterior Pigmented Layer)

- Double layer of epithelium lying apex to apex
- Derived from the neuroectoderm of the 2 layers of the optic cup
- Anterior layer
  - Lightly pigmented, adjacent to iris stroma, and associated with the muscular basal processes forming the dilator muscle
  - Continuous with the pigmented outer layer of the ciliary body epithelium
- Posterior layer
  - Composed of larger, cuboidal cells packed with melanin granules that face the posterior chamber
  - Continuous with inner nonpigmented layer of the ciliary body
  - The pigmented epithelium from the posterior iris extends slightly onto the anterior surface called the pupillary ruff.

Blood Supply

- Radial vessels from the major arterial circle in the ciliary body (formed from the 2 long posterior ciliary vessels and the 7 anterior ciliary)
- The endothelial layer of all vessels is nonfenestrated with tight junctions between cells and thick BM in order to maintain a blood-ocular barrier.
- Vascular supply of the major arterial circle of the iris

Nerve Supply

- Branches on long ciliary nerves (branches of nasociliary from V1)
  - Sensory nerves
  - SNS from superior cervical ganglion cause dilator muscle contraction and pupillary dilation (mydriasis).
- Branches from short ciliary nerves
  - Postganglionic parasympathetic nervous system (PSNS) nerves from ciliary ganglion
  - Originated in Edinger-Westphal nucleus (EWN) and cause sphincter constriction (miosis)

Ciliary Body

- 6-mm wide ring running around inside of anterior sclera
- Continuous with iris anteriorly and choroid posteriorly
- Extending from scleral spur back to ora serrata
- Externally, ciliary body extends from 1.5-mm posterior to corneal limbus to 7.5-mm behind limbus

Pars Plicata

- Anterior folded aspect of ciliary body
- Folds become the ciliary processes
- Zonules (zonular fibers) run between processes and turn centrally toward equator of lens, 0.5 mm away.

Pars Plana

- Smooth and flat, extending posteriorly from the pars plicata to the tooth-like edge of ora serrata of retina
- Given its relative avascularity and anterior location, it is an ideal region to allow entrance to the posterior segment of the eye.
- When injecting into the eye, a surgeon will measure 4 mm from the limbus (3.5 mm if pseudophakic) through this region in order to miss the vascular pars plicata anteriorly and avoid the delicate retina posteriorly.

Structure of Ciliary Body

Ciliary Epithelium

- Two layers of cuboidal cells, produce aqueous humor
- Nonpigmented

- Continuation of neurosensory retina
- BM faces inside to the posterior chamber (continuous with ILM)
- Apex oriented externally
- Continuation of the retinal pigment epithelium (RPE) layer
- BM faces outward to the ciliary body stroma (continuous with BM of RPE)
- The apex is separated from the apex of the nonpigmented layer by ciliary channels.

Ciliary Stroma

- Composed of bundles of loose connective tissue and blood vessels in which muscles are embedded
- The stroma extends into the ciliary process to create the core.
- Branches of long posterior ciliary arteries form a major arterial circle near the base of the iris.
- Capillary networks are fenestrate and lie close to the ciliary epithelium.

Ciliary Muscles

- These smooth muscles comprise the bulk of the ciliary body.
- Longitudinal (meridian)
  - The most anterior and external (closest to sclera) pass from trabecular meshwork to stroma of choroid.
- Oblique (radial)
  - Middle layer, radiate away from scleral spur
- Circular
  - Most internal, run around ciliary body like a sphincter
- Postganglionic PSNS nerves from ciliary ganglion enter via short ciliary nerve to supply the ciliary muscles. Contraction of the longitudinal and circular muscles moves the ciliary body forward and thus relieves tension on zonules to allow lens accommodation.
- Blunt trauma to the eye can allow tearing of anterior chamber angle into the ciliary body. The tear extends through the ciliary body at the oblique muscle layer, resulting in angle recession.

Choroid

- Thin vascular pigmented layer running from optic nerve to ciliary body
- Thicker posteriorly (220 µm) and thinner anteriorly (100 µm)
- Firmly attached to sclera at optic nerve (continuous with pia and arachnoid), vortex veins, and ciliary nerve and vessel openings
- Firmly attached to retina
- Loosely attached to other areas of sclera by sheets of connective tissue
- Highly pigmented, can be site of primary melanoma

Layers of Choroid

Vessel Layer

- External layer (closest to sclera)
  - Contains arterial branches of short posterior ciliary arteries and large veins that coalesce to form vortex veins

Choriocapillaris

- Middle layer, network of wide bore capillaries supplied and drained by the vessel layer
- The capillaries are lined by fenestrated endothelial cells

Bruch's Membrane

- Innermost layer, 2- to 4-µm thick
- Five layers of Bruch's
  - BM of capillary endothelium
  - Outer collagen layer
  - Elastic meshwork
  - Inner collagen layer
  - BM of RPE

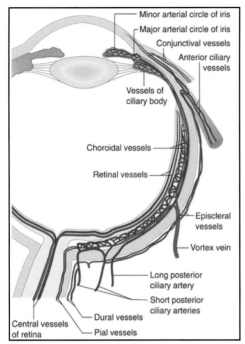

Figure 1-9. Vascular supply to the eye. All arterial branches originate with the ophthalmic artery. Venous drainage is through the cavernous sinus and the pterygoid plexus. (This figure was published in *Review of Ophthalmology*. Friedman NJ, Kaiser PK, Trattler WB. Copyright Elsevier [2005].)

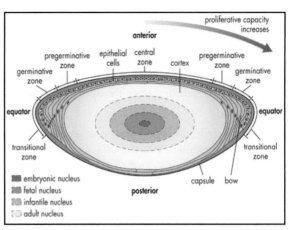

Figure 1-10. Gross anatomy of the adult human lens. (This figure was published in Saxby LA. Anatomy. In: Yanoff M, Duker JS, eds. *Ophthalmology*. Copyright Elsevier [1999].)

Blood Supply of Choroid

- Short ciliary and recurrent branches of the anterior ciliary both from the ophthalmic artery
- Very vascular and frequently the site of metastases (Figure 1-9)
- The potential space between the outer choroid and sclera can be the location for collection of blood or fluid (suprachoroidal hemorrhage or effusion).

Nerve Supply to Choroid

- Long ciliary nerves (from nasociliary of V1) (sensory and SNS)
- Short ciliary from the ciliary ganglion (PSNS and SNS)
  - After piercing sclera near the optic nerve, they run forward in perichoroidal space. Branches are given off to choroid to form plexuses that terminate in blood vessel walls.

Lens

- The lens (Figure 1-10) is the part of the refractive media, including the cornea and vitreous.
- 10-mm wide, 4-mm thick structure sitting behind the iris and pupil and anterior to the vitreous
- Lens equator is 0.5 mm away from the ciliary processes of the pars plicata and is held in place by suspensory zonules.
- The lens is biconvex with the anterior surface having less convexity (larger radius of curvature) than the posterior surface. This shape gives it a refractive index of 1.36 in the periphery and 1.40 in the inner zone.
- The lens accounts for 15 to 20 D of the eyes' 60 D total.

Lens Capsule

- An elastic BM formed by the lens epithelial cells
- Thicker on the sides (20 µm) and thinnest posteriorly (3 µm)

- Made of type IV collagen in 40 lamellae
- It can be stretched by 60% before tearing.
- The zonules from the ciliary processes attach onto the capsule at the equator.
- The main function of the capsule is to mold the shape of the lens in response to the pull of the zonules.
- The elastic pull of the capsule tends to form the lens into a globular (round) rather than a discoid shape.

Lens Epithelial Cells

- Cuboidal cells found only under the anterior surface of the capsule
- At the equator, the cells elongate into columnar cells, which become arranged in rows.
- The mitotic activity is maximal at the equator (germinal zone) as they transform them into lens fibers.
- The anterior lens epithelial cells function to transfer material to the lens interior and to produce the lens capsule.
- The equatorial lens epithelial cells function in dividing and differentiating into lens fibers.

Lens Fibers

- The fibers constitute most of the mass of the lens.
- At the equator, the epithelial cells elongate and thin.
- The apical and basal portions span the distance from the apical epithelial cells to the posterior capsule.
- Newer lens fibers compress older ones, continually pushing the lens inward on itself.
- The thinner anterior and posterior aspects of the fibers can move further than the thicker nucleated middle regions, so the lens fibers take on a U shape.
- The fibers can initially span the entire AP distance of the lens, resulting in the organized common insertion of the fibers of the fetal Y sutures.
- After years of continual growth, the fibers are unable to fully span the AP diameter of the lens, and the suture pattern becomes disorganized.
- The nucleus of the lens fibers slowly migrates anteriorly, progressing further than the nucleus of the more outside fiber.
- As the inner fibers become compacted, they create the harder central nucleus of the lens, with the less compacted exterior creating the softer cortex.
- The lens fibers contain numerous gap junctions, both between themselves and between the superficial lens epithelial cells, which allow survival of the deeply displaced cells.
- Many of the fibers lose their nuclei.
- The fibers create protein crystallins that increase the refractive index of the lens.
- The lens continues to grow throughout life. No cells are discarded. This results in a one-third increase in lens size in a 65 year old.

Suspensory Ligaments (Zonules)

- The zonules are fine delicate fibers formed in the epithelium of the ciliary processes.
- The fibers fuse to form 140 bundles that run toward the lens.
  - As they approach the lens, they break into fine fibers that fuse with the lens capsule.
- A larger anterior zonular sheet and smaller posterior zonular sheet is created.
- Parasympathetic nerve impulses via the long posterior ciliary nerves result in contraction of the circular muscle of ciliary body, allowing inward movement of the zonules and the relaxation of the pull on the equator of the lens.
- As the lens capsule contracts, the thickness of the lens increases, thereby increasing its dioptric power. Concomitantly, the contraction of the horizontal and radial muscles of the ciliary body moves the lens forward, adding to the increase in power.
- Constriction of the pupil also limits the entrance of light rays to the thick central lens. This process is called accommodation and can increase the power of the eye by 14 D in a young person.

Vitreous

- Volume
  - Two-thirds to four-fifths of globe, 4 mL
- Weight
  - 4 g
- Shape
  - Spherical with cup-shaped depression for lens (hyaloid fossa)
- Composition
  - Transparent gel composed of 99% water, salt, soluble proteins, hyaluronic acid, collagen fibers
- Function
  - Transmit light
  - Support lens
  - Assist holding neural retina to RPE

Attachments

Vitreous Base

- 6-mm wide attachment straddling ciliary epithelium of pars plana and peripheral retina
- Strongest attachment (avulsion indicates trauma)
- Collagen fibers fan into vitreous

Retina

- Collagen fibers of vitreous insert into BM of retina adjacent to optic nerve head

Lens

- Weigert's ligament fibers contact the BM (the lens capsule)
- The most posterior zonules from the ciliary body also attach here

Regions

Anterior Hyaloid

- Area anterior to vitreous base

Posterior Hyaloid

- All vitreous surfaces that are posterior to the vitreous base

Cortex of Vitreous

- Peripheral vitreous where collagenous fibrils and hyaluronic acid are in high density that coalesce and blend with the BM of the retina. This thickened cortex of the retina has been termed *hyaloid membrane*, but structurally it is just thickened vitreous cortex.
- The vitreous base is the area of strongest attachment and divides the hyaloid into anterior and posterior.

Cloquet's Canal

- Extends from the back of the lens to the optic disc (1- to 2-mm wide)
- Curved walls of canal form the hyaloid tract consisting of low-density vitreous, where hyaloid artery once ran.

Retina

- Size
  - Thickness
    - 100 µm at ora serrata
    - 560 µm near optic disc
    - Thinnest at fovea
  - Extends from optic disc to ora serrata, nasal side is shorter than temporal side

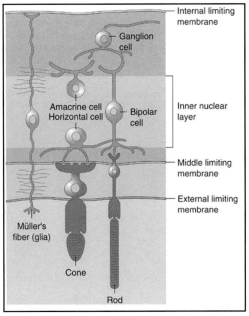

Figure 1-11. Neuronal connections in the retina and participating cells. (This figure was published in Schubert HD. Structure and function of the neural retina. In: Yanoff M, Duker JS, eds. *Ophthalmology*. Copyright Elsevier [1999].)

- Composition
  - 160 million rods
  - 6 million cones (40% to 50% in macula)
  - Müller's cells (only found in retina)
    - Extend from external limiting membrane (ELM) to internal limiting membrane (ILM)
    - Cell bodies in inner nuclear layer (INL)
    - Store glycogen and release glucose to retinal neurons
    - Insulate neurons
    - Forms BM around retinal vessels

Layers of Retina (Outer to Inner)

Retinal Pigment Epithelium

- Composition and function (Figure 1-11)
  - Monolayer of pigmented cuboidal (at ora)/columnar (at fovea) cells
  - Outer BM is the inner part of Bruch's membrane of the choroid.
  - Inner: Fingerlike villi interdigitate with photoreceptor outer segments
  - Anteriorly merges with pigmented (inner) epithelium of ciliary body
  - Zonula occludens (tight junctions) maintains blood-retinal barrier.
  - Absorb light and heat
  - Supply nourishment to outer retina
  - Turnover of photoreceptor outer segments
  - Storage of vitamin A, formation of rhodopsin
  - ATP pump maintains subretinal environment (dehydrated) and helps maintain retinal adhesion.

Layer of Rods and Cones

- Composition and function
  - Outer segments of photoreceptors (stacked discs or lamellae containing photoreceptor pigments)
  - Cilium connecting outer to inner segment, "stalk"
  - Absorb light, begin neural signal
  - One of the highest metabolic rates in the body because new lamellae (discs) must be constantly made

External Limiting Membrane

- Composition
  - ○ Not a true membrane but an illusion due to cell junctions (zonula adherens) between Müller's cells and photoreceptors
  - ○ Located external to photoreceptor cell bodies, but internal to their outer and inner segments

Outer Nuclear Layer

- Composition
  - ○ Outer photoreceptor fibers connecting inner segment to cell nucleus
  - ○ Cell body (nucleus) of photoreceptor
  - ○ Inner photoreceptor axons—heading to outer plexiform layer (OPL)
  - ○ Müller's cell processes

Outer Plexiform Layer

- Composition
  - ○ Inner cone fibers and their expanded termination or pedicle
  - ○ Inner rod fibers and their expanded termination or spherule
  - ○ Synapses between photoreceptor and horizontal cells and between bipolar cells and between other photoreceptors
  - ○ Müller's cell processes
  - ○ Middle limiting membrane
    - ▪ Name for area in OPL, given because of the strength caused by gap junctions and interweaving of fibers
    - ▪ Likely important during development in keeping retinal vessels from invading outer retina
    - ▪ Also a barrier for fluid accumulation from either side
    - ▪ Approximate junction of vascular inner retina and the avascular outer retina supplied by diffusion from choriocapillaris

Inner Nuclear Layer

- Composition and function
  - ○ Horizontal cell bodies, located closer to OPL, carries information laterally
  - ○ Bipolar cell bodies, located in middle of INL. Relay impulse from photoreceptor to ganglion cell.
  - ○ Müller's cells, provide glial support function for retina
  - ○ Amacrine cells, body located in inner side of INL, modify input of bipolar cells to ganglion cells
  - ○ Blood vessels (from here to vitreous blood supply is from retinal vessels)

Inner Plexiform Layer

- Composition and function
  - ○ Axonal endings of bipolar cells
  - ○ Dendrites of ganglion cells
  - ○ Processes of amacrine cells

Ganglion Cell Layer

- Composition
  - ○ Cell bodies of ganglion cells
  - ○ Vessels, astrocytes, Müller's cell processes
  - ○ Amacrine and bipolar processes that terminate on ganglionic cell body
  - ○ All ganglion cell axons nasal to the fovea will cross at optic chiasm.
  - ○ All axons temporal to fovea will not cross.

Nerve Fiber Layer

- Composition
  - ○ Ganglion cell axons
  - ○ No myelination in retina

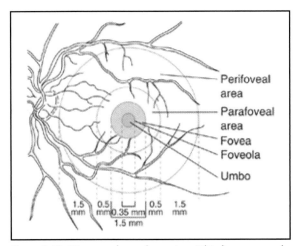

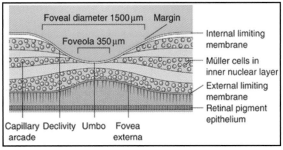

Figure 1-13. Foveal margin, foveal declivity, foveola, and umbo. (This figure was published in Schubert HD. Structure and function of the neural retina. In: Yanoff M, Duker JS, eds. *Ophthalmology*. Copyright Elsevier [1999].)

Figure 1-12. Diagram of macular region. (This figure was published in Schubert HD. Structure and function of the neural retina. In: Yanoff M, Duker JS, eds. *Ophthalmology*. Copyright Elsevier [1999].)

Internal Limiting Membrane

- Composition
  - o True BM contacting footplate of Müller's cells to the posterior hyaloid (condensation of cortical vitreous)
  - o Continuous with BM of inner nonpigment epithelium of ciliary body

Regions of Retina

"Anatomic" Structure of Macula

- Temporal to optic disc, within the arcade of temporal retinal vessels (Figure 1-12)
- 5 to 6 mm in diameter
- 4-mm temporal and 0.8-mm inferior to optic disc
- Foveola in center, 0.35 mm in diameter, contains yellow "macula lutea" (Figure 1-13)
- Fovea centralis, 1.5 mm in diameter (macular avascular zone)
- Parafovea
  - o Ring of 0.5-mm wide that surrounds fovea
- Perifovea
  - o Ring of 1.5-mm wide that surrounds parafovea

Posterior Pole

- Fovea lies 3-mm temporal and slightly inferior to optic disc
- Axons from macula pass directly to lateral aspect of disc
- Temporal axons bypass fovea and sweep around, forming superior and inferior arcuate bands
- Peripheral retina axons enter peripheral (outside) part of nerve
- More central axons enter the center aspect of the nerve

Foveola

- Only cones present (no rods)
- Cone nuclei are slanted outward
- OPL barely present as the cone fibers slant radially away from the center
- No other layers (INL, IPL, ganglion cell layer [GCL], nerve fiber layer [NFL]) so avascular
- ILM present but thin
- The presence of ganglion or bipolar cells marks end of foveola

Figure 1-14. Transition of neural retina to nonpigmented epithelium at the ora serrata. (This figure was published in Schubert HD. Structure and function of the neural retina. In: Yanoff M, Duker JS, eds. *Ophthalmology.* Copyright Elsevier [1999].)

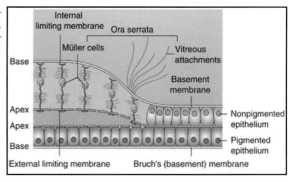

Fovea

- RPE cells taller, more pigmented, xanthophyll pigment present
- More cones than rods, 4 to 5 layers of cone nuclei in ONL
- Long cone fibers of OPL run horizontally, called Henle's layer, to allow the photoreceptor bodies to be displaced lateral from center.
- Ganglion cell layer is 6 layers thick.
- 35,000 cones in rod-free part of fovea, 1 million cones total
- Avascular foveola and part of fovea is 0.5 to 0.6 mm across.

Parafovea

- Greatest accumulation of nerve cells in retina (most in GCL and INL)
- Henle's fiber layer is very thick
- Cones in lower density than at foveola, and rods are present
- Average of 1 rod between any 2 cones
- Ganglion cell layer peaks at 7

Perifovea

- Average of 2 rods between any 2 cones
- Becomes peripheral retina when Henle's fiber layer disappears and GCL is one-layered

Ora Serrata of Peripheral Retina

- Located deep to insertion sites of recti muscles or about 6- to 7-mm posterior to corneal edge (limbus) or 6- to 8-mm anterior to equator
- 2.1-mm wide temporally and 0.7- to 0.8-mm nasally
- ILM becomes BM of nonpigmented ciliary epithelium (Figure 1-14)
- Müller's cells undifferentiated and become the nonpigmented epithelium of ciliary body
- RPE cells become the pigmented epithelium of the ciliary body and fuse with the changing Müller's cells as the center retinal layers disappear

Blood Supply of Retina

- Central retinal artery (CRA) supplies inner two-thirds of retina via branches from the ICA → ophthalmic artery → CRA (first branch) → arcades
- Cilioretinal arteries are found in 25% of eyes, arising from branches of short posterior ciliary arteries
- Choriocapillaris supplies outer one-third of retina (supplied by short and long posterior ciliary arteries)
- Watershed of the 2 regions is the OPL (middle limiting membrane)

Optic Nerve

- 50 mm from disc to chiasm
- Composed of 1.2 million nerve fibers (the axons of the retinal ganglion cells)
- 90% small (1 μm) from ganglion cells mostly associated with cones
- 10% large (2 to 10 μm) associated with rods in peripheral areas

- An afferent sensory nerve. The axons form into bundles called fascicles and are surrounded by support tissue (astrocytes).
- 1.5 mm in diameter, enlarges to 3.5 mm behind lamina cribrosa due to myelin

Optic Disc (Optic Nerve Head)

- Area that the optic nerve leaves the eye passing through sclera at lamina cribrosa, through 200 to 300 channels
- Located 3- to 4-mm nasal and 0.8-mm above fovea, which results in an absolute scotoma (blind spot) 15 to 20 degrees temporal and slightly inferior to fixation

Layers of the Optic Disc

Nerve Fiber Layer

- The axons from the macula enter at the temporal border of the disc, traveling as the maculopapular bundle.
- Axons, from areas of the retina more temporal to the fovea, sweep around the fovea and enter the disc at the superior and inferior temporal quadrants.
- Although the blood supply to the nerve fiber layer of the retina is from the CRA (and any cilioretinal artery supply in 15%), the intraocular portion of the optic nerves derives its blood supply from an anastomotic circle of Zinn (Haller) in the sclera, supplied by short posterior ciliary arteries.

Prelaminar

- The axons turn 90 degrees and enter the optic disc.
- Peripheral retinal axons occupy the peripheral part of the optic nerve.
- Axons from the central part of the retina run in a more superficial layer of the nerve fiber layer of the retina and enter the inner part of the optic nerve.
- The blood supply is primarily from short posterior ciliary arteries through the circle of Zinn.

Laminar

- The lamina cribrosa is composed of beams of connective tissue continuous with sclera, spanning the optic disc opening.
- There are 3 to 10 layers of connective tissue forming the lamina.
- The many trabeculae form a sieve of oval or round openings to allow the passage of the nerve fascicles and the central retinal vessels.
- The lamina is weaker than surrounding sclera and can "bow" posteriorly with high IOP.
- The blood supply to this layer is also short posterior ciliary arteries and the circle of Zinn.

Retro Laminar

- The axons become myelinated, and the nerve doubles in thickness.
- At this point, the orbital portion of the optic nerve begins.
- The blood supply to this portion of the optic nerve is from the short posterior ciliary nerves and some pial vessels.
- The branches of the short posterior ciliary arteries to the optic nerve head resemble other CNS and retinal vessels and are different from branches to the choroidal circulation. They do not leak as they are surrounded by pericytes, lack fenestrations, and have tight junctions. They also autoregulate.

Sections of Optic Nerve

Intraorbital Optic Nerve

- It is 25- to 30-mm long. This is 5 to 10 mm longer than the distance to the optic canal, giving the nerve a sinuous course that permits freedom of eye movement and some protection in the event of proptosis (Figure 1-15).
- Oligodendrocytes cover the nerve fibers with myelin sheaths.
- The entire nerve is covered with vascular pia, delicate arachnoid, and an outer layer of dense dura mater that blends with the sclera anteriorly and is continuous with the meninges of the brain. The subarachnoid space is continuous up to its termination at the eyeball.

Figure 1-15. The sections of the optic nerve. (This figure was published in Sadun AA. Anatomy and physiology. In: Yanoff M, Duker JS, eds. *Ophthalmology.* 2nd ed. Copyright Elsevier [2004].)

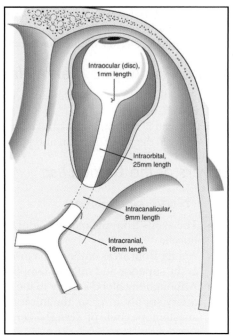

- Ten to 15 mm behind the eye, the CRA and vein pierce the dura sheath and cross obliquely to enter the nerve.
- The vascular supply to the intraorbital optic nerve is from the pial plexus of vessels, just external to the nerves that send small branches through septa to the nerve. These pial vessels are supplied from branches of the ophthalmic artery.
- High intracranial pressure (ICP) can be transmitted through the canal and forward along the nerve within the dura sheath up to the optic disc. This pressure can compress the anterograde axoplasmic flow of the nerve fibers, resulting in swelling of the optic nerve. Papilledema, by definition, is bilateral optic disc swelling due to increased ICP.

Intracanalicular Optic Nerve

- The optic canal lies with the lesser wing of the sphenoid bone and is 5- to 9-mm long.
- The dura sheath of the nerve fuses with the periosteum of the canal, fixating the nerve.
- The subarachnoid space is continuous through the canal. The ophthalmic artery and SNS fibers also run through the canal and are hence inside the subarachnoid space at this point.
- The blood supply to this area is from the pial plexus.
- The medial wall of the optic canal is made of thin bone separating the canal from the sphenoid and posterior ethmoid sinuses. Infection or mass in this area can cause compression of the optic nerve, which is fixed within the canal.

Intracranial Optic Nerve

- Within the intracranial subarachnoid space, the nerve heads medially, superiorly, and posteriorly to the optic chiasm in the floor of the third ventricle
- The pial plexus in these regions is supplied by branches of the ICA as well as ophthalmic and superior hypophyseal.

Visual Pathways

An overview of the remaining elements of the visual pathway will be provided in the neuro-ophthalmology section (Figure 1-16).

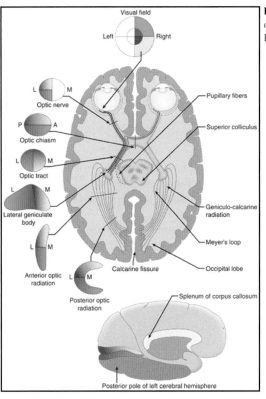

Figure 1-16. Visual pathway. (This figure was published in *Review of Ophthalmology.* Friedman NJ, Kaiser PK, Trattler WB. Copyright Elsevier [2005].)

Optic Chiasm

- The merging of optic nerves allows for the crossing of some fibers to facilitate topographic lateralization and the possibility of binocular fusion.
- The chiasm is located approximately 15-mm behind and slightly above the optic canal. The fused structure is 15-mm wide and 8-mm deep.
- The optic tracts exit the posterior corners, heading laterally and slightly up.
- The chiasm sits in the junction of the anterior wall and the floor of the third ventricle.
- The blood supply to the chiasm is from a pial plexus that is supplied by many adjacent vessels
- Location
  - Anteriorly
    - Anterior cerebral and anterior communicating arteries
  - Posteriorly
    - Tuber cinereum (near cavity of third ventricle and infundibulum)
  - Superiorly
    - Anterior wall of third ventricle
  - Inferiorly
    - Diaphragma sellae and the pituitary (10-mm below)
  - Laterally
    - ICA (after exiting cavernous sinus)

Optic Tracts

- The optic tracts emerge from the posterolateral aspect of the chiasm, flatten, and wind their way around the cerebral peduncle (the base of the brain and midbrain).
- Most of the nerve fibers terminate (and synapse) in the lateral geniculate nucleus (LGN).
- Ten percent of the fibers leave in a superior brachium entering the pretectal nucleus in the superior colliculus to become part of the pupillary light reflex arc.
- The blood supply to the tracts is from a pial plexus supplied by local arteries.
- The optic tract contains the retinal ganglion cell axons from the temporal retina of the ipsilateral eye (uncrossed) and the nasal retina of the contralateral eye (crossed).

Lateral Geniculate Nucleus

- Small ovoid swelling on the undersurface of the thalamus
- The LGN is made of 6 visible layers. The crossed retinal fibers project to layers 1, 4, and 6. The uncrossed retinal fibers go to layers 2, 3, and 5. The LGN is made up of 1 million neurons, approximately the number in the optic nerve.
- The blood supply to the LGN is from a branch of each of the middle cerebral posterior cerebral arteries.

Optic Radiations

- These postsynaptic nerve fibers originate in the LGN and terminate in the occipital cortex.
- The fibers exiting the lateral aspect of the LGN carry signal from the inferior retina.
- They loop laterally and inferiorly around the lateral horn of the ventricle, turn posteriorly, and terminate on the inferior bank of the calcarine fissure of the occipital cortex.
- The fibers from the peripheral retina sweep farther forward in the temporal lobe, creating Meyer's loop.
- The nerve fibers exiting the medial aspect of the LGN carry signal from the superior retina.
- They turn posterior, pass through the parietal cortex, and terminate on the superior bank of the calcarine fissure.

Occipital Cortex (Striate Cortex)

- The visual cortex may be divided into the following:
  - Primary visual area (Brodmann's Area 17)
    - Located on the medial surface of the occipital lobes, in and around the calcarine fissure, and extending posteriorly to encompass the occipital tips
    - Histologically, the cortex is thin and has a white stria (line) in the gray matter from the myelinated nerve fibers of the optic radiation ("striate cortex").
    - Topographically, the left occipital lobe receives input from the right visual field. The superior bank receives input from the inferior visual field. The occipital tip serves the central macular area and accounts for one-third of the visual cortex. The peripheral retina projects more anteriorly on the inner occipital lobe, with the area anterior to the calcarine fissure receiving the monocular input from the nasal retina of the contralateral eye (temporal crescent).
  - Secondary visual area (Brodmann's Areas 18 and 19)
    - The secondary visual centers (18, 19) surround the calcarine fissure (17)
    - Histologically, it is nonstriated.

Cranial Nerves

- The area receives input from Area 17, other cortical areas, and the thalamus and aids in the interpretation of visual data.
- Twelve pairs of nerves arise from the brain and leave through foramina or fissures (Table 1-2).
- All supply head and neck, except the 10th that also supplies thorax and abdomen.
- The orbit is directly involved with 5 of the 12 cranial nerves. An overview of all 12 will be provided followed by a detailed review of the 5 nerves of most importance to the orbit.

General Types of Nerves

Efferent

- Signal from brain to cause an "effect"
- General somatic (motor) efferent (to striated muscle)
- Special visceral efferent (striated muscles of branchial arch)
  - Signal from cerebral cortex synapses with motor nuclei in the brainstem
  - The axons thus make up the lower motor neurons.
  - Cerebral input crosses midline prior to midbrain.
  - Bilateral input is sent to all nuclei except those causing movement to the lower part of the face (CN VII) and protruding tongue (XII).

TABLE 1-2. CRANIAL NERVES

	NAME	FUNCTION	APPLICATION	ROUTE
I	Olfactory	Sensory	Smell	Cribriform plate
II	Optic	Sensory	Vision	Optic canal
III	Oculomotor	Motor	Eye movement, Constrict pupil (PSNS)	SOF
IV	Trochlear	Motor	Eye down and out	SOF
V	Trigeminal	Sensory	Cornea, forehead, scalp, eyelid, nose	SOF
V1	Ophthalmic	Sensory	Cornea, forehead, scalp, eyelid, nose	SOF
V2	Maxillary	Sensory	Cheek, upper teeth, nasal septum, maxillary sinus, palate	Foramen rotunda
V3	Mandibular	Motor / Sensory	Muscle of mastication, tensor tympani / Lower cheek, lower teeth, anterior tongue, mouth	Foramen ovale
VI	Abducens	Motor	LR	SOF
VII	Facial	Motor / Sensory	Muscles face and scalp, stapedius / Salivary and lacrimal glands / Taste anterior two-thirds of tongue	Internal acoustic meatus → facial canal → stylo-mastoid foramen
VIII	Vestibular-cochlear	Sensory	Hearing and position sense	Internal acoustic meatus
IX	Glosso-pharyngeal	Motor / Sensory	Swallowing and salivary (parotid) gland (PSNS), Taste (posterior 1/3), Carotid sinus (baroreceptor)	Jugular foramen
X	Vagus	Motor/sensory	Aorta, larynx, trachea, bronchi, lung, upper aspect GI tract, liver, kidney, pancreas	Jugular foramen
XI	Spinal accessory	Motor	Soft palate, pharynx, larynx, sternocleidomastoid, and trapezius	Jugular foramen
XII	Hypoglossal	Motor	Tongue	Hypoglossal canal

SOF = Superior orbital fissure; LR = Lateral rectus; GI = Gastrointestinal

- o Strokes can cause complete paralysis of the lower half of the face or half of the tongue, but a lower motor neuron lesion (ie, Bell's palsy) can paralyze the upper half also.
- General visceral efferent (PSNS → glands and smooth muscle)
  - o Example
    - Nuclei for oculomotor (III) are from EWN.

Afferent

- Signal to brain, perceives what "affects" the body
- General sensory afferent (general sensation, eg, touch)
  - o Nerve cell bodies of the sense organs originate outside the brain. Their axons enter brain and synapse in nuclei. Axons from nuclei then cross midline and pass to cerebral cortex.
- Special somatic afferent (hearing, balance, vision)
- General visceral afferent (viscera)
- Special visceral afferent (smell, taste)

Nerves of the Orbital Cavity

Motor Nerves

Oculomotor (CN III)

- Innervates all muscles of orbit except LR and SO
- CN III emerges from the anterior midbrain, passing into the subarachnoid space and between posterior cerebral and superior cerebellar arteries.
- It then runs parallel and lateral to the posterior communicating artery.
- It pierces the tentorium cerebelli and lateral to the clinoid process, perforates the dura, and comes to lie in the lateral wall of the cavernous sinus.
- It runs forward and receives a sensory branch from V1 and SNS branch off the carotid artery complex.
- It divides into superior (smaller) and inferior (larger) branches that both enter through the superior orbital fissure (SOF) within the tendinous ring.
- Superior division passes upward, lateral to optic nerve, then enters the SR muscle one-third forward from origin. Branches pass through (or occasionally around) SR and upward to the levator muscle.
- Inferior division divides into 3 branches.
  - The shortest passes medial to the optic nerve to enter MR.
  - The branch to IR runs forward on its upper surface and enters at one-third.
  - The longest branch, to IO, runs along the orbital floor before entering the posterior border of muscle. A short thick branch leaves this, sending fibers to the ciliary ganglion. These synapse and then form short ciliary nerves to supply sphincter pupillae and ciliary muscle.
- Motor nucleus to CN III
  - Located in midbrain anterior to aqueduct, at the level of superior colliculus
  - Both levator muscles are supplied by a single central group of cells (central caudal nucleus).
  - The SR muscle is supplied by the contralateral CN III nucleus.
  - The remaining muscles (MR, IO, IR) are supplied ipsilaterally.
- EWN lies posterior to the oculomotor nucleus, sends preganglionic nerve fibers to accompany CN III, heading for ciliary ganglion.
  - Receives input from pretectal nucleus, allowing the direct and consensual light reflex. Input from corticonuclear fibers allows accommodation.
- Clinical implications
  - CN III complete lesion → eye down and out (unopposed action of CN IV and VI)
    - Ptosis upper lid (paralysis of levator)
    - Dilated unreactive pupil (loss of sphincter constriction)
    - Loss of accommodation (loss of innervation to ciliary body)
  - CN III incomplete lesion
    - Loss of sphincter constriction and accommodation
    - External ophthalmoplegia (loss of EOM function)

Trochlear Nerve (CN IV)

- The thinnest CN supplies the SO muscle.
- Only CN to leave posterior surface of brainstem
- Nucleus in midbrain, anterior to aqueduct at level of inferior colliculus
  - Fibers head posteriorly around aqueduct and exit on the back surface where they cross to the contralateral side.
  - Nerve passes lateral and forward in subarachnoid space.
  - Pierces dura near posterior clinoid and passes in lateral wall of cavernous sinus (below CN III, above V1)
  - Enters orbit through SOF, but lies outside tendinous ring. Heads medial and enters top surface of SO muscle.
- Clinical implications
  - Midbrain lesion affecting both CN III and IV nuclei will cause EOM palsies on opposite sides as the CN IV decussates on the dorsal surface of midbrain.

Abducens Nerve (CN VI)

- Motor nucleus located in posterior pons, under the fourth ventricle
- Travels forward through pons, and then exits anteriorly (near junction with medulla oblongata)
- Runs up, out, and forward in subarachnoid space
- Pierces the dura and turns sharply over apex of petrous part of temporal bone (under petroclinoid ligament in Dorello's canal)
- Runs freely in the center of the cavernous sinus, inferolateral to ICA. Enters orbit through SOF within the tendinous ring.
- Passes forward to enter medial surface of LR
- In cavernous sinus, SNS fibers from ICA plexus join CN VI and then pass to CN III.
- Clinical
  - CN VI is a long and slender nerve sensitive to the stretch of trauma or compression of increased ICP, especially where it crosses over apex and enters canal.
  - While CN III, IV, V1, and V2 line the lateral wall of cavernous sinus and are susceptible to compression by a mass, CN VI runs in the center and will be resistant to compression. However, it is still sensitive to a vascular event or aneurysm.
  - Nuclei of CN III, IV, and VI receive bilateral input from cerebral cortex (the "higher centers"). Lesions of unilateral cortex affect both eyes and may limit movement of eyes away from damaged side (eyes turned to affected cortex), but limitation of the 2 eyes is equal, so there will be no diplopia.

Sensory Nerves

Trigeminal Nerve (CN V)

- Largest of all cranial nerves
- Sensory
- Motor fibers to muscles of mastication carried by mandibular division (V3).
- Nuclei of trigeminal nerve
  - Most of the cell bodies of trigeminal nerve are in the trigeminal ganglion. Touch and pressure nerves ascend to the main sensory nucleus of the pons.
  - Pain and temperature nerves ascend or descend to the spinal nucleus that is situated at various levels extending from the pons through the medulla oblongata and down to the upper spinal column (C2).
  - Proprioception impulses from facial and extraocular muscles are carried in unipolar cells that bypass the trigeminal nucleus and reside in the mesencephalic nucleus.

Trigeminal Nerve Divisions

Ophthalmic Division (V1)

- Divides off superior aspect of trigeminal ganglion, passing forward to enter the cavernous sinus (Figure 1-17)
- Joined by fine branches on SNS fibers from internal carotid. Gives off meningeal branch to supply the tentorium cerebelli.
- Exits cavernous sinus and divides into its 3 branches (lacrimal, frontal, nasociliary) prior to passing into the SOF

The 3 Divisions of V1

- Lacrimal nerve
  - The smallest branch. Enters orbit in SOF, outside the tendinous ring. It passes superior to the LR muscle.
  - Receives a PSNS branch from V2 (zygomaticotemporal branch of maxillary nerve), passing from the facial nerve (VII) and headed to the lacrimal gland
  - Enters lacrimal gland, sends branches to conjunctiva, and pierces orbital septum to supply forehead

Figure 1-17. Sensory nerves of the orbit, in lateral view. (This figure was published in *Atlas of Clinical and Surgical Orbital Anatomy.* Dutton JJ., Copyright Elsevier [1994].)

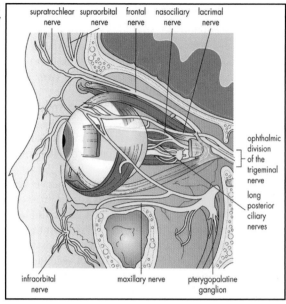

- Frontal nerve
  - ○ Enters orbit in SOF (outside ring) and courses forward above levator
  - ○ Divides into large supraorbital branch and smaller supratrochlear branch
  - ○ Supraorbital
    - ▪ Exits orbit via supraorbital notch
    - ▪ To skin and conjunctiva of upper lid, and forehead and scalp (back to the vertex), mucus membrane of frontal sinus
  - ○ Supratrochlear
    - ▪ A thin branch that passes to medial side of orbit to pass above trochlea of CN IV
    - ▪ Communicates with infratrochlear branch of nasociliary nerve
    - ▪ Exits orbit by piercing orbital septum, then turns upward to supply (sensory) orbicularis oculi and frontalis muscles. Supplies sensation to the upper eyelid and medial forehead.
- Nasociliary nerve
  - ○ Enters orbit in SOF inside the tendinous ring, between the superior and inferior branches of CN III
  - ○ Initially located lateral to the optic nerve, it later crosses medially with the ophthalmic artery, then anteriorly above the MR to end by passing through the anterior ethmoidal artery.
  - ○ From here, it is renamed the anterior ethmoidal nerve and travels with a corresponding branch of the ophthalmic artery, entering the cranium via the anterior ethmoidal air cells and then cribriform plate and ending by supply the tip of the nose.
  - ○ Four branches of the nasociliary nerve
    - ▪ Ramus communicans
      - ▫ Contains sensory nerves from the eye traveling via short ciliary nerves that pass through the ciliary ganglion to the ramus to join the nasociliary nerve
    - ▪ Long ciliary nerves
      - ▫ Usually 2 that exit as they cross optic nerve, they pass forward with short ciliary nerves from the ganglion. They enter the eye near optic nerve and pass forward deep to sclera to supply ciliary body, iris, and cornea. They contain SNS fibers to dilate the pupil and sensory fibers from the cornea.
    - ▪ Posterior ethmoidal nerve
      - ▫ Exits through the posterior ethmoidal foramen to supply the ethmoidal and sphenoidal air cells. Frequently missing.
    - ▪ Infratrochlear nerve
      - ▫ Arises at anterior ethmoidal foramen and is joined by a branch from the supratrochlear nerve. Continues forward and heads under the trochlea, pierces orbital septum to supply lacrimal sac, medial aspect upper and lower lids (skin and conjunctiva), and upper/lateral nose.

Maxillary Division of the Trigeminal Nerve (V2)

- After exiting the middle part of the trigeminal ganglion, it enters the lower lateral wall of the cavernous sinus.
- Exits skull via the foramen rotunda to enter pterygopalatine fossa sending 2 branches to pterygopalatine ganglion
- Continues lateral and forward and enters orbit through inferior orbital fissure
- Continues in floor of orbit in the infraorbital canal and exits through the infraorbital foramen
- Branches
  - Ganglionic
    - Two branches suspend the pterygopalatine ganglion and contain sensory fibers from orbital periosteum and mucus membrane of nose, pharynx, and palate.
    - Postganglion SNS fibers enter nerve from the ganglion and then exit via the zygomatic nerve heading to the lacrimal gland.
    - Zygomatic nerve
      - Arises from maxillary nerve and enters through inferior orbital fissure. Continues its superior course in lateral wall of orbit. Divides into 2 sections.
  - Zygomaticotemporal
    - Carries postganglionic nerve fibers that joined from the pterygopalatine ganglion. These pass to the lacrimal gland while termination of nerve exits orbit through canal in zygomatic bone to supply skin on the lateral side of the forehead.
    - Zygomaticofacial
      - Exits orbit through canal in temporal bone to supply skin on cheek
    - Infraorbital nerve
      - As the zygomatic nerve continues forward, it gives off alveolar nerves to the maxillary sinus and upper teeth.
      - As the maxillary nerve enters the infraorbital canal, it becomes the infraorbital nerve that leaves the orbit through the canal dividing into facial branches to the cheek and upper lip
- Clinical implications
  - Hutchinson's sign
    - Involvement of the eye with herpes zoster virus is likely if the tip of the nose is involved.
  - Supraorbital nerve exits orbit via notch (or foramen), which can be palpated in the orbital rim superior to the pupil. The supratrochlear will be one finger width nasal. Both can be blocked for forehead regional anesthesia.
  - Retrobulbar anesthesia will block movement of the eye (CN III and VI, but not IV) and all pain fibers (via long ciliary nerves) and cause the pupil to dilate.
  - The infraorbital foramen containing the infraorbital nerve (the continuation of the maxillary nerve) can be palpated just below the orbital rim in line with the pupil. Local anesthetic can be used to provide regional anesthesia to the lower lid, cheek, upper lip, and side of nose.

Extraocular Muscles

- General overview
  - Voluntary striated skeletal muscle
  - Greater vascularity than skeletal muscles in other areas of the body
  - Thin muscle fibers each run almost the distance of the entire muscle
  - Two types of muscles
    - Thin slow contracting type with grape-like motor end plates
    - Thicker fast contracting "twitch" type with classic motor end plate
  - Tendons
    - Made of parallel bundles of collagen fibers that merge and blend into sclera
    - Supported by elastic fibers that stop at insertion site
- Innervation of muscles
  - Myelinated nerves enter muscle body at junction of posterior and middle thirds.
    - These break into smaller branches that run distally and proximally between muscle bundles.

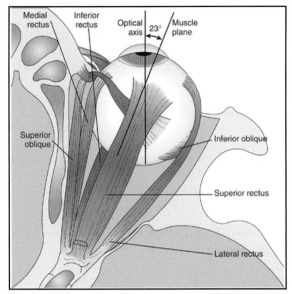

Figure 1-18. The extraocular muscles of the right eyeball in the primary position, seen from above. (The figure was published in Campolattaro BN, Wang FM. Anatomy and physiology of the extraocular muscles and surrounding tissues. In: Yanoff M, Duker JS, eds. *Ophthalmology.* 2nd ed. Copyright Elsevier [2004].)

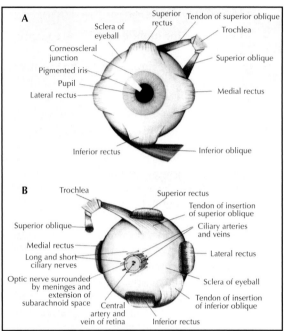

Figure 1-19. Right eyeball. (A) Anterior view, showing the attachment of the extraocular muscles. (B) Posterior view, showing the precise insertion of the superior and inferior oblique muscles. (*Clinical Anatomy of the Eye.* Snell RS, Lemp MA. Copyright © 1989. Reproduced with permission of Blackwell Scientific Publications.)

- Nerves to fast-twitch muscle have single classic motor end plate (neuromuscular junction) with ratio of one nerve to every muscle fiber. Nerves to slow contracting muscle may or may not be myelinated and have multiple "grape-like" end plates to multiple nerve fibers (one nerve to many muscles fibers).
  o Nerve feedback
    - Muscle spindles are located in the proximal and distal third of EOM and send feedback about muscle length (stretch).
    - Golgi tendon organs are located in tendons and are stimulated by squeeze, thus sending feedback concerning state of EOM tension.
- Extraocular muscles (Figures 1-18 and 1-19 and Table 1-3)
  o Four rectus muscles (medial, lateral, superior, inferior)
  o Arise from the common tendinous ring (the annulus of Zinn)
  o This is an oval thickening of periosteum at the orbital apex.
  o It encircles the optic foramen and the medial part of the SOF.
  o Rectus muscles arise from this tendinous ring and pass forward as a cone to insert in sclera of the globe.

Superior Rectus Muscle

- Arises from the superior aspect of the tendinous ring, partially attached to the dura of optic nerve. Passes forward and lateral at a 23-degree angle.
- Has oblique insertion 7.7 mm from limbus
- As muscle passes through Tenon's fascia, a sheath of fascia spreads posteriorly to cover muscle. This sheath is connected to the levator muscle to ensure the 2 muscles work synergistically. A fascial slip also passes to the superior fornix to help raise it in upgaze.
- Superior division of CN III enters SR at junction of posterior and middle one-third of muscle on inferior side. Branches continue through muscle to innervate levator.

TABLE 1-3. EXTRAOCULAR MUSCLES

Muscle	Origin	Insertion From Limbus	Tendon Length	Nerve	Action
Superior rectus (SR)	Superior tendinous ring	7.7 mm	5.8 mm	Superior division CN III	Elevation Incyclotorsion Adduction
Inferior rectus (IR)	Inferior tendinous ring	6.5 mm	5.5 mm	Inferior division of CN III	Depression Excyclotorsion Adduction
Lateral rectus (LR)	Lateral tendinous ring Greater wing of sphenoid	6.9 mm	8.8 mm	CN VI	Abduction
Medial rectus (MR)	Lateral tendinous ring	5.5 mm	3.7 mm	Inferior division of CN III	Adduction
Superior oblique (SO)	Sphenoid bone superior medial to optic nerve	Inserted posterior to equator, superolaterally	Long	CN IV	Incyclotorsion Depression Abduction
Inferior oblique (IO)	Maxillary bone (anterior orbit)	Posterior to equator, inferolaterally	None	Inferior division CN III	Excyclotorsion Elevation Abduction

Inferior Rectus Muscle

- Arises from inferior aspect of tendinous ring and passes forward and lateral at a 23-degree angle. Pierces Tenon's fascia and a Tenon's sheath likewise covers muscle and also connects to the IO muscle.
- Has connective tissue slip to lower eyelid
- Innervated by branch of inferior division of CN III that enters muscle on superior surface

Lateral Rectus Muscle

- Arises from the lateral portion of the tendinous ring as it bridges the SOF
- A separate smaller head arises from the greater wing of sphenoid bone, lateral to the fibrous ring.
- The muscle passes anteriorly in the lateral aspect of the orbit.
- Innervated by abducens nerve (CN VI) on the medial surface

Medial Rectus Muscle

- Largest of EOM
- Arises from medial tendinous ring and is attached to dura of optic nerve. It passes forward, close to the medial wall of the orbit. It has the shortest tendon and closest insertion to the limbus.
- The fascial sheath covering the muscle sends fibers toward the medial wall of the orbit from the medial check ligament.
- The branch of the inferior division of CN III enters on the internal (lateral) side of the muscle.

Superior Oblique Muscle

- Arises from sphenoid bone just superior-medial to the tendinous ring
- This long slender muscle passes forward and forms a round tendon.
- This tendon becomes covered by a synovial sheath and then passes through the fibrocartilage trochlea located in the trochlear fossa of the frontal bone.

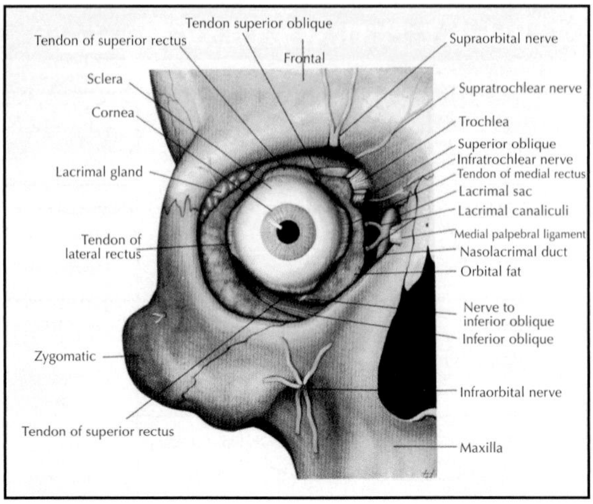

Figure 1-20. Right eye, showing the eyeball exposed from in front. Note the arrangement of the superior and inferior oblique muscles. (*Clinical Anatomy of the Eye*. Snell RS, Lemp MA. Copyright © 1989. Reproduced with permission of Blackwell Scientific Publications.)

- As the tendon exits, it turns downward, backward, and laterally (forming a 54-degree angle), piercing Tenon's fascial sheath to pass below the SR muscle.
- The tendon fans out to attach to sclera posterior to the equator.
- The fascial sheath covering the tendon extends anterior all the way to the trochlea.
- Innervated by the trochlear nerve (CN IV) on the superior surface, close to the insertion

Inferior Oblique Muscle

- It is the only orbital muscle to originate from the front of the orbit.
- Arises from the floor just inside the orbital margin and lateral to the nasolacrimal canal
- Extends posteriorly, superiorly, and laterally (at 51-degree angle) to pass below to inferior rectus muscle
- Attaches posteriorly on the globe, near macula, partially covered by the LR muscle.
- The fascial sheath covering is connected to the sheath of the inferior rectus muscle
- Innervated by a branch of the inferior division of the oculomotor nerve (CN III), entering on the superior surface at its midpoint
- Clinical
  o The oblique muscles lie inferior to the adjacent rectus muscles (Figure 1-20). The SO muscle is inferior to the SR, just as the IO is under the inferior rectus. Remember the old axiom, "Obliquity is inferior to rectitude."
  o The sheaths covering the 4 rectus muscles send connective tissue extension to create the intermuscular septum between the muscles. This creates an intraconal space inside this muscular cone and separates from the extraconal space.
- Spiral of Tillaux (Figure 1-21)
  o The spiral of Tillaux refers to the progressive increase in the distance of the insertion of the rectus muscles with respect to the limbus.
  o The spiral moves from the MR → IR → LR → SR.
  o The distances are approximations and will vary with individuals. The spiral roughly indicates the position of the ora serrata internally.

Orbital Blood Vessels

- Summary
  o There are no lymphatic vessels in the orbit (except draining lacrimal gland and lids).
- Blood supply (Figure 1-22)

Ophthalmic Artery

- The eye and orbit receive most of their blood supply from the ophthalmic artery.

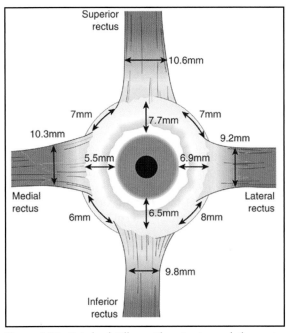

Figure 1-21. Spiral of Tillaux. The structure of the rectus muscle insertions. (The figure was published in Campolattaro BN, Wang FM. Anatomy and physiology of the extraocular muscles and surrounding tissues. In: Yanoff M, Duker JS, eds. *Ophthalmology.* 2nd ed. Copyright Elsevier [2004].)

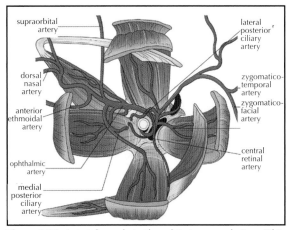

Figure 1-22. Arterial supply to the orbit, in coronal view. (This figure was published in *Atlas of Clinical and Surgical Orbital Anatomy.* Dutton JJ., Copyright Elsevier [1994].)

- First branch of ICA, as it emerges from cavernous sinus
  - Initially within the subarachnoid space, it runs forward and through the optic canal, lateral to the optic nerve.
- It then pierces the meningeal sheath to lie on the outside running inferolateral to the nerve. The artery then turns medially and crosses above the optic nerve (85% of time).
- After reaching the medial wall, it turns anteriorly, running between the MR and SO muscles. At the medial end of the upper eyelid, it divides into supratrochlear and dorsal nasal branches.

Branches of Ophthalmic Artery

Central Retinal Artery

- First branch of ophthalmic artery
- Runs forward under the optic nerve until 1.25 cm prior to globe, where it turns upward, piercing dura and arachnoid, then migrates to the center of the nerve.
- It passes through lamina cribrosa to enter the eye and then divides to supply the 4 quadrants of the eye.
- The blood supply to the inner two-thirds of the retina is from the CRA.
- In 15% of individuals, a cilioretinal artery exists. This branch from the choroid circulation passes up on the lateral side of the optic disc to supply a portion of retina that may include the macula. This can preserve some vision in the event of a cilioretinal artery occlusion. The cilioretinal artery does not anastomose with the CRA.

Lacrimal Artery

- Second branch of the ophthalmic artery
- Runs forward on the LR, supplies the lacrimal gland and continues to the lid
- Branches
  - Muscle branch to LR
  - Zygomatic branches to face
  - Terminal branches to lateral palpebral artery in lids

- Muscular branches
  - o Variable, but tends to follow branches of oculomotor nerve
  - o Each muscle has 2 anterior ciliary arteries (except LR which has one) that supply conjunctiva and sclera and then enter at the muscle insertion to supply the anterior eye, including the major circle of iris.

Ciliary Arteries

Long Posterior Ciliary Artery

- Arises when ophthalmic artery crosses over the top of the optic nerve
- Runs forward with the nerve and enters at 3 and 9 o'clock through sclera external to the ring of short posterior ciliary arteries
- Continues forward between sclera and choroid to the ciliary body, and divides to supply the iris, including the major arterial circle of iris (with branches of anterior ciliary artery), as well as recurrent branches to the anterior choroid

Short Posterior Ciliary Arteries

- Approximately 7 vessels leave the ophthalmic artery as it crosses the optic nerve.
- They divide into up to 20 branches and enter sclera around the optic nerve. They supply the choroid forward to the equator and merge with the flow from the recurrent long posterior artery supply.
- Small branches around the optic nerve join to form the Ring of Zinn and supply the nerve head.

Supraorbital Artery

- Leaves the ophthalmic artery and heads upward to the medial border of the SR
- Follows supraorbital nerve forward, on top of levator superioris muscle, exiting via the supraorbital notch to supply the upper eyelid, forehead, and skull

Posterior Ethmoidal Artery

- Arises from ophthalmic artery to reach the medial orbital wall
- Passes between MR and SO muscles to continue medial through the posterior ethmoidal canal to supply the ethmoidal sinus, dura, or anterior fossa and nasal mucosa

Anterior Ethmoidal Artery

- Larger than the posterior branch, it leaves the orbit through the anterior ethmoidal canal.
- It heads up into the anterior cranial fossa, back down through cribriform plate to the nose, and then out to the face.
- During this long course, it supplies the ethmoidal sinuses, meninges, frontal sinus, nasal cavity, and skin on the nose.

Meningeal Artery

Medial Palpebral Arteries

- Begin below the trochlear pulley and descend behind the nasal lacrimal sac to pierce orbital septum and exit above and below the medial palpebral ligament
- Pass laterally under the orbicularis muscle to enter the upper and lower lids, forming the peripheral and marginal arterial arches that anastomose with branches of lateral palpebral artery (off the lacrimal branch)

Supratrochlear Artery

- This terminal arises near the trochlear pulley, heading up to pierce orbital septum and exit orbit to supply skin to forehead and scalp.

Dorsal Nasal Artery

- This terminal branch pierces orbital septum above the medial palpebral ligament and supplies lacrimal sac and skin of the side of the nose.

Infraorbital Artery

- Arises from the maxillary artery in pterygopalatine fossa, entering orbit through the inferior orbital fissure to supply branches to the inferior rectus and IO muscles and to the lacrimal sac
- It then passes out of the inferior orbital canal to supply the face and upper jaw.

Nerve Supply to the Arteries of the Orbit

Sympathetic

- Postganglionic sympathetic nerves from the superior cervical ganglion supply CRA up to lamina cribrosa (but not beyond).
- Postganglion fibers passing through the ciliary ganglion supply the choroid and iris via the long and short ciliary arteries.

Parasympathetic

- Fibers from the inferior branch of the oculomotor nerve synapse in the ciliary ganglion.
- The resultant postganglionic nerve fibers then pass with the ciliary arteries to enter the eye.
- Their effect on the blood vessels is unknown.

Venous Supply of the Orbit

- The superior and inferior ophthalmic veins drain most of the orbit, emptying into the cavernous sinus (Figure 1-23).
- The central retinal vein empties into the superior ophthalmic vein or directly into the cavernous sinus.
- The veins are tortuous, have many anastomoses, and have no valves.
- Fistulas between the arterial blood and the cavernous sinus can allow higher pressure arterial blood to flow in a retrograde direction down the valveless orbital veins. Trauma may allow a high flow fistula between the carotid circulation and the cavernous sinus. Arterial disease (ie, high blood pressure) may cause a low flow fistula between dural arteries and the cavernous sinus. The retrograde flow will cause engorgement of veins and proptosis.

Superior Ophthalmic Vein

- Begins in the medial upper eyelid where the supraorbital vein and a branch of facial vein join
- Passes posteriorly above the eye in the orbital fat-receiving branches similar to the branches of the ophthalmic artery
- Drains the upper vortex veins
- Usually is joined by the CRA and inferior ophthalmic artery near the apex of the orbit
- Exits through the SOF and drains into the cavernous sinus

Inferior Ophthalmic Vein

- Begins as a plexus on the floor of the orbit
- Passes posteriorly on the inferior rectus, receiving branches from muscle and draining inferior vortex veins
- If it does not drain into the cavernous sinus, it may exit through the inferior orbital fissure and empty into the pterygoid venous plexus.

Central Retinal Vein

- The retinal veins join to form the central retinal vein, which passes through the lamina cribrosa adjacent to the CRA.
- It travels in the optic nerve, but exits 10 to 15 mm behind the eye.
- After passing through the dura sheath, it empties into the superior ophthalmic artery or directly into the cavernous sinus.

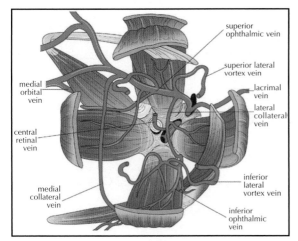

Figure 1-23. Orbital veins. Venous drainage from the orbit, in coronal view. (This figure was published in *Atlas of Clinical and Surgical Orbital Anatomy*. Dutton JJ., Copyright Elsevier [1994].)

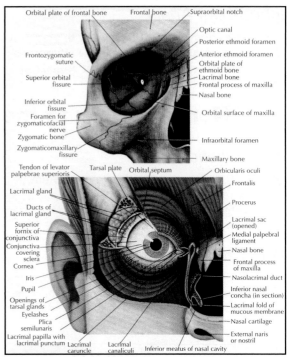

Figure 1-24. Right orbit and the eyelids. (A) Bones of the right orbit, anterior view. (B) Muscles of the eyelids. The lateral part of the upper lid has been removed to reveal the lacrimal gland and its relationship to the tendon of the levator palpebrae superioris muscle and the conjunctiva. (*Clinical Anatomy of the Eye*. Snell RS, Lemp MA. Copyright © 1989. Reproduced with permission of Blackwell Scientific Publications.)

Bones of the Orbit

- The orbital cavity is a pear-shaped bony socket with its apex directed posteriorly, medially, and superiorly (Figure 1-24).
- The media walls of the 2 orbits run parallel with each other in the sagittal plane (forward and backward).
- The lateral wall extends 45 degrees to the medial wall (and 90 degrees to the other lateral wall).
- The orbital margin is very strong and forms a quadrilateral shape.

Orbital Rim

Inferior Rim

- The infraorbital foramen opens 5 mm below the midpoint of the rim and contains the infraorbital vessels and nerve. This margin is quite sharp.

Medial Rim

- The lower half of the margin is distinct and easily palpable. The upper half becomes indistinct.

Superior Rim

- Rounded medial one-third and sharp lateral two-thirds. At the junction is the supraorbital notch (sometimes foramen) containing the supra-orbital vessels and nerve.

TABLE 1-4. ANTERIOR ORBITAL LANDMARKS

Rim	*Bone Structures Forming the Rim*
Inferior	Zygomatic bone Maxillary bone
Medial	Maxillary process of frontal bone
Superior	Lacrimal crest of the frontal process of the maxilla Frontal bone
Lateral	Frontal process of zygomatic bone Zygomatic process of frontal bone

TABLE 1-5. ORBITAL ANATOMY

Wall	*Bone Structure Forming the Wall*
Floor	Orbital plate of maxilla Orbital surface of zygoma Palatine
Medial	Frontal process of maxilla Lacrimal Orbital plate of ethmoid Body of sphenoid
Roof	Orbital plate of frontal Lesser wing of sphenoid
Lateral	Zygomatic Greater wing of sphenoid

Lateral Rim

- The strongest rim. A marginal tubercle, just inside rim, is the attachment for the lateral slip of the levator aponeurosis, the lateral palpebral ligament, and the lateral check ligament (see Table 1-4).

Orbital Walls

- The 4 walls of the orbit are made from 7 bones (Table 1-5).

Floor

- The thin floor separates the orbit from the maxillary sinus.
- Anteriorly, the wall is continuous with the lateral wall but is separated posteriorly by the inferior orbital fissure.
- The infraorbital groove extends forward on the maxillary bone. As it migrates anteriorly, it becomes a canal and then a foramen that opens below the rim onto the face.
  - The floor below the fissure is stronger than the thin bone on either side.

Figure 1-25. Orbital apex, superior and inferior orbital fissure, MR, IR, LR, SR, levator (L), and SO. Note that the trochlear nerve lies outside the muscle cone. (This figure was published in *Review of Ophthalmology.* Friedman NJ, Kaiser PK, Trattler WB. Copyright Elsevier [2005].)

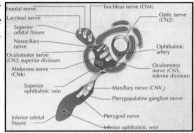

Medial Wall

- This wall is very thin.
- It separates the orbit from the ethmoidal air cells and the nose.
- Anteriorly, the lacrimal groove contains the nasolacrimal sac.
- This is bound by the anterior and posterior lacrimal crests and opens inferiorly as the nasolacrimal duct.

Roof

- Separates orbit from anterior cranial fossa containing the frontal lobe
- Above the anterior medial roof are the frontal air sinuses.
- Laterally, a concave fossa contains the lacrimal gland just inside the rim.

Lateral Wall

- This is the thickest wall.
- Anteriorly, the zygomatic bone separates the orbit from the temporal fossa.
- Posteriorly, the greater wing of the sphenoid separates the orbit from the middle cranial fossa containing the temporal lobe.
- The SOF divides the roof from the lateral wall in the posterior orbit.

Openings in the Orbit

Optic Canal

- Contained within the lesser wing of sphenoid bone
- It is 4- to 10-mm long and connects the orbit to the middle cranial fossa.
- The optic canal contains the optic nerve and its meningeal covering and the ophthalmic artery surrounding the sympathetic nerve plexus (Figure 1-25).

Superior Orbital Fissure

- Lying between the greater and lesser wings of the sphenoid bone, this fissure sits between the roof and the lateral wall.
- A small spine sits midway on the lower edge and allows the attachment of the origin of the LR muscle.
- The origins of the 4 rectus muscles form the circle, the common tendinous ring of Zinn, which surrounds the optic nerve and bisects the SOF.
- This ring is formed by a thickening of the periosteum of the associated bones.
- Structures in the SOF
  - Within Ring of Zinn
    - Superior and inferior divisions of oculomotor (III) nerve
    - Abducens nerve (CN VI)
    - Nasociliary nerve (branch of V1)
  - Lateral to Ring of Zinn
    - Lacrimal nerve (CN VI)
    - Frontal nerve (CN V1)
    - Trochlear nerve (CN IV)
    - Superior ophthalmic vein

Inferior Orbital Fissure

- Lies between greater wing of sphenoid and the orbital plate of the maxilla
- Connects the orbit to the pterygopalatine and infratemporal fossa
- Structures within the inferior orbital fissure
  - Maxillary nerve (subsequently called the infraorbital nerve) (CN V2)
  - Zygomatic nerve (CN V2)
  - SNS nerve from pterygopalatine plexus
  - Inferior ophthalmic vein

Zygomaticofacial and Zygomaticotemporal Foramina

- These small foramina lie in the lateral orbital wall and transmit the zygomaticofacial nerve to the face

- Clinical
  - The bony orbit is essentially a closed space. The posterior openings are filled with structures or covered by periosteum (inferior orbital fissure). Masses, swelling, inflammation, or bleeding will commonly result in proptosis.
  - The rim is very strong but can be fractured with significant force. A force directly on the eye can allow a "blow out fracture" that breaks the thin bones of the floor or medial wall. Inferior blow-out fractures can damage the infraorbital nerve, resulting in anesthesia of the cheek.
  - Sharp objects entering the orbit, in addition to ocular trauma, can pierce through the thin orbital roof into the anterior cranial fossa.
  - The close proximity of the important structures at the orbital apex makes them susceptible to compression by expanding pathologies. The symptoms and signs of such compression could include vision loss, motility impairment, and anesthesia of the cornea, forehead, and nose.

Embryology Overview

- Summary
  - Embryonic plate → neural plate → optic pit → optic stalk → optic vesicle → optic cup
- Fertilization leads to a blastocele (clump of cells)
  - Mass of inner layer cells (= embryo blast) that become the embryo
  - By day 16, the embryo blast differentiates into a trilaminar disc (3 layers in the center of the placenta).
  - The trilaminar disc refers to the 3 primary germ cell layers
    - Ectoderm
    - Mesoderm
    - Endoderm
- Only ectoderm and mesoderm involved in eye development
  - By the end of week 3, the ectoderm differentiates into the following:
    - Surface ectoderm
      - Covers outside
    - Neuroectoderm
      - This central area thickens and rolls inward, forming the neural tube (Figure 1-26). Portions of this migrate posteriorly to become neural crest tissue.
  - At the rostral (brain) end, the neural folds have not yet fused into the neural tube.
  - Thickening of neural ectoderm here produces optic primordium.
  - The optic primordium migrates outward (causing an optic pit when viewed from inside).
  - As this invagination elongates outward, the pit becomes the optic stalk.
  - The end of the stalk, the optic vesicle, contacts the outer layer, made of surface ectoderm.
  - Contact induces the surface ectoderm to thicken, becoming the lens placode (day 27).
  - The optic vesicle begins to fold in on itself, forming the optic cup.
  - The lens placode invaginates into the optic cup, separating from the surface ectoderm and becoming the lens vesicle (day 33).

Figure 1-26. Neural tube formation. (This figure was published in *Review of Ophthalmology*. Friedman NJ, Kaiser PK, Trattler WB. Copyright Elsevier [2005].)

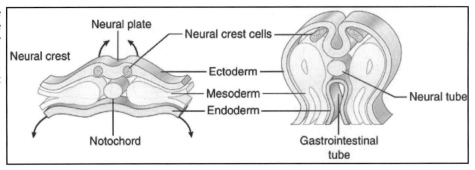

Figure 1-27. Components of the tunica vasculosa lentis. (Illustration by Christine Gralapp.) (This figure was published in *Review of Ophthalmology*. Friedman NJ, Kaiser PK, Trattler WB. Copyright Elsevier [2005].)

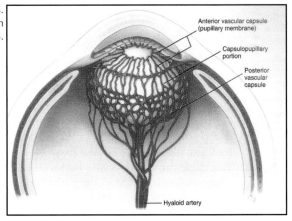

- A fissure develops on the inferior surface of the optic stalk and cup, called the optic (or choroidal) fissure.
- This allows the migration of mesoderm into the optic stalk that will become the hyaloid system (day 33).
- The hyaloid artery surrounds the lens and creates tunica vasculosa lentis (Figure 1-27).

Embryologic Structures and Origins

- Lens (Table 1-6 and Figure 1-28)
  - The lens cells (surface ectoderm) are oriented inward, forming an external BM that becomes the lens capsule.
  - The anterior cells (ie, front of lens) remain below the capsule while the posterior cells elongate, becoming lens fibrils, and lose their nuclei.
  - The primary lens fibers form the central embryonic nucleus. The epithelial cells at the equator of the lens elongate and become fibrils that extend to cover the nucleus. The ends of the fibrils have common attachments, forming the Y sutures anterior and posterior to the embryonic nucleus (Figure 1-29).
  - Clinical
    - The lens capsule surrounds the surface ectoderm-derived lens and isolates it immunologically from the remainder of the eye.
- Vitreous (Figure 1-30)
  - The primary vitreous develops from the hyaloid system (weeks 5 to 6).
  - This regresses to give Cloquet's canal.
  - It collapses to the center as the secondary avascular vitreous, made of collagen and vitreous gel from the retina, fills the eye (month 2).
  - The tertiary vitreous is the formation of collagen lens zonules between the lens equator and optic cup.

TABLE 1-6. EMBRYOLOGIC STRUCTURES AND ORIGINS

EMBRYOLOGIC STRUCTURE	ORIGIN
Retina	Neuroectoderm
RPE	Neuroectoderm
Optic nerve	Neuroectoderm
Choroid	
Endothelium	Mesoderm
Mesenchyma	Neural crest
Sclera	
Most	Neural crest
Temporal part	Mesoderm
Cornea	
Epithelium	Surface ectoderm
Remainder	Neural crest
Angle	
TM	Neural crest
Schlemm's canal	Mesoderm
Iris	
Epithelium	Neural ectoderm
Muscles	Neural ectoderm
Stroma	Neural crest
Lens	Surface ectoderm
Lids	Surface ectoderm
Muscles	Mesoderm
Bones	Neural crest
Fat	Neural crest
Lacrimal gland	Surface ectoderm

- Retina
  - The folding inward of the optic cup creates a double layer of neuroectoderm.
  - The inside thicker layer develops into the neurosensory retina.
  - The outside thinner layer becomes the retinal pigment epithelium later. It is separated from the inner layer by a transient "nerve fiber layer of Chievitz," which later becomes the inner plexiform layer. The retinal pigment epithelia are the first cells in the body to produce melanin. They have an inductive effect, as the underlying choroid and sclera do not grow appropriately in the absence of retinal pigment epithelium.
  - Clinical
    - The embryonic layer, the potential space between outer pigmented retina (RPE) and the inner neural retina can become separated by a retinal detachment.

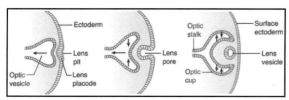

Figure 1-28. Optic cup formation. (Reprinted with permission from Friedman NJ, Kaiser PK, Trattler WB. *Review of Ophthalmology.* Philadelphia, PA: Elsevier; 2005.)

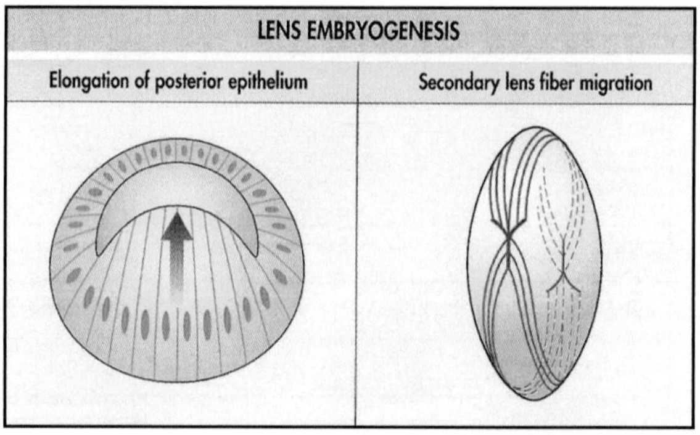

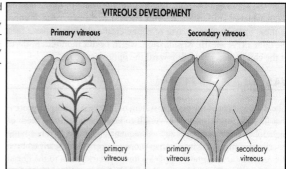

Figure 1-29. Lens embryogenesis. Elongation of the posterior epithelium results in obliteration of the lens lumen. Secondary lens fiber migration leads to the formation of the Y sutures. (This figure was published in Azar NF, Davis EA. Embryology of the eye. In: Yanoff M, Duker JS, eds. *Ophthalmology.* 2nd ed. Copyright Elsevier [2004].)

Figure 1-30. Vitreous development. The primary vitreous and hyaloid artery fill the optic cup. The primary vitreous retracts, and the hyaloids artery regresses, while the secondary avascular vitreous develops. (This figure was published in Azar NF, Davis EA. Embryology of the eye. In: Yanoff M, Duker JS, eds. *Ophthalmology.* 2nd ed. Copyright Elsevier [2004].)

- Optic nerve
  - In week 6, ganglion cells develop from the optic stalk and migrate toward the eye.
  - At week 7, pia, arachnoid, and dura differentiate from neural crest cells.
  - Myelination starts at chiasm in month 7 and ends at lamina cribrosa at 1 month after birth.
- Choroid
  - Made of mesenchymal tissue (neural crest) surrounding the vascular channels that are endothelial lined (mesoderm).
- Sclera
  - Most of sclera is neural crest.
  - The temporal section is mesoderm.
  - Develops later as it progresses from anterior (week 7) to posterior (week 12) as the neural crest cells migrate
  - The lamina cribrosa is made of neural crest cells that have penetrated the optic nerve.
- Cornea
  - Epithelium is surface ectoderm.
  - The other layers are from the neural crest, which pinched off the lens placode. Descemet's and Bowman's membranes develop in the third and fourth months.
- Anterior chamber and angle
  - Trabecular meshwork is made of neural crest cells.
  - Schlemm's canal is made of mesoderm. Cells from trabecular meshwork meet the iris at week 15. At birth, the angle is narrow and begins to deepen 3 months after birth.
- Iris and ciliary body
  - The pigmented epithelium is made of the neural ectoderm that was at the tip of the optic cup. It is continuous with the 2 layers of the retina/RPE.
  - The sphincter and dilator papillae muscle are also neural ectoderm from the RPE layer that moves forward, but the stroma is from neural crest cells that migrate inward.

- Eyelids
  - Surface ectoderm extends over the cornea and then fuses by week 10 to 12. They separate at month 6 when glandular structure and cilia develop.
- Vascular system
  - Ophthalmic artery develops at week 6.
  - Retina vascularization begins at the fourth month and reaches the nasal ora serrata at week 32. It completes the vascularization by reaching the temporal ora at term.
- Periocular tissues
  - Bones, cartilage fat, and connective tissue are all neural crest.
  - EOMs arise from mesoderm (week 5 to 7).
  - Lacrimal gland is surface ectoderm (week 6 to 7).
- Realignment of globes
  - Initially = 180 degrees
  - Month 3 = 105 degrees
  - Birth = 71 degrees
  - Adult = 68 degrees

Suggested Readings

Bron AJ, Tripathi RC, Tripathi BJ. *Wolff's Anatomy of the Eye and Orbit*, 8th ed. London, UK: Chapman & Hall; 2001.

Cibis GW, et al. *Fundamentals and Principles of Ophthalmology*, Section 2: Basic science and clinic course. San Francisco, CA: American Academy of Ophthalmology; 2003.

Freidman NJ, Kaiser PK, Trattler WB. *Review of Ophthalmology*. Philadelphia, PA: Elsevier Saunders Publishing; 2005.

Smith ME, Kincaid MC, West CE. *Basic Science, Refraction and Pathology*, the requisites. St. Louis, MO: Mosby; 2002.

Snell RS, Lemp MA. *Clinical Anatomy of the Eye*, 2nd edition. London, UK: Blackwell Science; 1998.

Stewart WB. *Surgery of Eyelid, Orbit and Lacrimal System*. Vol. 1-3. San Francisco, CA: American Academy of Ophthalmology; 1993.

Questions

1. Which of the following does not result from failure of the optic fissure to close?
   a. Optic nerve coloboma
   b. Lid coloboma
   c. Iris coloboma
   d. Choroidal coloboma

   The lid is formed by surface ectoderm, later in ocular development. The optic nerve, iris, and choroid are made of neuroectoderm and are completed when the optic (choroidal) fissure of the optic vesicle closes completely around the mesoderm that becomes the hyaloid artery.

2. The uveal tract (uvea) is attached at all of the following *except*:
   a. Scleral spur
   b. Ora serrata
   c. Vortex veins
   d. Optic nerve

   The retina attaches to the choroid at the ora serrata. The choroid is continuous with the ciliary body and attaches at the scleral spur, as well as at the optic nerve, entrances of the ciliary arteries, and exits of the vortex vein. An ultrasound can help differentiate a retinal detachment from a choroidal detachment using this anatomic knowledge.

3. What region of the retina is last to be vascularized?
   a. Temporal retina
   b. Equator
   c. Nasal periphery
   d. Posterior pole

   The nasal retina is shorter than the temporal retina due to the nasal side insertion of the optic nerve.

4. Which wall of the orbit is the thinnest?
   a. Superior
   b. Inferior
   c. Lateral
   d. Medial

The medial wall (lamina papyracea of the ethmoid bones).

5. Which of the following is *not* a branch of the ophthalmic division of the trigeminal nerve?
   a. Lacrimal
   b. Supratrochlear
   c. Long ciliary
   d. Zygomaticofacial

Zygomaticofacial and zygomaticotemporal are branches of the maxillary division of the trigeminal nerve.

6. Where does the nasolacrimal duct enter the nose?
   a. Superior meatus
   b. Under middle turbinate
   c. Inferior meatus
   d. Sphenoethmoidal recess

Under inferior turbinate in the inferior meatus.

7. Which muscle originates in the annulus of Zinn?
   a. Levator palpebrae
   b. Lateral rectus
   c. Superior oblique
   d. Inferior oblique

The annulus of Zinn is made up of the origins of the 4 rectus muscles.

8. Which extraocular muscle inserts the furthest posterior from the limbus?
   a. Superior rectus
   b. Medial rectus
   c. Inferior rectus
   d. Lateral rectus

Superior rectus (remember the spiral of Tillaux). The SO and IO insert even further posteriorly, behind the equator.

9. The inner plexiform layer of the retina contains all of the following *except*:
   a. Synapses of ganglion cells
   b. Axons of horizontal cells
   c. Axons of amacrine cells
   d. Axons of bipolar cells

The horizontal cells synapse in the OPL, sending photoreceptor information laterally.

10. All of the following are true concerning Müller's muscle (superior tarsus muscle) *except*:
    a. Horner's syndrome will cause a mild ptosis
    b. Hyperthyroidism can cause lid retraction
    c. Phenylephrine drops for dilation can increase the palpebral fissure width
    d. Fear and excitement lower the upper lid

Fear and excitement will ↑SNS and contract Müller's muscle, thereby elevating the lid. This is the mechanism of lid retraction with phenylephrine and hyperthyroidism (↑SNS). Horner's syndrome (↓SNS) can cause partial ptosis.

Ocular Examination

Peter Bergenske, OD

Outline

Probst LE, Tsai JH.
Ophthalmology: Clinical and Surgical Principles (pp. 53–90).
© 2012 SLACK Incorporated

The Case History

Chief Complaint and General History

- A problem-oriented approach is most practical, with focus on the chief complaint and any secondary complaints.
- The personal and family general health histories are also part of the comprehensive ocular examination.

History Specific to the Ocular Examination

- Patients may neglect to mention symptoms that they assume are normal or that they feel are not related to their eyes or vision.
- It is important to document timing, onset, duration, and any factors that relieve or exacerbate the symptoms or complaints.
- Patients often present for a routine eye examination with no, or minimal, symptoms.

Common Visual Complaints

Blurred Vision

- To inquire about distance vision, one might ask "Do you have difficulty reading road signs while driving?" or "Do you have trouble reading the board or overheads in school?"
- To inquire about near vision, one might ask if the patient has difficulty reading fine print such as the telephone book or medication labels.
- Patient responses to these questions help form preliminary diagnoses of refractive and other visual problems.
  - Blur for distance with no difficulty at near is indicative of myopia.
  - Minimal blur for distance, but increasing symptoms and blur at near may indicate hyperopia, or possibly a deficiency of accommodation or convergence.
  - Blur that is relatively distance independent may indicate astigmatic error or possible media opacity.

Headache

- Common primary or secondary complaint
- May be related to ocular conditions such as uncorrected refractive error or associated with visual symptoms, such as in migraine with visual aura, or may be unrelated to the visual system
- Headaches occurring in direct association with demanding visual tasks are likely due to uncorrected refractive error (hyperopia or anisometropia especially), accommodative insufficiency, or disorders of the binocular system.
- Vision-related headaches are typically dull, mild to moderate in severity, and are generally relieved by cessation of the visual task.
- Headaches due to accommodative stress are usually described as brow or frontal.
- Squinting to compensate for low degrees of uncorrected refractive error commonly leads to muscle tension-type headache.
- Headaches that cannot be related to use of the eyes are most likely due to other causes, and the ocular examination often serves to rule out visual problems from the long list of possible headache etiologies.

Ocular Discomfort (Asthenopia)

- Symptoms may include eye pain or ache, ocular fatigue, or general discomfort of the eyes and surrounding area.
- Although organic causes of these symptoms bear investigation, such symptoms can arise from refractive, accommodative, or binocular deficiencies as well.

Dry Eye

- Dry eye is a common ocular complaint.
- Patients will more commonly complain of sandy, gritty, or burning sensation rather than dryness.
- Although numerous objective tests have been developed to aid in the diagnosis of dry eye, the patient history is perhaps the most significant, as the patient's symptoms correlate with his or her level of discomfort.
- A variety of dry eye questionnaires have been developed and validated to assist in the identification of patients with different degrees of dry eye.

Important Elements of Ocular History

Current Refractive Correction

- Current spectacles should be analyzed completely.
  - The current lens power and add power if present
  - The type of multifocal
  - The presence of prism
  - Base curves

o For soft contact lenses, it is helpful if the patient is asked to provide the lens packaging, as this will contain information on the lens material, power, base curve, and diameter.
o In addition, the contact lens wearer should be asked about his or her current lens-wearing regimen, along with the following:
  ▪ Frequency of scheduled lens replacements
  ▪ Number of hours worn per day
  ▪ Frequency of overnight wear
  ▪ Lens care regimen

Family Ocular History

- The most common ocular and related conditions with strong hereditary influences include the following:
  o Refractive error
  o Color deficiency
  o Glaucoma
  o Diabetes
- Other, less common conditions with strong familial ties include the following:
  o Retinitis pigmentosa
  o Retinoblastoma
  o Nystagmus
  o Ocular coloboma

Medical History

- Common systemic conditions with ocular manifestations include the following:
  o Diabetes
  o Hypertension
  o Connective tissue disorders
  o Thyroid disease
  o Embolic conditions
  o HIV-AIDS
- Many systemic medications can have significant ocular effects.

The Ocular Examination

Visual Acuity

- Measure of the visual system's ability to resolve fine detail
- Typically measured using a chart with a series of letters of decreasing size
- Visual acuity is indicated as the smallest object read at the specified test distance. Good visual acuity implies the following:
  o Adequate optical correction
  o Normalcy of the ocular structures and visual pathway
- Reduced visual acuity is the most common reason for ocular examination and warrants systematic evaluation to determine its cause and possible amelioration.

Limitations of Visual Acuity

- Visual acuity is limited by the following:
  o Optical characteristics of the eye
  o Spacing of photoreceptors in the retina
- Illumination and contrast can also affect visual acuity measurement. Effort should be made to maintain constant conditions for acuity measurement to avoid apparent change that may simply be due to lighting conditions.

Units of Measurement

- The standard notation for visual acuity is the Snellen fraction.
- The numerator represents the testing distance. For distance vision, the standard in the United States is 20 feet. Elsewhere, it is commonly 6 meters.
- The denominator is the letter size, specified in terms of the distance at which the letter subtends 5 minutes of arc.
- Standard letters for visual acuity testing have a stroke width of 1 minute of arc.
- Visual acuity of 20/20 indicates the test was performed at 20 feet and the patient was able to resolve letters that subtend 5 minutes of arc at 20 feet.
- For patients with vision so poor that they cannot read any letters on the test chart at the standard distance, it may be necessary to move them closer to the chart until some letters can be read. In such case, the acuity is recorded as the test distance over the letters read. If the patient can read the 200 letters with the chart at 5 feet, the acuity is 5/200.
- When the acuity is too poor to resolve any letters regardless of distance, it is still useful to record an indication of quality of vision present. The common notations include the following:
  - Counting fingers (CF)
    - Patient is able to count fingers of examiner in front of patient's face.
  - Hand motion (HM)
    - Patient is able to tell the examiner is waving a hand in front of the patient.
  - Light perception (LP)
    - Patient is unable to detect the movement of a hand, but can discern if a light is being shone into the eye or not.
  - No light perception (NLP)
    - The patient is not able to sense light at all.

Measurement of Visual Acuity

- Visual acuity is usually measured with the patient seated in the examination chair.
- Lighting and chart conditions should ideally be standardized.
- Visual acuity testing may be conducted as follows:
  - Have the patient occlude one eye but keep both eyes open.
  - Measure acuity in one eye, then occlude that eye and measure acuity in the other.
  - Measure acuity with both eyes together.
  - Encourage the patient to keep trying once he or she stops reading letters.
  - Once he or she is missing about half the letters on a line, threshold has been reached.
  - The examiner should watch the patient to note if the patient is squinting, has abnormal head position, and to make certain the fellow eye is properly occluded.

Acuity Chart Design

- Acuity charts typically consist of approximately 10 lines of letters, or optotypes, that decrease in size from top to bottom (Figure 2-1).
- Within a line, letters are of equal stroke width and spacing.
- Letters should be of equal legibility.
- For pediatric and illiterate populations, special optotypes are used that require the subject to identify an object or an orientation.

Testing for Visual Acuity at Near

- Visual acuity measured at 20 feet that is not maintained at a near working distance is often caused by presbyopia.
- As for distance visual acuity, each eye should first be tested independently, then together.
- It is best to use test letters or text that follows rules similar to those used for distance testing. One such system is referred to as M notation, and the notations refer to meters at which the letter subtends 5 minutes of arc (Figure 2-2).
- Many methods of specifying print size are in common use: Jaeger's, point size, Snellen equivalent. All have limitations that make the M system preferable. The test distance should routinely be recorded.

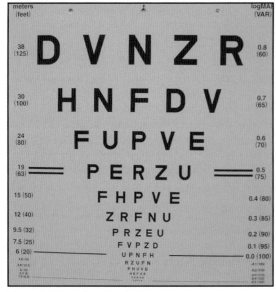

Figure 2-1. Visual acuity chart.

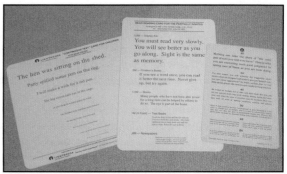

Figure 2-2. Cards for testing near visual acuity.

Acuity Testing With Pinhole

- Placing a pinhole in front of the eye reduces the effective pupil size and diminishes the blur circle at the retina.
- This simple principle makes the pinhole test useful in determining whether reduced acuity is likely due to refractive error or some other cause.
- If acuity improves with the pinhole, it is likely that the problem is refractive and that the eye can be corrected to the acuity achieved with the pinhole by spectacle correction or a contact lens.
- If acuity is not improved with the pinhole, the assumption is that the reduction in acuity is due to a problem with the ocular media, retina, or optic nerve.

Visual Acuity Standards

- There are numerous standards of visual acuity that individuals must meet in order to be eligible for certain privileges, occupations, or benefits.
- It is important to distinguish between visual acuity measured without correction (uncorrected) and acuity measured with best correction.
- A minimum of 20/40 in at least one eye (with or without correction) is commonly required for an unrestricted driver's license.
- Some occupations, such as police officers and firefighters, are required to have at least 20/40 acuity without correction.
- Entry into some military services, such as pilot training, often requires 20/20 acuity without correction.
- One specification for legal blindness is acuity of no better than 20/200 in the better eye with best correction.

Pupil Testing

Pupil Size

- Pupil size should be observed in both moderate and dim illumination, documenting the size of each pupil in the 2 conditions (Figure 2-3).
- Pupil sizes are typically equal, and differences greater than 1 mm or 20% are considered significant degrees of anisocoria.
- Anisocoria that is greater in the light than in the dark suggests a problem with innervation or function of the sphincter muscle of the eye with the larger pupil.
- Anisocoria that is greater in the dark suggests a problem with innervation or function of the dilator muscle in the eye with the smaller pupil.

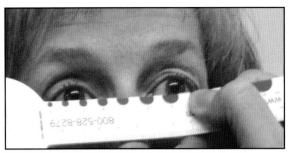

Figure 2-3. Pupil size can be estimated with a graduated ruler as shown.

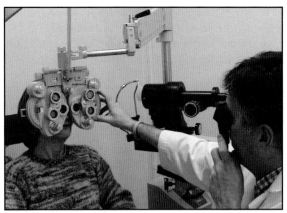

Figure 2-4. Retinoscopy.

Light Reflex

- Stimulating one eye with a bright light source should cause the pupils in both eyes to constrict.
- Removal of the light source should cause the pupils of both eyes to dilate.
- The response of the eye stimulated by the light is called the direct response.
- The response of the fellow eye is called the consensual response.

Swinging Flashlight Test

- The swinging flashlight test is useful in comparing the patency of the visual pathways in the 2 eyes.
- The light source illuminates one eye for several seconds and then is briskly moved to the other eye. Observation is made of the eye being illuminated.
- Continued constriction of each pupil is expected.
- Dilation of the stimulated pupil indicates that the consensual response is greater than the direct and that there is a relative afferent defect for this eye.
- Constriction of the stimulated pupil indicates that the direct response is greater than the consensual and that there is a relative afferent defect for the fellow eye.

Near Response

- The pupils should constrict with accommodative effort, regardless of accommodative amplitude.
- The magnitude of constriction should be similar to that which is observed with the light response.

Assessment of Refractive Error

Retinoscopy

- Retinoscopy (Figure 2-4) is a simple and effective means of objectively determining the refractive status of the eye.
- As not all patients can respond adequately to subjective tests or be adequately evaluated with automated devices, it is imperative that the ophthalmic clinician master the technique.
- Retinoscopy is based on the following principles:
  - The clinician shines the beam of light into the patient's eye and observes the resulting red reflex (which is the light imaged on the retina).
  - The clinician moves the light by tilting the head of the retinoscope and observes the movement of the reflex relative to the direction of movement of the light.
  - Movement in the same direction is called *with* motion and indicates the observed eye has a focal length that is longer than the examiner's working distance. Typical working distance is 67 cm, or -1.50 diopters (D). Thus, *with* motion indicates the eye is less than 1.50 D myopic (and may be emmetropic or hyperopic).
  - If motion is in the opposite direction, it is called *against* motion and indicates the focal length of the eye is less than the working distance.

o No motion of the observed reflex indicates neutrality and that the focal length of the eye is the same as the working distance.
- Determining refractive status of the eye by retinoscopy involves observation of the reflex and adjusting lenses in front of the patient's eye until neutrality is observed.
   o If *with* motion is observed, plus lenses are added.
   o If *against* motion is observed, minus lenses are added.
   o The working distance must be subtracted from the neutral point. That is, if neutrality is observed with a plano lens in front of the eye, the refractive status is -1.50 D. If neutrality is reached at +1.50, the refractive status is emmetropia. The adjustment made depends on the working distance, which is assumed here to be a standard 67 cm.
- For astigmatic eyes, neutrality must be found for both major meridians. The major meridians are determined using the retinoscope streak reflex to find the meridians in which the reflex aligns with the projected streak.
- Automated devices have been developed that will provide a retinoscopic finding with a high degree of accuracy in a majority of eyes. Their use is limited, however, in that they often provide unreliable findings in eyes with irregular astigmatism or media opacity and in uncooperative patients such as very young children.

Subjective Refraction

- Although retinoscopy and automated, objective methods are capable of determining the refractive status with a high degree of accuracy, subjective response from the patient is highly valuable in determining an acceptable and optimal correction (Figure 2-5).
- The process involves finding the optimal refraction for each eye independently, then balancing the 2 eyes for a final binocular endpoint.

Monocular Refraction

- The starting point for the refraction point will be the retinoscopy finding, the patient's previous spectacle correction, or the results of an autorefraction. The basic steps are the following:
   o Find the best sphere correction
   o Find the cylinder power
   o Find the axis
   o Refine the cylinder power
   o Refine the axis
   o Refine the sphere
- The process is one of providing a choice between 2 lens powers or axes while the patient views suprathreshold letters. The patient is to respond indicating which of the 2 choices gives the clearest and sharpest vision.

Spherical Refraction

- The size of steps between choices is a function of the patient's ability to notice difference. For example, 0.25 to 0.50 D changes are typical with normal acuity and sensitivity.
- Care must be taken to not "over-minus" the patient who is able to accommodate easily, as additional minus will not blur the vision.
- When additional plus power blurs the target and additional minus does not improve the acuity, the best sphere lens has been found.
- Astigmatism is similarly determined; however, it is useful to have a starting point to determine axis and power.
- The retinoscope finding and previous spectacles can be very helpful when available. In addition, the keratometer is useful. The keratometer measures radius of curvature of the cornea.
- As the cornea is the primary refracting element of the eye, corneal astigmatism is typically quite consistent with refractive astigmatism power and axis.
- Lenticular astigmatism most often creates error of approximately −0.50 diopters of cylinder (DC) x 90
- Javal's rule states the following:
   o Refractive astigmatism = (Corneal astigmatism + [-0.50 DC x 90])

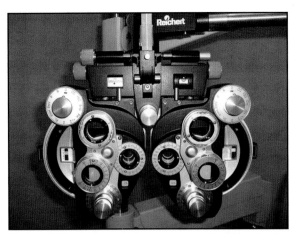

Figure 2-5. The phoropter is commonly used to determine the subjective refraction.

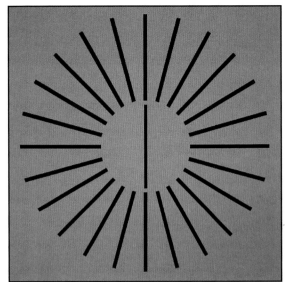

Figure 2-6. A fan dial chart for determining astigmatism.

Cylindrical Refraction

- Subjective determination of approximate cylinder power and axis can be achieved by having the patient observe a fan dial chart (Figure 2-6) through a modest amount of plus power.
- Starting with the entire fan dial blurred, the amount of plus is reduced until the patient reports that one line on the fan dial appears darker than the others.
- The darker line is perpendicular to the axis of the minus cylinder lens needed (referring to the lines as clock hours, the axis will be the clock hour multiplied by 30).
- Final cylinder power and axis determination is commonly and best arrived at through use of the Jackson flip crossed cylinder.
    o Cylinder power is determined in a manner similar to that of the sphere using the flip of the Jackson cylinder as the 2 choices.
    o The cylinder axis of the Jackson lens is marked in red for the minus cylinder axis and in white for the plus cylinder axis.
    o The axis is placed in alignment with the cylinder in the phoropter or trial frame, and the patient chooses the better of the 2 choices. If testing in minus cylinder, selecting the position with red aligned with the axis indicates a call for more minus cylinder power.
    o Axis is determined by bisecting the axis being tested. For minus cylinder testing, the axis is rotated in the direction indicated by the red markings of the preferred position, eventually bracketing to a final position.

Binocular Balance

- Once the monocular refraction is completed, procedures should be followed to ensure balanced accommodative demand whenever possible.
- The most common method is to use the von Graefe technique of equalizing blur under condition of prism-induced diplopia.
- The von Graefe technique assumes the 2 eyes have equal best-corrected acuities.
- A prism of power of approximately 4 prism diopters (PD) is placed base up before the right eye, thus displacing the image for this eye below the image of the left eye.
- Plus power of +0.50 to +0.75 is added to the monocular finding for each eye, creating a slight degree of blur.
- Viewing a suprathreshold line of letters (ie, a line or two larger than the smallest line the patient can read), the patient is asked to compare the two images.
- The sphere power(s) is adjusted to create equal degree of blur.
- Fusion is restored by removing the prism, and the sphere powers are then adjusted in tandem to give best binocular visual acuity.

Cycloplegic Refraction

- The pre-presbyopic hyperopic patient is often able to see well simply by exerting enough additional accommodation to compensate for the hyperopia.
- This habitual use of accommodation can result in a relatively high level of tonic accommodation.
- The clinician may find the patient accepts less plus power than the full amount of hyperopia.
- Cycloplegia, which temporarily inactivates the accommodative mechanism, is a useful tool in detecting the full amount of hyperopia.
- Cycloplegic agents are parasympatholytic agents that affect the iris sphincter and ciliary muscle, causing mydriasis and loss of accommodation.
- The most commonly used cycloplegic agent is 1% cyclopentolate, which causes nearly complete cycloplegia in 20 to 60 minutes with effects lasting 6 to 24 hours.
- The amount of plus accepted by routine (noncycloplegic) refraction is called the *manifest hyperopia*.
- *Latent hyperopia* is the difference in the amount plus accepted with cycloplegia compared to the manifest hyperopia.
- Cycloplegic findings are perhaps of greatest value in evaluation of infants and strabismic children; however, some degree of cycloplegia should also be employed in the preoperative workup of the refractive surgery patient.

Accommodation

- The process of accommodation allows the eye to temporarily change focal length, allowing diverging light from near objects to be focused on the retina.
- Contraction of the ciliary muscle allows relaxation of the zonular fibers and subsequent increase in convexity of the crystalline lens.
- Accommodation stimulus and response are commonly expressed in diopters, the reciprocal of the linear distance in meters from the object to the eye.
- The accommodative *far point* is the point for which the eye is in focus with accommodation fully relaxed.
- The accommodative *near point* is the point for which the eye is in focus with maximum accommodation.
- Accommodative *amplitude* is the dioptric equivalent of the distance between the far point and the near point.
- Accommodative amplitude typically declines with age in a fairly linear pattern.

Measurement of Accommodation

Amplitude of Accommodation

- Assuming the far point is established and the refractive error corrected, the amplitude of accommodation is measured subjectively.
  - A detailed target is slowly advanced toward the eye(s) as the patient attempts to keep the target in sharp focus.
  - A target is kept at a set distance (typically 40 cm), and minus lenses are added to change the demand.
  - The end point of measurement is when the patient first indicates slight, sustained blur of the target as accommodative demand is increased.

Accommodative Response

- The response of the eye to an accommodative stimulus may be accommodation that is equal to, greater than, or less than the stimulus. Assessment of the response can be accomplished in the following ways:
  - Crossed cylinder test, in which a near target of perpendicular lines is viewed through a ±0.50 crossed cylinder lens with the minus cylinder axis in the vertical meridian (Figure 2-7).
    - If the accommodative response is less than the demand, the horizontal line will be in sharper focus.
    - If the accommodative response is more than the demand, the vertical line will be in sharper focus.
    - Plus or minus lenses can be added to bracket a neutral point.

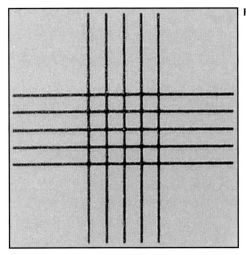

Figure 2-7. The near crossed cylinder target.

○ Objective measure of response can be determined by dynamic retinoscopy.
  ▪ Viewing through the distance correction, the patient views a target at his or her normal reading distance.
  ▪ If the retinoscope is in the same plane as the near target, and the accommodative response is correct for that distance, a neutral reflex will be noted.
  ▪ It is normal to find a "lag" of accommodation, resulting in observation of *with* motion of the reflex.
  ▪ The "lag" can be quantified either by adding plus lenses to neutrality or by altering the working distance of the retinoscope.

Relative Accommodation

- Positive and negative relative accommodation are measured by adding minus and plus lenses, respectively, to determine the amount the accommodation that can be increased or decreased by the patient while viewing a target at a fixed distance.
- For pre-presbyopic patients, this test is conducted with the distance correction in place.
- For presbyopic patients, this test is conducted with the near correction in place.

Correction of Presbyopia

- Age-related loss of accommodative ability leads to the need to prescribe optical correction for near that is different than the distance correction. This correction is always more plus (or less minus) than the distance correction.
- The difference between the distance and near correction is expressed as the "add" power. The optimal "add" for a patient is determined by any combination of several methods once the distance refraction is determined.
  ○ The crossed cylinder test for accommodative response often leads to an excellent starting point.
  ○ Simply adding plus lenses to the distance correction until the patient can read the near target indicates the limit of negative relative accommodation. Additional plus may be needed for comfortable and sustainable near vision.
  ○ The add power may be prescribed based on patient age, though this will lead to over-correction in many cases, and under-correction of others, so subjective verification is recommended.
  ○ The optimal "add" will typically be in the center of the positive and negative relative accommodation range.

Binocular Functions

- The binocular system is composed of sensory and motor functions, which, when functioning normally, allow the images from each eye to be combined into perception of a single image.
- Abnormal function of the motor components of binocular vision can lead to discomfort, diplopia, and eventually, suppression.

Ocular Motility

Monocular Eye Movements

- Movements of the eye, termed *ductions*, are rotary in nature, with each occurring about 1 of 3 axes: anteroposterior (coincident with the line of sight), vertical, and horizontal (both perpendicular to the line of sight)

Binocular Eye Movements

- In order for both eyes to direct the line of sight on the object of regard, binocular coordination is required. There are 2 types of binocular eye movements:
  - Versions are conjunctive movements that move both eyes in the same direction
  - Vergences are disjunctive movements that move the eyes in opposite directions

Eye Alignment

- When eye alignment is normal, the individual is able to maintain bifoveal fixation on the object of regard in any position of gaze.
- When eye alignment is maintained with both eyes viewing, but a deviation exists when one eye is covered, the condition is called heterophoria, or phoria.
- When eye alignment is not maintained when both eyes are viewing, the condition is called heterotropia, or strabismus.

Measurement of Eye Alignment and Movement

Observation

- Assessment of eye movement and alignment begins with observation of head position. Individuals with a paretic extraocular muscle often adapt a head posture to compensate.
  - A face turn indicates a paretic horizontal rectus muscle.
  - Chin elevation or depression indicates involvement of a vertical rectus muscle.
  - Head tilt indicates involvement of an oblique muscle.

Diagnostic Fields of Action

- Further evaluation is made by directing the patient to move the eye or eyes into each of the 6 diagnostic fields of action, allowing assessment of each muscle with minimal effect of the others.
  - The patient is directed to keep the head steady and in primary position.
  - The examiner moves a fixation target slowly in an "H" pattern, directing the patient to follow the target without moving the head.
  - Any deviation from alignment is noted, and the patient is asked to say if he or she experiences pain or diplopia in any of the directions.

Hirschberg Test

- For very young patients or other patients not capable of understanding or cooperating with the above test, the Hirschberg corneal light reflex test can be employed in the diagnostic fields of action as well as in primary gaze.
  - The examiner directs a penlight or similar light source at the patient viewing along the line connecting the light with the patient's eyes.
  - The patient is encouraged to look at the light as it is moved in the "H" pattern.
  - If binocular fixation is maintained, the corneal light reflexes will remain symmetrical throughout the test.
  - Deviation of one of the light reflexes relative to the other is indicative of loss of binocular fixation. The field(s) in which the deviation is noted is diagnostic of the muscle(s) involved.
  - Measurement of deviation is made by estimation (1-mm displacement of the light reflex representing approximately 21 PD) or by use of handheld prisms to bring the reflexes into symmetrical alignment (Krimsky modification).

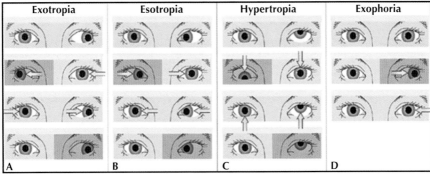

Exotropia	Esotropia	Hypertropia	Exophoria

Figure 2-8. Cover test for tropias and phorias. (A) For exotropia, covering the right eye drives inward movement of the left eye to take up fixation; uncovering the right eye shows recovery of fixation by the right eye and leftward movement of both eyes; covering the left eye discloses no shift of the preferred right eye. (B) For esotropia, covering the right eye drives outward movement of the left eye to take up fixation; uncovering the right eye shows recovery of fixation by the right eye and rightward movement of both eyes; covering the left eye discloses no shift of the preferred right eye. (C) For hypertropia, covering the right eye drives downward movement of the left eye to take up fixation; uncovering the right eye shows recovery of fixation by the right eye and upward movement of both eyes; covering the left eye shows no shift of the preferred right eye. (D) For exophoria, the left eye deviates outward behind a cover and returns to primary position when the cover is removed. An immediate inward movement denotes a phoria, and a delayed inward movement denotes an intermittent exotropia. (This figure was published in *Strabismus and Pediatric Ophthalmology.* Diamond G, Eggers H. Copyright Elsevier [1993].)

Cover Testing (Figure 2-8)

Unilateral Cover Test

- The unilateral cover test (Figure 2-9) is particularly useful and accurate in determining the presence of a strabismus. Unlike the previously described methods, it is readily performed for both distance and near fixation.
  - With the refractive correction in place, the patient is asked to fixate a target.
  - The examiner covers one eye, watching for any movement of the fellow eye.
  - If no strabismus is present, both eyes fixate on the target as long as both eyes remain uncovered.
  - Movement of the fellow eye indicates that this eye was not fixating along with the other, and thus it had to move to maintain fixation on the object of regard.
  - The test is repeated a number of times for each eye in order to determine the direction of deviation and the laterality of the strabismus if present.

Alternating Cover Test

- The alternating cover test is useful for determining the presence and direction of a heterophoria and for determining the magnitude of deviation of either a heterophoria or strabismus.
  - With the refractive correction in place, the patient is asked to fixate a target.
  - The examiner covers one eye for a few seconds, then moves the cover to the fellow eye, observing the motion of the eye just uncovered, which moves to pick up fixation of the target.
  - The movement is characterized based on the direction of movement observed:
    - If there is no movement, the posture is called *orthophoria.*
    - Horizontal movement in inducates exophoria or exotropia, depending on whether the unilateral test indicated a heterphoria or strabismus, respectively.
    - Horizontal movement out indicates esophoria or esotropia.
    - Downward vertical movement indicates hyperphoria or hypertropia, and upward movement indicates hypophoria or hypotropia.
  - The amount of movement can be quantified in PDs by finding the direction and amount of prism needed to neutralize the observed movement.

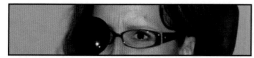

Figure 2-9. The cover test helps determine alignment of the eyes.

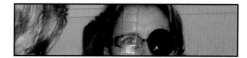

Figure 2-10. A prism bar is used to neutralize the motion of the eye.

○ Both the unilateral and alternating cover test can be performed for each of the diagnostic fields of action to determine consistency of a deviation throughout the fields.
  ▪ A deviation that remains consistent throughout the fields is termed *comitant*.
  ▪ When there is significant difference in the observed deviation in different fields of gaze, the deviation is termed *noncomitant*.

Subjective Measures of Alignment

- Assessment of heterophoria can be accomplished by subjective means, usually viewing through the phoropter. Alternatively, it can be measured through the use of loose prisms or prism bars (Figure 2-10).
- For the phoropter, the proper interpupillary distance and the patient's refractive findings should be in place.
- Testing is conventionally done for both distance (6 m) and near (40 cm) fixation.

Horizontal Phoria Measurement

- Approximately 6 D of base down prism is introduced in front of the right eye, creating diplopia with the right eye's image below the left eye's image.
- If the upper image is directly above the lower, orthophoria is indicated.
- If the upper image is displaced left or right of the lower, the rotary prism is introduced in front of the left eye such that base-in or base-out prism can be created.
- The left eye's image is occluded, then uncovered briefly, and the patient is asked to report the location of the image. Prism is increased gradually with each cycle of cover/uncover until the upper image appears directly above the lower.
- The direction and amount of prism required gives a measure of the direction and magnitude of the deviation.

Vertical Heterophoria Measurement

- Approximately 12 D of base-in prism is introduced in front of the right eye, creating diplopia with the right eye's image to the right of the left eye's image.
- Proceeding in a fashion similar to that previously described, base-up or base-down prism is introduced over the left eye until the images are in horizontal alignment with one another.

Associated Phoria and Fixation Disparity

- Measures of associated phoria and fixation disparity assess the alignment while both eyes are open and fixating.
- The methods of measurement of alignment discussed thus far assess what happens when fusion is disrupted by occlusion or prism dissociation. Just as with accommodation, where response can lag behind or exceed demand, so can vergence be greater or less than the demand.
- The difference between demand and actual vergence response is called the fixation disparity.
- The associated phoria is the amount of prism required to reduce the fixation disparity to zero.

Measurement of Vergence Amplitude

- The vergence response is largely reflexive, depending principally on the distance to the object of regard.
- Horizontal vergence movements are typically of greatest concern and can be convergent or divergent.
- Vertical and cyclovergences also exist but are less commonly of interest.
- Range of vergence amplitude is of interest in that a binocular system functioning at the limit of its ability is likely to cause the patient symptoms of strain, fatigue, and possibly diplopia.

Near Point of Convergence

- As an object is brought toward the eyes, the 2 lines of sight must converge in order to keep the object single. The ability to respond appropriately to such a stimulus is associated with convergence insufficiency.

Measurement of Convergence

- The examiner is seated in front of the patient, who should be wearing his or her full near correction.
- A near-point target is gradually advanced toward the patient's bridge, and the patient is asked to report when the object appears doubled.
- The examiner simultaneously watches the converging eyes for smoothness of response and for the point at which one eye deviates.
- The near point of convergence is the distance from the eyes at which fusion is lost
- Expected ranges vary but as a general rule should be the following:
  - 5 cm or less for pre-presbyopic patients
  - 9 cm or less for presbyopic patients

Loose Prism and Prism Bar Vergence

- Amplitude of any type of vergence can be determined for any fixation direction by use of loose prisms or a prism bar.
  - The patient, who should be wearing his or her full near correction, views the intended target.
  - A prism is introduced in front of one eye, and the examiner observes this eye for reflex movement to compensate the prism.
  - The amplitude is the maximum amount of prism for which the patient can rapidly recover fusion.

Risley's Prism

- A subjective method for measuring vergence amplitude can be accomplished using the rotary prisms in the phoropter. The phoropter should be set to the proper interpupillary distance, and the patient's refractive findings should be in place. Testing is conventionally done for both distance (6 m) and near (40 cm) fixation.
  - To measure the horizontal ranges, a target is fixated while viewing through the rotary prisms, both set at zero. The prisms are oriented such that base-in or base-out is created by rotating the prism dial.
  - For convergence range, the prisms are slowly and simultaneously increased in base-out direction.
  - The patient is asked to report the point at which the target becomes double. This is noted as the break point.
  - Often, the patient will report the target becoming blurry before fusion is lost. This indicates the patient is eliciting accommodative convergence to maintain a single image. The point at which blur is noted is the blur point.
  - Once diplopia is reported, the prisms are slowly reversed to decrease the amount of base-out effect, and the recovery point is noted.
  - The range is recorded in prism diopters indicating the blur/break/recovery.
  - A similar method using base-in prism is used to determine the divergence range.
  - Vertical range is determined by placing one of the rotary prisms in front of one eye, increasing the prism in first the base-up and then base-down direction, again noting when the patient reports diplopia.

Accommodative Convergence to Accommodation Ratio

- Accommodation and convergence are yoked such that accommodation serves as a stimulus to initiate positive vergence.
- The amount of convergence stimulated by accommodation is called accommodative vergence.
- If the amount of accommodative convergence is inadequate or too great for fusion, then fusional vergence must be further exerted to align the eyes.

- The amount of accommodation convergence created by a unit of accommodation is called the AC/A ratio.
- The AC/A ratio is measured by determining the change in the angle of phoria or strabismus between two levels of accommodation.
- The calculated method of determining the AC/A ratio is accomplished by changing the test distance to get the change in accommodation.
- The gradient method is accomplished by adding plus or minus lenses with the target at a constant distance.
- The AC/A ratio is clinically useful in both diagnosis and management of binocular disorders.
  - A high AC/A ratio will lead to esophoria or esotropia at near and is often best managed with plus lenses to decrease the convergence.
  - A low AC/A ratio will lead to exophoria or exotropia at near. Addition of minus lenses to stimulate accommodative convergence will be of little use, indicating the need for prism or perhaps convergence exercises to assist the fusional vergence system.

Sensory Fusion

- Sensory fusion of visual information from the 2 eyes is a complex phenomenon. Clinically, sensory fusion is broken down into 3 levels.
  - First-degree fusion refers to simultaneous perception of the images from both eyes. If motor fusion is aberrant, this will result in diplopia unless the patient suppresses the information from one eye.
  - Second-degree fusion refers to the ability to fuse the 2 images without diplopia or suppression.
  - Third-degree fusion refers to the ability to fuse the 2 images and have an appreciation of depth.

Stereopsis

- Tests for stereopsis are useful in that a finding of a threshold within normal ranges can generally be relied on to imply that sensory fusion and motor alignment are present.
- Most common are those using polarized lenses to isolate right and left eye images (Figure 2-11).
- A perception of depth is created by appropriate horizontal displacement of the images being viewed.
- Stereopsis is a useful screening test because for stereopsis to be normal:
  - A constant strabismus cannot be present
  - Vision in each eye must be present and relatively normal
  - There cannot be large differences in clarity or image size between the eyes

Second Degree Fusion Testing—Worth 4 Dot Test

- Patients who do not have normal stereopsis may still have some level of fusion.
- This is typically evaluated with the Worth 4 dot test (Figure 2-12).
- The test consists of 4 light sources arranged at the 12, 3, 6, and 9 o'clock positions.
- The light at 12 o'clock is red, those at 3 and 9 are green, and the one at 6 is white. In order to perform the test, the patient should have the refractive correction in place.
- A red filter is placed over one eye, and a green filter is placed over the other
- If the patient has normal second-degree fusion, he or she will report seeing 4 lights: 1 red, 2 green, and 1 that may appear white with a tinge of red or green
- Abnormal responses include reports of seeing 2, 3, or 5 lights.
  - If 2 or 3 lights are seen, the patient is suppressing one eye.
  - If 5 lights are seen, the patient is diplopic and but is demonstrating simultaneous perception.

Tears, Cornea, and External Examination

Precorneal Tear Film Evaluation

- The first refracting surface of the eye is formed by the precorneal tear film, the integrity of which is essential to ocular comfort and clear vision. Evaluation of the tear film is an important step in evaluation of patients with symptoms of dry eye or visual disturbance. Common clinical tests include tests of tear stability, flow, and volume.

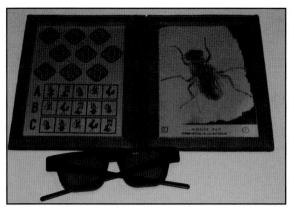

Figure 2-11. A common polarized stereopsis test.

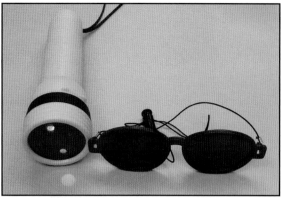

Figure 2-12. The Worth 4 dot test uses red, green, and white lights along with red-green glasses.

Tear Break Up Time

- The tears are a complex concoction consisting of lipid, aqueous, and mucin constituents.
- The mucin elements, produced primarily by the conjunctiva, serve to allow compatibility of the largely aqueous tears with the epithelium.
- Lipids are produced by the meibomian and other lid glands and serve to limit evaporation.
- Deficiency in either the lipid or mucin elements can lead to irregular tear film that does not wet and smooth the corneal surface properly.
- One test of the integrity of the tear film is the tear break up time (TBUT). The TBUT is assessed as follows:
  - Fluorescein is introduced to the tears by pipette or wetted strip.
  - The patient is instructed to blink 3 times and then keep the eye open.
  - Observing with the cobalt filter in the slit lamp, measure the time that elapses before areas of the tear film "break up," appearing as black areas in contrast to the fluorescence of the tear layer.
  - Normal tear break up time is 10 to 15 seconds. Significantly less than that is quite indicative of dry eye conditions.

Measures of Tear Flow and Volume

Schirmer's Test

- Though notoriously unreliable, the Schirmer's test (Figure 2-13) has persisted as a test for insufficient tear flow. It can be performed with or without instillation of a topical anesthetic to prevent reflex tearing.
  - A specially designed filter paper is folded at one end and inserted at the temporal lower eye lid.
  - The filter paper is left in place for 5 minutes.
  - The true dry eye patient is expected to wet less than 5 mm of the strip in 5 minutes.
  - The test is often contaminated by reflex tearing due to irritation caused by the strip.

Phenol Red Thread Test

- More recently, a similar test using a dyed cotton thread has been shown to be an improvement over the Schirmer's test.

Tear Prism Height (Tear Meniscus)

- The slit-lamp microscope can be used to observe the prism of tears that is normally present along the lower eyelid margin, either with or without fluorescein. Accurate measurement is difficult, and reflex tearing due to the illumination may contaminate the observation, but such simple observation can be useful in determining presence or absence of adequate tear volume.

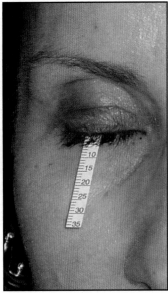

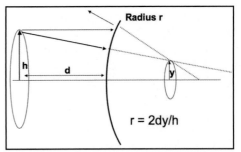

Figure 2-14. Determining radius using reflection. d and h are fixed. Measurement of y allows calculation of r.

Figure 2-13. The Schirmer's tear test measures tear flow.

Corneal Curvature

The corneal shape determines the principal refracting surface of the eye.
- Most often dictates the amount of astigmatic error and is of critical interest in both contact lens fitting and refractive surgery
- Irregular corneal shape is the source of many potential optical aberrations that can limit the visual acuity.
- Assessment of corneal curvature is accomplished quantitatively by measurement of images reflected by the front surface of the cornea and tear film. Qualitative assessment is made possible by observation of the quality and consistency of the reflected images.

Radius of Curvature

- The determination of radius is based on the reflective properties of the cornea, which acts like a diverging, convex mirror (Figure 2-14).
  - o An object with height (h), at distance (d) from the reflecting surface will create a virtual image of height (y).
  - o For reflection-based devices such as the keratometer or corneal topographer, h and d are fixed, and y is measured. Radius (r)can then be calculated as follows:
    $$r = 2dy/h$$
  - o Quantitative measures give the radius of curvature at the measured point, and this is often converted into a diopter value.
  - o An assumed index of refraction is used to convert the radius to the expected dioptric power of a surface with the measured radius having the assumed index. The standard index used is 1.3375. This is lower than the true index of the cornea, thus taking into account the fact that the negative-powered back surface is not otherwise considered.
  - o As these diopters are an estimation based on the assumed index, they are often referred to as diopters "k" to distinguish from true surface power. This becomes of particular importance in dealing with contact lenses, where the diopter "k" value is often used interchangeably with lens radius, but is in no way an accurate indication of actual lens surface power. The conversion is readily available in chart form or can be easily calculated using the following application of the following surface power formula:
    $$\text{Diopters ``k''} = (1.3375 - 1.00)/r$$

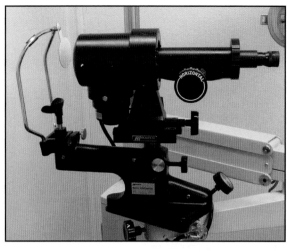

Figure 2-15. The keratometer can be used to measure central corneal curvature.

Keratometry

- The keratometer (Figure 2-15) uses a semisilvered mirror and a series of prisms to create an easy method for measuring the height of the reflected image in 2 meridians. Simple alignment of the mires as viewed through the instrument is all that is required.
  - The patient is positioned at the keratometer with the forehead and chin in contact with the rest. Occlude one eye.
  - Sighting from outside the instrument, the vertical and horizontal position is determined using the vertical alignment marker and the reflected glow of the illumination.
  - The patient views the reflected image of the eye being measured.
  - Viewing through the instrument, one will see 3 mire images. Focus the mires, and make fine adjustment to center the reticle in the lower right mire.
  - Rotate the instrument until the 2 cross to the left in line with one another (this rotational position determines the 2 principal meridians of the cornea).
  - Adjust the wheel on the left side of the instrument to superimpose the 2 crosses. The reading on this wheel gives the radius of the horizontal meridian.
  - Adjust the wheel on the right to superimpose the horizontal lines above the focusing mire. The reading gives the radius of the vertical meridian.
  - Readings are recorded, giving both the radius/diopter value and the axis (eg, 45.25 @ 10, 46.50 @ 100). Note also if mires are regular or distorted.
- Keratometer readings are generally limited to the central 3.50 mm of the cornea, although peripheral measurements can be obtained by having the patient fixate appropriately. For measurement of curvature outside the standard range of the instrument, adding +1.25 or -1.25 D lenses to the mire face can extend the range up or down, respectively. Conversion tables for this purpose are available in most contact lens texts.

Corneal Topography—Videokeratography

- Whereas the keratometer uses the reflection of a single circular mire, devices designed to provide qualitative information on corneal shape generally use multiple concentric rings (Figure 2-16). Subjective assessment of these complex reflected images is greatly enhanced by use of videokeratographers. These devices capture a video image of the reflected rings, and the image is analyzed by computer. Alignment of the patient is similar to the method described for the keratometer. Image capture is either controlled by the examiner or may be automatic.
  - Provide rapid evaluation of corneal shape
    - Particularly useful in the detection and diagnosis of corneal irregularity, such as keratoconus, and evaluation of the postrefractive surgery patient. They can be very helpful in design of contact lenses.
    - A corneal "map" is produced from the analysis of the captured image. Proper interpretation of the topographical map is important in order to avoid erroneous conclusions.

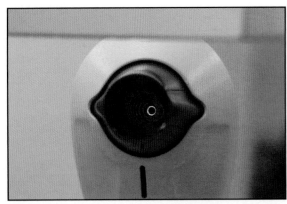

Figure 2-16. Videokeratographers reflect multiple rings to map the corneal curvature.

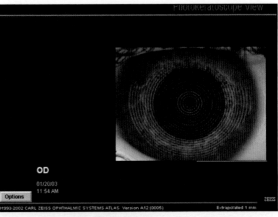

Figure 2-17. The raw image captured by the topographer.

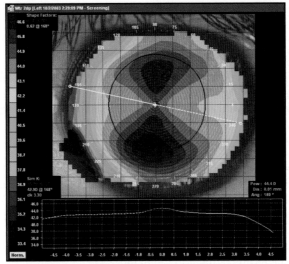

Figure 2-18. A corneal map showing with-the-rule corneal astigmatism.

o Examine the raw image of the reflected rings (Figure 2-17). This may reveal tear film irregularity or lid effects that may influence the map.

o Maps may be spherically biased axial maps or tangential. The axial map is usually considered more useful for contact lens fitting. The tangential map is a better representation of localized variations in shape, as may be of interest following refractive surgery.

o Maps are 2-dimensional and use a color scale whereby warmer colors indicate steeper radii, cooler colors the flatter radii (Figure 2-18).

o Scales may be normalized for the specific cornea or absolute based on average corneas. These can have significantly different appearances for nonaverage eyes.

• Topographers generate a number of numerical indices that are useful in diagnosis.

o Surface irregularity index (corneal irregularity measure) compares the best fit of a regular toric surface with the shape of the cornea. This gives an indication of irregular astigmatism. Normal eyes may have values up to a maximum of 1.0. This index often correlates well with visual acuity.

o Shape factor is a measure of the degree of flattening along the flattest meridian. Normal corneas are moderately prolate with gradual peripheral flattening. A perfect sphere has a shape factor of zero. Normal eyes are typically less than 0.5. Greater than 0.5 should lead to suspicion of an ectatic condition, such as keratoconus. A negative shape factor indicates an oblate shape and is indicative of previous refractive surgery.

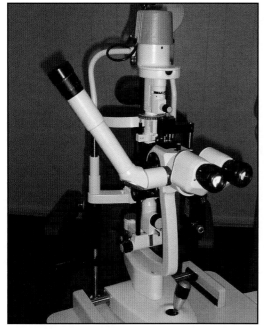

Figure 2-19. The slit-lamp biomicroscope.

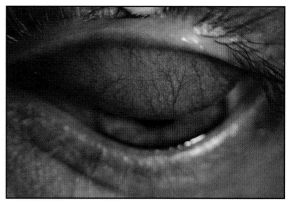

Figure 2-20. Eversion of the upper lid.

Examination of the Eye

Slit-Lamp Examination

- External examination of the eyes begins with observation under normal room illumination without magnification, allowing simultaneous view of both eyes. Normally, there is good symmetry of lid position, iris color, and degree of ocular redness. For a more detailed view, the slit-lamp biomicroscope is unsurpassed in allowing well-illuminated and magnified views of the external eye (Figure 2-19).

Examination of the External Eye

- The patient is positioned at the instrument with the forehead and chin resting as intended.
- The patient is asked to close the eyes, and the illumination and focus is adjusted. With the eyes still closed, the lashes and surface of the lids are examined with low magnification and full beam width.
- The patient is asked to open the eyes and fixate a target.
- The examination begins with the lashes and lid margins and proceeds systematically to include the bulbar and palpebral conjunctiva, the fornices, and canthi. In order to view the superior palpebral surface, the upper lid is everted (Figure 2-20).

Examination of the Cornea

- Due to the transparency of the cornea, the slit lamp is extremely useful in examination. Learning to use a variety of illumination techniques will allow observation of many subtle findings not apparent by other methods (Table 2-1).
- Begin with a 2-mm wide beam that straddles the limbus, creating a "sclerotic scatter," which provides internal illumination of the cornea. The cornea is observed outside the biomicroscope. This technique is useful in detecting corneal edema and foreign bodies.
- Observing through the biomicroscope under moderate magnification, the cornea is then scanned with the slit at 1- to 2-mm width and at maximal height
- Observation should be made of the directly illuminated area and the areas retroilluminated by reflection from the iris as well as areas proximal to the beam and the retroillumination.
- Fluorescein may be instilled after the eye has been examined with white light. With the cobalt filter in place, the slit-lamp illumination will cause fluorescence that varies with the concentration of the fluorescein. Fluorescein temporarily dyes the tear film and stains mucus and missing areas of the surface epithelium. It also pools in depressions and spaces between papillae and conjunctival folds.

TABLE 2-1. SLIT-LAMP ILLUMINATIONS

Illumination	*View*	*Method*
Sclerotic scatter	Cornea: edema or opacity	2-mm beam at limbus, view from outside instrument
Diffuse	External structures	Wide beam, 8X to 10X magnification
Direct	Cornea, conjunctiva	Full beam height, 12X to 25X
Parallelopiped	Cornea, lens, vitreous	1- to 2-mm beam width
Optic section	Cornea, lens, to judge depth	Slit beam, high illumination
Conic section	Anterior chamber for cells and flare	Beam 1 mm x 1 mm
Specular	Corneal endothelium	Microscope and light at 60 degrees
Indirect		
Proximal	Cornea	1- to 2-mm slit. Observe next to directly illuminated area.
Retroillumination	Cornea, iris, lens	Observe backlighting from iris (for cornea), from fundus for lens and iris

Corneal Sensitivity

- When neurotrophic keratitis or herpetic keratitis is suspected, assessment of corneal sensitivity can be accomplished clinically by using a Cochet-Bonnet esthesiometer, or by applying a fine cotton wisp to cornea and observing for response (Figure 2-21). A sterile cotton-tipped applicator is used.
  - If one eye is suspected of being hypoesthetic, test the normal eye first.
  - Gently touch the cornea with the wisp, trying to keep the examiner's hand out of view.
  - Test the fellow eye, and note difference in responses.

Corneal Thickness

- Measurement of central corneal thickness has become commonplace because of its role in risk assessment of glaucoma patients and its importance in presurgical evaluation of the refractive surgery candidate. Several ultrasound devices are available.
  - The cornea is anesthetized with a topical anesthetic.
  - The ultrasound probe is applied perpendicular to the cornea, and a reading is obtained (Figure 2-22).
  - Corneal thickness can also be measured optically with the Orbscan (Bausch and Lomb, Rochester, NY) or the Pentacam (OCULUS, Lynnwood, WA).

Anterior Segment Evaluation and Measurement of Intraocular Pressure

- Slit-lamp evaluation of the anterior chamber and measurement of intraocular pressure are part of a routine eye examination and serve primarily to aid in the detection of risk factors for narrow-angle and open-angle glaucoma.

Anterior Chamber Angle Depth

- A simple slit-lamp technique of grading the peripheral angle agrees well with gonioscopic measurement. As the estimation technique is far simpler and less invasive, it is the standard technique for screening for narrow angles that warrant further evaluation.
- With the slit-lamp magnification at approximately 15X and the microscope 60 degrees to the lamp, a thin slit beam is angled so it is perpendicular to the temporal limbus.
- The beam is moved so that it just illuminates a thin area of the iris and creates an optic section of the cornea.

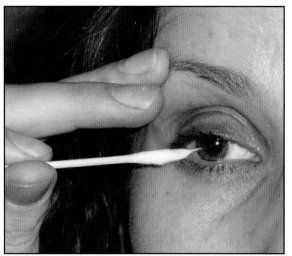

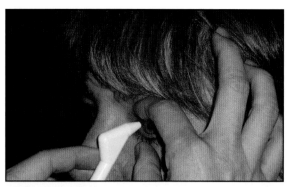

Figure 2-22. Ultrasound pachymetry is commonly used to measure corneal thickness.

Figure 2-21. Use of cotton wisp to test for corneal sensitivity.

- A clear space, which represents the anterior chamber depth (Figure 2-23), is observed and compared with the apparent thickness of the cornea. The comparison is repeated at the nasal angle.
- The following grading scale is used. Most eyes will be graded as 3 or 4. If the angles are graded 2 or less, gonioscopic evaluation is indicated.
  - Grade 4
    - The clear space is at least as wide as the corneal thickness, and the chance of angle closure is practically zero, with exception of a plateau iris.
  - Grade 3
    - The clear space is between one-quarter and one-half the thickness of the cornea section. Risk of angle closure is extremely low.
  - Grade 2
    - The clear space is one-quarter the thickness of the cornea section. Such an angle is capable of angle closure.
  - Grade 1
    - The clear space is less than one-quarter the thickness of the cornea section, indicating a very narrow angle. Angle-closure risk is high.

The Iris

- The iris should be examined carefully for evidence of pigment dispersion, pseudoexfoliation, rubeosis, and synechia. Presence of postsurgical iris defects, iris atrophy, nevi, and heterochromia should be noted. The following sequence may be followed:
  - Note the contour of the iris, which should be relatively flat. Tenting or bowing of the iris (iris bombé) can indicate synechiae. Localized elevation may indicate ciliary body cyst or tumor.
  - Observe distribution of pigment on the iris surface. Areas of depigmentation are consistent with iris atrophy.
  - Retroilluminate the iris by decreasing the slit-beam height to send light just through the pupil. Transillumination defects of the peripheral iris in a spoke-like pattern are indicative of pigment dispersion syndrome. Transillumination of the sphincter region is typical of exfoliation syndrome.

The Aqueous

- The aqueous should be evaluated for presence of cells or flare, which are indicators of active inflammation. Room lights should be dimmed, and the intensity of the slit beam should be at the highest setting.
  - The slit beam is reduced to a conical beam. The light source should approach the eye obliquely.
  - The focus is moved from posterior cornea to anterior lens and iris.

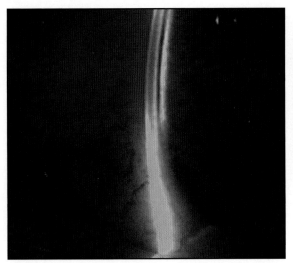

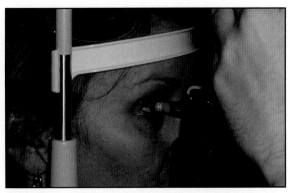

Figure 2-24. Goldmann's tonometry.

Figure 2-23. Estimating the anterior chamber depth with the slit lamp.

- o Cells appear as discrete objects floating in the aqueous.
- o Flare causes a general clouding of the aqueous that renders the light beam visible as it passes through the aqueous.

Measurement of Intraocular Pressure

- Intraocular pressure is routinely measured as part of the risk assessment for glaucoma and to monitor the efficacy of pressure-lowering medications. A number of devices are in common use for measuring intraocular pressure.
  - o The standard instrumentation is the Goldmann's tonometer, which is typically attached to the slit-lamp biomicroscope. The procedure for Goldmann's tonometry (Figure 2-24) is as follows:
    - Anesthetize the cornea with a fluorescein/anesthetic combination drop designed for this purpose.
    - The tonometer tip should be clean, dry, and positioned in the instrument. The arm containing the tip is swung into place, and the tonometer is swung into the click-stop position. With the cobalt filter in place, the slit beam should be widened and angled to fully illuminate the tonometer tip.
    - Set the tonometer scale at the 1 position, representing 10 mm Hg.
    - The patient is positioned in the slit lamp with the forehead and chin against the respective rests. The patient is instructed to blink several times and then to try to keep the eyes wide open. If necessary, the examiner or an assistant may need to hold the upper lid out of the way. Care must be taken to not apply any pressure to the globe as this will result in spuriously high readings.
    - Viewing outside the microscope, bring the tonometer tip toward the eye until it begins to touch the cornea. A circumcorneal glow should be apparent.
    - Viewing through the microscope, the mires are adjusted to center them over the corneal apex. Proper position is indicated by a pair of symmetrical half circles.
    - The tonometer is gradually advanced (by means of the joystick) until the inner edges of the 2 half circles align.
    - The pressure is noted by multiplying the scale reading by 10.
    - It is good practice to take 2 to 3 readings and average them. In addition to recording the pressure, the time of day is also noted. For patients on antiglaucoma medications, the time since the last dose of medication should also be noted.
    - The tonometer tip should be disinfected following each use. A 10-minute soak in 3% hydrogen peroxide is considered standard for this.

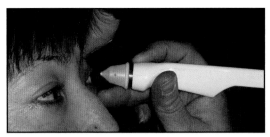

Figure 2-25. The Tono-Pen.

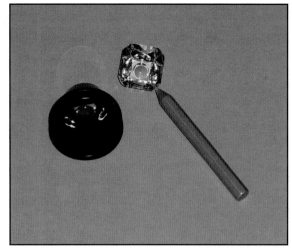

Figure 2-26. Gonioscopy lenses.

○ Numerous other types of tonometers are in common use.
  ▪ Hand-held tonometers are of particular value for patients for whom positioning in the slit lamp is problematic (ie, Perkins tonometer, Tono-Pen AVIA [Reichert Technologies, Buffalo, NY]; Figure 2-25).
  ▪ Noncontact tonometers are useful as screening devices and have advantages in that the anesthetic is not needed and there is minimal contamination risk.
○ Patients who have thinner-than-normal corneas will give falsely low readings with all of these devices. History of refractive surgery should alert the practitioner that the tonometer reading is likely inaccurate. Conversely, thicker than normal corneas will yield falsely high readings. Unfortunately, there is no simple nomogram to provide accurate conversion of readings with atypical corneal thickness.

Gonioscopy

• Gonioscopy, which allows detailed inspection of the anterior chamber angle structures, is performed when there is suspicion of either angle-closure potential or the existence of some other process or condition that may compromise outflow through the trabecular meshwork. Lenses allow the examiner to use the slit-lamp biomicroscope to attain an indirect view of the angle structures.
  ○ Gonioscopy lenses (Figure 2-26) neutralize the optical effect of the cornea and allow view into the angle via mirrors oriented to provide the intended view. There are 2 general types of lenses:
    ▪ The Goldmann's-style lens is relatively large and requires use of a viscous gonioscopic fluid to maintain appropriate interface with the cornea. In order to view all quadrants, the lens needs to be rotated on the eye. Although relatively unpleasant for the patient, it is easy to use and handle.
    ▪ The Zeiss- or Posner-style lens is smaller and is simply held against the anesthetized cornea without use of additional fluid. As there are 4 mirrors, all 4 quadrants can be viewed without moving the lens. An additional benefit is the ability to use the lens to apply pressure to the eye allowing one to differentiate synechial closure from simple apposition closure.
  ○ In either case, the procedure is similar.
    ▪ With the cornea anesthetized, the patient is positioned at the slit lamp.
    ▪ If using a Goldmann's lens, the lens is held concave side up and is carefully filled with gonioscopic fluid, taking care to avoid bubbles in the solution.
    ▪ Have the patient look down, position and hold the upper lid against the superior orbital rim.
    ▪ Have the patient look up, and apply the gonioscopic lens directly to the cornea
      □ For the Goldmann's lens, begin by applying the edge opposite the mirror to the lower cornea and tilt the lens up as the patient looks straight ahead. Maintain position by lightly holding with the thumb and first 2 fingers and bracing the other fingers on the patient's cheek.

- The Zeiss is applied similarly, but without use of the additional fluid. It is held in place with light but steady force against the cornea while again bracing the ring and little finger on the cheek.
  - The angle is graded and recorded. The Schaffer system is used to grade the angle between peripheral iris and the trabecular meshwork using the following gradations:
    - Grade 4
      - Angle is 35 to 45 degrees
    - Grade 3
      - Angle is 20 to 35 degrees
    - Grade 2
      - Angle is 10 to 20 degrees
    - Grade 1
      - Angle is less than 10 degrees
    - Slit
      - Angle is open slightly but much less than 10 degrees
    - Zero
      - Angle is closed

Crystalline Lens

- Although the principal instrument for examination of the crystalline lens is the slit-lamp biomicroscope, lens opacities can be first detected by qualitative evaluation of the reflex from the fundus that is seen with the retinoscope or direct ophthalmoscope. Routine use of this observation will provide the examiner with the ability to quickly assess the light-blocking effect of any opacity and aid in estimation of the degree of visual loss that may be attributed to it.
- Biomicroscopic examination is best accomplished with the pupil dilated in order to detect peripheral and incipient opacities, although assessment of an opacity affecting the visual axis may not necessitate it. The standard technique involves careful examination with parallelopiped or widened optic section (Figure 2-27).
- The light source is positioned at a 30-degree angle to the microscope to begin and then is slowly swept across the lens from 30 degrees temporal to 30 degrees nasal, focusing on first pass on the anterior surface of the lens and subsequently on the posterior surface, all the while observing for opacities.
- The nucleus is illuminated by slightly widening the beam, and the color, degree of clarity, and presence of vacuoles are noted.
- The lens can be retroilluminated by placing the light source just slightly off click-stop (about 5 degrees) such that the red fundus reflex is observed. Observe and note any opacities, their position, and the degree to which they appear to block light.
- Grading systems for lens opacities are useful in standardizing and monitoring change; however, the principal determinants for degree of severity involve assessment of visual function. These include measurement of low- and high-contrast visual acuity and effects of glare on acuity.

Posterior Segment

- Evaluation of the posterior segment begins with slit-lamp examination of the anterior vitreous. This can be accomplished in concert with, and as continuation of, the examination of the crystalline lens. Observation of the vitreous should include its relative mobility and the presence and density of the cobweb-like strands of which it consists. The presence of a distinct posterior face, beyond which there is essentially empty optical space, is indicative of posterior vitreous detachment.
- The majority of emphasis on posterior segment examination is placed on the various regions and methods of viewing the ocular fundus. It is assumed that the reader is generally familiar with the relevant anatomy.

Optic Nerve Head

- The optic nerve head (Figure 2-28) is routinely evaluated due to its significance and diagnostic value in a wide variety of ophthalmic and neurological conditions. Evaluation includes observation of the following:

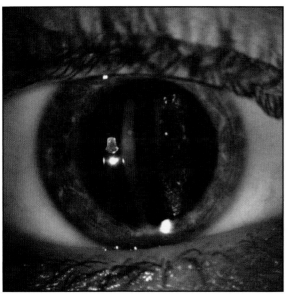

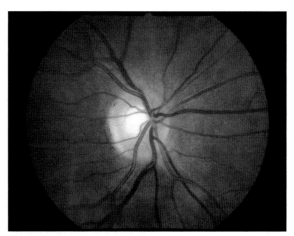

Figure 2-28. A normal optic disc.

Figure 2-27. The crystalline lens as viewed though the slit lamp with an optic section. (Reprinted with permission of Nada Lingel, OD, MS.)

- o Ratio of physiological cupping to overall disc diameter (cup to disc or C/D ratio)
- o Relative thickness of rim tissue
- o Disc perfusion and color
- o Location/displacement of vessels entering the disc
- o Degree to which the disc margins are distinct and/or elevated

Cup to Disc Ratio

- Typically, a depression, termed the *physiological cup*, exists in the center of the optic disc. This area is devoid of optic nerve fibers and is often proportional to overall disc size. Of particular concern are conditions in which nerve tissue is lost and the cupped area enlarges, as is typical in glaucoma and ischemic optic neuropathies. Accurate notation of the C/D ratio is useful in both the detection and monitoring of such ocular conditions.
- The process of estimation involves determination of the location of the borders of the disc and the cup. Such evaluation is greatly improved with stereoscopic examination, as the border of the cup is easily mistaken for variations in coloration rather than variation of elevation.
  - o Note is made of the ratio of the horizontal diameter of the cup area compared to the horizontal diameter of the entire disc.
  - o Similar observation is made of the vertical diameter ratio. Both are recorded in tenths (eg, 0.5 horizontal X 0.6 vertical).

Rim Tissue

- As the true concern is with presence or lack of neural tissue, it is often considered that the importance placed on C/D ratio is perhaps overemphasized.
- Observation of existent rim tissue may be at least equally important.
- This "donut versus hole" issue supports recommendation that evaluation of the rim tissue is at least equally important.
- The normal rim tissue will vary in thickness based on location around the rim.
- The inferior rim tissue should be widest, followed by the superior, nasal, and temporal aspects (ISNT). This relationship has given rise to the ISNT acronym that reminds clinicians of these relative relationships. Significant variation from the ISNT thickness arrangement should be considered in risk assessment of ocular disease affecting the optic nerve.

Disc Perfusion and Color

- Disc color is typically taken to reflect disc perfusion.
- Observation of many normal discs is useful for the clinician to develop a good sense of normal versus abnormal.
- With clear media, the disc color is normally a light yellow to pink.
- Media opacities can alter this perception and make judgment based on color circumspect.
- Frank pallor of portions of the disc or the entire disc are typical in cases involving poor or incomplete perfusion.

Vessel Location

- The central retinal artery and vein and their major branches typically emerge from or enter into the disc near the center of the disc and cup.
- As tissue is eroded in diseases affecting nerve fiber density, vessels are progressively displaced toward the temporal rim.
- Vessels normally pass over the rim into the cup supported by nerve tissue.
- Erosion of nerve tissue can lead to an undermining of vessels entering the disc, and vessels that seem to disappear over the rim and reappear deeper in the cup should give rise to suspicion of loss of normal tissue.

Disc Margins

- The margins of the normal disc are typically quite flat and easily distinguished from the surrounding sensory retina. Indistinct or elevated disc margins should cause suspicion of a variety of possible etiologies, each of which warrants further investigation to determine significance:
  - o Nerve head drusen
  - o Pseudotumor cerebri
  - o Systemic hypertension
  - o Space-occupying cranial lesion

Nerve Fiber Layer

- Defects in the nerve fiber layer in the region of the disc have been correlated with visual loss in glaucoma.
- Funduscopic detection can be difficult, and devices employing scanning layer technology have been developed to make this interpretation repeatable and accurate.
- Use of a red-free filter may enhance the ability of the examiner to observe defects in the nerve fiber layer with conventional funduscopic techniques.

Retinal Vascular System

- The central retinal artery bifurcates into superior and inferior branches and further into nasal and temporal branches. Beyond this, there are additional bifurcations.
- At each of these junctures, the vessels become smaller, and these sites are prone to blockage by emboli. Observation of emboli or frank blockage of a branch artery indicates need for prompt medical work-up for vascular occlusive disease.
- The arteries and veins of the retina travel in pairs that are prone to cross at random intervals, typically with the artery crossing the vein. These crossings should be observed for evidence of systemic hypertensive disease, which can manifest itself by a compression of the underlying vein.
- As the larger veins approach the optic disc, they coalesce into the central retinal vein. The change in direction that occurs as this vessel plunges into the cup is prone to create a pulsation that will be observed in many normal individuals, suggesting that the intraocular pressure is greater than the diastolic venous pressure in this vessel.
- Conversely, spontaneous pulsation of the central retinal artery is an abnormal finding that indicates either elevated intraocular pressure or poor perfusion of the central retinal artery. In either case, further evaluation and intervention are indicated.

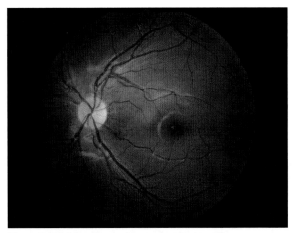

Figure 2-29. A healthy and normal posterior pole.

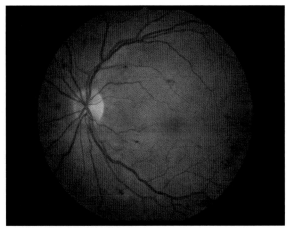

Figure 2-30. Fundus view showing early diabetic changes.

Posterior Pole

- The posterior pole (Figure 2-29) is considered delineated by the superior and inferior temporal vascular arcades. Within this area is the macula, the center of which is the fovea.
- As the most sensitive area of the retina and responsible for central vision, this area should be carefully examined for defect.
- The fovea appears as a small concavity devoid of vasculature.
- The internal limiting membrane covering this concave shape acts as a mirror, giving rise to a bright reflective pinpoint spot that identifies the center of the fovea.
- This reflex is readily observed in younger eyes and is present in many older eyes, although the brilliance may be quite diminished.
- Funduscopic examination centers on even distribution of pigment that gives a homogenous appearance to the fovea and macula.
- Exudate or pigmentary disturbance in this region is typical of macular degeneration in older patients and of macular disease or dystrophy in patients of younger age.

Diabetic Fundus Examination

- Among the severe debilitating effects of diabetes mellitus are the ocular complications affecting the ocular fundus (Figure 2-30). This fact, in combination with the development of effective treatment for some forms of the condition, prompts many diabetic patients to have routine fundus examinations. Examiners should be aware of the classifications and findings for nonproliferative and proliferative retinopathy.

Retinal Periphery

- For purposes of examination, the peripheral retina is divided somewhat artificially into 4 quadrants as well as geographic regions delineated by both specific anatomical landmarks and by the geometry of the globe. In addition, clock hours (referenced to the examiner's view) are used in recording and communicating findings. These give rise to the fundus mapping system illustrated in Figure 2-31.
  - In addition to the obvious anatomical area of the ora serrata, a principal "landmark" is the equator, the location of which is considered to be at the greatest circumference of the globe.
  - Other useful landmarks are the ampullae of the vortex veins, which are typically located one per quadrant, and the long and short posterior ciliary nerves.
  - The long ciliary nerves enter the eye at the 3 and 9 o'clock positions and are visible funduscopically in the region between the equator and the ora serrata.
  - The short ciliary nerves are more random in their location and orientation, often appearing in the region of the vortex ampullae.

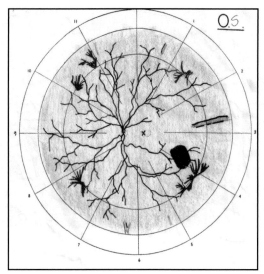

Figure 2-31. Sample fundus drawing. (Reprinted with permission of Nada Lingel, OD, MS.)

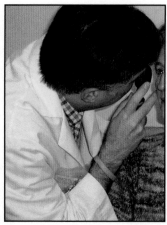

Figure 2-32. The direct ophthalmoscope.

Instrumentation and Method of Fundus Examination

Examination of the fundus requires simultaneous illumination and observation of the retina. This is accomplished through a variety of methods, the most common being described here. It is almost always beneficial to dilate the pupil prior to examination, and in fact, it is essentially impossible to observe peripheral structures or to achieve a stereoscopic view with an undilated eye. Most commonly, the pupils are dilated with a combination of 0.5% to 1.0% tropicamide and 2.5% phenylephrine.

Direct Ophthalmoscopy

- The direct ophthalmoscope (Figure 2-32) was invented in the late 19th century by Helmholtz and was the first such device to allow satisfactory examination of the fundus. Still commonly used by general medical practitioners, it has fallen from favor of ophthalmic practitioners due to some of its limitations. It is, however, simple and portable and allows for a highly magnified view of the posterior pole. The procedure for its use is as follows:
  - ○ To examine the right eye, the instrument is held before the examiner's right eye. This is reversed for the left eye.
  - ○ Start with +3.00 in the diopter wheel of the instrument, and observe the eye from about 30 cm away. The fundus reflex should be apparent.
  - ○ Slowly advance toward the patient, adjusting the diopter wheel to obtain and maintain focus on the retinal vessels.
  - ○ Follow a vessel as it increases in caliber to locate the optic nerve head.
  - ○ Examine the optic nerve head, the vascular branches out several bifurcations, and finally the macula.

Binocular Indirect Ophthalmoscopy

- The binocular indirect ophthalmoscope (Figure 2-33) provides a bright and wide field of view and allows examination of the entire fundus. The instrument consists of a head-mounted light source along with a lens and prism apparatus that optically reduces the examiner's interpupillary distance. This is used in combination with a biconvex condensing lens. It is an extremely flexible instrument allowing varying degrees of magnification and field of view by use of different power-condensing lenses. Practice is required to obtain proficiency with this instrument and to adapt to the view, which is reversed and inverted.

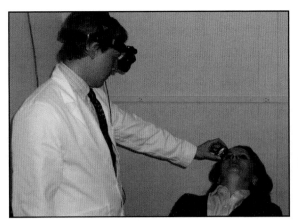

Figure 2-33. The binocular indirect ophthalmoscope.

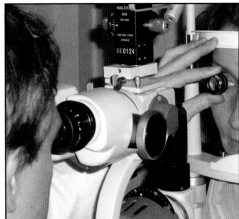

Figure 2-34. Use of a high-plus lens to observe the fundus at the slit lamp.

- Scleral indentation allows the examiner to view the peripheral fundus in a dynamic fashion. This is particularly useful in evaluation of retinal degeneration or breaks.
  - The patient may be seated or reclined. The reclined position allows for the most complete view and is also more comfortable for the patient and the examiner for prolonged examination.
  - The headset is adjusted so that the eyepieces allow the examiner to fuse at 40 cm.
  - The light setting is adjusted appropriately, understanding that the brighter illumination will allow better view, but is less well tolerated by the patient.
  - The examiner should be at arm's length from the patient's eye. The light should be directed into the patient's pupil.
  - The condensing lens is held with the thumb and forefinger and brought into the beam close to the patient's eye. The white ring on the lens denotes the patient side of the lens.
  - The initial view will include the fundus and the ocular adnexa. As the lens is drawn away from the patient's eye, the view of the fundus expands to fill the lens.
  - Drawing the lens further from the patient's eye will cause the examiner to again see the ocular adnexa in the condensing lens. When this occurs, the lens is moved closer to the patient's eye again to obtain the best and most complete fundus image.
  - Maintaining an arm's length distance with the lens, the patient is directed to look in each field of gaze to allow view of the different regions of the retina. To view the superior retina, the patient is instructed to look up and so on.
  - Systematic examination typically starts with superior retina, then superior-nasal, nasal, and so on around the periphery and ends with examination of the posterior pole.
  - Scleral indentation is accomplished by first having the patient look in the opposite direction of that which is to be viewed. The indentation instrument is placed on the lid at the inner border of the tarsal plate. The patient is then asked to slowly look in the direction of interest, and the examiner follows the eye movement with the indenter.

Slit-Lamp Funduscopy With High-Plus Lenses

- The slit lamp can be used in a fashion very similar to binocular indirect ophthalmoscopy, using a high-plus condensing lens to image the fundus (Figure 2-34). Lenses range in power from +60 to +90. The higher the lens power, the less the magnification and the greater the field of view. This technique allows a highly magnified and stereoscopic view of the posterior pole and optic nerve head.
  - The pupils are dilated, and the patient is positioned at the slit lamp.
  - The slit beam is reduced in dimension both vertically and horizontally.
  - The biomicroscope is positioned as far back from the patient as possible, and the beam is directed into the pupil of the eye to be examined.
  - The high-plus lens is introduced into the beam, and the slit lamp is advanced toward the patient until retinal details are in focus.

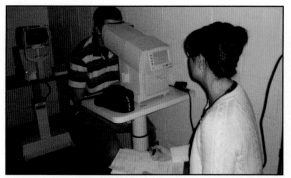

Figure 2-35. The Frequency Doubling Technology (FDT) visual field screener.

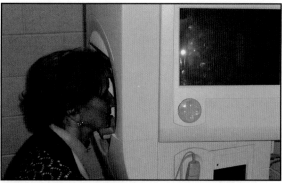

Figure 2-36. The Humphrey visual field analyzer.

○ The slit lamp and lens can then be manipulated to view the posterior view in great detail. As with the direct ophthalmoscope, start with evaluation of the optic nerve head, then follow several vessels out beyond 2 or more bifurcations and then end with the macula.

Slit-Lamp Funduscopy of the Peripheral Retina

- The slit lamp can be used to great advantage to view the peripheral retina with high magnification, but the techniques require use of mirror-containing lenses that contact the eye in the same manner as gonioscopic lenses. The angle of the mirror will dictate the portion of the fundus that can be examined.

Visual Field Testing

Just as visual acuity is used in assessment of central visual function, visual field testing is used to assess the function of peripheral vision. This is particularly useful in detecting loss of visual function that may not be apparent to the patient. The pattern of visual field loss and the relationship between the visual field findings of the 2 eyes can provide invaluable diagnostic information.

Screening Tests

- Numerous visual field tests examine for the presence or absence of a visual field defect, that is, to determine if the field is normal or abnormal. These tests compare the field tested with data regarding the normal visual field. Such suprathreshold testing is quick and efficient, but provides little or no quantitative data (Figure 2-35).

Quantitative Tests

- When specific information regarding the degree of sensitivity loss is required, a quantitative test becomes necessary (Figure 2-36). Such tests are much more specific than screening tests in terms of area and depth of loss of function. Most modern quantitative tests are performed using automated devices with assistance from a qualified technician. Quantitative tests can be generally classified into kinetic and static categories.
  ○ Kinetic tests plot fields that show the limits of equal sensitivity, or isopters.
    - A target of fixed size, color, and luminance is moved gradually from the area of nonseeing to seeing, and the point at which the patient first detects the target is recorded.
    - The procedure is repeated for different meridians to plot the complete field for this stimulus.
      □ This process is then repeated for a number of other stimuli.
      □ Areas of nonseeing, called scotomas, are also plotted with respect to various stimuli.
  ○ Static perimetry uses a stationary target that gradually increases in visibility. The level at which the stimulus is first noted is recorded.
    - Testing is repeated at numerous locations in a grid pattern.
    - Sensitivity is plotted using a gray-scale pattern. Areas of high sensitivity are plotted in light gray, and areas of low sensitivity in dark gray or black, indicating no detectable sensitivity at this locale.

Interpreting Automated Visual Field Information

- A systematic assessment of visual field printouts (Figure 2-37) starts with a review of ancillary information that may affect the findings:
  - o Pupil size should be noted. A small pupil in a patient with media opacities will artificially limit the visual field.
  - o Refractive correction must be correct for the fixation distance required for the test, as blur can cause sensitivity to be reduced. For corrections beyond ±6.00 D, a contact lens correction should be considered.
  - o The patient's visual acuity should be noted, as this may account for general sensitivity reduction and for fixation loss during testing.
- Patient reliability indices are helpful in determining the usefulness or significance of the test data. The patient's willingness and ability to respond can vary with a number of factors and have significant influence on test results.
  - o Fixation errors are detected by occasional and random placement of a suprathreshold stimulus in an area of the physiological blind spot.
  - o False-positive errors occur when the patient responds, but there is no stimulus.
  - o False-negative errors occur when the patient fails to respond to a suprathreshold stimulus appearing in an area in which sensitivity has been established.
  - o These errors, in addition to short-term fluctuations in response, are compared with age-matched normal control subjects.
- Automated perimeters provide a number of statistical indices that are useful in determining the degree of loss of visual field.
  - o The average deviation from age-matched normal controls for each tested location is summarized as the mean defect or deviation (MD) and gives an indication of the overall loss.
  - o The pattern standard deviation (PSD), or loss variance (LV), is corrected for the MD and gives an index of degree of localized field loss. This takes into account the normal slope of change across the field and detects significant localized variance. This index may also be corrected for the individual patient's short-term fluctuations.
  - o The glaucoma hemifield test (GHT) is specifically designed to test for sensitivity loss that occurs with glaucoma. It compares points above and below the horizontal midline that correspond to the loss in the regions of the nerve fiber bundle that are characteristic of glaucoma. A designation of abnormal with this test indicates a difference greater than that would be found in less than 1% of normals.
- Probability plots represent a comparison of the patient's findings with age-matched normal values for each area tested, thus displaying the amount of deviation from normal on a point-by-point basis.
  - o The total deviation plot uses different degrees of shaded boxes to indicate the degree of deviation from normal limits.
  - o The pattern deviation plot uses the same system of shaded boxes but takes into account overall deviation.
  - o If there is little difference between the total and pattern deviation plots, this indicates the loss is predominately localized.
  - o If the pattern deviation appears much less pronounced than the total deviation, a generalized loss is indicated.

Confrontation Visual Field

- The most basic visual field test is the confrontation test, which compares the examiner's field of vision with that of the patient (Figure 2-38). It is quick to administer and should be done as part of a standard eye examination. It is capable of detecting only moderate to advanced visual field defects and cannot be relied upon to detect early defects. A number of automated screening tests are available that are substantially more sensitive.
  - o The examiner sits facing the patient.
  - o The eye not being examined is occluded. The examiner closes his or her own eye that is opposite that of the patient's occluded eye.
  - o The patient and examiner maintain fixation on each other's open eye.
  - o A small target is slowly moved from outside the patient's field of view, and the patient is to report when the object is just seen.

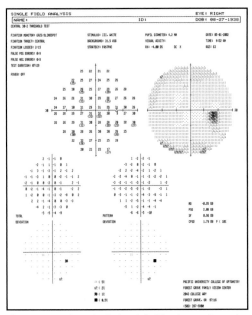

Figure 2-37. A typical visual field printout from the Humphrey field analyzer. (Reprinted with permission of Nada Lingel, OD, MS.)

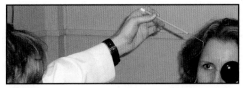

Figure 2-38. Performing the confrontation visual field.

- o The examiner notes the limit of the field in comparison with his or her own field.
- o The process is repeated in several meridians in each quadrant.
- o The normal monocular field is 95 degrees temporal, 75 degrees inferior, 60 degrees nasal, and 60 degrees superior from fixation.

Amsler Grid Central Field Testing

- When macular disease is suspected, the Amsler grid provides a quick test of the visual field of the macular region (Figure 2-39).
  - o The patient wears his or her near correction for the test.
  - o The grid is well-illuminated and held 30 cm from the patient.
  - o The eyes are tested one at a time. It is often best to test the "better" eye first if there is a known or suspected difference.
  - o With one eye occluded, the patient is asked to maintain fixation on the center white dot.
  - o While fixating the center, the patient is asked the following:
    - If all 4 corners are visible
    - If the lines are complete and straight
    - If all the squares appear to be the same size
  - o Record any abnormal responses. If possible, have the patient draw the defects on a recording form.

Color Vision Testing

Color vision testing is performed to screen for the presence and grade the severity of color vision anomalies. Most color vision deficiencies are congenital, and due to being x-linked, they are about 20 times more common in males than females.

- Some form of color deficiency affects up to 8% of North American males and about 0.5% of females.
- Normal color perception relies on a system of 3 cone types, each with different but overlapping sensitivity curves. This trichromacy allows finely graded distinction of colors over the range of the visible spectrum.
- Color vision deficiencies typically occur when 1 of the 3 cone types is weak or absent.
  - o The cones with peak sensitivity in the reds are referred to as the protan system.
  - o Those with peak in the greens are the deutan.

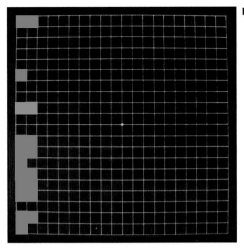

Figure 2-39. Amsler grid for testing the central field.

- o Those in the blue end are the tritan.
- o Deficiency in either the protan or deutan will give rise to red-green confusion, while tritan defects result in blue-yellow confusion.
- o Individuals who have all 3 cone types, but in which 1 of them is less sensitive than normal are referred to as anomalous trichromats.
- o Those who have only 2 cone types are called dichromats.
- o Dichromats have relatively extreme color deficiency while trichromats can present with various levels of difficulty ranging from very mild to nearly as severe as those found in dichromats.
- Congenital color defects are always bilateral and symmetrical, while acquired defects typically are either unilateral or asymmetrical.
  - o For purposes of screening for congenital defects, binocular testing is acceptable. If an acquired defect is suspected, monocular testing should be employed.
  - o With the exception of the anomaloscope, which is internally illuminated, all color vision tests are intended to be presented under a standard illumination provided by the Macbeth lamp. When the lamps are unavailable, standard indoor lighting with a 100-watt light bulb will suffice for most circumstances. Fluorescent lighting and direct sunlight should be avoided.

Anomaloscope

- Considered the "gold standard" for color vision testing, this relatively expensive and complex device can distinguish the dichromat from the anomalous trichromat and give a continuous grading of the degree of defect.
- Due to its expense and the need for an experienced examiner, the test is not in common use. Simpler tests that provide adequate information are typically employed.

Pseudoisochromatic Plates

- The most common color vision test uses one form of the pseudoisochromatic plates, which contain figures within patterns of crowded dots, the colors of which are chosen to confuse the color-deficient patient (Figure 2-40).
- There is typically a first demonstration, or "malingerer's" plate, which should be easily passed regardless of the color vision status.
- Subsequent plates include numbers that are either seen as different or not at all by the color-deficient patient.
- Normal patients will see the numbers correctly in all but the 2 plates that have hidden numbers visible only to some color-deficient patients.
- In addition to the numbers, there are also plates with a pathway that are to be followed. These are intended for children or illiterate patients.
- The patient should not be allowed to touch the colored plates, as this will spoil the plates after just a few such instances.

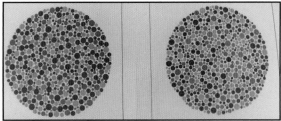

Figure 2-40. Pseudoisochromatic plates for color vision testing.

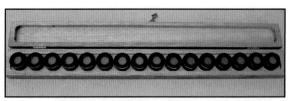

Figure 2-41. The Farnsworth D-15 test.

- There are many sets of plates available, the most common being the Ishihara series. Each set contains its own specific pass/fail criteria.
- Although some plate sets attempt to grade degrees of deficiency and determine deutan versus protan deficiency, their main value lies in their usefulness as sensitive and rapid screening tests.

Color Sorting Tests

- Color sorting using swatches of dyed wool was one of the first methods employed for identifying color vision defects. Modern tests use colored papers based on the Munsell system of color specification. The most common test is the Farnsworth D-15 test (Figure 2-41). This test is not suitable for screening as it will "pass" many mildly color-deficient individuals, but it is highly useful in sorting those likely to have an occupational limitation from the milder cases and, in the former, provides a means of distinguishing deutan from protan and to elicit tritan defects. Tritan defects are very rare as congenital defects, but can be an important diagnostic finding in acquired defects.
  - The Farnsworth D-15 test consists of colored papers mounted in black circular caps.
  - One cap is fixed in the test tray, and the others are removed and placed in random order.
  - The task is to pick the colored cap that most closely matches the reference cap. Once that cap is placed, it becomes the reference, and so forth until all 15 caps have been arranged in the tray.
  - Turning the tray over reveals the sequence numbers for the caps. The test is scored by plotting the pattern of the cap placement on the score sheet. The specific errors and their orientation yield information about the nature of the color-perception defect.

Contrast Sensitivity

Contrast sensitivity testing provides information regarding visual function that goes beyond that which can be determined by standard visual acuity testing. As such, it has become increasingly common in clinical use. Many types of charts exist, each with their own method, criteria, and reliability. Contrast sensitivity testing has the following uses:

- Screening for visual pathway disorders, such as optic neuritis, in which ophthalmoscopic appearance of the eye may be normal
- Assessing symptoms of poor vision in patients who appear to have otherwise normal findings. This can be of use in both the preoperative cataract work-up and in the evaluation of the postrefractive surgery patient.

Glare Testing

Glare testing, which assesses the impact of a light source on visual acuity or contrast sensitivity, can be used to determine the degree of disability caused by scatter due to media opacity. Such testing can be useful in determining the need for glare-reducing tinted spectacles or for cataract surgery.

Potential Acuity Testing

In patients with dense cataract, it is of use to have an indication of the acuity that can potentially be achieved by removal of the cataract. This is in order to avoid unnecessary procedures and to prevent disappointment by the patient undergoing the surgery. Several methods exist. Some devices project a grating target onto the retina while others use a version of a Snellen acuity chart. Grating targets tend to overestimate the acuity of amblyopic eyes or those with maculopathies. The Potential Acuity Meter (PAM) tends to underestimate acuity in normal eyes if the opacity is very dense.

Potential acuity testing is a useful augmentation to other preoperative tests, particularly when media obscure the view of the posterior pole.

Electrodiagnostic Testing

Visual Evoked Potential

- The electrical activity of the brain that is initiated by a visual stimulus is referred to as the visual evoked potential (VEP). The activity can be measured by placing electrodes on the scalp over the occipital cortex and presenting the visual system with specific patterns as stimuli. The VEP is useful in diagnosis of optic nerve disorders, particularly optic neuritis and ocular albinism, as well as in the evaluation of presumed psychogenic vision loss. It is also of use in assessing vision function in newborns and infants and thus is an important tool in the early diagnosis of amblyopia.

Electroretinogram

- The electroretinogram (ERG) measures electrical activity from several types of cells in the sensory retina. The ERG is obtained by placing an electrode at the surface of the cornea with a contact lens. A second electrode serves as a reference and is attached to the forehead or in the speculum holding the contact lens, and a ground electrode is placed in an electrically neutral location, such as the ear. Specific stimuli are used with the eye both dark-adapted and light-adapted. The electrical potential between the 2 electrodes is amplified, and both wave amplitude and time factors are analyzed.
- The ERG is useful in differentiation and diagnosis of a number of retinal disorders, such as retinitis pigmentosa and its related disorders, choroideremia, and gyrate atrophy (see also Chapter 9).

Suggested Readings

Carlson N, Kurtz D. *Clinical Procedures for Ocular Examination*. 3rd ed. New York, NY: McGraw-Hill; 2004.
Zadnik K. *The Ocular Examination—Measurements and Findings*. Philadelphia, PA: Saunders; 1997.

Questions

1. If visual acuity is tested at 10 feet and the patient read the 40-foot letter, this is equivalent to 20-foot acuity of
   a. 10/20
   b. 20/10
   c. 20/40
   d. **20/80**

2. If visual acuity is 20/200 and does not improve with a pinhole, the most unlikely explanation for reduced acuity is
   a. Media opacity
   b. **Uncorrected refractive error**
   c. Macular degeneration
   d. Optic atrophy

3. If no motion is detected when the retinoscope is 50 cm from the eye, the refractive error of the eye is
   a. 1.00 D
   b. 1.50 D
   c. **2.00 D**
   d. 2.50 D

4. The keratometer reading of an eye is 44.00 at 180 degrees and 42.50 at 90 degrees. Javal's rule would predict the refractive astigmatism to be
    a. -1.00 x 90
    b. -1.00 x 180
    c. -2.00 x 180
    d. **-2.00 x 90**

5. The unilateral cover test is principally used to
    a. **Determine presence of strabismus**
    b. Determine presence of heterophoria
    c. Determine magnitude of strabismus
    d. Determine magnitude of heterophoria

6. If the phoria measured through a plano lens is 2 PDs exophoria and the phoria measured though a -2.00 lens is 8 PDs esophoria, the AC/A ratio is
    a. 3
    b. **5**
    c. 8
    d. 10

7. Tests for volume of tear flow include all except
    a. Schirmer's
    b. Phenol red thread
    c. Tear prism height
    d. **TBUT**

8. The keratometer and videokeratographer are used to measure
    a. **The front surface radius of the cornea**
    b. The front surface power of the cornea
    c. The radius of the peripheral cornea
    d. The index of refraction of the cornea

9. In observation of the optic disc, it is expected that the rim tissue
    a. Will be thinnest inferior
    b. Will be thickest temporal
    c. Will be thicker nasal than superior
    d. **Will be thickest inferior**

10. For a patient for whom there is suspicion of angle closure, the following pair of tests would be most relevant to making the diagnosis:
    a. Pachymetry and tonometry
    b. Tonometry and visual field
    c. **Gonioscopy and tonometry**
    d. Slit-lamp estimation of angle and pachymetry

11. An advantage of the binocular indirect ophthalmoscope is the
    a. **Wide field of view**
    b. High magnification
    c. Erect image
    d. Ease of use

12. In analysis of automated visual field findings, the Pattern Standard Deviation is an indicator of degree of
    a. Overall loss
    b. Difference between overall loss and localized loss
    c. Loss in the nerve fiber bundle regions
    d. **Localized loss**

Optics and Corrective Lenses

Peter Bergenske, OD

Outline

Probst LE, Tsai JH.
Ophthalmology: Clinical and Surgical Principles (pp. 91–112).
© 2012 SLACK Incorporated

Introduction

The human eye, among many other things, is an optical device that follows the laws of physics. Fortunately, most of the optical phenomena associated with the eye fall under the very basic rules of fundamental geometrical optics, the basics of which are summarized here.

Refraction

- Uninterrupted, a single ray of light travels in a straight line until it strikes either a reflecting surface or a transparent surface.
  - The change in direction of a light ray transmitted through a transparent surface is called refraction.
  - The change in direction of a light ray depends on the angle at which the ray strikes the surface (angle of incidence) and the optical density of the entered medium (index of refraction).

Index of Refraction

- Light travels through some materials faster than others. Except for the special circumstance of a vacuum, light travels fastest through air. To quantify the optical density of a material, the speed of light through air is compared to the speed of light through the material. This ratio is called the optical index, or index of refraction.

$$\frac{\text{speed of light in air}}{\text{speed of light in the material}} = \text{index of refraction of the material}$$

Snell's Law

- If light strikes a surface of a material of a different index of refraction at an angle other than 90 degrees, it changes direction (Figure 3-1).
  - The amount of change in direction is a function of the angle of incidence (relative to normal) and the change in index of refraction, following Snell's law: if the ray is traveling in a medium of index "n" and enters a second medium of index "n'" at angle "I," one can compute the change in direction (to angle I') using the sines of the angles:

$$n \sin I = n' \sin I'$$

  where I is the angle of incidence and I' is the angle of refraction relative to the normal.
- Simple calculation will reveal that light entering a medium of higher index will deviate toward the normal and light traveling from a higher to a lower index will deviate away from the normal.

Prisms and Prism Diopters

- If a light ray enters a medium of higher index, it slows down. If the material, such as a slab of glass or plastic, has parallel surfaces, the light ray, though temporarily slowed, is not altered in direction because the refraction at the 2 surfaces cancel one another. If the 2 surfaces are not parallel, however, the angle of incidence at the 2 surfaces are not equal and do not cancel one another and the direction of the ray is changed. This is the principle behind a prism:
  - A slab of glass with nonparallel surfaces will have a base (the thickest edge) and an apex (the thinnest edge).
  - A light ray passing through a prism will be deviated toward the base.
  - For an individual viewing through the prism, it will appear that the object viewed is shifted toward the apex (Figure 3-2).
  - The amount of deviation depends on the angle between the 2 sides and the index of refraction of the material.
  - The units of prism displacement are called prism diopters, which are expressed as centimeters of displacement per meter of distance traveled.
  - A light ray that is displaced 1 cm over a distance of 1 m is deviated by 1 prism diopter.
  - Prism can be used in ophthalmic lenses to either cause or allow the eye to turn in a specific direction and is commonly used to alleviate problems involving misalignment of the eyes.

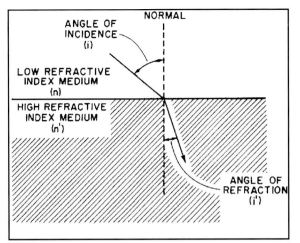

Figure 3-1. Snell's law: If light strikes a surface of a material of different index of refraction at an angle other than 90 degrees, it changes direction. (Reprinted from *System for Ophthalmic Dispensing.* 2nd ed. Brooks C, Borish I. Copyright [1996], with permission from Elsevier.)

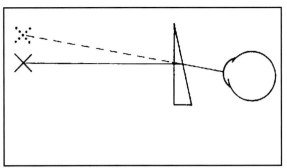

Figure 3-2. An object viewed through a prism appears displaced. (Reprinted from *System for Ophthalmic Dispensing.* 2nd ed. Brooks C, Borish I. Copyright [1996], with permission from Elsevier.)

Focal Length

- Unlike simple prisms, which have flat surfaces, lenses have one or more curved surfaces. As a result, the angle at which a given ray strikes the curved surface will vary depending on how close or far the point of entry is from the center of the lens.
  - A ray striking the geometrical center of the lens at a 90-degree angle will not change direction.
  - The further the point of entry is from the center of the lens, the greater the angle of incidence, and thus the greater the angle of refraction.
  - For a convex curved surface, parallel light rays will converge to the focal point (Figure 3-3).
  - For a concave surface, rays are diverged away from a virtual focal point (Figure 3-4).
  - The distance from the lens to the focal point is called the focal length.

Lens Power

- Lens powers are most conveniently expressed in units of the inverse of focal length, called diopters (D).
  - For converging lenses, diopters are positive, and for negative lenses, diopters are negative.
  - The units of focal length are meters, and diopters are inverse meters
    $$D = 1/\text{focal length}$$
  - A lens of zero power has infinite focal length. Such a lens is referred to as having plano power.

Surface Power

- Each surface of a lens contributes power to the lens. This power is a function of the change in index of refraction (air to lens or lens to air) and the radius of curvature of the surface.
- Surface power is calculated in this manner:
  Where:
  $$F = \frac{n^1 - n}{r}$$
  F is the surface power
  n′ is the index of the lens material
  n is the index from which the light enters the material (if air, n = 1)
  r is the radius of curvature of the surface (meters)
- If the lens is thin, the total power of the lens is simply the sum of the front surface power and the back surface power
  $$F1 + F2 = F(\text{Total})$$

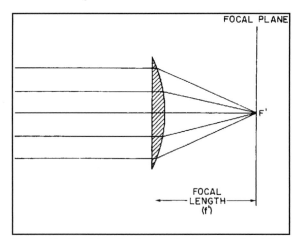

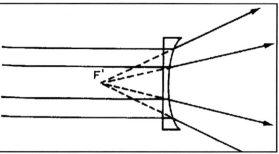

Figure 3-4. Focal length of a negative lens. (Reprinted from *System for Ophthalmic Dispensing.* 2nd ed. Brooks C, Borish I. Copyright [1996], with permission from Elsevier.)

Figure 3-3. Focal length of a positive lens. (Reprinted from *System for Ophthalmic Dispensing.* 2nd ed. Brooks C, Borish I. Copyright [1996], with permission from Elsevier.)

Vergence

- If light rays are diverging from a point, they are said to have negative vergence.
- If they converge toward a point, they have positive vergence.
- Vergence and diopters can be added algebraically to solve simple optical problems. For example, light rays with –5.00 of divergence striking a +5.00 D lens will result in parallel rays having zero vergence.
- Vergence is expressed in diopters or inverse meters. Light diverging from 0.40 m away has $1/-0.40 = -2.50$ D of divergence.

Spherical Lenses

- A lens with a single point focus is a spherical lens, the simplest form of ophthalmic lens (Figure 3-5). The radius of curvature for each surface is symmetrical such that rotational orientation of the lens is of no consequence.

Cylindrical Lenses

- Many ophthalmic lenses require nonsymmetrical optics to correct astigmatic refractive errors. In this case, one or more of the lens surfaces has the geometrical shape of a torus.
    - Toric surfaces are characterized by having a meridian of greatest curvature and least curvature perpendicular to one another. This shape is similar to a cylinder, although both surfaces are curved. A section of a bicycle tire or a bagel is perhaps illustrative.
    - As surface power is a function of curvature, this asymmetry results in a nonsymmetrical focus that is orientation-specific.
    - A toric lens can be specified by its meridian of greatest power, its meridian of least power, and the orientation, or axis.
    - Cylinder lens specification can reference the maximum and minimum power meridians in either order
    - Depending on the order, the lens will be specified as either plus cylinder or minus cylinder. This has no relation to the actual form the lens will be made in. (Virtually all ophthalmic lenses are manufactured with a convex spherical, plus power, front surface, and a concave, negative power, back surface that is either spherical or toric. Technically, this is considered a minus cylinder.)
    - The orientation of a cylinder lens is specified by the axis. For a plus cylinder lens, the axis is the meridian of least plus, or most minus, power. For a minus cylinder lens, the axis is the meridian of least minus, or most plus, power (Figure 3-6).

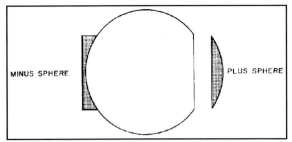

Figure 3-5. The shape of a spherical lens. (Reprinted from *System for Ophthalmic Dispensing*. 2nd ed. Brooks C, Borish I. Copyright [1996], with permission from Elsevier.)

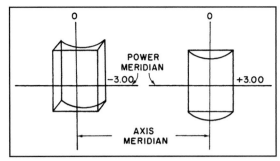

Figure 3-6. General shape of a plus or minus cylindrical lens. Note one meridian is flat and thus has plano power. (Reprinted from *System for Ophthalmic Dispensing*. 2nd ed. Brooks C, Borish I. Copyright [1996], with permission from Elsevier.)

Spherocylindrical Lenses

- Many, if not most, ophthalmic lenses can be thought of as being a combination of a sphere and a cylinder. Such lenses are considered spherocylindrical.
  - If specified as plus cylinder lenses, the least plus meridian is specified as the sphere, and the difference between this and the most plus meridian is specified as the cylinder, with the axis being the meridian of least plus power.
  - If specified as minus cylinder lenses, the least minus meridian is specified as the sphere, and the difference between this and the most minus meridian is specified as the cylinder, with the axis being the meridian of least minus power.
- In order to construct this optical configuration, one may select a spherical lens from the trial case and combine it with a plus or minus cylinder at the appropriate axis. Ophthalmic lenses are manufactured to combine these effects in a single lens.

Lens Formulas

- The formula for a spherocylindrical lens is written in a format that relates both components.
  - Sphere (combined with) cylinder and axis (the meridian of the sphere power)
  - A lens with power of +2.00 in the 180 meridian and +3.00 in the 90 meridian can be specified in plus cylinder form as +2.00 sphere with +1.00 cylinder. The axis is the meridian of the sphere and thus is 180. The lens formula would be written as follows:
        +2.00 +1.00 x 180
        Sphere Cylinder Axis
  - The same lens could be specified in minus cylinder form. In this case, the sphere is +3.00, the cylinder is -1.00, and the axis is 90. The lens formula would be written as follows:
        +3.00 -1.00 x 90
        Sphere Cylinder Axis

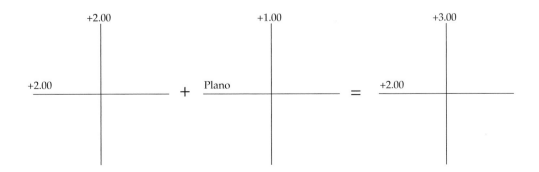

- To illustrate, these lens powers can be depicted on a power cross that identifies the 2 principal meridians. Note the power between the principal meridians varies continuously from the minimum to maximum power, such that the power in the 45 and 135 meridians is +2.50.

Lens Formula Transposition

- It is often convenient to transpose from one written cylinder form to the other. One method is to draw the lens powers on a power cross, such as in the illustration, and make the determination as described above. It is also convenient to use a set strategy that can be easily memorized:
    - Add the sphere and cylinder power algebraically. This is the new sphere power.
    - Change the sign of the cylinder power from minus to plus or plus to minus.
    - Change the axis by 90 degrees (respecting the convention that axis is between 1 and 180 degrees).

Refractive Error

- Determination of the refractive status of the eye is a routine element of the ocular examination. Errors of refraction represent the vast majority of ocular problems.

Emmetropia and the Ametropia

- The ideal human eye, at rest, is in focus for infinite distance such that parallel rays of light are focused precisely and uniformly at the level of the photoreceptors of the retina.
    - Emmetropia is the condition in which the eye is naturally in focus for light approaching with zero vergence.
    - For this to occur, there must be a match between the optical components and the axial length of the eye.
    - When this condition is not met, the eye is said to have a refractive error, or ametropia. Ametropias occur when the focal power of the eye is too great (myopia), too slight (hyperopia), or nonsymmetrical (astigmatism).

Myopia

- The most common refractive error is myopia, commonly referred to as nearsightedness. Myopia occurs when the optical power of the eye has too much converging power for the length of the eye, causing light rays to focus in front of the retina.
    - When the eye is of normal length, the occurrence of myopia is considered secondary to an error in power of the cornea and crystalline lens and is termed *refractive myopia*.
    - Axial myopia is said to occur when the principal deviation from normal is excessive axial length of the eye, which can be associated with higher rates of open angle glaucoma and retinal tears.
    - Optical correction of myopia is accomplished with lenses of appropriate negative power.

Hyperopia

- Hyperopia, or farsightedness, occurs when the optical components of the eye are too weak for the length of the eye, and thus light converges beyond the retina.
    - As with myopia, hyperopia can be considered as refractive or axial.
    - Highly hyperopic eyes are often of shorter axial length, making them more prone to angle closure.
    - Optical correction of hyperopia is accomplished with lenses of appropriate positive power.

Astigmatism

- When the optical system of the eye is not spherical, the eye will have astigmatism.
    - Most often, astigmatism can be attributed to a cornea that is more curved in one meridian than the others. If this is the case, the eye is said to have corneal astigmatism.

o If the cornea is spherical but one or both surfaces of the crystalline lens are toric, the result is lenticular astigmatism.
o The meridians of greatest and least power are called the principal meridians.
o In regular astigmatism, the meridian of greatest power is 90 degrees away from the meridian of least power.
o For most astigmatic eyes, the vertical meridian is of greater power than the horizontal. This kind of astigmatism is classified as *with-the-rule*.
o When the horizontal meridian is of greater power than the vertical, it is classified as *against-the-rule*.
o If the only refractive error is the astigmatism and one principal meridian is focused on the retina, the error is called simple astigmatism, which can be either myopic or hyperopic.
o If both meridians are focused in front of the retina, it is called myopic astigmatism, and if they are focused beyond the retina, it is hyperopic astigmatism.
o Mixed astigmatism occurs when one meridian is focused in front of the retina and the other behind.
o Optical correction of astigmatism is accomplished with cylindrical or spherocylindrical lenses.

Irregular Astigmatism and Higher Order Aberrations

- Irregular astigmatism occurs when the principal meridians of an astigmatic error are not 90 degrees apart. In addition, nonuniformity of the optical system can occur in many variations. These variations have been classified into a hierarchy of aberrations, which can be separated mathematically into many classes beyond the common divisions of spherical and astigmatic error. Examples include spherical aberration, trefoil, quatrefoil, and secondary astigmatism.
  o Higher-order errors of refraction are orientation-specific and pupil size-dependent.
  o The correction of such errors is beyond the capability of spherical and spherocylindrical lenses.
  o In some cases, a contact lens can neutralize many of these errors.

Anisometropia

- Anisometropia is the condition when the refractive errors of the 2 eyes are different. High degrees of anisometropia can lead to amblyopia, and its spectacle correction can create problems due to different prismatic and magnification effects of the lenses.

Accommodation and Presbyopia

- The emmetropic eye, or the corrected ametropic eye, is in focus for parallel light rays (zero vergence). To view an object that is more proximal than optical infinity, additional converging power must be employed to neutralize the divergence of the rays from the object. This is normally accomplished by a change in the power of the crystalline lens via the process of accommodation.
  o Accommodation increases the converging power of the eye; however, the ability to do so decreases with age.
  o This decline in accommodative ability is referred to as *presbyopia*.
  o Optical correction of presbyopia is accomplished with lenses of appropriate positive (or less negative) power. Such lenses allow for precise focus for near objects, but consequently will cause a myopic blur of distant objects. The optical solution to this dilemma is one of the many variations on multifocal lenses, which provide one focus for distant objects and one or more foci for nearer objects.

Prescribing Refractive Error

Spectacle Lenses

- As mentioned in the previous sections, the most common remedy for alleviation of problems related to refractive error is the prescription of spectacle lenses.
  o In order to be practical, spectacle lenses must be mounted in a spectacle frame that is properly sized and fitted for the patient by the optician.
  o Proper alignment of the lenses is important, as misalignment can cause numerous visual problems even if the lens prescription itself is correct.

- Spectacle lenses are made in the lens form called a meniscus.
  - In a meniscus lens, the front curve is convex and the back curve is concave.
  - The relation between these 2 surfaces dictates whether this is a plus or minus power lens.
- Spherocylindrical lenses have one curve that is spherical and one that is toric.
  - When the front surface is toric, the lenses are called plus cylinder lenses.
  - When the back surface is toric, the lenses are called minus cylinder lenses.
  - As plus cylinder lenses are cosmetically and optically inferior as ophthalmic lenses, virtually all modern ophthalmic lenses are made as minus cylinder lenses.
- The front surface curve of an ophthalmic lens is called the base curve.
  - The base curve contributes substantially to the magnification or minification caused by the lens.
  - It is important that base curves are comparable between right and left lenses and from one pair to the next for the same patient in order to avoid adaptation and perceptual difficulties.

Single-Vision Lenses

- Single-vision lenses provide uniform refractive correction throughout the lens such that the correction compensating the eye is the same regardless of direction of gaze or object distance. Spherical or spherocylindrical single-vision lenses are commonly prescribed for use by nonpresbyopic patients or presbyopes who prefer separate lenses for distance and near tasks.

Multifocal Lenses

- Multifocal lenses provide more than one focal length through different parts of the lens such that the user must position the lens or the object in a specific orientation in order to match the focal length with the object distance.
  - Common multifocal lenses are bifocals, trifocals, and progressive addition lenses.
  - Bifocals are generally prescribed such that the upper portion of the lens provides correction for distance viewing. The lower portion is prescribed for close viewing. The upper portion is specified the same as that which would be prescribed for distance single-vision lenses.
  - The lower portion of a bifocal is specified simply by the diopter change between the upper and lower portion (as cylinder and axis remain the same throughout). The difference between the upper and lower is called the add power.
  - Because it is the amount added to the distance correction to create greater convergence (less divergence), the add is always a plus power.
- When the add power required becomes relatively high (over +2.00), patients may find they have "no man's land" of focus between the range covered by the upper lens and lower lens.
  - Trifocal lenses are similar to bifocals with the addition of an intermediate range portion situated just above the lower, near portion.
  - Nearly all trifocal designs set this intermediate lens at half the add power.
- Progressive addition lenses provide a continuous variation in focal length and are commonly used due to several advantages over conventional bifocal and trifocal lenses.
  - In progressive addition lenses, the lens power varies continuously from the distance correction set directly in front of the pupil and the add power, positioned inferior and slightly nasal (medial) to allow for convergence of the lines of sight.
  - This provides a constant and continuous range of focus absent of the optical "jump" that occurs with conventional bifocals.
  - Progressive lenses are also cosmetically superior due to the absence of the dividing lines characteristic of bifocals and trifocals.
  - Progressive addition lenses (Figure 3-7) are typically more costly and require greater precision in fitting and manufacturing, yet their optical and cosmetic benefits are preferred by many patients.

Vertex Distance

- Spectacle lenses are positioned some finite vertex distance from the principle optical planes of the eye. Once light leaves the lens and prior to approaching the eye, there is some change in the vergence of the light. In lower power lenses (less than 5.00 D), this difference is typically trivial.

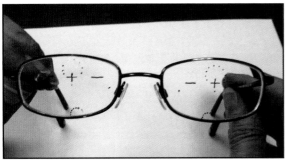

Figure 3-7. Progressive addition lens with optical center identified.

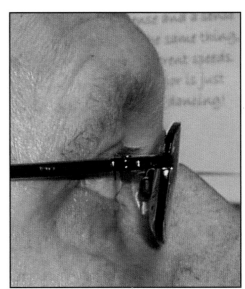

Figure 3-8. Vertex distance between the lens and the eye can influence power needed.

o As lenses increase in power, the distance between the lens and the eye (the vertex distance) can become significant (Figure 3-8).
o For high-plus corrections, more plus power is needed as the lens moves closer to the eye.
o For high-minus correction, less minus power is needed as the lens moves closer to the eye.
o Physical fit of the spectacles can have significant impact, and it is important that the refractionist pay heed to the vertex distance of test lenses when prescribing for high-power lenses.
o Change in vertex distance is of particular concern when prescribing contact lenses based on a spectacle lens refraction.

Prism

- The optical axis of a lens passes through the optical center. At this point, the front and back surfaces are parallel, and light does not change direction.
  o For light rays passing through the lens at points remote from the optical center, the amount of deviation is a function of the lens power and the distance from the center.
  o This deviation is called the prismatic effect of the lens.
- If the line of sight (a line connecting the fovea with the object of regard) passes through the optical center of a lens, the image is not displaced. If the line of sight is directed at some portion of the lens not on the optical center, the image will be displaced.
  o The amount of displacement follows Prentice's Rule that states the following:
    ▪ The prism diopters (cm/m) of displacement is equal to the distance from the optical center in centimeters (c) multiplied by the diopter power of the lens (F).
  o Thus, viewing 1 cm off center of a 2-D lens induces 2 prism diopters of displacement of the image.
    ▪ Prism displacement is of no consequence when lenses are of relatively equal power.
    ▪ In conditions of high anisometropia differential, prism displacement can be uncomfortable and visually disturbing.
    ▪ Prism is useful in spectacle lenses to remediate some problems of ocular misalignment and is commonly prescribed for these conditions.
  o In order to specify a prism, one must include not only the prism power, but the direction of displacement.
    ▪ Displacement of light traveling through a prism is toward its base.
    ▪ Although prism orientation can be in any direction, ophthalmic prisms are always specified in vector manner with a combination of base in, out, up, or down.

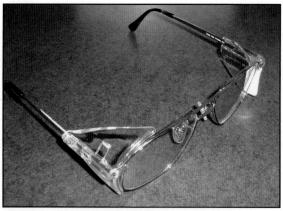

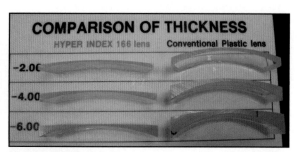

Figure 3-10. Choice of lens material can influence final thickness of the lens.

Figure 3-9. Industrial safety eyewear with side shields attached.

Impact Resistance and Safety Eyewear

- All ophthalmic lenses must, by law, meet minimum requirements for impact resistance.
    - In some circumstances, it is considered standard of care to specify lenses that meet even higher standards. Such circumstances include prescriptions for use in sports or by children and those intended for use as industrial safety eyewear.
    - All safety prescriptions should specify lenses be made of the most highly impact-resistant material, polycarbonate.
    - Industrial safety eyewear prescriptions should also include the specification that frames are to include side shields (Figure 3-9).

High-Index Materials

- The index of refraction of the lens material will dictate the thicknesses required to achieve the prescribed lens power.
    - The higher the index of refraction, the less difference is required between the front and back surfaces and thus the less thickness.
    - Often, there is a tradeoff between index of refraction and specific gravity, such that thinner lenses are not always lighter in weight.
    - Another drawback can be greater chromatic dispersion with higher index, causing "rainbow" fringes on lights viewed peripherally through some high-index lenses.
    - Modern high-index lenses can be thinner and lighter with minimal chromatic dispersion and offer significant advantage to patients requiring high degrees of refractive correction (Figure 3-10).

Aspheric Lenses

- Another strategy for making high-power lenses thinner is the use of aspheric surfaces. This is of particular value in higher plus corrections and has added benefit of reducing some lens-induced aberrations.

Photochromic Lenses

- Photochromic lenses include elements that undergo a photochemical transformation when exposed to ultraviolet light, causing the lenses to darken. Both glass and plastic lenses are available with this feature.

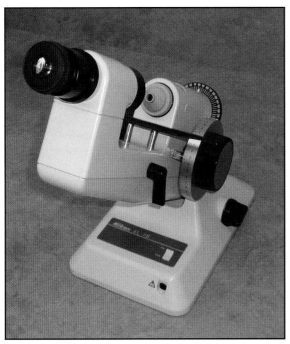

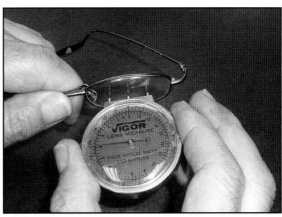

Figure 3-12. The lens clock is used to measure the base curve of the spectacle lens.

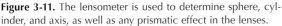

Figure 3-11. The lensometer is used to determine sphere, cylinder, and axis, as well as any prismatic effect in the lenses.

Other Tints

- Lenses can be tinted to a wide variety of degrees of transmittance and spectral absorption. This can be used to an advantage for many ocular conditions to improve contrast and visual performance or comfort.

Lens Measurement

- The focal length of a lens, including the sphere, cylinder, and axis, can be readily determined with a lensometer. Both manual and automatic versions are commonly used.
  - ○ The lensometer can also be used to determine the optical center and prismatic effect of a lens as well as the add power of a multifocal lens (Figure 3-11).
  - ○ By marking the optical centers of both lenses mounted in a spectacle frame, one can also determine the distance between the centers, which in most cases should equal the patient's interpupillary distance (IPD).
- The base curve of a spectacle lens is determined using a device called the lens measure, or lens clock (Figure 3-12). The lens measure operates on the principle of sagittal depth, measuring the depth of a given segment of a circle. From this, the radius of curvature of the lens surface is determined.

Contact Lenses

- Contact lenses provide an alternative to spectacles that have specific advantages.
  - ○ Because a contact lens maintains its position relative to the eye regardless of direction of gaze, peripheral lens distortion and induced prismatic effects are eliminated.
  - ○ Reducing the vertex to the plane of the cornea also greatly diminishes magnification difference between lenses of different power.
  - ○ For many athletic or occupational applications, the presence of the spectacle frame is a hindrance and potential hazard.

- o Spectacle lenses fog with temperature change and become difficult to use in rain or marine conditions.
- o Many patients prefer the freedom from the annoyance of wearing spectacle frames or simply feel they look better without glasses.
- As contact lenses are worn directly on the eye, prescribing contact lenses requires several considerations that are not of concern when prescribing spectacles.
    - o The contact lens must physically fit the eye in order to be comfortable. Some patient adaptation may be required even if the lens fits well.
    - o The presence of a contact lens can have a number of impacts on the normal ocular environment.
    - o The lens interacts with the blinking mechanism and must be nonirritating to the palpebral conjunctiva as well as the ocular surface.
    - o The contact lens represents a semipermeable membrane that must transmit oxygen and carbon dioxide in order for the avascular cornea to carry on normal respiration.
- A number of complications can occur that, although not unique to contact lens wear, are significantly more common. The fitting of contact lenses requires additional vigilance and responsibility to monitor and manage potential complications.

Oxygen Transmission of Contact Lenses

- The anterior cornea is dependent on oxygen dissolved in the tear film. In the open eye, this oxygen comes from the atmosphere and in the closed eye from the palpebral conjunctival vasculature. The presence of a contact lens imposes a barrier to this supply.
    - o All modern contact lens materials allow some transmission of oxygen through the lens.
    - o The amount of oxygen transmitted is directly related to the permeability of the material and inversely related to the thickness of the lens.
    - o Oxygen permeability is a characteristic of the lens material and is defined as the product of its diffusion coefficient (D) and the solubility factor (k) for oxygen. It is common to refer to this permeability as the Dk of the material.

$$\text{Permeability} = Dk$$

    - o The amount of oxygen that can be transmitted through a given lens is specified as the transmissivity, which is determined by dividing the Dk by the thickness (t) at any given point of the lens. The Dk/t is often quoted for lenses, but one must realize that the number quoted is typically for the center of a -3.00-D lens, and the number is optimistic relative to other lens thicknesses.

$$\text{Transmissivity} = Dk/t$$

    - o A great deal of effort has been directed at developing materials of higher Dk, as there are numerous limits to how thin a lens can be.

Types of Contact Lenses

- Contact lenses are broadly divided into categories of flexible (soft) lenses and rigid (hard) lenses. Lenses are also divided into categories based on intended use, based both on recommended wearing schedule and replacement frequency.

Flexible (Soft) Lenses

- The most common type of contact lens is the soft hydrogel.
    - o These lenses are made of hydrophilic plastics and are often differentiated by their percent water content.
    - o For hydrogel lenses, water content is directly related to Dk.
- Silicone hydrogel lenses are rapidly replacing the conventional soft hydrogel lens.
    - o Silicone hydrogel lenses have substantially higher Dk values and still offer all of the advantages of soft hydrogels.
    - o For silicone hydrogels, water content is inversely related to Dk because water content goes down as silicone content goes up.
- Pure silicone lenses exist; however, application is very limited due to material compromises that make them unacceptable in most instances.

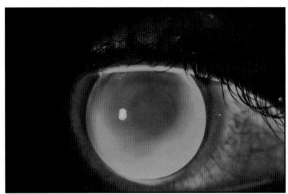

Figure 3-13. A rigid gas-permeable lens in situ. Fluorescein is used to assess the relationship of the lens to the eye.

- Due to their flexibility, soft contact lenses conform to the shape of the cornea and do not mask astigmatism. In order to correct astigmatism with a soft lens, a toric surface is applied, and the lens must be designed and fit to be rotationally stable.
- Most soft contact lenses are designed to be replaced fairly frequently.
  - ○ Replacement frequency can range from daily up to about 1 year.
  - ○ Most commonly, lenses are designated to be replaced every 2 to 4 weeks, but this is largely dictated by cost, and with improved manufacturing, the trend has been toward shorter replacement intervals.
  - ○ There is good evidence that more frequent replacement is associated with fewer complications.

Rigid (Hard) Lenses

- There are significant optical advantages to a nonflexing contact lens, particularly with regard to correction of corneal astigmatism.
  - ○ When the astigmatism manifest in the eye's refraction is attributable to corneal toricity, a rigid lens placed on the cornea will neutralize the astigmatism.
- A rigid lens adheres to a thin tear layer (Figure 3-13) but does not conform to the topography of the cornea as a soft lens does. This is of advantage not only for regular corneal astigmatism, but also in instances of irregular corneal astigmatism.
  - ○ Aberrations due to corneal disease, trauma, or degenerations such as keratoconus are often managed with rigid contact lenses.
- In some cases, the corneal toricity is too great to allow a stable fit of a spherically curved rigid lens.
  - ○ A lens with a toric back curve is used to improve the physical fit of the lens in circumstances of high corneal toricity.
  - ○ A toric back surface will often induce unwanted cylindrical correction, and a compensating cylinder power is placed on the front surface. This type of rigid lens is called bitoric.
- There are many rigid lens materials in a spectrum of Dk values. Rigid lenses tend to be rather durable and thus are replaced infrequently in comparison with soft lenses.

Fitting Procedures

- Contact lens fitting involves achieving an acceptable physical fit of a lens that optimally corrects the refractive error, is comfortable for the patient to wear, and interferes minimally with the physiology of the cornea and tear film. Although somewhat of an art, most contact lens fitting is readily accomplished using modern lens materials and designs.
  - ○ Contact lens manufacturers provide fitting guides that are typically well-tested. The novice fitter can achieve high degrees of success by simply following these guides.
- Factors affecting the physical fit of the lens include shape and sagittal height of the cornea and the apposition of the lids.
  - ○ Corneal shape is assessed by determining the corneal topography and by measuring the diameter of the cornea.

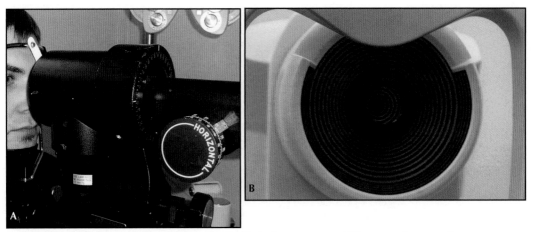

Figure 3-14. Corneal shape can be determined with (A) the keratometer and (B) a corneal topographer.

- o Corneal topography is best determined with the use of a computerized videokeratoscope that will provide measurement of central as well as peripheral corneal shape. Often, this is determined with the keratometer, which gives accurate measure of the central cornea only (Figure 3-14).
  - o The corneal diameter is readily estimated by measuring the horizontal visible iris diameter (HVID) (Figure 3-15).
  - o Combining the shape information from the keratometer or topographer with the HVID measurement gives reliable determination of the sagittal height of the cornea.
  - o Measuring curvature alone can be misleading as larger corneas have significantly greater sagittal height than do smaller corneas such that difference in HVID can quickly neutralize differences in measured curvature.
- • When available, it is nearly always advantageous to place a trial lens on the eye. Most soft contact lenses are made available in a full range of powers, curves, and diameters as diagnostic lenses. Rigid lenses more commonly are made to order, and trial fitting is accomplished using a limited set of diagnostic lenses designed to determine best fit regardless of lens power.
- • Soft contact lens fit is assessed by observing centration and movement of the lens on the eye.
  - o The well-fitted lens will center over the pupil and completely cover the entire limbus.
  - o The ideal soft lens diameter will allow 1- to 1.5-mm overlap beyond the limbus. Movement with the blink should typically be 0.25 to 1 mm.
  - o With the eye in upgaze, the lens should drop slightly but remain over the entire cornea.
  - o With the eye in primary gaze, a slight push on the lens should allow the lens to move easily, and once released, the lens should reposition with the next blink.
  - o Patient comfort is expected, although a lens that is too tight is often comfortable initially.
- • Rigid lenses are typically 2 to 2.5 mm smaller than the HVID and move 1 to 2 mm with the blink. Exact centration is desirable but often not necessary. As the rigid lens does not conform to the shape of the eye, the bearing relation between lens and the cornea must be assessed.
  - o Sodium fluorescein is instilled in the tears, and the eye is observed using the cobalt filter at the slit lamp.
  - o The fluorescein allows visualization of the tear layer between the lens and the eye. Points of touch and areas of clearance can be readily identified by observing the pattern of fluorescence beneath the lens.
  - o Although comfort is a good indicator of fit in experienced rigid lens wearers, it is common to use a topical corneal anesthetic to allow initial assessment of fit in the inexperienced wearer who is yet to adapt to the presence of the lens.
- • Special rigid lenses of very large diameters are sometimes used in the management of extreme corneal conditions that do not allow for typical fitting patterns. Such lenses may be so large as to cover the entire cornea (intralimbal lenses) or to rest over the sclera (scleral lenses).

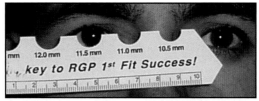

Figure 3-15. Corneal diameter measurement.

Wearing Schedules

- In addition to lens fitting dimensions and optical correction, the prescribing of contact lenses also includes instructions for use. A principal consideration is the wearing schedule, which dictates primarily how the lenses are worn.
  - ○ *Daily wear* refers to the condition in which the lenses are worn during waking hours only. This is the most common schedule, and all contact lenses are approved for this use.
  - ○ *Extended wear* refers to the condition in which the lenses are worn both waking and sleeping for one or more days. More recently, extended wear has been reserved for use with overnight wear for up to 7 days.
  - ○ The term *continuous wear* refers to overnight wear for more than 7 days. The current maximum number of continuous days recommended for any lens type is 30 days.
  - ○ Extended and continuous wear schedules apply only to certain lenses designed and approved for these schedules.

Lens Care

- With the exception of lenses designated to be replaced after each use, all contact lenses require care to keep them in a safe and usable condition.
  - ○ Contact lens care products must clean and disinfect the lenses, yet not be harmful to the lens or the eye.
  - ○ The functions of lens care products include cleaning, rinsing, and disinfecting.
  - ○ Many modern products are used for all 3 functions and are referred to as multipurpose solutions.
- Cleaning is accomplished commonly with the inclusion of surfactant ingredients. Rubbing the lens with the solution is effective, as is prolonged rinsing. A brief rinse is necessary following the cleaning. This can be done with the multipurpose solution or a sterile saline.
- Disinfection is normally achieved by preservative agents known to be effective against most ocular pathogens. Alternatives to preservative-based solutions include solutions containing hydrogen peroxide and devices that use ultraviolet or heat as the disinfecting mechanism.

Complications of Contact Lens Wear

- Contact lens wear is generally very safe, and the incidence of sight-threatening complications is very low. On the other hand, contact lenses interact directly with the eye and can act as a mechanical irritant, expose the eye to chemical toxicity, alter the ocular environment in ways that lead to inflammatory events, and predispose the eye to infectious processes. Contact lens wear can also act as a confounding variable in ocular diagnosis, in that ocular conditions that occur concurrent with contact lens wear may be incorrectly assumed to be secondary to the contact lens.

Mechanical Complications

- The physical presence of the contact lens can lead to a variety of complications.
  - ○ A poorly fitted lens can irritate the palpebral conjunctiva or abrade the cornea. Such complications tend to be self-limiting as the patient normally ceases wearing an irritating lens.
  - ○ A foreign body can become lodged between the lens and eye. This can cause a superficial disruption of the corneal epithelium that will stain with fluorescein. Often, the patient will present after the foreign body has been dislodged and the only evidence is the epithelial defect (Figure 3-16).

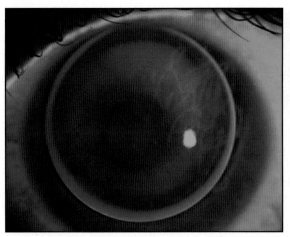

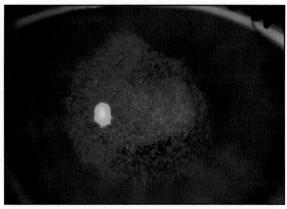

Figure 3-17. Toxic keratitis can result from exposure to inappropriate lens care products. (Reprinted with permission of Patrick Caroline.)

Figure 3-16. Foreign-body track beneath a rigid contact lens. (Reprinted with permission of Patrick Caroline.)

- Lens fit can also lead to a break in the epithelium, presumably due to interaction of the lens surface with the epithelium.
  - Such defects are typically arcuate in shape and are either in the superior or inferior location.
  - A type of mechanical arcuate break that has been particularly noted with the silicone hydrogel lenses is termed *superior epithelial arcuate lesion* (SEAL)

Toxic Complications

- Contact lenses can absorb chemical substances, and when they do, they can also facilitate prolonged contact time with the eye, such that normally benign substances can cause ocular irritation.
  - Patients should be advised to refrain from putting any medication in the eye while lenses are worn.
  - Waiting 5 minutes to insert contact lenses after instilling an eye medication is typically sufficient to avoid lens absorption and prolonged contact.
- Contact lens care products can cause varying degrees of irritation in some patients (Figure 3-17).
  - In any case in which a contact lens patient has otherwise unexplained signs or symptoms of ocular irritation, the care products should be considered suspect.
  - Trial with nonpreserved lens products or elimination of care products through use of single-use lenses is advised.

Inflammatory Complications

- Corneal infiltrates
  - Corneal infiltrates may be induced as part of the response to bacterial toxins, viruses, and inflammatory stimuli from contact lens solution preservatives.
    - Corneal infiltrates are relatively uncommon in contact lens wear.
    - When observed, infiltrates are usually within 2 mm of the limbus.
    - Although they may be observed in otherwise quiet and white eyes, the presence of infiltrates should give rise to suspicion of underlying corneal infection, blepharitis, or lens soilage (Figure 3-18).
  - A special case of corneal infiltrate that occurs almost exclusively with overnight wear of lenses is the contact lens peripheral ulcer (CLPU) (Figure 3-19).
    - At acute presentation, there is anterior stromal infiltrate with loss of overlying epithelium.
    - CLPUs are differentiated from infectious keratitis by characteristics of their peripheral location, small size (<2 mm), nearly perfect circular shape, minimal symptoms, and relative absence of concurrent signs.
    - Often, the patient is minimally symptomatic and does not seek attention, only to present at a later time with a residual scar at the location of the infiltrate.

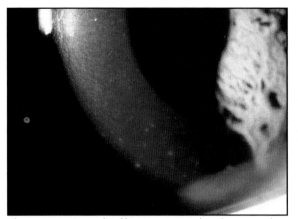

Figure 3-18. Corneal infiltrates associated with contact lens wear. (Reprinted with permission of Patrick Caroline.)

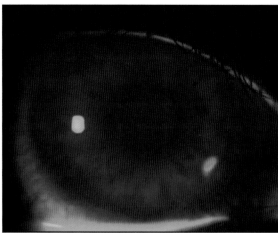

Figure 3-19. Contact lens peripheral ulcer. (Reprinted with permission of Patrick Caroline.)

- The CLPU is culture-negative and is thought to be a response to exotoxins of gram-positive organisms.
- There is no evidence that CLPU predisposes the patient to infectious keratitis.
- Recurrence is likely and is best prevented by cessation of overnight wear of contact lenses.
- Neovascularization
  - Hypoxia, compression of vessels by tight fitting lenses, and toxic and inflammatory stimuli may all cause corneal vascularization. Injection of the limbal vessels is thought to be a precursor.
    - Hypoxia appears to be the primary causative factor in contact lens-induced neovascularization (Figure 3-20).
    - Refitting with lenses of higher oxygen transmission is usually adequate to prevent further encroachment.
    - Once adequate oxygen levels are achieved, neovascular vessels cease to fill and remain only as ghost vessels.
- Contact lens-induced acute red eye (CLARE)
  - Some patients wearing lenses on an overnight basis will experience an acute inflammatory event termed *CLARE* (Figure 3-21).
    - Most often, the patient experiencing an episode of CLARE is awakened with unilateral ocular pain, redness, and photophobia.
    - Typically, symptoms improve upon removal of the contact lens, and the patient presents with limbal and conjunctival injection, diffuse peripheral infiltrate, but no evidence of epithelial break.
    - Although a tight-fitting lens is nearly always associated with CLARE, it is believed that the inflammatory response is associated with the presence of gram-negative organisms.
    - There is a high incidence of recurrence, and patients experiencing CLARE are often best advised to limit contact lens wear to waking hours only.
- Contact lens-induced superior limbic keratoconjunctivitis (Figure 3-22)
  - Soft contact lens wearers can develop an inflammatory condition that mimics superior limbic keratoconjunctivitis, but has no association with thyroid disease. It is thought to be associated with reaction to care product preservatives, although a mechanical mechanism has also been suspected.
    - Signs include intense hyperemia of the superior bulbar conjunctiva. Vessels and infiltrate may radiate in a wedge-shaped pattern into the cornea.
    - There, cornea and limbus typically stain with fluorescein.
    - Management consists of discontinuance of lens wear until resolved, refitting into new lenses, and avoidance of preservative-based lens disinfection systems.

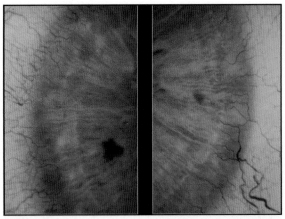

Figure 3-20. Neovascularization secondary to contact lens-induced hypoxia. (Reprinted with permission of Patrick Caroline.)

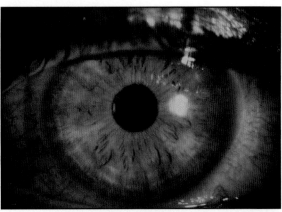

Figure 3-21. Contact lens-induced acute red eye. (Reprinted with permission of Patrick Caroline.)

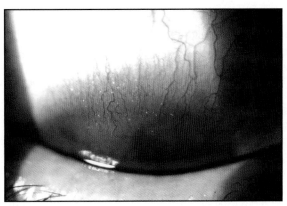

Figure 3-22. Contact lens-induced superior limbic keratoconjunctivitis.

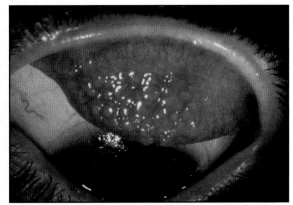

Figure 3-23. Contact lens-induced papillary conjunctivitis. (Reprinted with permission of Patrick Caroline.)

- Contact lens-induced papillary conjunctivitis (Figure 3-23)
  - A papillary response resulting in formation of large and irregular papillae can be seen in a variety of conditions that cause irritation of the upper tarsal conjunctiva. Giant papillary conjunctivitis has been reported with ocular prostheses, exposed sutures, and both flexile and rigid contact lenses.
    - Symptoms of itching, mucoid discharge, and decreased lens tolerance accompany the finding of large elevations on the upper tarsal conjunctiva.
    - The etiology appears to be a combined mechanical and hypersensitivity reaction associated with denatured tear proteins on the lens surface.
    - Improved lens maintenance and more frequent lens replacement are helpful.

Infectious Complications

- Although rare, microbial infection of the cornea is the most severe potential complication of contact lens wear. A contact lens acts as barrier to oxygen that can lead to metabolic changes in the epithelium and stroma. With inadequate oxygen, the epithelium loosens, glycogen levels drop, and the ability of some micro-organisms to adhere to the epithelium increases. Viral, fungal, and protozoan infections occur, but the majority of contact lens-related infectious keratitis is associated with bacterial infection.
  - Risk factors appear to be overnight wear of lenses, inadequate oxygen supply to the cornea, and poor compliance with wear and hygiene protocols.
  - Other risk factors for contact lens-associated infection include epithelial trauma, concurrent use of steroid eye medications, smoking, and swimming.

- Infection with the protozoan *Acanthamoeba*, although rare, is of particular note due to the devastating nature of the condition and its high association with contact lens wear, particularly in conjunction with contaminated water.
- Prompt response, diagnosis, and appropriate management are essential in limiting the degree of ocular damage and loss of vision. Because of the increased risk of infectious complications, epithelial defects associated with contact lens wear should not be patched.

Therapeutic Applications of Contact Lenses

- Contact lenses have a variety of applications in the treatment of ocular disease. These include uses as a bandage for corneal conditions, a reservoir and vehicle for delivery of ocular medications, and for cosmetic treatment of disfigured eyes.

Bandage Contact Lenses

- Many types of soft contact lenses are used as bandage materials, although most applications now employ one of the silicone hydrogel lenses due to their superior oxygen transmissibility and relative stiffness.
  - The presence of the lens can provide substantial pain relief and promote healing by limiting lid interaction with the corneal surface and preventing drying of the surface.
  - Applications for bandage lenses include treatment of a wide variety of epitheliopathies including recurrent erosion, corneal abrasion, and filamentary and Thygeson's keratitis.
  - A bandage lens is used routinely in the postoperative management of the photorefractive keratectomy patient.
  - A bandage contact lens can lessen pain and protect the cornea in conditions such as ocular pemphigoid and Stevens-Johnson syndrome.

Contact Lenses as a Drug Delivery Device

- Due to the ability of a soft contact lens to absorb many medications, interest exists in using contact lenses to deliver medications to the eye. Such a system could have significant advantage when continuous treatment is needed. Development of methods to bind medication to the contact lens materials with specific programmed release is under investigation and will likely have numerous applications.

Cosmetic

- Specially designed contact lenses can be used to improve appearance as well as vision of disfigured eyes. An artificial iris can improve light control and appearance of eyes with aniridia or coloboma. Opaque-tinted lenses are used for otherwise blind and disfigured eyes to provide better appearance.

Contact Lens Specification and Measurement

Base Curve

- The back surface radius of curvature of a contact lens is called the base curve. It should be noted that this is in contrast to the use of the same term to specify the front curve of a spectacle lens.
  - The base curve of a contact lens is most often specified in millimeters, but is also commonly converted to diopters using the standard keratometer index of 1.3375.
  - Note this is not the true surface power of the lens, as the refractive index of the lens material is typically between 1.40 and 1.50, depending on the makeup of the plastic. The convention of using the "diopters-K" arises from the practicality of using the keratometer reading of the cornea to determine lens fit.
    For base curve of a contact lens, r = 1/diopters-K, and
    Diopters-K = 1/r, where r is in meters
- The base curve of a rigid lens is readily measured with the radiuscope (Figure 3-24) and can also be measured with the keratometer using a special adapter to hold the lens in place. The base curve of a soft contact lens cannot be measured practically.

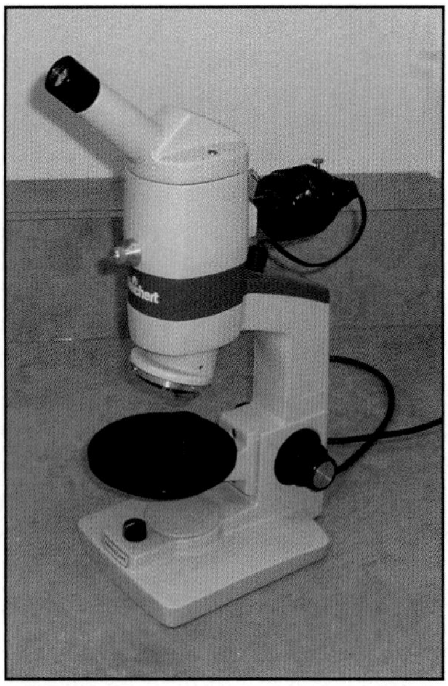

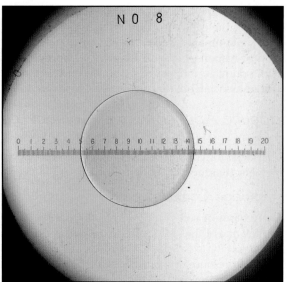

Figure 3-24. The radiuscope is used to measure the base curve of a rigid contact lens.

Figure 3-25. A reticule magnifier can be used to measure the diameter of a rigid or soft contact lens.

Diameter

- Contact lenses are also specified by their overall diameter.
  - Typical diameters for rigid lenses are 8.5 to 10.0 mm, although larger and smaller lenses may be used.
  - Soft contact lenses range from 12.0 mm for pediatric applications to 15.0 mm or greater for special application lenses.
  - The typical soft lens diameter is 13.8 to 14.2 mm.
- Rigid and soft lens diameters can be measured using a reticule magnifier (Figure 3-25).

Sagittal Depth and Lens Fit

- Diameter and base curve combine to establish the overall sagittal depth of a lens, which dictates the fit of the lens on the eye.
  - A lens that is too tight has too great a sagittal depth and can be corrected by making the lens smaller or the base curve flatter (ie, longer radius).
  - A lens that is too loose can be tightened by specifying a larger diameter or steeper base curve (ie, shorter radius).

Power

- Focal power of the lens is specified in diopters, which is readily measured on the lensometer for rigid lenses. Soft contact lenses present a greater challenge to measure power, although it is possible to do with the lensometer.

Suggested Readings

Brooks C, Borish I. *System for Ophthalmic Dispensing.* 2nd ed. Boston, MA: Butterworth-Heinemann; 1996.
Keating M. *Geometric, Physical and Visual Optics,* 2nd ed. Boston, MA: Butterworth-Heinemann; 2002.
Silbert JA. *Anterior Segment Complications of Contact Lens Wear,* 2nd ed. Boston, MA: Butterworth-Heinemann; 2000.

Questions

1. The direction a light ray will take when it enters a transparent medium is dependent on the index angle of incidence and which of the following?
    a. Angle of reflection
    b. Index of refraction
    c. Speed of light in air
    d. Sine of the angle

2. Parallel rays striking a convex curved surface
    a. Diverge
    b. Remain parallel
    c. Converge to a focal point
    d. Are shifted toward the apex of the surface

3. A spherocylindrical ophthalmic lens
    a. Combines 2 cylinders to form a sphere
    b. Combines 2 spheres to form a cylinder
    c. Has 2 cylindrical surfaces
    d. Has 1 spherical surface and 1 cylindrical surface

4. The plus cylinder form of -1.00 -1.00 x 90 is
    a. -2.00 +1.00 x 180
    b. -2.00 +1.00 x 90
    c. +1.00 +1.00 x 180
    d. Plano +2.00 x 90

5. For an eye with against-the-rule astigmatism
    a. The vertical meridian is the meridian of least power
    b. The horizontal meridian is the meridian of least power
    c. A contact lens is not an option
    d. The cylinder is always corneal

6. The curve of the front surface of a spectacle lens is which of the following?
    a. Meniscus
    b. Cylinder
    c. Add
    d. Base curve

7. If a patient's refraction for distance is -5.00 and for near is -3.50, the "add" power that will be specified is
    a. +1.50
    b. +2.00
    c. +2.50
    d. +3.50

8. If a patient's line of sight passes through a point 0.5 cm above the optical center of a +5.00 lens, the induced (base down) prism is
    a. 1 prism diopter
    b. 1.5 prism diopters
    c. 2 prism diopters
    d. 2.5 prism diopters

9. For the following contact lens characteristics, which lens will have the lowest oxygen transmissivity?
    a. Dk = 175, thickness = 0.10 mm
    b. Dk = 140, thickness = 0.08 mm
    c. Dk = 110, thickness = 0.07 mm
    d. Dk = 85, thickness = 0.05 mm

10. A principal role for a bandage contact lens is which of the following?
     a. Correction of the refractive error
     b. **Management of pain**
     c. Delivery of more oxygen to the cornea
     d. Reversing neovascularization of the cornea

Ocular Pharmacology

Paul Rafuse, PhD, MD, FRCS(C)

Outline

Basic Principles

- Drugs can be delivered to target tissues of the eye and orbit by a variety of means.
  - Direct (topical)
  - Enteral
  - Parenteral
- Absorption from the gastrointestinal (GI) tract is subject to the "first pass effect" of hepatic metabolism reducing the effective dose of active ingredient reaching the eye.
- By avoiding the liver, intravenous or intramuscular injections can both hasten and heighten the effect of a medication.
- The most direct route of drug administration is topical application of a drop, ointment, or gel.

Probst LE, Tsai JH.
Ophthalmology: Clinical and Surgical Principles (pp. 113–132).
© 2012 SLACK Incorporated

- Due to the dense sensory innervation of the cornea, the pH and tonicity of the solution or suspension becomes important. The multilayered construction of the cornea, with a lipophilic epithelium, hydrophilic stroma, and again lipophilic endothelium, serves as a significant barrier to drugs entering the eye.
  - Intraocular penetration of the active agent requires it to be principally lipophilic.
  - If it is supplied in an aqueous vehicle, the concentration of the solution becomes limited by the solubility of the chemical.
  - Alternatively, the drug is mixed in water as an emulsion or suspension.
- Generally, topical agents intended for intraocular structures (eg, glaucoma medications acting on the structures of the iridocorneal angle) are very concentrated.
  - Highly concentrated agents may be toxic systemically.
  - Only a small percentage of an eye drop makes its way into the eye. At least 80% of the volume of a single drop passes into the lacrimal drainage system if it isn't lost as spillage.
  - Drugs entering the nasolacrimal drainage system are absorbed systemically by crossing the nasal mucosa directly into the venous blood stream, bypassing the first pass effect of the liver.
    - Example of the amount of drug in one drop and its potential effect: Atropine sulfate 1% is 10 mg/mL (weight/volume). If there are 50 μL in one drop (ie, 20 drops in 1 mL), there is 0.5 mg of atropine in one drop. Potentially, 80% of this 0.5 mg is absorbed across the nasal mucus into the blood stream. This intravenous dose of atropine, delivered unintentionally by placing one drop in one eye, approximates the dose given intravenously to a patient during cardiac resuscitation for asystole.
  - Passage of topical ophthalmic drugs into the nasolacrimal drainage system and systemic circulation can be minimized by pressing and holding a finger over the inner canthus for 5 minutes.
  - Because blinking pumps tears down the lacrimal system, simple eyelid closure for 5 minutes has a similar effect.

Diagnostic Agents

Anesthetics

Local Anesthetics

- Local anesthetics are tertiary amines linked by either ester or amide bonds to an aromatic residue. They are all supplied as hydrochloride salts.
- All local anesthetics provide analgesia by disrupting electrical nerve conduction in sensory fibers. Specifically, they block voltage-sensitive sodium channels and the rapid depolarization of the membrane potential during an action potential.
- The topical agents are ester types.
  - Cocaine
  - Proparacaine (0.5%)
  - Tetracaine (0.5%)
  - Benoxinate (0.4%) in combination with 0.25% fluorescein (Fluress)
- Esters have a higher lipophilicity than amides allowing faster and better corneal penetration—corneal and conjunctival anesthesia is achieved within 30 seconds and can last 30 minutes or more.
- Topical anesthetics are essential to the eye exam. They allow for applanation tonometry, diagnostic contact lens placement, corneal scrapings for microbial culture, and removal of superficial corneal and conjunctival foreign bodies.
- Some therapeutic uses: Topical anesthesia is routinely used for multiple laser and incisional surgical procedures—therapeutic contact lens placement for anterior and posterior segment laser procedures, corneal surgery by laser or scalpel, cataract surgery, glaucoma surgery.
- Recently, viscous lidocaine has been used for topical cataract surgery despite its slower onset of action because it has a longer duration of action than proparacaine and is less toxic to the corneal epithelium than tetracaine.

Regional Anesthetics

- Surgery requiring regional (ie, retrobulbar, peribulbar, periocular) anesthesia involves injection of an amide-type agent.

TABLE 4-1. MYDRIATIC AND CYCLOPLEGIC PROPERTIES OF THE TOPICAL ANTIMUSCARINIC DRUGS

Drug	Concentration (%)	*Mydriasis*		*Cycloplegia*	
		Onset (min)	Offset (days)	Onset (min)	Offset (days)
Atropine	1.0	30 to 40	7 to 10	60 to 180	6 to 12
Scopolamine	0.25	20 to 30	3 to 7	30 to 60	3 to 7
Homatropine	2.0 to 5.0	40 to 60	1 to 3	30 to 60	1 to 3
Cyclopentolate	0.5 to 1.0	30 to 60	1	25 to 75	¼ to 1
Tropicamide	0.5 to 1.0	20 to 40	¼	30	<¼

Adapted from Gilman A, Goodman LS, Rall TW, Nies AS, Taylor P. *Goodman and Gilman's The Pharmacological Basis of Therapeutics.* 6th ed. New York, NY: McGraw-Hill; 1990:161.

o In order of increasing duration of action: lidocaine (0.5% to 2%), mepivacaine (1% to 3%), bupivacaine (0.25% to 0.75%)

o Amides are preferred over the ester injectables because they have a longer duration of action and are less allergenic. Esters are quickly inactivated by the serum pseudocholinesterases while amides require hepatic metabolism.

o The duration of action of injectable amide anesthetics can be prolonged with adjuvant low-dose epinephrine (1:50,000 to 1:200,000) for vasoconstriction. While useful for lid surgery, lidocaine with epinephrine is not recommended for retrobulbar blocks in patients with compromised retrobulbar circulations such as in advanced glaucoma.

Dilators (Mydriatics)

- The autonomic innervation of the iris involves both sympathetic and parasympathetic pathways.

Adrenergic Agonists

- The radially oriented neuroepithelial dilator muscle is physiologically activated by endogenous norepinephrine. Alpha-1 adrenoceptors can also be stimulated by exogenous agonists such as phenylephrine 2.5% to facilitate dilation of the pupil.
- Phenylephrine and other sympathomimetics such as apraclonidine can activate alpha-1 receptors residing in other structures of the eye and orbit.
- Blood vessel constriction causes whitening of the conjunctiva, and stimulation of the sympathetically innervated Müller's muscle in the upper lid results in lid retraction.
- Care must be taken with concentrated phenylephrine (10%) in patients with labile hypertension. With unobstructed nasolacrimal outflow, the systemic absorption can be enough to cause a hypertensive crisis.

Cholinergic Antagonists

- The pupillary sphincter muscle is supplied by the parasympathetic nervous system. Muscarinic receptors are normally stimulated by acetylcholine to constrict the pupil.
- The eye is under parasympathetic tone, meaning the dominant autonomic effect is due to the cholinergic stimulation.
- Antimuscarinic agents such as atropine cause relaxation of the pupil sphincter and mydriasis. They also paralyze the ciliary body (ie, cycloplegia), which is useful in determining the nonaccommodative refraction for an eye (Table 4-1).
- Some therapeutic uses
  - o Dilation
    - For examination of structures posterior to the pupillary plane. Short-acting agents such as tropicamide or cyclopentolate are often combined with phenylephrine to achieve rapid and maximal dilation.

- ○ Cycloplegia for refraction
  - Particularly important in children and young adults with high accommodative range. In children with esotropias, the portion of the deviation due to accommodative convergence needs to be determined.
- ○ Cycloplegia for comfort and reduction of inflammation
  - In uveitis, keratitis and inflammatory types of glaucomas
- ○ Treatment of hypotony
  - Long-acting cycloplegic agents are also used following traumatic cyclodialysis and filtering surgery for glaucoma to discourage ciliary and choroidal detachment.
- ○ Cycloplegia for amblyopia penalization
  - Useful in hyperopic and very young patients to blur their near vision in the nonamblyopic eye
- Care must be taken with small babies to limit the systemic absorption of atropine. Central and peripheral nervous system toxicity (fever, flushing, tachycardia, and delirium) can readily occur due to their small volume of distribution.

Diagnostic Dyes

Fluorescein

- A fluorescent hydroxyxanthone dye used for a variety of purposes; activation of the fluorescein molecule with blue light of 480 nm causes an electron shift with resulting emission of light at a longer yellow-green wavelength of 520 nm or more.
- Some of the diagnostic uses for fluorescein include assessment of corneal abrasions, aqueous leaks through the cornea and conjunctiva (the Seidel test), measurement of intraocular pressure (IOP) by applanation tonometry, angiography of the anterior and posterior segment, and investigation of the patency of the lacrimal drainage system.

Rose Bengal

- A vital stain specific for devitalized cells and mucin. This red dye directly stains damaged epithelial cells of the cornea and conjunctiva, making it useful for the investigation of tear deficiency states.

Indocyanine Green

- A tricarbocyanine dye, indocyanine green (ICG) is a much larger molecule than fluorescein, which keeps it within the lumen of fenestrated blood vessels such as those found in the choroid. It can be visualized directly through the retinal pigment epithelium, unlike fluorescein, making it useful for evaluation of diseases of the choroidal vasculature. ICG can also be used to stain the anterior capsule during cataract surgery and to stain epiretinal membranes for posterior segment procedures.

Trypan Blue

- This is a cheaper alternative to ICG for staining the lens capsule to facilitate anterior capsulotomy during cataract surgery.

Therapeutic Agents

Anti-Inflammatories

Steroids

- Glucocorticoids are used to treat both idiopathic and secondary inflammations in the eye. They are administered topically, by local injection, and systemically, both orally and intravenously. Table 4-2 lists a number of common ocular inflammations and routes of steroid administration..
- Steroids are relatively insoluble in water and therefore are often prepared as suspensions to obtain the highest possible effective dose for topical administration
  - ○ Some of the commonly used topical agents are prednisolone acetate 0.12% and 1% (suspensions), prednisolone phosphate 1% (solution), dexamethasone 0.1% (solution and ointment), fluorometholone acetate 0.1% (suspension), loteprednol etabonate 0.5% (suspension), rimoxolone 1% (suspension), and difluprednate (emulsion).

TABLE 4-2. ROUTES OF STEROID ADMINISTRATION FOR OCULAR INFLAMMATION

INFLAMMATION	STEROID ROUTE
Episcleritis	Topical
Scleritis	Systemic
Keratitis	Topical
Anterior uveitis	Topical
Posterior uveitis	Peribulbar, intravitreal, systemic
Endophthalmitis	Intravitreal, periocular, systemic
Chronic cystoid or diabetic macular edema	Periocular, intravitreal
Optic neuritis	Systemic (intravenous → oral)
Cranial arteritis	Systemic
Sympathetic ophthalmia	Topical, periocular, systemic

TABLE 4-3. PRINCIPAL OCULAR SIDE EFFECTS OF TOPICAL OR PERIOCULAR STEROIDS

Elevation of IOP due to reduced trabecular outflow leading to glaucoma
Cataracts—posterior subcapsular type (due to altered lens metabolism)
Local immunosuppression, which facilitates bacterial and viral (especially herpetic, fungal, and mycobacterial) infections
Mydriasis due to enhanced sympathetic tone
Scleral and conjunctival thinning
Thinning of eyelid skin
Ptosis secondary to weakening of levator muscle

- ○ Some of the more frequently used injectable agents are betamethasone sodium phosphate (4 mg/mL), dexamethasone acetate (8, 16 mg/mL), triamcinolone acetonide (3, 10, 40 mg/mL), and methylprednisolone acetate (20 to 80 mg/mL).
- ○ The most common oral corticosteroid used by the ophthalmologist is prednisone, which is supplied either in tablet form (1, 5, 20 mg) or as a syrup (1 mg/mL).
- Steroids exert cell-specific effects on a multitude of cell types including lymphocytes, macrophages, neutrophils, vascular endothelial cells, and fibroblasts.
- They stabilize intracellular membranes and inhibit the release of hydrolytic enzymes and other inflammatory mediators such as histamine, bradykinins, and platelet-activating factor.
- Their most important anti-inflammatory action may be the inhibition of phospholipase A2, which releases free arachidonic acid from phospholipids. This is the first step of the cascade of events in the metabolism of prostaglandins and other inflammatory mediators.
- The capacities of corticosteroids to save sight are nearly matched by their potential for ocular and systemic side effects. Ocular side effects are most likely with prolonged direct application (Table 4-3). Systemic adverse events are more often seen with systemic administration (Table 4-4).

TABLE 4-4. SIDE EFFECTS OF SYSTEMIC STEROIDS

Systemic hypertension due to mineralocorticoid effect and sodium retention
Suppression of the pituitary-adrenal axis
Systemic immunosuppression with predisposition to infection and reactivation of dormant infection (especially tuberculosis)
Aggravation of peptic ulcers
Hyperglycemia with exacerbation of pre-existing diabetes mellitus or manifest diabetes development in those with borderline blood sugar control
Muscle weakness and wasting
Central nervous effects—euphoria, agitation, insomnia, psychosis, and appetite stimulation
Centripetal redistribution of body fat—truncal obesity and "buffalo hump"
Aseptic necrosis of the femoral head

- The most significant ocular side effect of directly applied corticosteroids is the potential for elevation of IOP and glaucoma. Regular monitoring of IOP for all patients on local steroid therapy is critical, but especially for those on high-dose, frequent application, long-term regimens and those with glaucoma or a positive family history for the disease.
- Fluorinated compounds, such as fluorometholone, penetrate the cornea to a lesser extent and therefore cause less of a rise in IOP. Unfortunately, they are also less potent in their anti-inflammatory properties than the nonfluorinated drugs.
- Perforation of the globe can occur with corneal and/or scleral thinning, particularly in association with herpetic infections and rheumatoid arthritis treated with topical steroids.
- Patients at risk for compromising side effects of systemic steroid therapy (eg, diabetics, those with a history of tuberculosis, peptic ulcers, and labile hypertension) should be cautioned about the risks and comanaged with a general practitioner or internist. Rare, but devastating, events such as aseptic necrosis of the hip should be specifically addressed.

Nonsteroidal Anti-Inflammatory Drugs

- Nonsteroidal anti-inflammatory drugs (NSAIDs) exert their anti-inflammatory action by inhibiting the enzyme cyclooxygenase, which converts free arachidonic acid to prostaglandins.
    - Recognizable oral forms include aspirin (acetylsalicylic acid), indomethacin, ibuprofen, naproxen, and diclofenac. Systemically, this class has antipyretic and analgesic properties as well.
    - The systemic use of this class of drug is limited. There have been a few reports using indomethacin for inflammatory orbital diseases, as well as scleritis and posterior uveitis.
- Systemic NSAIDs show some promise as adjunctive agents in the treatment of posterior uveitis, secondary vasculitis, and chronic anterior uveitis (eg, juvenile rheumatoid arthritis-associated iridocyclitis).
    - Oral NSAIDs have been associated with a variety of GI and renal adverse effects. The GI effects range from stomach upset to bleeding ulcers and secondary anemia.
    - Renal blood flow is reduced with these agents, such that patients with compromised glomerular filtration can go into acute renal failure. They all prolong bleeding time due to their anti-platelet effects, which is a concern for patients undergoing surgery.
- The topical NSAIDs are flurbiprofen 0.03% (Ocufen), diclofenac 0.1% (Voltaren), ketorolac 0.5% (Acular), ketorolac 0.4% (Acular LS), ketorolac 0.45% (Acuvail), nepafenac 0.1% (Nevanac), and bromfenac 0.09% (Xibrom).
    - The on- and off-label uses of these medications continue to increase.

o Topical NSAIDs have been shown to be of value for inhibition of miosis during cataract surgery. Diclofenac and ketorolac have been used to control the inflammation and pain following cataract, glaucoma, laser, and PRK surgery. Both are used in the management of cystoid macular edema (CME). Ketorolac is approved for the treatment of seasonal allergic conjunctivitis.

o Aside from transient burning and stinging, topical NSAIDs are generally well-tolerated. There have been a few reports of corneal melting, and even perforation, with the use of diclofenac and ketorolac. These cases were usually associated with patients having diabetes and/or ocular surface diseases.

o Topical NSAIDs are contraindicated in patients with active herpes keratitis.

Antihistamines, Mast Cell Stabilizers, and Decongestants

- Both oral and topical histamine (H-1) receptor blockers can provide relief from the itch, redness, and swelling of ocular allergic disease: seasonal blepharoconjunctivitis, atopic keratoconjunctivitis, vernal keratoconjunctivitis, giant papillary conjunctivitis, and drug-induced allergic conjunctivitis.
  o Oral agents are often necessary but are all plagued to varying degrees with the side effect of sedation.
  o The topical H-1–specific receptor antagonists are emedastine difumarate 0.05% (Emadine), levocabastine 0.05% (Livostin), and azelastine 0.05% (Optivar). Immediate amelioration of allergic symptoms is possible with these agents.
- For the prophylactic management of Type I hypersensitivity allergy, topical mast cell stabilizers play an important role. These agents prevent mast cells from releasing histamine and other mediators (eg, prostaglandins, leukotrienes, bradykinins, and chemotactic factors) of conjunctival injection and swelling.
  o The 3 agents available in this class are sodium cromoglycate 2% (Opticrom) or 4% (Crolom), lodoxamide tromethamine 0.1% (Alomide), and pemirolast (Alamast). These drugs are particularly indicated in vernal keratoconjunctivitis. Due to their mechanism of action, a therapeutic benefit may not be apparent until after 2 or more weeks of treatment.
- Recently, a few combination mast cell stabilizers H-1 antagonists have become available.
  o Olopatadine hydrochloride 0.1% (Patanol), olopatadine hydrochloride 0.2% (Pataday), ketotifen fumarate 0.025% (Zaditor), nedocromil sodium, and azelastine (Optivar) fall in to this group, which has proven to be very effective in providing quick relief for seasonal allergic conjunctivitis.
- The popular over-the-counter preparations for nonspecific (ie, undiagnosed) itchy, red eyes generally consist of preparations containing an antihistamine and vasoconstrictor (ie, decongestant). There is a multitude of combinations of antazoline or pheniramine with oxymetazoline or naphazoline. These products are intended for short-term use only because prolonged and frequent use of decongestant-containing medications can lead to habitual use and chronically injected eyes.

Immunosuppressants

- Systemic drugs that cause generalized immunosuppression and are used to treat an eye disease are reserved for serious sight-threatening and/or life-threatening diseases.
- Eye conditions and systemic diseases with ocular inflammatory features in this category would include Behçet's disease, sympathetic ophthalmia, Vogt-Koyanagi-Harada syndrome, necrotizing rheumatoid keratitis/scleritis, Wegener's granulomatosis, polychondritis with scleritis, ocular cicatricial pemphigoid, bilateral Mooren's ulcer, or juvenile rheumatoid arthritis-associated iridocyclitis refractory to conventional treatment.
- Patients requiring systemic therapy of this nature would be comanaged with a rheumatologist or clinical immunologist.
- Some examples of systemic immunosuppressive medications include the following:
  o Azathioprine is a prodrug for 6-mercaptopurine, a purine analog, which acts as an antimetabolite by interfering with DNA metabolism. It is widely used as a steroid-sparing drug. It causes bone marrow suppression, which can lead to secondary infections.
  o Cyclophosphamide is an alkylating agent that interferes with DNA replication. It is the treatment of choice for Wegener's granulomatosis and polyarteritis nodosa and supplements other immunosuppression agents in the treatment of many other serious conditions. It is noted for causing hemorrhagic cystitis and myelosuppression.

o Methotrexate is a folic acid analog and antimetabolite inhibitor of DNA and RNA synthesis. Myelosuppression is the major dose-limiting toxicity.

o Chlorambucil is another alkylating agent that cross-links DNA, impairing its replication. It is a second- or third-line agent used in the treatment of inflammatory syndromes recalcitrant to conventional therapies. Hematologic toxicity, gonadal dysfunction, and secondary malignancies (usually an acute leukemia) temper its widespread use.

o Cyclosporine is a noncytotoxic agent that exerts its immunosuppressive effects through inhibition of T-helper cell activation. Its relative safety at low to moderate doses, combined with its impressive efficacy, has led to its use in an increasingly wide array of inflammatory syndromes. Nephrotoxicity and hypertension are risks with high-dose, long-term regimens.

o A new topical ophthalmic emulsion of cyclosporine 0.05% (Restasis) has appeared for the treatment of keratoconjunctivitis sicca. Topical cyclosporine has also been used in the management of corneal transplant rejection and vernal keratoconjunctivitis.

Anti-Infectives

Antibacterials

- Penicillins and cephalosporins are the usual starting point for a discussion on antibiotics.
  o There are a number of synthetic compounds now, but the original sources were the mold *Penicillium notatum* for penicillin and the fungus *Cephalosporium acremonium* for cephalosporins.
  o Both are bactericidal in activity by virtue of their destructive effect on the bacterial cell wall. They are referred to as "β-lactam antibiotics" because of the presence of a characteristic ring in their chemical structure, which is also a target of the β-lactamase enzymes, which inactivate these antibiotics.
  o Most early-generation drugs in this class are effective against gram-positive bacteria (eg, *Staphylococcus aureus* and *S. epidermidis*, α-hemolytic streptococcus), gram-negative cocci (eg, *Neisseria meningitides, N. gonorrhoeae*), anaerobic gram-positive cocci, and spirochetes such as syphilis and Lyme disease.
  o The second-, third-, and fourth-generation cephalosporins and more recent penicillins (ie, carbenicillin, ticarcillin and piperacillin) are more broad-spectrum with enhanced activity against gram-negative organisms, such as *Enterobacter, Proteus, Klebsiella and Pseudomonas.*
  o To circumvent the penicillinases (ie, β-lactamase for penicillin) of some organisms, many penicillins are semisynthetic penicillinase-resistant, such as methicillin and cloxacillin. They may also be mixed with a β-lactamase inhibitor such as clavulanic acid.
  o This class is limited in ophthalmology to systemic administration and regional or topical injection of parenteral solutions.
- Sulfonamides are structurally similar to para-aminobenzoic acid and competitively inhibit the bacterial synthesis of folic acid. This makes sulfonamides bacteriostatic against an array of organisms including *S. pneumoniae, H. influenzae, Actinomyces*, and *C. trachomatis.*
  o The application of this class in ophthalmology is essentially restricted to topical sulfacetamide solution (10% to 30%) or ointment (10%) to treat mild bacterial conjunctivitis or provide prophylaxis against conjunctivitis in patients with filtering blebs (often streptococcus species).
  o Sulfonamides cannot be used in patients with sulfa allergies, and this class has been associated with toxic epidermal necrolysis (ie, Stevens-Johnson syndrome).
- The aminoglycosides include gentamicin, tobramycin, and amikacin. They exert their bactericidal action by binding the 30 S and 50 S ribosomal subunits to interfere with the initiation of protein synthesis.
  o Enzymatic degradation and difficulty penetrating the cell wall of bacteria limit the effectiveness of these drugs against some organisms. Co-administration with a penicillin, to break down the cell wall, can have a synergistic effect.
  o Topical gentamicin and tobramycin are effective against anaerobic, gram-negative bacilli, as well as gram-positive *Staphylococcus aureus* and *S. epidermidis.*
  o Systemic toxicities of parenteral therapy include vestibular dysfunction and renal failure. Topical agents are noted for their corneal and conjunctival irritation. A bacterial conjunctivitis has been followed by a chemical conjunctivitis in a few overzealously treated instances.

- The "tetracyclines" include tetracycline, doxycycline, and minocycline. They inhibit protein synthesis by binding to the 30 S ribosomal subunit and are thus bacteriostatic.
  - Tetracyclines are active against a broad-spectrum of gram-positive and gram-negative organisms. They are not very soluble in water and in ophthalmology have been used principally to treat chronic Staphylococcal blepharitis, especially associated with acne rosacea.
  - Oral tetracyclines are generally well-tolerated aside from mild gastric irritation and skin photosensitivity. They chelate calcium, and their deposition in and discoloration of developing teeth makes them contraindicated in children and pregnant women.
- Chloramphenicol is another broad-spectrum antibiotic that inhibits protein synthesis by binding to the 50 S ribosomal subunit.
  - This well-tolerated and effective drug has limited use now because it has been associated with an idiosyncratic and sometimes lethal aplastic anemia. It has been formulated as a 0.5% solution and a 1% ointment.
- Fluoroquinolones are fluorinated derivatives of nalidixic acid. They are bactericidal due to their ability to inhibit DNA gyrase (bacterial topoisomerase II).
  - The available topical agents include norfloxacin, ciprofloxacin, ofloxacin, levofloxacin, moxifloxacin, and gatifloxacin.
  - Ciprofloxacin is available in several forms: ciprofloxacin HCl tablets (Cipro 250 mg, 500 mg, 750 mg), ciprofloxacin HCl IV solutions, ciprofloxacin HCl ophthalmic solution 0.3% (Ciloxan), and ophthalmic ointment.
  - Topical ofloxacin 0.3% (Ocuflox) is more lipophilic than Ciloxan and may allow higher aqueous concentrations when the corneal epithelium is intact.
  - Bacterial resistance to fluoroquinolones can occur by mutational changes to the DNA gyrase or reduced transport into the bacterial cell.
  - Both of these fluoroquinolones provided excellent coverage against gram-negative and most gram-positive organisms. They are relatively less effective against Streptococcus species.
  - The latest generation of compounds in this class includes gatifloxacin 0.3% (Zymar), gatifloxacin 0.5% (Zymaxid), moxifloxacin 0.5% (Vigamox), levofloxacin 1.5% (Iquix), and besifloxacin 0.6% (Besivance). They inhibit both topoisomerase II and IV, which enhances the spectrum of antimicrobial coverage to include *Streptococcus pneumoniae*, atypical micro-organisms, and anaerobes.
  - These agents have become the drugs of choice for monotherapy of corneal ulcers and recalcitrant bacterial conjunctivitis.
  - All of the topical fluoroquinolones are well-tolerated. There have been reports of white crystalline corneal deposits with frequent application of norfloxacin and ciprofloxacin.
- Macrolide antibiotics are bacteriostatic and bind to the P site of 50 S ribosomal subunit and interfere with protein synthesis.
  - Azithromycin 1% (AzaSite) is available in topical form.
    - While AzaSite is currently approved for bacterial conjunctivitis, many physicians are using it to treat blepharitis due to its antibacterial and anti-inflammatory properties.
- Vancomycin is a bactericidal agent that exerts its effects on gram-positive bacteria through inhibition of glycopeptide polymerization in the cell wall.
  - It is most often used to treat individuals with allergies to penicillin and cephalosporins and those with methicillin-resistant infections. It is used for the empiric treatment of endophthalmitis before culture and sensitivity results are available.

Antivirals

- Acyclovir is a synthetic guanosine that, upon sequential phosphorylation within the virus-infected cell, inhibits viruses in 3 ways.
  - Acyclovir triphosphate acts as a competitive inhibitor of viral DNA polymerases.
  - Insertion of the triphosphate into a growing strand of viral DNA causes chain termination.
  - Irreversible binding between the viral DNA and the interrupted chain causes permanent inactivation.
- Acyclovir (Zovirax) is available in topical (dermatologic and ophthalmic), oral, and intravenous forms.

TABLE 4-5. TREATMENTS FOR PARASITIC INFECTIONS

PARASITIC INFECTIONS	DRUGS OF CHOICE
Toxoplasmosis	Sulfadiazine, pyrimethamine, clindamycin
Trachoma + inclusion conjunctivitis	Tetracycline, erythromycin, sulfonamides
Trypanosomiasis	Suramin
Onchocerciasis	Ivermectin
Cysticercosis	Albendazole (surgical removal of intraocular parasites)
Filariasis and loiasis	Diethylcarbamazine
Strongyloidiasis	Thiabendazole

- Topical ganciclovir (Zirgan) inhibits DNA polymerase and incorporates into the viral DNA.
- Topical acyclovir and trifluridine 1% (Viroptic) serve as the mainstays of treatment for herpes simplex type I keratitis. Acyclovir is better tolerated with less corneal toxicity.
- Oral acyclovir, as well as valacyclovir (Valtrex) and famciclovir (Famvir), are indicated for the treatment of herpes zoster infections. Relief from the acute signs and symptoms, and the severity and duration of the postherpetic neuralgia can be achieved if prompt treatment is instituted.
- Parenteral ganciclovir and foscarnet have been used with some success to treat cytomegalovirus (CMV) retinitis. The renal toxicity of these agents can be obviated with the use of a ganciclovir sustained-release intravitreal implant.

Antifungals

- The polyene antibiotics used to treat fungal infection of the eye and orbit are amphotericin B and natamycin. These drugs bind to sterols in the cell membrane of fungi, rendering them leaky. Concomitantly administered antifungal or antibiotic agents can then gain access to the interior of the cell to achieve a synergistic effect.
- Natamycin is preferred for the filamentous fungi including *Aspergillus*, *Cephalosporium*, *Fusarium*, and *Penicillium*, while amphotericin B is the better choice for the yeast *Candida albicans* and orbital *Mucormycosis*.
- Filamentous and yeast-like fungi can also be treated with oral, intravenous, and local (topical, subconjunctival, and intravitreal) imidazoles (ketoconazole and miconazole), triazoles (fluconazole and itraconazole), and flucytosine.

Antiparasitics and Anti-Acanthamoeba Medications

- In addition to surgical débridement, a constellation of agents and classes have been used topically and systemically with varying success in the treatment of ocular and orbital parasitic infections (Table 4-5).
- Adjuvant systemic and topical corticosteroids are often administered with systemic antiparasitic medications to control the profound inflammatory and allergic reactions to the antigenic load caused by the dead and dying organisms.
- Acanthamoeba is a ubiquitous amoeba that can invade the corneal stroma and survive simple drug regimens as both trophozoites and double-walled cysts. Eight different species have been associated with keratitis.
- A list of anti-acanthamoeba medications (topical and systemic) would include the biguanide and diamidine classes, as well as neomycin, paromomycin, natamycin, ketoconazole, itraconazole, clotrimazole, and fluconazole.

Glaucoma Medications

- Modern definitions of glaucoma describe an optic neuropathy characterized by cupping and associated with paracentral visual field loss. Elevated IOP is often referred to as a risk factor for the disease, as opposed to an obligatory characteristic. Nonetheless, the only proven means of slowing the progression of glaucoma involves lowering IOP.
- All of the approved antiglaucoma medications lower IOP by reducing the inflow (production) of aqueous and/or by facilitating its outflow through the 2 outflow pathways (trabecular or uveoscleral).

Parasympathomimetics (Miotics)

- Pilocarpine and carbachol are the remaining drugs in this class.
- Both exert their IOP-lowering effects by stimulating muscarinic receptors, which lead to contraction of the ciliary body and enhancement of trabecular outflow.
- They are shortacting (prescribed 3 to 4 times daily) with negligible systemic effects at normal dosing.
- The ocular side effects of these 2 medications are significant.
- Spasm of the ciliary body can lead to an ocular or periorbital ache and a myopic shift in refraction. The resulting miosis can cause nyctalopia in patients with cataracts.
- On a more long-term basis, miotics use can cause chronic low-grade intraocular inflammation, resulting in the formation of posterior synechiae and a fixed miosis, which can be a complicating factor at the time of cataract surgery.
- Pupillary block and chronic contracture of the ciliary muscle can lead to chronic "creeping" angle closure.
- Tugging on the pars plana and peripheral retina can potentially open retinal holes in areas of thinning, resulting in retinal detachment.
- The principal indications for the use of parasympathomimetic agents are primary open-angle glaucoma and glaucomas associated with exfoliation, pigment dispersion syndrome, and uncomplicated pseudophakia. Pilocarpine also plays a role in the initial management of acute angle-closure glaucoma.
- Poor indications for the use of miotics include neovascular and uveitic glaucomas. Idiopathic chronic angle-closure and malignant glaucoma can be aggravated with this class as well.
- Pilocarpine and carbachol are commercially available as hydrochloride solutions by a number of manufacturers. Pilocarpine can be obtained in concentrations ranging from 0.25% to 6%, and carbachol is available in concentrations from 0.75% to 3%.
- Indirectly acting cholinesterase inhibitors, such as the carbamate inhibitor, physostigmine, and organophosphate inhibitor, echothiophate, had been used in the past. The latter agent was significantly cataractogenic, caused iris pupillary cysts and was associated with the development of pseudopemphigoid.

Beta-Blockers

- It was a serendipitous discovery that oral β-blockers lower IOP.
- Topical β-blockers are useful in the treatment of all primary and secondary, open- and closed-angle varieties of glaucoma. They are least useful in treating patients progressing at normal IOP ranges (ie, normal pressure glaucoma) and for patients already on a systemic β-blocker.
- Topical timolol maleate (0.25% to 0.5%) can lower IOP by 30%.
  - The nonselective β-blockers timolol, levobunolol, carteolol, and metipranolol all act as aqueous suppressants (Table 4-6). Reductions in cyclic adenylate monophosphate (cAMP) appear to be involved in the mechanism of action.
  - There is some evidence that betaxolol, the only β1-receptor antagonist, may work via a β-receptor-independent pathway and increase chloride conductance and/or act as a calcium channel blocker.
  - Topical propranolol cannot be used clinically because it has a local anesthetic effect.
  - Topical β-blockers are generally well-tolerated from an ocular standpoint. Allergies are rare; dry eye symptoms are the most common side effects.
  - All of the products are intended to be used on a twice-daily schedule except Timoptic-XE, which is a once-daily product. Beta-blockers are relatively long-acting drugs, and many ophthalmologists will prescribe the nonselective solutions for once-a-day use to minimize systemic toxicity.

TABLE 4-6. COMMERCIALLY AVAILABLE BETA-BLOCKERS

Betaxolol hydrochloride 0.25% suspension (Betoptic S)
Levobunolol hydrochloride 0.25, 0.5% solutions (Betagan)
Carteolol hydrochloride 1% solution (Ocupress)
Metipranolol hydrochloride 0.3% solution (Optipranolol)
Timolol maleate 0.25, 0.5% solutions (Timoptic)
Timolol maleate 0.25, 0.5% gel-forming solutions (Timoptic-XE, Timolol Maleate Ophthalmic)
Timolol hemihydrate 0.25, 0.5% solutions (Betimol)

TABLE 4-7. ABSOLUTE* AND RELATIVE CONTRAINDICATIONS TO THE USE OF TOPICAL BETA-BLOCKERS

Asthma*
Chronic obstructive pulmonary diseases (eg, emphysema, chronic bronchitis)*
Greater than first-degree heart block*
Sinus bradycardia (especially in the elderly)
History of syncopal events
History of life-threatening depression
Brittle insulin-dependent diabetes (ie, frequent insulin reactions)
Impotence

- Systemically, topical β-blockers can be absorbed to a significant enough extent that they can reduce β-receptor–mediated events throughout the body (eg, reduce cardiac rate and contractility, cardiac output, and blood pressure).
- Topical β-blockers are not necessarily contraindicated in patients with congestive heart failure because systemic drugs in this class are frequently used now to treat this condition. While both topical and oral β-blockers can raise serum levels of triglycerides and lower high-density lipoproteins, oral agents in this class are used routinely following myocardial infarction and have been shown to increase survival (Table 4-7).
- It is important that patients are instructed on lid closure or how to perform nasolacrimal occlusion for 5 minutes following instillation of topical β-blockers.

Adrenergic Agonists

- Epinephrine has been used to treat glaucoma for more than 100 years. Its use has dwindled in recent years because of its unfavorable local and systemic safety profile and the introduction of much more efficacious and tolerable classes.
- Epinephrine is a nonselective agonist of all the adrenergic receptor subtypes ($\alpha 1$, $\alpha 2$, $\beta 1$, $\beta 2$). Stimulation of some of these receptors can increase aqueous production, decrease aqueous production, and increase both trabecular and uveoscleral outflow. The net effect is a reduction in IOP.
- The ocular side effects of epinephrine include conjunctival injection, adrenochrome deposits, follicular conjunctivitis, mydriasis, and CME in aphakia. Systemic absorption can lead to elevated blood pressure and extrasystoles.

TABLE 4-8. ORAL AGENTS MOST LIKELY ASSOCIATED WITH COMMON CARBONIC ANHYDRASE INHIBITOR SIDE EFFECTS

Metabolic acidosis	Acetazolamide
Paresthesias of the extremities	Acetazolamide
Urolithiasis	Acetazolamide
Potassium depletion	Acetazolamide
Aplastic anemia	Acetazolamide
Anorexia and weight loss	Methazolamide
Malaise and depression	Methazolamide

- Topical epinephrine hydrochloride has been available as solutions from 0.5% to 2% (Epifrin, Glaucon). It was intended for 3 times daily dosing.
- The development of the epinephrine prodrug dipivefrin (dipavalyl epinephrine) allowed a lower concentration solution with reduced ocular irritation and systemic toxicity. Dipivefrin hydrochloride 0.1% (Propine) is a relatively lipid soluble ester, which, on passage through the cornea, is hydrolyzed to epinephrine.

Alpha-2 Agonists

- The 2 agents in this class, apraclonidine and brimonidine, activate α2-adrenoceptors to reduce levels of cAMP, which leads to a reduction in aqueous production and a lowering of IOP. Brimonidine also causes a small increase in uveoscleral outflow.
- Apraclonidine hydrochloride 0.5% and 1% (Iopidine) also stimulates α1-receptors, which accounts for the mydriasis, upper lid retraction (secondary to activation of Müller's muscle), and conjunctival blanching seen with this drug.
  - Tachyphylaxis is noted with chronic use.
  - The principal reason chronic use is limited with apraclonidine is that at least 50% of users develop a severe allergic blepharoconjunctivitis with a median onset of 5 months. For this reason, apraclonidine is mainly used to treat IOP spikes following laser trabeculoplasty, laser iridotomy, anterior segment surgery, and for short-term adjunctive medical therapy.
- Brimonidine tartrate 0.2% (Alphagan) and 0.1% without benzalkonium chloride (BAC) (Alphagan-P) are highly selective α2-agonists, which demonstrate significantly less tachyphylaxis than apraclonidine with equal efficacy (25% to 30% IOP reduction).
  - Brimonidine tartrate 0.2% is better tolerated than apraclonidine and can be used longer term, but discontinuation due to redness still occurs at a rate of 30% or more after 2 to 3 years. Initial studies have shown that the lower concentration of 0.1% in Alphagan-P, coupled with it having a different preservative (Purite—a stabilized oxychloro complex from chlorite, chlorate, and chlorine oxide), further reduces the red eye rate.
  - The most frequent systemic side effects associated with brimonidine are dry mouth and fatigue. Both brimonidine products are meant to be used 3 times daily, although in practice they are commonly used twice daily.
  - There are in vitro and laboratory animal studies that suggest that, in addition to having an IOP-lowering effect, brimonidine may exert an IOP-independent neuroprotective effect. Clinical validation of this property remains to be established.

Carbonic Anhydrase Inhibitors

- Oral acetazolamide (Table 4-8) has been used clinically to treat glaucoma for almost 50 years. It was followed a number of years later with methazolamide and much later by 2 topical agents, dorzolamide and brinzolamide.

TABLE 4-9. RELATIVE CONTRAINDICATION TO THE USE OF ORAL CARBONIC ANHYDRASE INHIBITORS

Adrenal insufficiency
Hepatic failure
Chronic respiratory acidosis
Renal failure
Any metabolic acidosis (eg, hyperchloremic, diabetic ketoacidosis, excessive salicylate use)
Repeated episodes of kidney stones

- Oral carbonic anhydrase inhibitors (CAIs) have been used outside the treatment of glaucoma in ophthalmology for such disparate conditions as CME, retinitis pigmentosa, and pseudotumor cerebri.
- CAIs are structurally related to sulfonamides, and allergic cross-reactivity is possible.
  - All 4 agents lower IOP by inhibiting the enzyme carbonic anhydrase (isozyme II), which is involved in the secretion of aqueous by the ciliary epithelium.
  - The oral agents are generally more efficacious in lowering IOP (25% to 35%) than the topical agents (15% to 22%). Unfortunately, both acetazolamide and methazolamide are poorly tolerated systemically, sometimes for different reasons.
  - Methazolamide is not actively secreted by the kidneys and is less protein-bound than acetazolamide, allowing use of lower doses
  - Systemic CAIs can cause an acute myopic shift in refraction
  - An absolute contraindication to the use of acetazolamide is sickle cell disease. The acidosis created by this agent can exacerbate the sickling of red blood cells.
  - Oral CAIs (Table 4-9) are available as acetazolamide 125- or 250-mg tablets (Diamox) or 500-mg slow-release capsules (Diamox Sequels) and methazolamide 25-mg or 50-mg tablets (Neptazane)
  - Acetazolamide tablets need to be taken 4 times daily, while stable serum levels of drug can be achieved with twice-daily administration of the capsules.
  - Methazolamide tablets can be taken either twice daily or 3 times daily.
- Both the oral and topical CAIs can be used for any IOP-lowering application. The topical agents are relatively safe and can be used in patients in whom β-blockers are contraindicated. Oral acetazolamide is the most frequently used CAI when immediate IOP reduction is necessary, such as in the event of an angle-closure attack.
- Topical CAIs, dorzolamide and brinzolamide, circumvent the majority of the systemic adverse effects suffered with the oral agents.
  - The ocular side effects of topical CAIs include stinging, allergy, superficial punctuate keratitis, and transient myopia.
  - Dorzolamide hydrochloride 2% solution (Trusopt) is relatively short-acting, requiring 3-times-daily dosing to maintain adequate trough effects. It is often used twice daily in conjunction with other aqueous suppressants such as topical β-blockers.
  - The less thoroughly studied brinzolamide 1% suspension (Azopt) appears to be equally effective to dorzolamide and may be associated with less stinging. It is used twice daily.

Prostaglandins

- This new class of ocular hypotensive is represented by 4 agents: latanoprost, bimatoprost, travoprost, and unoprostone. With the exception of unoprostone, these topical drugs are generally regarded as being slightly more effective than timolol in lowering IOP.
- This class shares a unique mechanism of action to lower IOP: enhancement of the uveoscleral outflow pathway, which bypasses the trabecular pathway and the episcleral venous pressure (EVP) of 8 to 10 mm Hg.

- ○ Improved passage of aqueous through the muscle bundles of the ciliary body could occur either by relaxation of the ciliary muscle or by remodeling the extracellular matrix. The latter mechanism may involve increased expression of matrix metalloproteinases.
- ○ Conceptually, the hypotensive lipids work like a "chemical cyclodialysis."
- ○ Theoretically, IOP levels of less than EVP can be achieved, particularly when the starting IOP is in the normal range.
- ○ The side effects of the prostaglandins are unique. Systemically, they may be inert because they are supplied in very low concentrations and the amount reaching the blood stream is less than endogenous prostaglandin serum levels. As with other classes, ocular irritation with conjunctival injection is more commonly reported with some prostaglandins than with others.
- ○ As a class, these drugs appear to be very long-acting. Apart from unoprostone, which is administered twice daily, the other 3 are dosed once daily, setting a new standard for patient acceptance and compliance.
- ○ The prostaglandin-unique ocular side effects include the following:
  - Increased iris and periocular skin pigmentation: due to up-regulation of tyrosinase activity in melanocytes, which leads to an increase in cellular melanin content. Iris darkening is more common in eyes with light brown and green/brown irides as opposed to those that are blue/gray in color.
  - Eyelash lengthening and thickness: due to stimulation of the growth phase of the hair follicle
  - Reactivation of corneal herpes simplex keratitis (isolated case reports)
  - Increased intraocular inflammation—isolated case reports
  - CME has been reported in patients with other risk factors for CME such as following complicated cataract surgery and chronic uveitis.
  - Ocular itch with nocturnal use
  - Orbital fat atrophy has been observed in some patients and can be particularly noticeable with uniocular treatment.
- Latanoprost 0.005% (Xalatan) is the best studied agent of the group.
  - ○ It is an isopropyl ester, which is hydrolyzed by corneal esterases to the active free acid to bind with the FP receptor (receptor for endogenous prostaglandin PGF2α).
  - ○ Latanoprost 0.005% lowers IOP by 27% to 34%.
  - ○ Xalatan has the highest concentration of BAC (0.02%) in the class. Despite this, it is one of the better-tolerated preparations.
- Travoprost 0.004% (Travatan) is another isopropyl ester pro-drug. Its free acid has the highest affinity for the FP receptor.
  - ○ Travoprost 0.004% lowers IOP by 25% to 33%.
  - ○ Studies with this prostaglandin have shown excellent diurnal IOP control.
  - ○ BAC 0.015% has recently been replaced with another preservative, Sofzia (a boric acid/polyol system).
- Bimatoprost (Lumigan) is structurally somewhat dissimilar to the preceding two compounds. It has been classified by some as a prostamide, the endogenous versions of which are endocannabinoids. Bimatoprost is hydrolyzed by the cornea to a lesser extent than the other prostaglandins, which suggests it may act on another, or additional, as yet to be identified receptor.
  - ○ There is some evidence that bimatoprost lowers IOP by enhancing both uveoscleral and trabecular outflow. It lowers IOP by 25% to 35%.
  - ○ In order to mitigate the most significant red eye rate in the class, the concentration of the active ingredient has been lowered from 0.03% to 0.01%. The BAC concentration has been increased from 0.005% to 0.02% to improve corneal penetration.
- Unoprostone isopropyl 0.15% (Rescula) is a docosanoid, a 22-carbon lipid molecule. Unoprostone 0.12% was introduced in Japan with modest IOP lowering effects of 11% to 23%.
  - ○ It may be the best tolerated of the group, but it has a much less impressive IOP-lowering capability compared to the other 3 lipid agents.

TABLE 4-10. PRECAUTIONS WHEN USING SYSTEMIC HYPEROSMOTICS

Diuresis in men with prostatic obstruction
Volume overload in patients in renal failure
Pulmonary edema and cardiac failure with fluid overload
Hyperosmolar nonketotic coma in diabetics (glycerin only)

- Most studies on the prostaglandins have involved patients with open angles: primary open-angle glaucoma (POAG) and ocular hypertension. There is evidence that this class is also effective in lowering IOP in chronic closed-angle and some pediatric glaucomas.
- They are not recommended for inflammatory glaucomas and other instances when CME is a possible outcome.

Topical Fixed Combination Agents

- In some parts of the world, fixed combinations of timolol-pilocarpine and epinephrine-pilocarpine are still available.
- In Europe and North America, fixed combinations of timolol maleate 0.5%-dorzolamide hydrochloride 2% (Cosopt), timolol maleate 0.5%-brimonidine 0.2% (Combigan), timolol maleate 0.5%-latanoprost 0.005% (Xalatan), timolol maleate 0.5%-travoprost 0.04% (DuoTrav), and timolol maleate 0.5%-bimatoprost 0.03% (Ganfort) are found.
- Fixed combinations of 2 (or more) topical antiglaucoma preparations offer a number of enticing advantages.
  - o There is the obvious convenience of fewer drop applications.
  - o Compliance can improve with fewer drop applications to forget.
  - o There is potentially less wash-out effect from 2 or more drops, applied too soon after one another.
  - o Cost savings should be achieved with reduced manufacturing, packaging, shipping, and storage expenditures.
  - o Fixed-combination products should be safer with less volume of solution/suspension applied to the tear film and reduced exposure to the nasolacrimal system.
  - o There is some evidence that allergy rates of individual components are reduced when they are incorporated in fixed combinations (ie, Combigan).

Hyperosmotics

- Oral or intravenous hyperosmotic agents are believed to lower IOP by drawing water from the vitreous, thereby shrinking its volume in the globe. Other effects on the central nervous system and ciliary epithelium may play a role (Table 4-10).
- The following preparations are now used for ocular hypertensive emergencies only:
  - o Oral glycerin (Osmoglyn) is administered at a dose of 1 to 1.5 g/kg body weight as a 50% mixture in a tart citric fruit drink. Maximum IOP effect is achieved in approximately 30 minutes. Nausea and vomiting from the drink and the high IOP can render this treatment less than fully effective.
  - o Intravenous mannitol (Osmitrol) is a more reliable way to lower IOP quickly. It is given at a dose of 1 to 2 g/kg in a 20% or 25% solution. It crystallizes below body temperature, and unless it is kept warm, it needs to be run through a filter, which greatly slows its delivery. Mannitol is not metabolized and is safe for use in diabetics.
- Topical hyperosmotic agents include the following:
  - o Glycerin, which is useful to reduce corneal epithelial edema during acute glaucoma to allow adequate visualization of the angle (ie, gonioscopy) for diagnostic purposes or to clear the view enough to perform laser iridotomy
  - o Hypertonic sodium chloride 5% (Muro 128), which can be helpful in dehydrating the corneal epithelium and stroma in the treatment of endothelial dystrophies or recurrent erosion syndromes

Other Ocular Medications

Antimetabolites

- Fluorouracil (5-FU) is a pyrimidine nucleoside analog that interrupts DNA and RNA synthesis by blocking the production of thymidylate.
  - Its inhibitory effect on rapidly growing cells may explain its effectiveness in the topical treatment of warts and conjunctival intraepithelial neoplasia (CIN). It is also used during (topically) and after (by subconjunctival injection) glaucoma filtering surgery to slow the proliferation of fibroblasts and the formation of episcleral scar tissue.
  - The principal local toxicity of this agent is to the corneal and conjunctival epithelium.
- Mitomycin C is an alkylating agent that inhibits DNA replication.
  - Like 5-FU, mitomycin C can be used during a trabeculectomy to limit healing. It is much more potent than 5-FU, and a single intraoperative application is usually sufficient to halt fibroblast growth.
  - Mitomycin C has also been used to inhibit cell growth in the treatment of CIN, pterygium recurrence, and corneal haze in photorefractive (PRK) procedures.
  - Due to its cytotoxic properties, mitomycin C can lead to melting phenomena involving the cornea, sclera, and conjunctiva. It is very toxic to the corneal endothelium and cannot be allowed to enter the eye.

Coagulation Modifiers

- Fibrinolytic agents
  - Tissue plasminogen activator (TPA), urokinase, and streptokinase are fibrinolytic agents that have been used in the management of cardiac thromboembolism.
    - TPA has been used for intraocular injection in the management of fibrin clots following vitrectomy and anterior segment surgery, particularly glaucoma-filtering procedures
  - Thrombin
    - Intravitreal thrombin has been reported to be useful to control bleeding during vitrectomy.
- Antifibrinolytic agents
  - Tranexamic acid and ε-aminocaproic acid inhibit the activation of plasminogen, which is necessary for fibrinolysis.
    - This clot-stabilizing property has been exploited to treat recurrent bleeding in severe hyphemas.
    - Because these agents are most effective when administered orally, contraindications include risk of diffuse intravascular coagulation, pregnancy, and patients with coagulation disorders and hepatic or renal compromise.

Dry Eye Medications

- Keratitis sicca occurs in association with a multitude of pathologies (ie, vitamin deficiencies, rheumatologic diseases, functional or anatomic eyelid deficiencies), and blepharitis-related or aqueous-deficiency dry eye symptoms become more prevalent with age.
- With an enormous population of users has emerged a great variety of artificial tear preparations and emollients, the active ingredients of which include hydroxypropyl cellulose, hydroxyethylcellulose, hydroxypropyl methylcellulose, and carboxymethylcellulose
  - Many of these occlusive agents are supplied as "preservative-free" in single-dispenser ampoules. Multimode preparations require a preservative such as BAC, potassium sorbate, chlorobutanol, Polyquad, sodium perborate, sorbic acid, and Purite.
  - Recently, a preservative-free topical cyclosporine emulsion 0.05% (Restasis) has become available. Twice-daily application of this product has provided symptomatic relief, and biopsy specimens have shown repopulations of goblet cells, a decrease in conjunctival epithelial cell turnover, and reduced numbers of lymphocytes.
  - The emollient forms of dry eye therapy are ointments prepared with petrolatum, liquid lanolin, mineral oil, methylparaben, and polyparaben. Most are used for night-time coverage.

Vitamin A Analogs

- Vitamin A metabolism plays an important role in retinal photoreceptor biochemistry.
  - ○ The retinal function, as measured by cone electroretinography (ERG), of some patients was found to be slowed with the oral administration of vitamin A palmitate 15,000 IU/day. Liver function studies should be followed when high doses of vitamin A are used chronically.
  - ○ Beta carotene 15 mg, a vitamin A precursor, in combination with vitamin C 500 mg, vitamin E 400 IU, zinc oxide 80 mg, and cupric oxide 2 mg was found to slow the decline of vision in a cohort of patients with moderate to severe age-related macular degeneration (AMD).
  - ○ A number of vitamin supplements specifically formulated to treat AMD have duplicated, or approximated, the above combination and doses used in the Age-Related Eye Disease Study (AREDS).
  - ○ Smokers should avoid beta carotene-containing preparations because this vitamin A precursor has been associated with an increased risk of developing lung cancer.

Suggested Readings

Allingham RR, Moroi, SE, Eds. *Shields Textbook of Glaucoma*. Philadelphia, PA: Lippincott Williams & Wilkins; 2005.

Cibis GH. *Fundamentals and Principles of Ophthalmology. Section 2: Basic Science Course*. San Francisco, CA: American Academy of Ophthalmology; 2005.

Fraunfelder FT, Roy FH, Randall J, Eds. *Current Ocular Therapy 5*. Philadelphia, PA: WB Saunders Company; 2000.

Gilman AG. *Goodman & Gilman's: The Pharmacological Basis of Therapeutics*, 8th ed. New York, NY: Pergamon Press; 1990.

Morrison JC, Pollack IP, Eds. *Glaucoma: Science and Practice*. New York, NY: Thieme; 2003.

Stamper RL, Lieberman MF, Drake MV, Eds. *Becker-Shaffer's Diagnosis and Therapy of the Glaucomas*. St. Louis, MO: Mosby; 1999.

Zimmerman TJ, Kooner KS, Eds. *Textbook of Ocular Pharmacology*. Philadelphia, PA: Lippincott-Raven; 1997.

Questions

1. One drop (50 µL) of phenylephrine 10% contains how much drug?
   a. 0.2 mg
   b. 0.5 mg
   c. 2 mg
   d. 5 mg
   e. 10 mg

2. Which of the following best describes how local anesthetics produce analgesia?
   a. Blocking the postsynaptic action of acetylcholine at the neuromuscular junction
   b. Blocking the release of neurotransmitter at the sensory nerve ending
   c. Blocking voltage-sensitive sodium channels in the sensory neuronal axons
   d. Blocking the propagation of an action potential by preventing calcium influx
   e. Blocking the repolarization of the action potential in the sensory neurons

3. Topical corticosteroids following cataract surgery can cause which of the following?
   a. Upper eyelid ptosis
   b. Miosis
   c. Thickening of eyelid skin
   d. Posterior capsule opacification
   e. Optic disc cupping without elevating IOP

4. Which of the following antibiotic classes has been associated with calcium chelation and discoloration of developing teeth?
   a. Aminoglycosides
   b. Tetracyclines
   c. Penicillins
   d. Fluoroquinolones
   e. Sulfonamides

5. What is the first drug of choice in the treatment of onchocerciasis?
   a. Suramin
   b. Ivermectin
   c. Sulfadiazine
   d. Erythromycin
   e. Tetracycline

6. Which of the following conditions is **not** an absolute contraindication to the use of topical β-blockers?
   a. Emphysema
   b. Congestive heart failure
   c. Chronic bronchitis
   d. Greater than first-degree heart block
   e. Asthma

7. Which of the following glaucoma medications would be a poor choice for the treatment of neovascular glaucoma?
   a. Pilocarpine hydrochloride 4%
   b. Timolol maleate 0.5%
   c. Dorzolamide hydrochloride 2%
   d. Acetazolamide
   e. Brimonidine 0.1%

8. All of the following ocular side effects have been associated with prostaglandins **except**
   a. CME
   b. Reactivation of herpes simplex keratitis
   c. Eyelash lengthening
   d. Darkening of periocular skin
   e. Dysplasia of iris nevi

9. Which of the following hypotensive agents is a docosanoid?
   a. Unoprostone
   b. Bimatoprost
   c. Brimonidine
   d. Latanoprost
   e. Travoprost

10. Which of the following drugs has been used to dissolve blood clots and fibrin in the anterior chamber?
    a. Tranexamic acid
    b. Thrombin
    c. TPA
    d. ε-aminocaproic acid
    e. Mitomycin C

SECTION II

CLINICAL SCIENCES

Oculoplastics

Jemshed A. Khan, MD

Outline

Probst LE, Tsai JH.
Ophthalmology: Clinical and Surgical Principles (pp. 135–198).
© 2012 SLACK Incorporated

Introduction

The subspecialty of oculofacial and orbital surgery includes the disorders and treatment of the eyelid, the orbit, and the lacrimal system as well as cosmetic surgery of the face.

Eyelid

Eyelid Evaluation

- Introduction
  - Evaluation of the periocular region involves soft tissues spanning from the forehead to the mid-face.
- Eyebrow
  - The mobile eyebrows function to signal facial expression and protect the eyes from forehead sweat.
  - The brow is normally positioned about 1 cm above the orbital rim.
  - The brow is elevated by the frontalis muscle and depressed by the orbicularis oculi, corrugator supercilii, and procerus muscles.
  - Men have a flatter brow contour, while women's brows arch, peaking directly above the lateral limbus.
  - With aging, the brow may droop, and compensatory contraction of the frontalis muscle may produce horizontal forehead rhytids.
- Eyelid
  - The eyelids protect the eye and orbit, produce the oily and mucinous tear components, assist in tear distribution, and contribute to the lacrimal outflow pump.
  - In primary gaze, the upper eyelid margin rests 1 to 2 mm below the upper corneal limbus.
  - The highest point of the upper eyelid marginal contour lies slightly nasal to the pupil.
  - The lower eyelid margin is positioned at the inferior corneal limbus.
  - The eyelid skin, among the thinnest of the body, tends to become redundant (dermatochalasis) with age or distend with edema.
  - The upper lid skin crease represents attachments from the levator aponeurosis to the orbicularis oculi muscle and dermis.
  - The upper lid crease lies 7 to 10 mm from the lid margin and is typically higher in women than men.
  - The orbicularis oculi protracts (closes) the eyelid. Overactivity (spasticity, blepharospasm, hemifacial spasm) and weakness (Bell's palsy, facial nerve paresis, chemodenervation) should be noted.
- Levator muscle-aponeurosis complex
  - The upper eyelid excursion from downgaze to upgaze (Figure 5-1) is termed *levator function* (LF) and normally measures 11 to 15 mm or more.
  - Upper eyelid position is measured via the margin reflex distance (MRD)—the distance between the central upper eyelid margin and the corneal light reflex.
  - The normal MRD (Figure 5-2) ranges between 2.5 and 4 mm.
  - An excess MRD suggests eyelid retraction, and a diminished MRD suggests blepharoptosis.
  - Pseudoptosis may be due to dermatochalasis, contralateral lid retraction, or hypotropia.
  - The capsulopalpebral fascia retracts the lower eyelid. Its histology and origin/insertion, however, are decidedly different from the levator complex.
  - Sympathetically innervated Müller's muscle also retracts the upper eyelid, but its range of motion is only 4 to 5 mm and denervation results in 1 to 2 mm of ptosis.
  - The undersurface of the tarsus may be examined by everting the eyelids. For the upper lid, eversion requires a narrow instrument, such as a cotton-tipped applicator to apply posterior and inferior pressure above the lid crease. With the patient looking downward, the eyelashes can be grasped, and the tarsal segment of the lid everted. If the eyelid is everted over a Desmarres retractor, the retractor handle can then be rotated posteriorly, thereby producing double eversion.

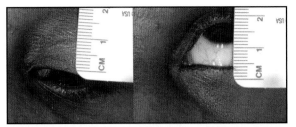

Figure 5-1. Levator function. Levator superioris motor activity is frequently represented by the measured range of upper eyelid excursion from extreme downgaze to extreme upgaze. It is important to block any active brow movement during this measurement.

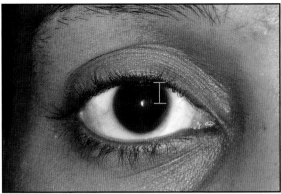

Figure 5-2. The MRD is the distance from the true eyelid margin to the central corneal light reflex. It is typically measured in primary gaze.

- Eyelashes
  - Abnormally directed (trichiasis), abnormally arising (distichiasis), depigmented (vitiligo), and broken and absent (madarosis) lashes should be noted.
  - The glands of Zeis are specialized sebaceous glands located at the eyelash base. Acute inflammation or infection of these glands produces an external hordeolum.
  - The nasal lid margin should be assessed for punctal stenosis or eversion. Localized inflammation medial to the punctum may be caused by canaliculitis.
  - Eyelid lymphatic drainage is checked by palpating the preauricular and submandibular lymph nodes.
  - Ethnic considerations
    - Heritable differences between Asian and other racial groups are quite pronounced in the eyelids.
    - In Asians, there is frequently an absence of the upper lid crease, the palpebral fissure is more obliquely slanted and narrowed, and an epicanthal fold (tarsalis variant) may be present.

Disorders of the Eyelid

Entropion

- Definition
  - Entropion is an inward rotation of the eyelid margin usually affecting the lower eyelid.
- Signs/symptoms
  - Eyelid margin inversion results in eyelash contact with the conjunctiva or cornea, producing symptoms of foreign-body sensation, tearing, discharge, ocular irritation, and redness.
  - Ophthalmic signs include superficial punctate keratopathy, corneal infection, and corneal scarring.
- Differential diagnosis
  - Entropion must be differentiated from other causes of eyelash contact with the ocular surface including the following:
    - Trichiasis, an acquired misdirection of the eyelashes without a concomitant inward rotation of the eyelid margin
    - Distichiasis, extra eyelashes emanating from the meibomian gland orifices to touch the globe
    - Epiblepharon, most often seen in Asian children, where an excess horizontal fold of pretarsal orbicularis muscle and skin ride above the eyelid margin to turn eyelashes vertically or against the globe, although the lid margin itself is not rotated inward
- Evaluation
  - Entropion is generally classified into 3 groups:
    - Congenital
    - Involutional (spastic and age-related, most common) (Figure 5-3)
    - Cicatricial (from scarring of the conjunctiva)

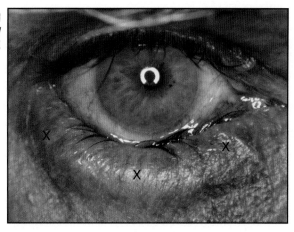

Figure 5-3. Involutional entropion of the lower eyelid. (Reprinted with permission from Lipham WJ. *Cosmetic and Clinical Applications of Botulinum Toxin.* 2nd ed. Thorofare, NJ: SLACK Incorporated; 2008.)

- A complete history, including past eyelid procedures, is vital.
- Careful examination of the eyelids and palpebral and bulbar conjunctiva will help to differentiate between entropion classifications (Table 5-1).
- Intermittent entropion may be elicited by having the patient forcefully squeeze the eyelids closed while looking downward.
- Treatment
  - Directed toward ocular irritation, secondary conjunctivitis, or keratopathy
  - Temporary measures
    - Artificial tears
    - Lubricating ointment
    - Bandage contact lens
    - Lid taping to rotate the anterior lamella away from the globe
    - These measures are often used for patients awaiting surgery or those too ill to undergo surgery.
  - Longer-term temporizing measures
    - Quickert sutures, in which 3 chromic sutures are placed full-thickness from the inferior conjunctival fornix to the skin at the eyelid margin and tied tightly to induce scarring in the anterior lamella and outward rotation of the eyelid margin
  - Surgical correction of involutional entropion addresses the underlying
    - Horizontal eyelid laxity
    - Disinsertion of the lower eyelid retractors
    - Overriding preseptal orbicularis oculi muscle
  - Surgical techniques of entropion repair
    - In the transconjunctival entropion repair, dissection is carried out through conjunctiva and retractors. Then, a small 3-mm strip of preseptal orbicularis is excised, the retractors are reattached to the inferior tarsus, and a lateral tarsal strip procedure is used for horizontal tightening.
    - Surgical approaches for cicatricial entropion address the posterior lamella shortening. In the Wies procedure, the lower eyelid is incised full-thickness from skin to conjunctiva 3-mm below the eyelid margin; sutures are then placed from cut edge of tarsus inferiorly out through skin superiorly and anteriorly and tied tightly, thus causing an anterior rotation of the eyelid margin.
- Prognosis
  - Generally good for involutional entropion, cicatricial entropion is more challenging.

Ectropion

- Definition
  - Ectropion is an eyelid margin eversion that may be congenital or acquired.
  - When due to gravity, it most commonly affects the lower eyelid.

TABLE 5-1. ENTROPION CLASSIFICATION

Type	Etiology	Eyelid Examination
Congenital	Lower eyelid retractor dysgenesis Structural defects in tarsal plate Relative shortening of posterior lamella	Overriding skin and orbicularis
Involutional	Horizontal eyelid laxity Medial canthal tendon laxity Lateral canthal tendon laxity Lower eyelid retractor disinsertion Preseptal orbicularis override	Eyelid easily distracted from globe Punctum laterally displaced 2 mm with lid tension Laxity after medial canthal tendon tuck White retractors found inferior to tarsus with intervening pink band of orbicularis between tarsus and retractor Poor downward excursion of eyelid in downgaze
Cicatricial	Vertically shortened posterior lamella by a cicatricial conjunctival process	Symblepharon Shortened fornices

- Signs/symptoms
  - o The poor eyelid-to-globe apposition may be asymptomatic or may lead to visual loss, ocular discomfort, photophobia, epiphora, and conjunctivitis/keratitis from cornea and conjunctival exposure (Figure 5-4).
  - o Surgery is indicated when corneal and conjunctival exposure or ocular irritation occurs.
- Evaluation
  - o Many tests can be performed to assess the ectropion etiology (Table 5-2). The snap test is performed by gently distracting the eyelid away from the globe and estimating the snap back time and millimeters of eyelid distraction from the globe. When laxity is present, the eyelid does not immediately return to the globe. Sluggish snap tests occur in involutional and paralytic ectropions.
    - ▪ Evaluation of eyelid closure is performed by having the patient gently and forcibly close the eyelids while the examiner applies a retracting force to open them. Poor eyelid closure and lagophthalmos result when the orbicularis has an atonic state secondary to a neurogenic process (seventh nerve palsy) or cicatricial changes (shortened anterior lamellae). In the former, minimal protracting force is present.
    - ▪ With cicatricial changes, the examiner will be unable to elevate the lower eyelid to the mid-pupil level, eyelash eversion on upgaze will be present, and normal skin tension lines will be absent.
- Treatment
  - o Eyelid ectropion may be medically and surgically treated to avoid visual loss, ocular discomfort, photophobia, epiphora, and conjunctivitis/keratitis.
  - o Supportive care with lubrication, removal of noxious stimuli, and eyelid manipulation (taping) may delay the need for urgent surgical intervention.
  - o With appropriate ectropion classification, surgical repair may be tailored to the individual patient. A combined surgical approach may be necessary for complex ectropions when more than one etiologic factor of ectropion is present. Main complications of surgery include over- and undercorrections.
  - o Surgical options
    - ▪ Involutional ectropion, an age-related process, can be managed by horizontally tightening the lower eyelid and re-inserting dehisced eyelid retractors.

Figure 5-4. Involutional ectropion with exposure of the palpebral conjunctiva. (Reprinted with permission from Agarwal A. *Handbook of Ophthalmology.* Thorofare, NJ: SLACK Incorporated; 2006.)

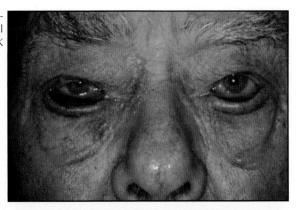

TABLE 5-2. ECTROPION CLASSIFICATION

TYPE	ETIOLOGY	EYELID EXAMINATION
Involutional	Horizontal eyelid laxity Medial canthal tendon laxity Horizontal tarsal laxity Lateral canthal tendon laxity Eyelid retractor recession	Eyelid easily distracted from globe Punctum laterally displaced with lid tension Eyelids easily evert on closure (floppy eyelid) Laxity after medial canthal tendon tuck Recessed capsulopalpebral fascia Ectropion with lateral eyelid tension
Cicatricial	Insufficient vertical eyelid skin	Eyelid retraction (often with scleral show) Eyelash eversion on upgaze Absent skin tension lines
Paralytic	Orbicularis oculi weakness	Loss of orbicularis tone on eyelid closure Lagophthalmos Eyelid retraction Possible loss of brow rhytids Possible lip droop
Mechanical	Excessive lid bulk	Tumor; edema

- In patients with floppy eyelid (tarsal instability), large full-thickness eyelid resections and reconstructions are performed.
- Cicatricial ectropion, a vertical shortening of the anterior or middle lamellae, may result from skin diseases (ichthyosis, actinic sun damage), allergy/atopy, infection (ie, herpes zoster), previous surgery or trauma, or congenital anterior lamellar deficiency as seen in blepharophimosis ptosis syndrome, Treacher Collins, and clefting syndromes. It can be managed by hard palate grafting to the posterior lamella and lateral canthal tightening and cheek resuspension, which is often aesthetically preferable to skin grafting.
- Paralytic ectropion, often resulting from Bell's palsy, should be managed conservatively with topical lubrication and eye drops. A temporary tarsorrhaphy may be performed to prevent corneal erosion and subsequent ulceration and to prophylax against ocular discomfort from corneal exposure keratopathy and lagophthalmos. As an alternative, the eyelid may be taped with lateral traction. To correct permanent orbicularis atony and eyelid laxity, a lateral tarsal strip procedure with fascia lata resuspension from medial to lateral canthal regions is often indicated.

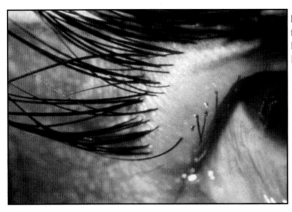

Figure 5-5. Distichiasis, ie, abnormal posterior eyelash origin from a meibomian gland orifice. (Reprinted with permission from Leal AG, Rodriguez PM. *The Atlas of Ophthalmology.* Thorofare, NJ: SLACK Incorporated; 2002.)

- ▪ Treatment of mechanical ectropion resulting from excess eyelid bulk (tumor), acute proptosis, conjunctival chemosis, periocular edema, or glasses pushing the eyelid down is directed toward the primary cause, often in conjunction with horizontal eyelid tightening.
- Prognosis
  - ○ Generally good for involutional ectropion, cicatricial ectropion is more challenging.

Trichiasis and Distichiasis

- Definition
  - ○ Trichiasis is a misdirection of lashes such that they curl toward and touch the eyeball rather than away from the globe.
  - ○ Distichiasis is an abnormal emergence of eyelashes from the meibomian gland orifices rather than the more anteriorly located lash line (Figure 5-5).
- Etiology
  - ○ Both conditions may be acquired, although distichiasis can also be congenital. When acquired, the cause is often underlying trauma, surgery, or inflammatory conditions. There may be an associated entropion.
- Signs/symptoms
  - ○ All are secondary to eyelash malposition and include foreign-body sensation, corneal irritation or keratopathy, epiphora, and mucus discharge.
- Evaluation
  - ○ Aided by the slit lamp to determine whether the lashes emerge from the lash line (trichiasis) or the meibomian gland orifices (distichiasis)
- Management
  - ○ Temporary (ie, plucking of the eyelashes [epilation])
  - ○ Permanent destruction of the eyelash follicle (eg, radiofrequency needle, electroepilation, cryotherapy, laser, or rarely radiation therapy). In severe cases, surgical excision, mucus membrane grafting, or lid-splitting with cryotherapy may be useful.
- Prognosis
  - ○ Generally good because these conditions respond to treatment
  - ○ Exceptions are trachoma and pemphigoid, which can progress despite treatment.

Ptosis

Congenital Ptosis

- Definition
  - ○ Congenital ptosis is a drooping of the upper eyelid or eyelids noted at birth or in early childhood.
- Etiology
  - ○ There are several etiologies of congenital ptosis.
  - ○ The most common type of congenital ptosis is myogenic ptosis. This is the result of a poorly developed levator muscle in which the normal muscle is replaced with fat or fibrous tissue.
  - ○ Less commonly, congenital aponeurotic ptosis results from a poor insertion of the aponeurosis onto the tarsal surface or may be associated with birth trauma.

- o Congenital neurogenic ptosis is associated with innervational defects that occur during embryologic development. This type of ptosis may be associated with congenital third nerve palsy, double elevator palsy, Horner syndrome, or Marcus Gunn's jaw-winking syndrome.
- o A mechanical congenital ptosis may be caused by a congenital neoplasm such as a hemangioma.
- o Several syndromes may manifest ptosis including blepharophimosis and Goldenhar's syndrome
- Signs/symptoms
  - o These will vary depending on the degree and type of ptosis. Patients with moderate to severe ptosis may manifest an elevated brow or a chin-up position in an effort to peer out from beneath the ptotic lid.
  - o Congenital myogenic ptosis may manifest lagophthalmos and some elevation of the eyelid in downgaze.
  - o Jaw winking is manifest by variation in the amount of ptosis with jaw muscle or extraocular muscle (EOM) movements (synkinesis).
- Evaluation
  - o A history, including possible birth trauma and family history of ptosis, should be taken
  - o The physical examination should include an evaluation of fissure height, LF, MRD, and upper eyelid crease position. Additionally, note should be made of head position, lagophthalmos, synkinetic movements, EOM function, pupillary examination, as well as any associated periocular findings, such as epicanthus inversus, telecanthus, phimosis, epibulbar dermoids, preauricular dermoids, etc.
  - o Most importantly, in all cases of congenital ptosis, visual function and refractive error must be assessed to identify those children at risk for amblyopia from anisometropia, strabismus, or occlusion of the pupil.
- Management
  - o The timing of surgical intervention in congenital ptosis is dependent on the degree of ptosis and the risk of amblyopia development.
  - o Additionally, social issues may motivate families to elect for the surgical repair of mild to moderate ptosis in the preschool period.
  - o The amount and type of ptosis as well as the LF are the determining factors in the choice of surgical procedure.
  - o In cases of mild ptosis, Horner syndrome, or those responsive to a drop of phenylephrine 2.5%, a Müllerectomy may be performed.
  - o External levator resection or advancement procedure is selected when the patient has mild to moderate ptosis (2 to 4 mm) with good to excellent LF (5 to 15 mm).
  - o In cases of severe ptosis (4 mm or greater) and poor LF (<5 mm), recruitment of the adjacent frontalis muscle with a tarsofrontalis suspension procedure would be indicated. Several types of suspension materials are available (autogenous or banked fascia lata, gore-tex, silicone slings, etc), the selection of which is dependent on patient age, surgeon, and parental preference.
- Prognosis
  - o In general, the prognosis for patients achieving an acceptable cosmetic and functional lid position is good in cases of mild to moderate ptosis or bilateral severe congenital ptosis (Figure 5-6).
  - o However, amblyopia occurs in 20% of cases of congenital ptosis, attributable to the ptosis itself in 4% of cases.

Acquired Involutional Ptosis

- Definition
  - o Involutional ptosis, the most common type of acquired ptosis (Figure 5-7), results from stretching, dehiscence, or disinsertion of the levator aponeurosis.
  - o Risk factors include age, ocular surgery, contact lenses, edema, blepharochalasis syndrome, pregnancy, and trauma.
- Signs/symptoms
  - o Patients with ptosis may complain of decreased vision in the superior visual field from the ptotic eyelid.
  - o Others will report difficulty in the reading position when the ptosis is accentuated in downgaze, owing to frontalis relaxation.

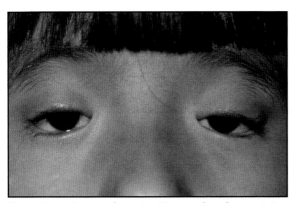

Figure 5-6. Congenital ptosis. (Reprinted with permission from Leal AG, Rodriguez PM. *The Atlas of Ophthalmology.* Thorofare, NJ: SLACK Incorporated; 2002.)

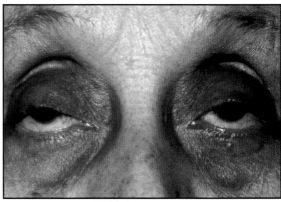

Figure 5-7. Acquired ptosis with characteristic high lid crease. (Reprinted with permission from Leal AG, Rodriguez PM. *The Atlas of Ophthalmology.* Thorofare, NJ: SLACK Incorporated; 2002.)

- o Patients may also note brow ache from excessive frontalis recruitment.
- o Reduction of the vertical palpebral fissure height (ie, drooping of one or both upper eyelids) is observed along with elevated or multiple creases on the affected side.
- o Frontalis compensation may elevate the brow on the affected side, and an abnormally high contralateral eyelid may be noted due to Hering's law.
- o Extreme thinning of the eyelid tissues may occasionally permit visualization of the dark shadow of the iris through a pale attenuated eyelid.
- Differential diagnosis
  - o The differential diagnosis includes the following:
    - Involutional ptosis
    - Horner syndrome
    - CN III palsy
    - Myasthenia gravis
    - Chronic progressive external ophthalmoplegia (CPEO)
  - o Causes of pseudoptosis include the following:
    - Dermatochalasis
    - Eyelid edema
    - Nanophthalmos
    - Microphthalmos
    - Phthisis bulbi
    - Enophthalmos (orbital floor fracture, metastatic breast cancer)
    - Hypertropia
    - Contralateral eyelid retraction
    - Proptosis seen in thyroid ophthalmopathy
- Evaluation
  - o A history should assess the age of onset, degree of visual impairment, associated symptoms, history of trauma, use of anticoagulants, thyroid status, or prior ocular surgery.
  - o Variability or fatigability suggests myasthenia gravis.
  - o Evaluation with clinical measurements may include vertical interpalpebral fissure height, MRD, upper eyelid crease position, LF, lagophthalmos, presence of Hering's law, Bell's phenomenon, Schirmer's testing, corneal sensation, pupils, and motility. Ptosis is often defined as an MRD of 2 mm or less.
  - o A high eyelid crease in the setting of normal LF is characteristic of involutional ptosis.
  - o During testing for LF, the frontalis muscle should be neutralized by manually immobilizing the brow to prevent inaccurate measurements.
  - o Visual field testing before and after eyelid taping can document the degree of visual field impairment.
  - o Measurement of the MRD before and after instillation of phenylephrine is useful for surgical planning.

- ○ Rest testing, the ice pack test, and edrophonium chloride (Tensilon) administration can be used to diagnose myasthenia gravis.
- Management
  - ○ As a temporizing measure, the ptotic eyelid may be taped up, but the definitive treatment of ptosis is surgical (Figure 5-8).
  - ○ The choice of operation is guided by the LF.
    - For LF more than 11 mm: Müllerectomy, tarsoaponeurectomy, levator aponeurotic repair and/or resection
    - For LF 6 to 10 mm: levator resection (internal and external)
    - For LF less than 5 mm: Frontalis suspension using either silicone rod or fascia lata
- Prognosis
  - ○ Prognosis with acquired involutional ptosis is excellent.

Acquired, Nonaponeurotic Ptosis

- Definition
  - ○ Acquired nonaponeurotic ptosis is any noncongenital ptosis due to causes other than simple attenuation or disinsertion of the levator aponeurosis.
- Etiology
  - ○ Several interesting diagnostic categories fall under the aegis of acquired, nonaponeurotic ptosis.
    - Neurogenic ptosis is due to decreased nerve stimulation of the lid protractors (levator aponeurosis or Müller's muscle). Causes include third nerve palsy (compressive or vasculopathic), Horner syndrome (decreased sympathetic innervation marked by a triad of miosis, ptosis, and anhidrosis), multiple sclerosis, tumors, and inflammatory states.
    - Myogenic ptosis is the result of a decrease in levator muscle function. Common causes include myasthenia gravis (due to antibodies to acetylcholine receptors at the neuromuscular junction), chronic progressive external ophthalmoplegia (slowly progressive paralysis of the lids and EOMs, which may demonstrate mitochondrial inheritance), myotonic dystrophy, oropharyngeal muscular dystrophy, and iatrogenic due botulinum toxin blockade of acetylcholine release.
    - Mechanical ptosis is due to extrinsic forces on the lid (eg, tumors, cicatrization).
- Signs/symptoms
  - ○ Sudden-onset ptosis is suspicious for third nerve palsy.
  - ○ Ptosis primarily present in the evening, along with diplopia, is suspicious for myasthenia gravis.
  - ○ Diplopia with systemic weakness, dysarthria, or dysphagia is suspicious for myogenic ptosis.
  - ○ A high lid crease on the ptotic lid is a sign of aponeurotic ptosis.
  - ○ Ptosis with miosis worse in the dark is indicative of Horner syndrome (Figure 5-9). Lack of dilation after ocular instillation of cocaine (4%) confirms the diagnosis of Horner syndrome.
  - ○ In third nerve palsy, a dilated pupil is an important sign of compression due to a tumor or enlarging aneurysm and requires emergency neurosurgical consultation. Extraocular motility may be affected in neurogenic and myogenic ptosis, and orbicularis function may be diminished in myogenic ptosis.
  - ○ Characteristics of myasthenia gravis include Cogan's lid twitch (a brief upward overshoot of the upper lid when the eye returns to primary gaze after downgaze), a positive ice test (decreased ptosis after application of ice for 2 minutes), and fatigability (increased ptosis after sustained upgaze).
- Differential diagnosis
  - ○ Pseudoptosis must be ruled out.
  - ○ Common causes of pseudoptosis include the following:
    - Dermatochalasis
    - Brow ptosis
    - Lid edema
    - Contralateral lid retraction
    - Hypotropia
    - Hypoglobus
    - Axial anisometropia

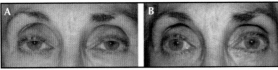

Figure 5-8. (A) Preoperative photograph of involutional ptosis. (B) After levator advancement surgery, the normal eyelid position is restored.

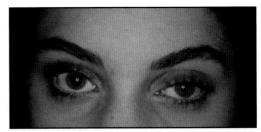

Figure 5-9. Horner syndrome of left eye. Note left miosis, left upper lid ptosis, and left lower lid reverse ptosis.

  - ▪ Enophthalmos
  - ▪ Microphthalmos
  - ▪ Phthisis
- Evaluation
  - o In pupil-sparing third nerve palsy, it is important to monitor the patient for development of pupillary involvement.
  - o In pupil-involving third nerve palsy (or pupil-sparing third nerve palsy that does not resolve in 6 months), neuroimaging is necessary to rule out nerve compression by a tumor or aneurysm.
  - o A positive Tensilon test can confirm myasthenia gravis. During this test, ptosis improves after injection of Tensilon. Vital sign monitoring is necessary during the test to detect cholinergic crisis. Serologic testing for acetylcholine receptor antibodies also confirms myasthenia gravis.
  - o Chest x-ray or computed tomography (CT) scanning for tumors or thymoma and carotid angiogram for carotid dissection may be indicated in Horner syndrome.
  - o EKG to rule out heart block and retinal evaluation for pigmentary changes are useful in identifying Kearns-Sayre syndrome. Muscle biopsy for ragged red fibers may also be used to clinch this diagnosis.
- Management
  - o Ptosis due to third nerve palsy should be followed until stable for 6 months. Even then, strabismus surgery should precede ptosis surgery, and ptosis repair should be reserved for patients with single binocular visual acuity.
  - o In patients with myasthenia gravis, pyridostigmine (Mestinon) is an oral anticholinesterase that may improve LF. Systemic steroids or immunosuppressives and thymectomy in patients with a thymoma may also bring nonsurgical improvement. Patients with ocular myasthenia should be followed for signs of systemic involvement.
  - o Ptosis due to botulinum toxin (BTX) will resolve as the toxin's effect wanes and responds to administration of a topical adrenergic agonist such as Naphcon A or Iopidine in the interim.
  - o Repair of myogenic ptosis involves caution due to limited orbicularis function, EOM function, and Bell's phenomenon. Treatment of myogenic ptosis involves treatment of the underlying cause.
- Prognosis
  - o Systemic manifestations may develop in 85% of patients who present with ocular myasthenia gravis.

Benign Eyelid Lesions

- Definition
  - o There are many lesions of the lid that should be differentiated from those that are malignant.
- Signs/symptoms
  - o Symmetric shape
  - o Regular borders
  - o Consistent color, whereas malignancies may show telangiectasias
  - o Loss of eyelid structures and lashes suggests a destructive lesion
  - o Ulceration
  - o Signs of melanoma
  - o Bleeding is common with basal cell carcinoma.
  - o Most benign eyelid lesions are treated by excision.

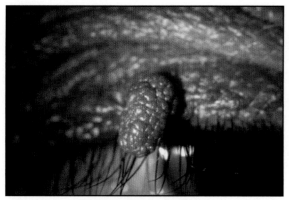

Figure 5-10. Squamous papilloma. (Reprinted with permission from Leal AG, Rodriguez PM. *The Atlas of Ophthalmology.* Thorofare, NJ: SLACK Incorporated; 2002.)

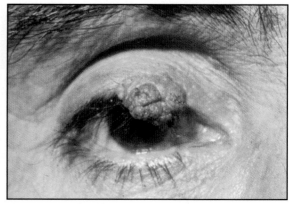

Figure 5-11. Seborrheic keratosis. (Reprinted with permission from Leal AG, Rodriguez PM. *The Atlas of Ophthalmology.* Thorofare, NJ: SLACK Incorporated; 2002.)

- Types of benign eyelid lesions
  - Squamous papilloma (acrochordon) (Figure 5-10)
    - Most common eyelid lesion
      - An epithelial hyperplasia, it is raised, flesh-colored, and irregular.
      - May be sessile or pedunculated ("skin tag")
  - Seborrheic keratosis (Figure 5-11)
    - Another example of epithelial hyperplasia
    - Waxy, stuck on appearance
    - Pigmented, lobulated, or pedunculated
    - Rare before middle age
  - Verruca vulgaris
    - Rare form of epithelial hyperplasia due to human papillomavirus infection
    - Classically elevated with a papillomatous surface
    - Best treated by excision, but cryotherapy may also be used to prevent recurrence
  - Epidermal inclusion cyst (sebaceous cyst)
    - Benign keratin-filled epithelial cyst
    - Arises from the upper segment of hair follicles and may be spontaneous or due to trauma
    - Epidermal inclusion cysts are yellow-white, raised, and smooth.
    - A central pore may be observed.
    - Treatment is excision or marsupialization.
  - Molluscum contagiosum (Figure 5-12)
    - A benign epithelial mass due to viral infection
    - Commonly seen on the lid margin of children, but may be associated with HIV infection
    - Typically nodular with central umbilication
    - Viral particles released into the tear film often cause a follicular conjunctivitis.
    - Treatment is by excision or cryotherapy.
  - Syringomas
    - Benign tumors of the eccrine sweat glands that arise from the deep dermis
    - Small, yellow, often multiple lesions typically found on the lower eyelids
    - Commonly treated by excision or carbon dioxide (CO_2) laser
  - Apocrine hidrocystoma (sudoriferous cyst)
    - Tumor of the glands of Moll
    - Raised translucent cystic lesion typically found along the eyelid margin and transilluminates
    - May grow when the patient sweats
    - Treated by excision or marsupialization
  - Nevi or "moles"
    - Raised lesions derived from melanocytes
    - May be pigmented or flesh-colored and may sprout hair
    - Pigmented nevi tend to lose pigmentation in the elderly.

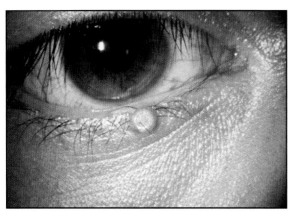

Figure 5-12. Molluscum contagiosum. Note central umbilication. (Reprinted with permission from Leal AG, Rodriguez PM. *The Atlas of Ophthalmology.* Thorofare, NJ: SLACK Incorporated; 2002.)

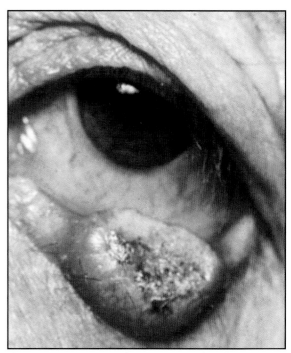

Figure 5-13. Keratoacanthoma. (Reprinted with permission from Leal AG, Rodriguez PM. *The Atlas of Ophthalmology.* Thorofare, NJ: SLACK Incorporated; 2002.)

- With age, nevi progress from the dermal-epidermal junction (junctional) to involve the junction and the dermis (compound) and finally occupy only the dermis (dermal).
- Junctional and compound nevi may rarely undergo malignant transformation.
- Intradermal nevi are commonly found on the eyelid margin. They are smooth, and the posterior surface often molds to the surface of the globe.
- Keratoacanthoma (Figure 5-13)
  - Rapidly growing dome-shaped nodule that rapidly develops a central crater, which is usually filled with keratin
  - Usually seen in patients of middle age or older
  - May be confused with squamous cell carcinoma and has been considered to have some potential for malignant transformation
  - Although this lesion may involute, it is best treated by excisional biopsy.
- Actinic keratosis
  - Premalignant lesion of sun-exposed skin and may transform into squamous cell carcinoma at a rate of 0.24% per year (1/417 lesion/yr)
  - Waxing and waning scaly red, round plaque with a rough texture
  - May spontaneously regress, but the number may increase with sun exposure
  - Treated by topical agents, excision, or cryotherapy
- Treatment
  - Guidelines for biopsy of benign lesions are as follows:
    - Because clinical features may be misleading, a biopsy is often useful in confirming a diagnosis.
    - For biopsy, the lesion is injected with local anesthetic with epinephrine.
    - Excisional biopsies remove the entire lesion, whereas incisional biopsies remove a portion of the lesion.
    - Small lesions with low suspicion for malignancy are often removed by excisional biopsy, while larger lesions or those suspicious for malignancy may be treated by incisional biopsy, which leaves residual tumor to identify the biopsy site should further treatment be necessary.

- Although superficial lesions may be removed by a shave biopsy, it is important not to use shave biopsies for pigmented lesions, because obtaining a full-thickness skin sample will provide the penetration depth of a melanoma, an important prognostic factor.
- It is important to provide a specimen with minimal crush artifact by minimizing handling of the tissue and using toothed forceps.
- When excising lesions of the eyelid margin, care must be taken to avoid or shield the globe.
- Bleeding may be treated with hand-held cautery, and a steroid-antibiotic combination ophthalmic ointment may be used for several days.

Malignant Eyelid Tumors

- Definition
  - Malignant eyelid lesions have a variety of presentations.
- Signs/symptoms
  - Eyelid malignancies often present as nontender, nonhealing skin ulcerations or nodules with irregular borders, usually after the fourth decade of life and often with lash loss and disruption of the lid margin architecture.
  - Ultraviolet radiation and pale skin are the major risk factors for basal cell carcinoma, squamous cell carcinoma, and melanoma.
  - Basal cell nevus syndrome and xeroderma pigmentosum are rare familial predispositions for basal cell carcinoma.
- Types of malignant eyelid lesions
  - Basal cell carcinoma (BCa) (Figure 5-14)
    - It accounts for 90% of all lid malignancies and arises from the basal cell layer of the epithelium, most often in the lower lid and medial canthus.
    - The classic nodular BCa is a "rodent ulcer" with central excavation and pearly, translucent telangiectatic borders.
    - The tumor margins of fibrosing/morpheaform BCa are difficult to clinically distinguish.
    - Occasionally, BCa has a misleading cystic appearance, is pigmented, or mimics chronic inflammatory disease.
    - The prognosis for completely excised BCa is excellent, and BCa does not usually metastasize.
    - Longstanding or recurrent BCa, especially in the medial canthus and vertical midface, may spread to the orbit or cranium.
  - Squamous cell carcinoma (SqCa) (Figure 5-15)
    - It is the second most common eyelid malignancy, about 1/40th as common as BCa.
    - SqCa arises from the squamous layer of the epithelium, and, as such, hyperkeratosis is more frequently seen with SqCa than BCa.
    - SqCa is more aggressive than BCa and may spread hematogenously, to lymph nodes, or along peripheral nerves (neurotrophic spread).
    - The prognosis for SqCa, though not as good as BCa, is usually optimistic unless the lesions have metastasized.
  - Keratoacanthoma
    - A crater-like, rapidly growing lesion that is increasingly regarded as an intermediate form of SqCa
  - Sebaceous adenocarcinoma
    - This arises from the meibomian glands, glands of Zeis, or periocular sebaceous glands, and is more common in the upper lids.
    - Sebaceous carcinoma is an uncommon but aggressive tumor that may masquerade as recurrent chalazion, blepharitis, or other ocular inflammations.
    - The deep-seated eyelid lesions may be yellow due to their lipid content.
    - Sebaceous carcinoma can spread to the conjunctiva where the lesions may be multiple and noncontiguous.
    - If the diagnosis is suspected, a full-thickness lid biopsy is required, and the pathologist should be alerted ahead of time so that lipid stains can be performed on the specimen.
    - The prognosis for sebaceous carcinoma is guarded because it is an aggressive, potentially multicentric lesion that is relatively radioresistant and tends to metastasize.

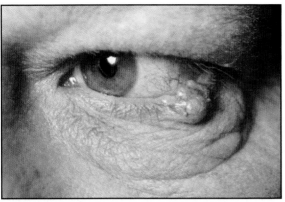

Figure 5-14. Basal cell carcinoma. (Reprinted with permission from Leal AG, Rodriguez PM. *The Atlas of Ophthalmology.* SLACK Incorporated: Thorofare, NJ; 2002.)

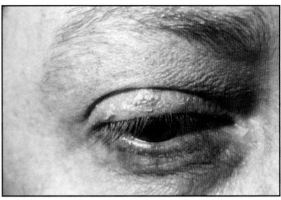

Figure 5-15. Squamous cell carcinoma. (Reprinted with permission from Leal AG, Rodriguez PM. *The Atlas of Ophthalmology.* SLACK Incorporated: Thorofare, NJ; 2002.)

- o Malignant melanoma (Figure 5-16)
    - A highly lethal tumor that classically presents with the "ABCD" of Asymmetry, Border irregularity, Color variegation, and Diameter greater than 6 mm.
    - Lentigo malignant melanoma and nodular melanoma are the most common eyelid melanomas.
    - Melanoma that has not extended beyond 0.75 mm depth has a 98% survival rate.
    - Because melanoma can metastasize widely to the lymph nodes, lung, and liver, a metastatic workup is recommended for tumor thickness greater than 1.5 mm.
- o Rare malignant eyelid tumors
    - Metastases (eg, lung, breast), cutaneous T-cell lymphoma (mycosis fungoides), Kaposi's sarcoma (often related to HIV), and Merkel cell tumor (a rare neuroendocrine tumor)
- Management
    - o The preferred management of all the aforementioned lid tumors (except the rare malignant eyelid tumors) is complete excision with tumor-free surgical margins established by frozen section, permanent section, or Mohs' surgery (lamellar micrographic analysis).
    - o With frozen section techniques, BCa and SqCa should be excised with 2- to 3-mm margins. Sebaceous carcinoma and melanoma should have up to 5-mm margins when possible.
    - o When the diagnosis is in doubt, an incisional biopsy can be taken at the border of normal and abnormal-appearing skin.
    - o The role of sentinel lymph node biopsy in sebaceous carcinoma and melanoma remains under evaluation.
    - o Eyelid reconstructive techniques must maintain a moist and protected mucosal covering for the cornea.
    - o Radiation, electrofulguration, and cryotherapy are adjunctive/palliative treatment modalities that have lower cure rates and are not advocated as primary treatment techniques unless the patient is too sick to tolerate surgery or the lesions are too widespread.
    - o Imiquimod cream has applications in superficial BCa, but is not approved for ophthalmic use.

Chronic Blepharitis

- Definition
    - o Blepharitis means inflammation of the eyelid.
    - o This common condition occurs at all ages, although more frequently in the elderly.
- Etiology
    - o The causes are numerous and overlapping, including anterior lamellae problems of infection by staphylococcus and seborrhea with accumulation of dead cells at the eyelash base.
    - o Posterior lamellae problems include inflammation of the meibomian glands (meibomianitis).
- Signs/symptoms
    - o Meibomianitis tends to produce symptoms and ocular irritation exceeding what one sees clinically.
    - o Due to the eyelid inflammation, the lids and/or eyes feel irritated.

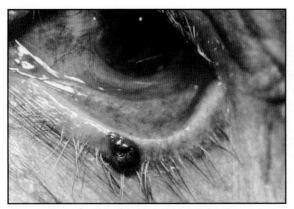

Figure 5-16. Malignant melanoma. (Reprinted with permission from Leal AG, Rodriguez PM. *The Atlas of Ophthalmology.* Thorofare, NJ: SLACK Incorporated; 2002.)

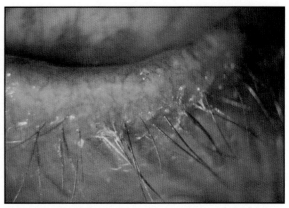

Figure 5-17. Blepharitis. (Reprinted with permission from Agarwal, A. *Handbook of Ophthalmology.* Thorofare, NJ: SLACK Incorporated; 2002.)

- o The tear film can be disrupted causing dry eye symptoms of burning, irritation, epiphora, and foreign-body sensation.
- o The lids are reddened and inflamed with varying degrees of thickening. Dead skin cells clumping at the base of the eyelashes are called *collarettes* or sleeves (Figure 5-17).
- o In more severe cases, especially with eyelid infections, breakdown of the skin with frank ulceration can occur.
- • Differential diagnosis
  - o It is important to distinguish blepharitis from carcinoma such as basal cell, squamous cell, or sebaceous cell.
  - o Sebaceous cell carcinoma is the great imitator. Any persistent condition that is not classical for blepharitis should be biopsied for diagnosis.
  - o If there is loss of eyelashes, nodular changes, or ulceration, biopsy is required.
- • Evaluation
  - o Usually straightforward with biomicroscopy to visualize the collarettes, margin inflammation, and mild discharge
  - o When meibomianitis is involved, one sees "pouting" of the meibomian gland orifices frequently with a thick whitish discharge similar to the consistency of toothpaste.
- • Treatment
  - o Chronic conditions, blepharitis and meibomianitis are controlled, not cured.
  - o Routine management of blepharitis requires careful eyelid scrubs on a daily or weekly basis, depending on the severity.
    - ▪ These are performed using either straight warm water or a mildly soapy solution of 3 drops of Johnson's baby shampoo (must be baby shampoo) stirred into a glass of warm water.
    - ▪ The patient then uses a cotton swab or washcloth wrapped around his or her fingertip to dunk into the solution and gently scrub at the base of the lashes.
    - ▪ In cases with potential bacterial infection, an antibiotic eye drop is instilled after the eyelid scrub. Eye drops do not clog the gland openings like ointments.
  - o If the patient also has meibomianitis, then a different protocol aimed at emptying the thickened secretion from the gland is required.
    - ▪ The patient is instructed to place steady warmth onto the closed lids for 10 minutes, and the glands are gently expressed toward the eyelid margin.
    - ▪ Eyelid scrubs are performed.
    - ▪ A variety of antibiotics and steroids have been tried in the past to control the meibomianitis with mixed results.
    - ▪ A recent advance is the use of cyclosporine-A drops applied topically twice daily for a minimum of 4 months. If the amount of gland pouting, secretion, and discomfort are diminished and the tear film breakup time is improved, then the drops can be continued either on a daily basis or reduced to 1 vial of cyclosporine-A, 4 doses per week.

TABLE 5-3. DIFFERENCES BETWEEN STYE, CHALAZION, AND INTERNAL HORDEOLUM

FEATURES	STYE (EXTERNAL HORDEOLUM)	CHALAZION	INTERNAL HORDEOLUM
Onset	Acute	Chronic	Acute
Involved gland	Zeis gland	Meibomian gland	Meibomian gland
Type of inflammation	Suppurative	Granulomatous	Suppurative
Classic signs	Localized, hard, pus, and tender swelling near the lid margin	Hard swelling away from the lid margin	Yellow point seen on everting the lids
Symptoms	Acute pain and swelling	Painless disfigurement	Severe pain
Treatment	Hot formentation, antibiotic, and removal of eyelash	Vertical incision and drainage	Antibiotic, analgesic, and vertical incision and drainage

Adapted from Agarwal A. *Handbook of Ophthalmology*. Thorofare, NJ: SLACK Incorporated; 2006.

- Prognosis
  - As these are chronic conditions, the patient must understand that treatment is aimed at control not cure.
  - For the majority of patients, with treatment, the symptoms are significantly reduced.

Chalazion and Hordeolum

- Definition
  - Chalazia result from inflammation of the meibomian gland.
- Etiology
  - They may be secondary to staphylococcal infection of the gland, producing inflammation and meibomianitis with eventual chalazion formation.
  - Internal and external hordeola are infectious processes, either an abscess of the gland of Zeis or an acute and rapid staphylococcal infection of the meibomian gland (Table 5-3).
- Signs/symptoms
  - The clinical appearance of a chalazion and hordeolum can be indistinguishable. Both appear as lid bumps varying in size from discrete to quite large and uncomfortable (Figure 5-18).
  - Chalazia are evaluated under the biomicroscope with lid eversion to determine if the lesion is coming to a head either internally or along the gland orifice.
  - The degree of erythema varies.
  - Small lesions can be fairly flat, and larger ones can be very distended.
  - The spacing between lashes can appear stretched due to the distension, but frank loss of cilia is unusual except with marked and prolonged inflammation or a masquerading malignancy.
- Differential diagnosis
  - Differentiation can be difficult between chalazion and hordeolum, although an acute history and painful eyelid margin location are more suggestive of hordeola.
  - Incision and drainage allows one to examine the contents, which can suggest the etiology.
  - If there is ulceration of the lesion or loss of lashes, malignancy should be suspected and tissue sent for biopsy.
  - If what appears to be a chalazion keeps recurring in the same location requiring multiple repeat incision and drainage procedures, one should suspect a sebaceous cell carcinoma masquerading as a chalazion. These frequently drain on their own with medical assistance.

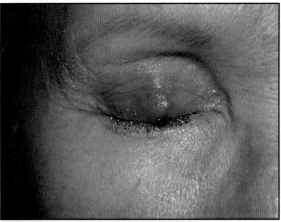

Figure 5-18. Internal hordeolum. (Reprinted with permission from Agarwal A. *Handbook of Ophthalmology.* Thorofare, NJ: SLACK Incorporated; 2002.)

- Treatment
  - ○ Warm compresses to the lesion for 15 minutes 4 times daily preceded by topical antibiotic application of drop or ointment
  - ○ The author prefers drops over ointments because of the higher antibiotic concentration and lack of blocking of gland openings.
  - ○ If the lesion does not drain on its own with 2 weeks of compliant treatment, then the physician can incise and drain in the office.

Xanthelasma

- Definition
  - ○ Xanthomas are yellow-orange lipid-filled nodules, papules, or plaques of the skin.
  - ○ When seen in the eyelid, they are termed *xanthelasma palpebrarum*.
  - ○ Lesions are generally situated medially in the upper or lower eyelids of middle-aged or older people, more commonly women (1.1%) than men (0.3%).
  - ○ Small at first, they may gradually enlarge to several centimeters in size.
- Etiology
  - ○ Xanthelasma may be an indicator of hypercholesterolemia in 50% of all cases.
  - ○ Familial dyslipidemias are common—especially type IIa (hyperbetalipoproteinemia), as well as higher rates of atherosclerosis and cardiovascular disease. Even normolipidemic patients with xanthelasma may have higher low-density lipoprotein (LDL) and lower high-density lipoprotein (HDL) cholesterol levels than controls. Patients under age 40 are at significant risk, and systemic lipid levels should be assessed. The combination of corneal arcus and xanthelasma indicates an even higher risk for significant lipid disorders.
  - ○ Xanthelasma have also been associated with liver or biliary disease, diabetes mellitus, hypertension, hypothyroidism, leprosy, multiple myeloma, Hand-Schüller-Christian disease, and reticulohistiocytoma cutis.
- Histological findings
  - ○ Perivascular lipid-laden foamy histiocytes in the superficial dermis, sometimes surrounded by fibrosis and/or inflammation
  - ○ Xanthelasma lipid is esterified cholesterol with replacement of normal unsaturated essential fats with saturated fatty acids, which are poorly metabolized.
- Evaluation
  - ○ Apparent on clinical examination alone and rarely requires biopsy
- Treatment
  - ○ Done for cosmetic reasons as the recurrence rate has been reported as high as 40%
  - ○ Surgical excision may be direct or via a blepharoplasty incision.
  - ○ Defects are often left to heal by granulation, although skin grafting or tissue advancement may be necessary for larger defects.

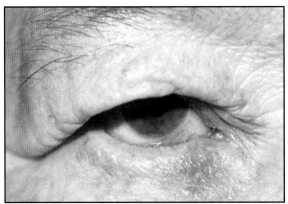

Figure 5-19. Dermatochalasis. (Reprinted with permission from Leal AG, Rodriguez PM. *The Atlas of Ophthalmology.* Thorofare, NJ: SLACK Incorporated; 2002.)

○ A staged approach may be taken for larger lesions with care taken to avoid lagophthalmos or ectropion.
○ CO_2 and Er:Yag laser ablation have been successfully applied.
○ Trichloroacetic acid (TCA) 50% to 100% treatment often requires multiple applications over several months.
○ Laser and TCA may cause hyperpigmentation or scarring.

Dermatochalasis

- Definition
  ○ Dermatochalasis is redundancy and laxity of the eyelid skin and occasionally orbicularis muscle, which may be associated with fat herniation (steatoblepharon) (Figure 5-19).
- Etiology
  ○ Dermatochalasis usually affects the elderly due to age-related loss of skin elasticity and weakening of the connective tissue of the eyelid.
  ○ Familial predisposition, Graves's ophthalmopathy, trauma, Melkersson-Rosenthal syndrome, and Ehlers-Danlos syndrome are conditions that may contribute to earlier onset of dermatochalasis.
- Signs/symptoms
  ○ Patients often complain of eyelid wrinkles and "bags" and may note a tired or aged appearance.
  ○ In addition to cosmetic changes, overhanging upper lid skin may obstruct vision, especially when the patient looks down to read. There is often improvement in vision when the patient uses a finger to elevate the upper eyelid skin.
  ○ Patients may notice a sensation of heaviness from the excess lid tissue and fatigue or headache from frontalis overaction.
  ○ Presbyopes with lower lid dermatochalasis sometimes have difficulties if excess skin smudges the bifocal segment.
  ○ Upper lid dermatochalasis can obstruct the superior field of vision, and temporal overhang of the upper lid skin (temporal hooding) may cause a pseudobitemporal hemianopsia. The visual field defects of dermatochalasis resolve when the eyelids are taped up.
  ○ There may be an associated eyelash ptosis, compensatory frontalis overaction, or compensatory chin-up head posture.
- Differential diagnosis
  ○ Brow ptosis and blepharoptosis should be distinguished from dermatochalasis.
  ○ Blepharochalasis is a rare condition characterized by recurrent episodes of eyelid edema usually in young patients, which causes thinning of the eyelid skin and may be a form of angioneurotic edema.
- Evaluation
  ○ Identify pre-existing blepharoptosis, brow ptosis, lacrimal gland (LG) prolapse, or horizontal lid laxity. Evert the lids to exclude underlying pathology.

- o Lateral bulging of the upper lid should be recognized as the LG, rather than mistaken for a fat pad.
- o If there is horizontal lower lid laxity, this must be corrected prior to lower lid skin excision or else postoperative ectropion may result.
- o In patients undergoing functional blepharoplasty, medical insurance usually requires perimetry documenting improvement of the superior field when the upper lids are taped up.
- Management
  - o Blepharoplasty entails excision of excess skin, orbicularis, and appropriate fat sculpting.
  - o Surgery can be performed with scalpel, radiosurgery, or laser technique and combined with laser skin resurfacing. Transconjunctival blepharoplasty can be performed for fat excision in the lower lid.
  - o The lid crease and skin incisions are marked prior to the injection of local anesthetic. Achieving symmetric upper lid creases is very important for aesthetics. In Asian patients, avoid creation of a high lid crease or excess debulking.
  - o The upper lid skin can be pinched to determine the appropriate amount of skin that can be excised without impairing eyelid closure.
  - o Aggressive fat removal should be avoided because a hollow "skeletonized" appearance may result.
  - o In lower lid blepharoplasty, it may be advantageous to reposition fat into the hollow "tear trough" area overlying the orbital rim.
- Prognosis
  - o Results are usually good when proper diagnosis and surgical technique are used.
  - o Possible problems following blepharoplasty include hemorrhage, infection, worsening of dry eye, corneal exposure from lagophthalmos or lower lid ectropion, asymmetric or irregular eyelid creases, residual redundant skin, and rounding of the lateral canthus.
  - o Retrobulbar hemorrhage
    - ▪ Following blepharoplasty can cause blindness and is a feared complication of blepharoplasty
    - ▪ When a patient presents with hematoma, excessive pain, and a relative afferent pupillary defect in the immediate postoperative period, then the blepharoplasty sutures should be opened to allow hematoma drainage.
    - ▪ If the orbit remains tense, canthotomy and cantholysis may be required.
    - ▪ Permanent diplopia after blepharoplasty is uncommon and is usually attributed to injury of the inferior oblique muscle during lower lid blepharoplasty.

Eyebrow Ptosis

- Definition
  - o *Eyebrow ptosis* is defined as drooping of the eyebrows and forehead.
- Etiology
  - o Eyebrow ptosis most often results from involutional changes of the forehead.
  - o Facial nerve palsy may also produce eyebrow ptosis.
- Signs/symptoms
  - o Eyebrow ptosis may become severe enough to decrease the superior visual field.
  - o Due to chronic frontalis muscle compensation, the patient may complain of brow ache, headache, or deep horizontal forehead rhytids.
  - o External evaluation will reveal the eyebrow below the superior orbital rim.
  - o Absence of horizontal forehead rhytids often occurs in cases due to seventh nerve palsy.
  - o Visual field testing may reveal a decreased superior field of vision that improves with manual elevation or taping of the eyebrows.
- Differential diagnosis
  - o The differential diagnosis includes involutional changes, facial nerve palsy, and dermatochalasis.
- Evaluation
  - o Measurement of the distance between the central brow and the superior orbital rim documents the degree of eyebrow ptosis.
  - o Frontalis muscle function is tested by asking the patient to elevate the brows.

- The examiner observes for coexistent dermatochalasis of the eyelids by manually elevating the eyebrows.
  - The forehead and hairline should be evaluated in order to determine the optimal technique for surgical repair.
- Management
  - Treatment depends upon the degree of ptosis, frontalis muscle function, presence of forehead furrows, height of the hairline, density of brow cilia, and patient tolerance for visible scarring.
  - The endoscopic brow lift allows for concealed endoscopic scars. Scars are placed behind the hairline, and the dissection proceeds along the subperiosteal plane to release the brow from its attachments along the superior orbital rim. The brow is then elevated and fixated.
  - The coronal forehead lift uses an incision that arches from ear to ear and is less desirable in patients with a high hairline. Incisions can also be placed near the hairline.
  - The midforehead lift uses a deep forehead crease for incision placement.
  - Excising a crescent-shaped segment of skin at the temporal hairline can elevate the lateral brow.
  - Direct brow elevation uses crescent-shaped incisions at the superior eyebrow edge, but it may result in conspicuous scarring or an unacceptable arch.
  - BTX injection can address mild to moderate eyebrow ptosis.
  - Recently, the use of suspension sutures has been advocated as a less invasive method for brow elevation.
- Prognosis
  - Because a variety of techniques may successfully address eyebrow ptosis, the choice of technique should be decided upon by the patient and surgeon after explanation of all options.

Floppy Eyelid Syndrome

- Definition
  - Floppy eyelid syndrome (FES) was described by Culbertson and Ostler in 1981 as an uncommon and often underdiagnosed cause of chronic unilateral or bilateral papillary conjunctivitis due to loose eyelids that lose contact with the globe during sleep.
- Etiology
  - Both histopathologic and mechanical factors play important roles in FES.
  - FES is most common in middle-aged, obese men, especially those with sleep apnea syndrome.
  - When these individuals sleep face down or on one side, unilateral conjunctivitis occurs on the preferred sleeping side.
  - The tarsal conjunctiva and cornea rub against the adjacent bedding (mattress or pillow).
  - Over time, the loose and easily everted eyelids become even more lax and rubbery.
  - There may be associated tear film abnormality, poor lid to globe apposition, LG prolapse, and rarely keratoconus.
- Signs/symptoms
  - Patients often present with nonspecific chronic irritation, redness, burning, tearing, and ropy mucus discharge.
  - Patients have seen several physicians before the correct diagnosis was recognized.
  - In addition to a "velvety" superior tarsal papillary conjunctivitis, these patients will exhibit unusually pliant and rubbery upper eyelids that are easily everted (Figure 5-20).
  - There may be associated eyelash ptosis, blepharoptosis, and loss of eyelash parallelism.
  - Slit-lamp examination often shows tear-film abnormalities and a superficial punctate keratopathy.
- Differential diagnosis
  - The differential diagnosis includes any cause of superior tarsal papillary conjunctivitis including giant papillary conjunctivitis (GPC), vernal conjunctivitis, superior limbic keratoconjunctivitis (SLK), and toxic keratoconjunctivitis.
  - Chronic bacterial conjunctivitis, blepharitis, dacryocystitis, canaliculitis, or molluscum contagiosum may also produce a chronic unilateral conjunctivitis with mucus discharge.
- Diagnosis and evaluation
  - The pathognomonic diagnostic finding is that simple traction on the upper eyelid will cause the eyelid to readily evert (see Figure 5-20).

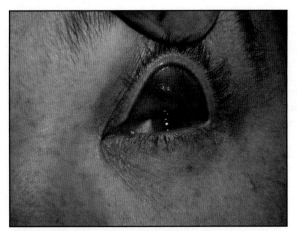

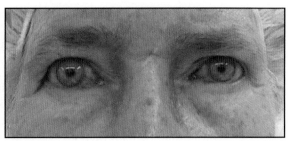

Figure 5-21. Bilateral eyelid retraction associated with thyroid-related ophthalmopathy.

Figure 5-20. Loose rubbery and easily everted eyelids of floppy eyelid syndrome.

- o The inflamed upper tarsal and palpebral conjunctiva will be red, velvety, and demonstrate confluent large papillae.
- o Slit-lamp examination of conjunctiva and cornea should be performed, and ancillary tests of the tear film are often helpful.
- Management and prognosis
- o Conservative management with a protective eye shield or patch at night, avoidance of eyelid rubbing, and topical lubricants will sometimes help.
- o Patients are encouraged to change their sleeping posture, but this is rarely successful.
- o Definitive treatment consists of horizontal eyelid shortening, which often alleviates symptoms.
- o Obese patients with a history of daytime sleepiness, loud snoring, and disruptive sleep should be evaluated for sleep apnea syndrome.

Eyelid Retraction

- Definition
- o Retraction results from shrinkage or fibrosis of the eyelid retractor muscles (levator palpebrae muscle of upper lid and capsule-palpebral head and fascia of the lower eyelid), which retracts the eyelid and exposes the sclera above the superior pole or below the inferior pole of the limbus (Figure 5-21).
- Etiology
- o Usually from thyroid eye disease, but may arise from metastatic breast cancer, trauma, or idiopathic causes
- Signs/symptoms
- o May include exposure of the globe, cornea, and conjunctiva; dry eye symptoms; photosensitivity.
- o Eyelid retraction, eyelid signs related to thyroid eye disease, stare, lid twitch, setting sun sign, lagophthalmos, and lack of eyelid closure during sleep
- Differential diagnosis
- o Orbital mass lesion (hemangioma, tumor, lacrimal mass, lymphoproliferative lesions), post-traumatic scar bands, symblepharon, and idiopathic
- Evaluation
- o Thyroid function test, thyroid stimulating immunoglobulin (TSI) level, CT scan, or magnetic resonance imaging (MRI) scan
- Management
- o When lubricants and medical management fails, recession of the eyelid retractors may be performed.
- o Recession may be coupled with placement of spacer materials such as AlloDerm, autogenous fascia lata, or temporalis fascia graft.

- ○ The ratio of degree of recession to end result should be at least 2.5X to 3X (for example, to get a 3-mm recession, one needs to recess back the levator at least 8 to 9 mm).
- Prognosis
  - ○ Poor surgical predictability in that only about two-thirds of patients achieve a satisfactory lid height after the first surgical recession.

Facial Nerve Palsy

- Definition
  - ○ Central or upper motor neuron seventh nerve palsy relatively spares the upper face, and eyelid closure due to bilateral innervation of the "upper" facial nerve nucleus.
  - ○ Peripheral or lower motor neuron seventh nerve palsy affects the ipsilateral upper and lower facial muscles. Peripheral facial palsy is usually due to a lesion of the ipsilateral facial nerve, but can occur with lesions of the ipsilateral facial nucleus or the facial nerve in the pons.
- Etiology
  - ○ Bell's palsy is the most common cause of peripheral facial nerve palsy and is likely the result of herpes simplex-related (HSV-1) swelling of the facial nerve in the long confined space of the osseous fallopian canal. Risk factors include diabetes, arteriosclerosis, pregnancy, and family history of facial nerve palsy.
  - ○ Infectious causes include herpes zoster oticus (Ramsay Hunt syndrome), Lyme disease, otitis media, HIV, infectious mononucleosis, other viral illness, and perhaps postimmunization.
  - ○ Inflammatory causes include sarcoidosis.
  - ○ Trauma and various neoplasms including acoustic schwannoma or other cerebellopontine angle tumor, brainstem glioma, metastasis, and parotid tumor can cause facial nerve palsy.
  - ○ Other causes include Möbius syndrome, hemifacial microsomia, and birth trauma.
- Signs/symptoms
  - ○ Sudden onset suggests Bell's palsy or infection.
  - ○ Insidious onset suggests tumor (eg, in the parotid gland).
  - ○ Patients may complain of corneal irritation, blurry vision, and tearing.
  - ○ Retroauricular pain is not uncommon in acute facial nerve palsy.
  - ○ There may be hyperacusis if the stapedius reflex is lost.
  - ○ Taste in the anterior tongue may be impaired, and patients may complain of drooling.
  - ○ Lower facial weakness is detected by asking patients to show their teeth, rather than smile.
  - ○ Central and peripheral facial nerve palsies are usually unilateral and show weakness of the lower face with loss of the nasolabial fold.
  - ○ Upper facial weakness can be detected by asking patients to wrinkle their brows and close the eyelids. Central seventh nerve palsies will show relative preservation of the brow furrows and lid closure. Peripheral seventh nerve palsies will show weakness of the frontalis, often with brow ptosis, decreased eyelid closure (lagophthalmos), loss of the spontaneous blink, and lower lid ectropion.
  - ○ There may be decreased tear production if the nervus intermedius (sensory and parasympathetic root of the facial nerve) is involved.
  - ○ Epiphora may be due to reflex tearing from corneal irritation, dysfunctional eyelid tear pump, or aberrant seventh nerve regeneration.
  - ○ Examination for lagophthalmos, Bell's phenomenon (globe elevation on forced lid closure), corneal integrity, Schirmer's test, and corneal sensation are important.
  - ○ Optic canal vesicles may aid in the diagnosis of herpes zoster.
  - ○ Palpation of the parotid gland through the mouth can be performed.
- Differential diagnosis
  - ○ Patients with Bell's palsy may believe they have suffered a stroke. With recurrent or bilateral facial nerve palsy sarcoidosis, Lyme disease, Möbius syndrome, -Rosenthal syndrome, and Guillain-Barré syndrome should be considered. Uncommon mimics of bilateral facial nerve palsy include myasthenia gravis and myotonic dystrophy.
- Evaluation
  - ○ Central facial nerve palsy should be evaluated with MRI.
  - ○ Workup of peripheral seventh nerve palsy depends on the suspected etiology (eg, a history of tick bite or erythema chronicum migrans requires testing for Lyme disease).

- o Baseline diabetes screening may be useful. In patients with complete loss of voluntary facial function, electroneurography performed at 4 to 14 days postparalysis may help predict recovery.
- o If facial nerve function does not improve after a month, neuroimaging should be performed.
- Management
  - o Ocular lubrication is essential for all facial nerve palsies with corneal exposure. Lubricating drops can be used during the day, and ointment instilled at night. When drops are required more than 6 times per day, preservative-free preparations are better tolerated.
  - o Moisture chambers, taping the lids closed, and digitally closing the lids may help.
  - o Cochrane database review supports the use of systemic steroids (eg, 60 mg prednisone x 5 days with taper) in Bell's palsy. The utility of additional antivirals has been questioned.
  - o Tarsorrhaphy should be performed early in patients with peripheral seventh nerve palsy and corneal anesthesia. Usually, the lateral third of the lids are sutured together.
  - o Other options include lower lid tightening, upper lid weights, and midface lifts. For severe lower lid retraction, a posterior lamellar graft or midface lift may be required. Upper lid weights work by gravity. Temporary external upper lid load weights are adhered with double-sided tape. Permanent gold weights are surgically implanted. Brow ptosis can be repaired if the patient can achieve adequate lid closure. Facial re-animation techniques such as hypoglossal-facial re-anastamosis are available.
- Prognosis
  - o In patients with absent Bell's phenomenon, absent corneal sensation, or dry eye, the cornea may be seriously damaged.
  - o The prognosis for Bell's palsy is good, even without treatment, and 84% of patients have almost full recovery after a few months.
  - o Facial nerve function following acoustic schwannoma surgery may vary with tumor size and surgical manipulation.

Essential Blepharospasm, Facial Dystonia, and Hemifacial Spasm

- Definition
  - o Essential blepharospasm represents bilateral involuntary spasms of the orbicularis oculi, corrugators, and procerus muscles while awake.
  - o Oromandibular dystonia occurring with essential blepharospasm is called Meige syndrome.
  - o Hemifacial spasm is characterized by unilateral intermittent synchronous contractures of the orbicularis oculi and other facial mimetic muscles.
- Etiology
  - o Essential blepharospasm occurs in isolation without other evidence of neurologic or ocular disease.
  - o Many patients show evidence of brainstem dysfunction, and the basal ganglia play a central role in the etiology of this dystonia.
  - o Hemifacial spasm results from pulsatile compression of the facial nerve at the root entry zone by aberrantly located or dolichoectatic vessels.
- Signs/symptoms
  - o Patients with essential blepharospasm show frequent squeezing and blinking, often in response to stimuli such as sunlight, wind, noise, movement, or stress.
  - o Patients may complain of inability to open the eyes, termed *apraxia* of eyelid opening.
  - o Hemifacial spasm typically begins in the orbicularis oculi and then spreads over time to involve the lower facial muscles.
  - o Voluntary facial movements, fatigue, stress, or anxiety may cause or worsen spasms.
  - o Patients often complain of a tight or pulling sensation along the affected side.
  - o EMG studies may show abnormalities in essential blepharospasm, and Charcot's sign is a characteristic lowering of the brow.
  - o Patients with hemifacial spasm may exhibit ipsilateral facial nerve weakness.
- Differential diagnosis
  - o Essential blepharospasm should be distinguished from reflex blepharospasm, ocular blepharospasm, blepharospasm associated with tardive dyskinesia, and other conditions such as facial tics, Tourette's syndrome, nonorganic blepharospasm, and focal seizures.
- Evaluation
  - o The patient with essential blepharospasm should be evaluated for apraxia eyelid opening and Meige syndrome.

- o Secondary causes for ocular blepharospasm such as ocular surface disease should be excluded.
- o Most cases of hemifacial spasm are caused by vascular compression from otherwise normal arteries or veins, abnormal vascular structures. However, aneurysms or arteriovenous malformation (AVM) may cause hemifacial spasm. Workup for hemifacial spasm often includes MRI in order to exclude pathologic compression of the facial nerve at the root entry zone.
- Management
  - o Medical therapies such as carbamazepine, diphenylhydantoin, and dimethylaminoethanol have shown disappointing results.
  - o BTX temporarily chemodenervates the dystonic facial muscles.
  - o Myectomy surgery can effectively control refractory essential blepharospasm for up to 5 years in most patients.
  - o Posterior fossa microvascular decompression may cure hemifacial spasm in up to 90% of cases.
- Prognosis
  - o Both essential blepharospasm and hemifacial spasm typically cause chronic spasms that significantly decrease quality of life.
  - o However, repeated BTX injection or surgery often effectively manages symptoms.

Syndromes With Eyelid Features

- Amyloidosis
  - o Familial amyloidosis may be autosomal dominant.
  - o Orbital infiltrates and marked dermatochalasis with cutaneous infiltration
  - o Dominant corneal dystrophy characterized by amyloid accumulation
- Ankyloblepharon
  - o Partial or complete fusion of the eyelids by webs of skin
  - o Lateral ankyloblepharon more common than medial
- Apert's syndrome (Acrocephalosyndactyly)
  - o Similar to Crouzon's, but with syndactyly
  - o Autosomal dominant
  - o Ptosis with antimongoloid slant
- Blepharophimosis syndrome
  - o Autosomal dominant
  - o Telecanthus, epicanthus inversus, phimosis of the lids and ptosis
  - o Lower lid ectropion and retraction may occur.
  - o Medial canthal tendons are abnormally long.
  - o Ptosis is usually associated with little or no demonstrable LF.
  - o Correction of the epicanthus and telecanthus is followed by ptosis repair.
- Chronic progressive external ophthalmoplegia
  - o Mitochondrial myopathy: Diagnosis by muscle biopsy or polymerase chain reaction testing
  - o Progressive bilateral ptosis followed by ophthalmoparesis
  - o Bell's phenomenon is often absent. Ptosis surgery should be conservative. Use of frontalis slings is reversible and usually the preferred technique.
- Coloboma
  - o Cleft usually in medial upper eyelid; lower lid colobomas usually temporal
  - o May be associated with other facial clefts (Pierre Robin syndrome), lacrimal deformities, and Goldenhar's syndrome
  - o Large colobomas may be caused by amniotic bands.
  - o Avoid using lid-sharing procedures (Hughes, Cutler-Beard) to repair colobomas in infants and children, which may lead to occlusion amblyopia.
- Congenital fibrosis
  - o Autosomal dominant or sporadic
  - o Ptosis, restriction of EOMs, fibrous replacement of the muscles
  - o Poor Bell's phenomenon
- Crouzon's syndrome (Craniofacial dysostosis)
  - o Premature craniosynostosis of the coronal, sagittal, and lambdoid sutures, hypoplastic midface
  - o Autosomal dominant with complete penetrance
  - o Proptosis secondary to shallow orbits may cause exposure keratitis, exotropia, optic atrophy (in 50%), keratoconus, ectopia lentis, iris coloboma, superior rectus hypoplasia, parrot's beak nose.

- Cryptophthalmos
  - Partial or complete absence of the eyebrow, palpebral fissure, eyelashes, and conjunctiva, with fusion of the partially developed adnexal structures to underlying globe
  - Globe is usually malformed and microphthalmic.
  - May be part of an autosomal recessive syndrome associated with dyscephaly, syndactyly, genitourinary abnormalities
- Distichiasis
  - Congenital or acquired extra row of eyelashes present in place of the openings of meibomian glands
  - Congenital form is dominantly inherited; it may be associated with ptosis and strabismus.
  - Acquired distichiasis may be caused by severe chemical burns, Stevens-Johnson syndrome (SJS), pemphigoid or chronic blepharoconjunctivitis.
  - Initial treatment includes ocular lubricants and soft contact lenses.
  - Surgical treatments
    - Cryotherapy
    - Lid splitting with cryotherapy
    - Excision of the involved tarsal plate with mucosal graft
- Ehlers-Danlos syndrome
  - Marked dermatochalasis may be present.
  - Type VI (autosomal recessive) may present with retinal detachments, microcornea, myopia.
- Epicanthus
  - Medial canthal skin fold
  - Fold most prominent in the upper lid
  - Fold most prominent in the lower lid
  - Fold equally distributed between the upper and lower lids
- Epiblepharon
  - Excess pretarsal orbicularis muscle and skin override the eyelid margin to turn eyelashes vertically or against the globe.
  - The lid margin itself is not rotated inward as in entropion.
  - Over time, this resolves in many children.
  - Surgical repair is sometimes necessary—a strip of skin and orbicularis are excised just below or above the eyelid margin, and the defect is closed.
- Euryblepharon
  - Widening of palpebral fissure caused by horizontal lengthening of the temporal portion of the lower eyelid and vertical skin shortening
  - May be autosomal dominant
  - Lateral canthal tendon is often inferiorly displaced.
  - Surgical repair includes a full-thickness block resection of the involved eyelid, repositioning of the lateral canthal tendon, and full-thickness skin graft to the area of vertical shortening.
- Familial hypercholesterolemia
  - Autosomal dominant
  - May present with xanthelasma in eyelids but most patients with xanthelasma do not have familial hypercholesterolemia
- Fetal alcohol syndrome
  - Caused by drinking alcohol during pregnancy: 0.2 to 1.5 per 1000 live births
  - Abnormal facial features, growth deficiencies, and central nervous system (CNS) problems
  - Ptosis, microphthalmia, strabismus, short palpebral fissures, epicanthic folds, blepharophimosis, myopia, cataracts, glaucoma, retinal coloboma
  - Hypertelorism, midface hypoplasia, short, upturned nose, wide philtrum, thin upper lip, cleft palate, posterior rotation of ears
- Goldenhar's syndrome (Oculoauriculovertebral dysplasia)
  - Sporadic in most cases
  - Lid colobomas, preauricular skin tags, limbal dermoids, vertebral anomalies, mandibular hypoplasia, microstomia. Ptosis, microphthalmia, cleft palate/lip (in 10% of cases).
- Gorlin's syndrome (Basal cell nevus syndrome)
  - Autosomal dominant cancer syndrome: genetic locus for Gorlin's syndrome is on chromosome bands 9q22.3-q31. Forty percent are new mutants.

- o Propensity to develop BCa and medulloblastoma
- o Marked sensitivity to ionizing radiation and sunlight
- Guillain-Barré syndrome
  - o Subacute primarily motor neuropathy; often occurs after a viral illness
  - o Bilateral ophthalmoplegia and ptosis may occur, pupils dilated and poorly reactive, facial diplegia.
  - o Cerebrospinal fluid (CSF) shows an elevated protein with few cells.
- Hemicraniofacial microsomia
  - o Low-set ears, short mandibular ramus, micrognathia, chin deviation, zygomatic arch deformities, lateral canthal displacement, side of the face hypoplastic or vertically short
  - o Mandibular hypoplasia
- Horner syndrome
  - o Signs produced when sympathetic innervation to the eye is interrupted
  - o Mild-to-moderate ptosis because of denervation of Müller's muscle, slight elevation of lower lid, miosis and dilation lag, iris heterochromia may occur in longstanding cases and in cases that occur younger than 2 years
- Hypertelorism (Greig's syndrome)
  - o Orbits and contents shifted laterally by a midline cleft or excessive ethmoid sinuses
  - o Antimongoloid slant of the eyelids, flat nasal bridge
- Marcus Gunn's syndrome (Jaw-winking syndrome)
  - o Ptosis with lid becoming retracted when patient opens the mouth and contracts the external pterygoid muscle
  - o Less commonly, lid retracts when patient clenches teeth and uses the internal pterygoid muscle.
  - o Caused by abnormal innervation of the levator muscle by the fifth nerve
- Myotonic dystrophy
  - o Autosomal dominant
  - o Bilateral ptosis, orbicularis weakness, poor blinking, chromatic cataracts
  - o Testicular atrophy, diabetes mellitus, first-degree heart block, frontal alopecia, temporal wasting, prolonged contraction of muscles
- Neurofibromatosis 1 (NF1)
  - o Disorder of the neuroectodermal system resulting in benign hamartomatous tumors of the skin, the eyes, and the nervous system
  - o Fifty percent are autosomal dominant; 50% are spontaneous mutations.
  - o Prevalence is 1 in 3000
  - o Café au lait spots, diffuse hyperpigmentation, hypopigmentation, cutaneous neurofibromas
  - o Optic nerve and optic chiasm gliomas in NF1 and NF2
  - o Meningiomas more common in NF2
  - o Lisch nodules on iris (benign hamartomas)
  - o Plexiform neurofibromas of the eyelid causing an S-shaped deformity
  - o Prominent corneal nerves, congenital glaucoma
  - o Absence of the greater wing of the sphenoid bone may lead to pulsatile proptosis
- Oculopharyngeal dystrophy
  - o Autosomal dominant; many have French Canadian ancestry
  - o Begins after age 40; slowly progressive ptosis with dysphagia and dysarthria
- Parinaud's syndrome
  - o Dorsal midbrain syndrome associated with bilateral upper lid retraction (Coller sign)
- Telecanthus
  - o Widened intercanthal distance with a normal interpupillary distance
  - o Soft tissue abnormality; bony orbits are normal
  - o May be associated with blepharophimosis or may be isolated
- Treacher Collins syndrome (Mandibulofacial dysostosis)
  - o Autosomal dominant with variable penetrance
  - o Bilateral condition that affects the first and second arch structures
  - o Malar hypoplasia, micrognathia
  - o Antimongoloid slant of the palpebral fissures, colobomas of the lower lids, absence of eyelashes medially, face may be fishlike
  - o Deafness and mental retardation may be present.

- Turner syndrome
  - ○ Occurs in females: have only 44 autosomes and one sex chromosome
  - ○ Webbed neck, cubitus valgus, ovarian agenesis, dwarfism, lower hairline, mandibular deformity, webbed elbows and knees, hypertension, lymphedema of hands and feet
  - ○ Ptosis, strabismus, cataracts, epicanthal folds, red-green color blindness
  - ○ Diagnosis by doing a buccal smear
- Waardenburg syndrome
  - ○ Autosomal dominant with variable penetrance
  - ○ Sensorineural deafness, widely spaced medial canthi, synophrys (confluent eyebrows), poliosis (white forelock) occurs in 20% to 40% and heterochromia irides in 30%
  - ○ Craniosynostosis, blepharophimosis, and glaucoma
- Xeroderma pigmentosum
  - ○ Autosomal recessive
  - ○ Hypersensitivity to ultraviolet radiation. It causes defects in DNA repair and synthesis, resulting in BCa, SqCa, and melanoma.
  - ○ SqCa of the conjunctiva is more common.

Principles of Eyelid Reconstruction

- General principles
  - ○ Basic principles of eyelid reconstruction are applicable regardless of the etiology of the defect, although the choice of technique will depend on the nature and size of the defect, age of patient, availability and mobility of adjacent tissue, and surgeon experience and preference.
  - ○ The basic rules ensure that form follows function.
  - ○ The goals of a reconstructive procedure are to provide for complete eyelid closure and globe protection, an epithelial anterior lamella, a smooth mucus membrane posterior lamella, a stable lid margin that hugs the globe, and adequate lid height without undue vertical tension.
  - ○ All of this is achieved while maximizing symmetry and cosmesis.
  - ○ The adherence to several basic principles will allow for an optimal outcome.
    - Prior to initiating reconstruction, narrow the defect as much as possible with horizontal tension and possible canthal lysis.
    - Use the simplest, least invasive technique possible to perform the reconstruction.
    - Select graft tissues to maximize symmetry and cosmesis.
    - Reconstruct the anterior or posterior lamella with a graft, but not both unless creating a blood supply for one graft.
    - Maximize horizontal tension and minimize vertical tension
    - If you encounter a defect, you cannot close, stop, patch the eye, and seek subspecialist consultation. As long as the eye is protected, the reconstruction can be delayed. An optimal result is more likely when the tissues available for reconstruction have not been previously used.
- Partial-thickness eyelid defects
  - ○ These may be repaired by direct closure, flaps, or grafts.
  - ○ The preferred donor skin graft sites are the contralateral or opposing eyelid (blepharoplasty), postauricular, or supraclavicular skin.
  - ○ Care must be taken to avoid vertical tension, leading to potential lagophthalmos or ectropion with resultant exposure keratopathy in both the donor and recipient eyelids.
  - ○ When full-thickness defects involve the lid margin, reconstruction depends on the size of the defect and whether the upper or lower eyelid is involved.
- Upper eyelid full-thickness defects involving the lid margin
  - ○ The reconstructive continuum is as follows:
    - Small defects (<one-third of the lid margin): Direct closure, possible lateral canthotomy, and superior cantholysis. Ensure that the tarsal surface is smooth without buckling. This may require the resection of a small amount of residual tarsus.
    - Moderate defects (up to one-half of the lid margin): Lateral canthotomy, superior cantholysis with mobilization of a lateral canthal flap (inverse Tenzel semicircular rotation flap), or tarsal mobilization from adjacent remaining tarsus with sliding or free skin flap

- Large defects (>one-half of the lid margin): Full-thickness opposing eyelid pedicle flap from the lower lid (Cutler- Beard), median forehead rotation flap, lower lid to upper lid marginal rotation flap, free tarsal graft covered by a sliding skin, muscle flap
- Lower lid full-thickness defects involving the lid margin
  - The reconstructive continuum is as follows:
    - Small defects (<one-third of the lid margin): Direct closure, possible lateral canthotomy, and inferior cantholysis
    - Moderate defects (up to one-half of the lid margin): Tenzel semicircular rotation flap, periosteal rotational flap, tarsoconjunctival opposing eyelid pedicle flap (Hughes)
    - Large defects (>one-half of the lid margin): Hughes reconstruction, cheek rotation flap (Mustarde)
    - Regardless of the size of the defect or the lid that is involved, the reconstructive techniques all adhere to the principles mentioned above.
    - Adherence to these principles will allow for a functional lid with an acceptable aesthetic outcome.

Eyelid Trauma

- Definition
  - Eyelid injuries may be categorized as blunt or sharp, clean or contaminated, and involving or not involving the lid margin.
- Etiology
  - Blunt injuries are often due to falls, motor vehicle accidents, and blows from blunt objects such as fists or balls, whereas sharp injuries result from stab wounds, glass, metal fragments, tree branches, or dog bites.
- Signs/symptoms
  - Victims of eyelid lacerations will have pain, tearing, and blurred vision.
  - Often, there is a laceration, swelling, ecchymosis, hemorrhage, and tearing.
- Evaluation
  - After a complete history stressing the mechanism of trauma, the first priority is to check the underlying globe for injuries and to rule out occult foreign bodies.
  - The visual acuity, extent of the lid injuries, and an assessment of LF and integrity of canthal tendons should be performed.
  - The presence of orbital fat increases the likelihood of damage to the levator muscle, aponeurosis, and underlying globe.
  - Medial lid margin lacerations may involve the canaliculus.
  - Radiologic imaging studies should be obtained in cases of a suspected foreign body or fracture.
- Management
  - In the absence of a serious eye injury or a life-threatening injury, primary plastic repair should ensue; however, in many cases surgery can be delayed for 48 hours without affecting the long-term results.
  - Foreign materials such as dirt and wood should be removed, but eyelid wounds should not be excessively débrided because even marginally viable eyelid tissues often survive given their excellent blood supply.
  - The tissues should be thoroughly irrigated and tetanus prophylaxis given if indicated.
  - Repair of full-thickness lid margin injuries requires a precise anatomical eyelid realignment to provide the best function and appearance.
  - Lacerations away from the lid margin should be closed tension-free to avoid broad scars. It is best to avoid deep sutures. Skin grafts and flaps are rarely necessary.
  - When tissue segments are missing or if the levator muscle or canaliculus is involved, patients should be referred to an oculoplastic surgeon skilled in complex eyelid repair.
  - Secondary repair to address cicatricial changes and ptosis may be necessary in some cases.
  - Broad-spectrum systemic antibiotics should be prescribed if the wound is contaminated in case of bites or if repair is delayed. The vision should be monitored and topical antibiotic ointment and dressings should be applied as necessary.
- Prognosis
  - With a sound understanding of eyelid anatomy, proper wound management and meticulous primary repair, the prognosis is excellent for both function and appearance.

Orbit

Evaluation of the Orbit

- The orbit is systematically evaluated using the mnemonic of the "6 Ps"
    - Pain
    - Progression
    - Proptosis
    - Palpation
    - Pulsation
    - Periorbital changes
- Painful orbital processes usually have an underlying infectious or inflammatory disease, acute retrobulbar hemorrhage, or malignant LG tumor. Sudden onset usually points to an infectious, inflammatory, or aggressive neoplastic process such as orbital cellulitis, nonspecific orbital inflammation, or rhabdomyosarcoma. Conditions that develop over weeks to even years include dermoids, pleomorphic adenomas (PAs) of the LG, and cavernous hemangiomas.
- *Proptosis* and *exophthalmos* are terms used to describe protrusion of the eye.
    - Hertel exophthalmometry measurements measure the protrusion distance in millimeters from the lateral orbital rim to the anterior corneal surface (Figure 5-22).
    - Relative proptosis is best seen when the examiner looks up from below with the patient's head tilted back (ie, "frog's eye view").
    - The direction of globe displacement helps to localize the lesion.
        - Axial or forward displacement is caused by retrobulbar, intraconal tumors directly behind the globe, such as optic nerve gliomas (OGs) and meningiomas.
        - The globe can be displaced upward by tumors originating from the maxillary sinus or downward by frontal sinus mucoceles or frontal bone tumors.
        - Large orbital floor fractures can also allow the globe to settle inferiorly.
        - Inferomedial displacement is most commonly caused by lacrimal tumors or dermoid cysts that arise from the frontozygomatic suture.
    - Both unilateral and bilateral proptosis in adults is most often caused by thyroid associated orbitopathy (TAO) and less frequently by other inflammation or neoplasms.
    - In children, bilateral proptosis may be caused by metastatic neuroblastoma, leukemia, or nonspecific orbital inflammation, whereas unilateral proptosis is most likely caused by orbital cellulitis.
    - *Enophthalmos* is a term used to describe a globe that is sunken into the socket and may be caused by sclerosing tumors, such as metastatic breast cancer or large orbital bone fractures.
- Palpation of the orbital rims in trauma is important to identify bony step-offs representing fractures. Palpation around the globe may reveal the presence of a mass in the anterior orbit, especially if there is LG enlargement or a dermoid cyst. Lesions in the superonasal area can include mucoceles or encephaloceles. One tests for retropulsion by gently pressing on the globe and feeling for resistance. Increased resistance to retropulsion is a nonspecific abnormality from either a retrobulbar tumor or diffuse inflammation.
- Pulsations of the eye are caused by transmission of the vascular pulse through the orbit. Bruits may be detected with a stethoscope or subjectively described by patients. Pulsation without bruits may be transmitted from the cranial vault to the orbit when there is absence of intervening orbital bone as may be seen in neurofibromatosis, meningoencephaloceles, or surgical removal of the orbital roof. Pulsation with bruits is most likely detected in a high-flow carotid cavernous fistula.
- Periorbital changes associated with thyroid-related ophthalmopathy (TRO) include retraction of the upper and lower eyelids, upper eyelid lag on downgaze, and vascular congestion over the rectus muscles. Other typical clinical signs include a salmon-colored conjunctival mass in lymphoma, an S-shaped lid in neurofibromatosis, and black-crusted cutaneous or nasal mucosal lesions in mucormycosis.

Disorders of the Orbit

Congenital Orbital Conditions

- Embryology
    - The orbit begins developing in the fourth through eighth gestational week.

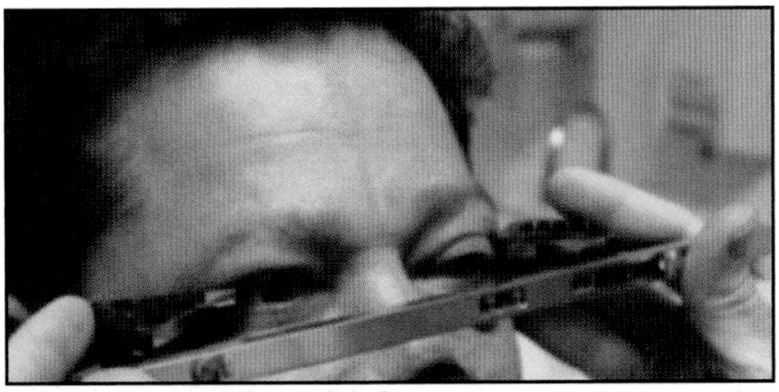

Figure 5-22. Hertel exophthalmometer measuring protrusion distance in millimeters from the lateral orbital rim to the anterior corneal surface.

- o Bone development is finalized during the fourth gestational month after the anteromedial rotation of the eyes.
- o Soft tissue development ends with the separation of lid fusion in the seventh month.
- o The mostly cartilaginous fetal cranium begins formation during week 7.
- Synophthalmia
  - o True cyclopia, or a single eye, is extremely rare.
  - o Synophthalmia, the fusion of both eyes into a single midline cavity, occurs more commonly.
  - o The degree of fusion is variable and is secondary to failed development and descent of the embryologic nasal process.
  - o A proboscis-like projection rests in the facial midline above the fused eye.
  - o Coexistent brain and ocular anomalies frequently occur.
- Anophthalmia
  - o True congenital anophthalmia is rare and due to failure to form a primary optic vesicle.
  - o Most cases are sporadic and can be unilateral or bilateral.
  - o Associated ocular findings can include an absence of EOMs, a reduced optic canal diameter, and poorly formed conjunctival fornices.
- Microphthalmia
  - o Microphthalmia is much more common than true anophthalmia.
  - o Severe cases can be mistaken as clinical anophthalmia.
  - o It may be sporadic or heritable, and the degree of visual dysfunction varies.
  - o Predominantly unilateral
  - o When bilateral, other organ system anomalies are often found.
  - o Microphthalmia is frequently accompanied by an attached cyst that forms due to failed closure of the fetal/choroidal fissure.
  - o Associated ocular findings include microcornea, cataract, aniridia, and persistent hypertrophic primary vitreous.
  - o Systemic associations can occur such as in microphthalmia dermal aplasia sclerocornea (MIDAS) syndrome.
  - o Genetic anomalies (13q deletion syndrome, trisomy 18) have been detected.
  - o Microphthalmia may induce a secondary hypoplasia of the orbit that requires aggressive socket expansion (serial acrylic conformers, dermis fat graft, soft tissue expanders).
  - o In cases with a coexistent cyst, cystic expansion helps induce orbital bone and eyelid development.
  - o Some cysts are managed by simple observation; others may require needle aspiration or surgical excision.
- Cryptophthalmia
  - o Failed formation of the ocular adnexa
  - o Patients present with partial or complete absence of the eyebrows, palpebral fissure, eyelashes, and conjunctiva (Figure 5-23).
  - o The malformed ocular adnexa may be fused to the globe and associated with ocular surface and intraocular defects.
  - o The condition can be unilateral or bilateral and can demonstrate an autosomal recessive inheritance.
  - o Syndactyly and genitourinary anomalies have been reported.

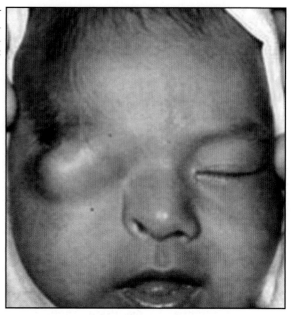

Figure 5-23. Cryptophthalmia. Patients present with partial or complete absence of the eyebrows, palpebral fissure, eyelashes, and conjunctiva. (Reprinted with permission from Leal AG, Rodriguez PM. *The Atlas of Ophthalmology*. Thorofare, NJ: SLACK Incorporated; 2002.)

- o Pseudocryptophthalmos is failure of the lids to separate from the globe but with an underlying intact globe.
- Hypertelorism
  - o Present when the 2 bony orbits are widely separated
  - o This differs from telecanthus (a widened medial canthus) and exorbitism (an angle of orbital divergence greater than 90 degrees).
  - o Primary hypertelorism results from the failed development of the embryologic maxillary process.
  - o Ocular defects may include exodeviations, microphthalmia, microcornea, and optic atrophy.
- Craniosynostosis
  - o Results from the premature closure of one or more dural sutures.
  - o Closure of a suture halts bone growth while growth parallel to the suture continues.
  - o Single-suture closure produces characteristic cranial dysmorphisms (coronal suture—brachycephaly; sagittal suture—scaphocephaly; lamboidal suture—plagiocephaly; metopic suture—trigonocephaly).
- Crouzon's syndrome (Craniofacial dysostosis)
  - o Presents as the triad of craniofacialsynostosis, midface hypoplasia, and exophthalmos
  - o Premature closure of multiple sutures results in a cranial dysmorphism that is unclassifiable.
  - o Restricted cranial growth limits central nervous system development and requires the surgical opening of the fused sutures.
  - o Midface hypoplasia results in shallow orbits and exophthalmos requiring ocular surface exposure management.
  - o Other ocular findings include hypertelorism, exorbitism, and strabismus.
- Apert's syndrome (Acrocephalosyndactyly)
  - o Presents with craniosynostosis and symmetric syndactyly of the hands and feet
  - o The coronal suture (brachycephaly) is most commonly affected, and syndactyly is often of the second, third, and fourth digits.
  - o Ocular findings are similar to Crouzon's syndrome, but less severe, and many patients have cardiac and visceral anomalies.

Orbital Infections

- Bacterial infections of the orbit or periorbital soft tissues are divided into preseptal versus orbital cellulitis. Orbital involvement arises through direct spread from adjacent sinusitis, direct inoculation following trauma, and skin infection or bacteremic spread from an endogenous site.

- Preseptal cellulitis
  - Definition
    - Inflammation and infection limited to the eyelids and periorbital structures anterior to the orbital septum
  - Etiology
    - The most common pathogens include *Streptococcus* species and *Staphylococcus aureus.*
    - Although *Haemophilus influenzae* was the most prevalent organism in preseptal and orbital cellulitis in the pediatric age group, it has become much less common since the introduction of the HiB vaccine in 1985.
  - Signs/symptoms
    - Clinical signs include eyelid edema and erythema without involvement of more posterior structures.
    - Visual acuity, pupil reactivity, and ocular motility are normal, and there is no pain on eye movement.
    - It is important to identify a local site of infection such as a stye, insect bite, or dacryocystitis.
  - Treatment
    - Treatment of preseptal cellulitis includes an oral antibiotic such as cephalexin or amoxicillin/clavulanate to cover the most common pathogens.
    - Imaging studies help to locate underlying sinusitis or orbital abscess when no obvious external source of infection is present or when no improvement is seen after 24 to 48 hours on oral antibiotics.
    - When extensive sinus disease is identified, intravenous antibiotics may be considered, and an ear, nose, and throat doctor should be consulted to consider sinus drainage. Surgical incision and drainage may be necessary if preseptal cellulitis progresses to a localized superficial abscess.
- Orbital cellulitis
  - Definition
    - Most orbital cellulitis arises in conjunction with preseptal cellulitis and sinusitis (Figures 5-24 and 5-25).
    - Orbital cellulitis involves infection of the soft tissue structures posterior to the orbital septum.
  - Signs/symptoms
    - Clinical findings include fever, proptosis, chemosis, ocular motility restriction, and pain on eye movement.
    - Decreased vision and pupil abnormalities suggest involvement of the orbital apex and require aggressive and rapid intervention.
    - Delay in treatment may result in cavernous sinus thrombosis, empyema, blindness, and even death.
  - Evaluation/treatment
    - Evaluation of the sinuses by CT scan is required, and broad-spectrum intravenous antibiotics such as ampicillin/sulbactam should be started.
    - If an abscess is noted with imaging, surgical drainage is usually necessary in adults.
    - If no abscess is identified, patients may be cautiously observed for improvement on antibiotic therapy for 24 hours.
    - If there is no improvement, patients should be re-imaged to look for a target for surgical exploration.
- Special forms of orbital infections
  - Orbital cellulitis in infants
    - Requires rapid, urgent, and aggressive diagnosis and treatment because of the rapidity with which infection may overwhelm the infantile immune system and result in sepsis, meningitis, or death.
    - Diagnosis often involves infectious disease consultation, as well as blood cultures and CSF studies.
  - Subperiosteal abscess
    - Results from accumulation of purulent material between the periorbital and orbital bones, and usually occurs as a result of bacterial sinusitis

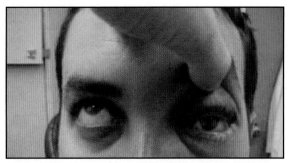

Figure 5-24. Thirty-three-year-old patient with left orbital cellulitis secondary to ethmoid and maxillary sinusitis with edema and erythema of left upper eyelid, proptosis, and limited extraocular motility.

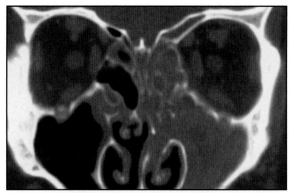

Figure 5-25. Orbital CT scan showing the marked ethmoid and maxillary sinusitis leading to the orbital cellulitis of the previous patient.

- In children, single gram-positive organisms are usually present, whereas in adults, polymicrobial infections are commonly observed.
- Subperiosteal abscesses in children typically resolve with antibiotic therapy alone, although intravenous antibiotics are typically needed initially.
- As extensions of sinus disease, subperiosteal abscesses tend to resolve if the sinusitis responds to treatment. If the sinus is drained, the orbital process will resolve without separate drainage.
  - ○ Mucormycosis and aspergillus
    - Common fungi involving the orbit
    - Mucor invades the orbit via sinuses or the nasal cavity causing an often fatal necrotizing vasculitis and thrombosis.
    - Patients are often acidotic, systemically ill, or immunosuppressed.
    - Diagnosis is made by biopsy of the involved blue-black necrotic tissue.
    - Aspergillosis can present acutely with fulminant sinusitis and secondary orbital invasion or as a chronic indolent infection. The sinuses can also harbor a chronic localized noninvasive aspergillosis described as a "fungus ball."
    - Allergic aspergillis sinusitis has been described in immunocompetent patients with nasal polyposis and chronic sinusitis.
    - Treatment involves aggressive surgical débridement, control of the underlying metabolic abnormality, and appropriate antifungal therapy.

Orbital Foreign Body

- Etiology
  - ○ Injuries are often work-related, but may occur in motor vehicle accidents, explosions, or gunshot wounds.
- Signs/symptoms
  - ○ The clinical presentation depends on the size, velocity, type, and location of the missile.
  - ○ Small, high-speed projectiles produce a small entrance wound with little discomfort.
  - ○ With larger foreign bodies, there may be pain, diplopia, and loss of vision.
  - ○ Presenting signs range from a minute eyelid or conjunctival entrance wound to large wounds with ecchymosis, hemorrhage, edema, loss of vision, impaired eye movement, or visible foreign body (Figure 5-26).
  - ○ An afferent pupillary defect signals optic nerve dysfunction.
- Differential diagnosis
  - ○ The differential diagnosis includes orbital hemorrhage, orbital fracture, orbital cellulitis, ruptured globe, and carotid-cavernous sinus fistula.
- Evaluation
  - ○ A history of the circumstances of the injury (eg, hammering metal on metal) is essential.
  - ○ A detailed search for an otherwise overlooked entrance wound is important, and ocular penetration must be ruled out.

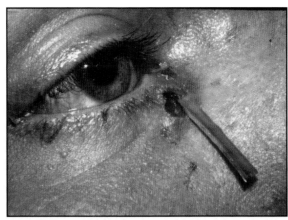

Figure 5-26. A wooden foreign body penetrating the orbit.

- ○ Examination should include visual acuity, pupillary responses, ocular motility, slit-lamp examination, and dilated ophthalmoscopy.
- ○ CT will provide information as to size, shape, and location of a metallic foreign body and any associated orbital floor fractures while MRI is more reliable in detecting vegetable foreign bodies and may cause dangerous migration of metal foreign bodies.
- Management
  - ○ Treatment of most orbital foreign bodies is conservative and expectant.
  - ○ Entrance wounds should be cultured and prophylactic antibiotics administered.
  - ○ Inorganic, inert, smooth posterior orbital foreign bodies do not need to be removed.
  - ○ Glass, stone, and plastic can be tolerated for many years.
  - ○ Conversely, organic foreign bodies such as wood and soil can cause an acute suppurative infection or chronic draining fistula and should be removed promptly.
  - ○ Foreign bodies are also usually removed if they are anterior in the orbit, easily accessible, or have sharp edges.
- Prognosis
  - ○ Management depends on the size, composition, entry site, and velocity of the orbital foreign body.
  - ○ Visual loss may occur immediately or be delayed.
  - ○ Surgical removal of inert, posterior orbital foreign bodies may be harmful and counterproductive.

Orbital Fractures

- Definition
  - ○ Blunt or penetrating orbital injuries may result in fractures, hemorrhage, and damage to the globe, EOMs, optic nerve, paranasal sinuses, and brain.
- Etiology
  - ○ Blunt objects with a diameter larger than the orbital rim such as fists, elbows, and baseballs may cause fractures of the orbital walls. Forceful trauma to the lateral cheek results in tripod fractures of the zygoma.
- Signs/symptoms
  - ○ Pain, decreased vision, diplopia, nausea, and numbness of the cheek, side of the nose, and upper gumline
  - ○ Eyelid ecchymosis, edema, subconjunctival hemorrhage, restriction of eye movement, and vertical diplopia are common (Figure 5-27).
  - ○ Enophthalmos may occur early or late.
  - ○ Infraorbital hypesthesia and eyelid crepitus are reliable signs that an orbital wall has been fractured.
  - ○ Patients with displaced tripod fractures will have flattening of the cheek and zygomatic arch, inferior displacement of the lateral canthus, and trismus.

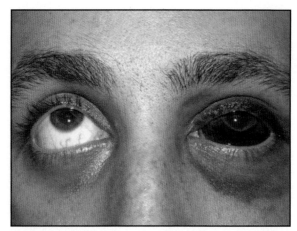

Figure 5-27. Eyelid ecchymosis, edema, subconjunctival hemorrhage, restriction of eye movement, and vertical diplopia seen with blowout fracture.

- Differential diagnosis
  - Other causes of vertical diplopia and vertical gaze restriction include fourth nerve palsy, inferior rectus palsy, EOM damage, orbital hemorrhage and edema, skew deviation, and Brown's syndrome.
- Evaluation
  - A careful history and eye examination should precede evaluation of the orbit.
  - Visual acuity, pupillary responses, ocular motility, intraocular pressure (IOP), slit-lamp biomicroscopy, and funduscopic examinations are essential.
  - Following Hertel exophthalmometry, the contours of the orbital rims, zygoma, and maxilla should be inspected and palpated. The cheek is tested for sensory loss.
  - Forced duction testing is helpful in evaluating entrapment of the inferior rectus muscle.
  - CT scanning with coronal views will demonstrate the size and location of the fractures (Figure 5-28).
- Management
  - Surgical repair of orbital fractures is indicated when the following are present:
    - Persistent vertical diplopia in a functionally important field of gaze
    - Cosmetically deforming enophthalmos (ie, >2 mm) hypoglobus
    - Large fractures likely to lead to enophthalmos
  - Otherwise, patients should be observed and treated with cold compresses. Avoidance of nose blowing and sleeping with the head elevated should be encouraged.
  - Tripod fractures need not be repaired unless there is significant bone displacements causing flattening of the malar eminence or depression of the zygomatic arch, enophthalmos, restriction of eye movements, trismus, or malocclusion.
- Prognosis
  - When fracture repair is properly timed and technically precise, most patients do well with resolution of diplopia and correction/prevention of enophthalmos.
  - Early intervention in properly selected patients leads to a high rate of visual preservation, cosmesis, and function.

Orbital Hemorrhage

- Definition
  - Orbital hemorrhage is bleeding into the confined space bound by the orbital bones, globe, and orbital septum.
  - A limited increase in volume is afforded by proptosis of the globe and anterior displacement of the septum.
  - Once this capacity is exceeded, hemorrhage results in elevated intraorbital and IOP.

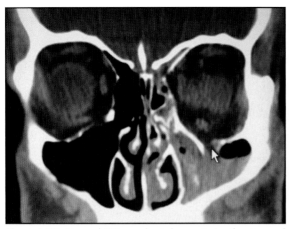

Figure 5-28. Coronal CT scan best demonstrates the size and location of the fracture.

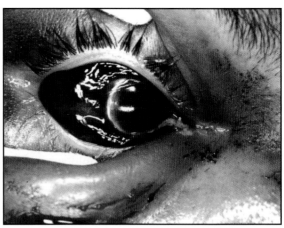

Figure 5-29. Orbital hemorrhage with proptosis, chemosis, subconjunctival hemorrhage, and ecchymosis of the eyelid.

- Etiology
  - Most orbital hemorrhages follow retrobulbar anesthetic injections for cataract or retinal surgery, blepharoplasty, craniofacial reconstruction, orbital fracture repair, rhinoplasty, or trauma.
  - Spontaneous hemorrhages may result from unsuspected lymphangiomas, varices, or malignant tumors.
  - Hypertension, leukemia, atherosclerosis, and hemophilia are associated with orbital hemorrhage.
- Signs/symptoms
  - Sudden onset of pain, nausea, diplopia, and visual loss are the typical symptoms.
  - With long-standing hemorrhages (hematic cyst), pain may not be a prominent feature.
  - Signs of orbital hemorrhage include variable degrees of proptosis, ocular motility disturbance, chemosis, and ecchymosis of the eyelid, subconjunctival hemorrhage, and elevated IOP (Figure 5-29).
  - An afferent papillary defect will be present in cases of optic nerve compromise.
  - Fundus exam may show optic disc edema, pulsations of the central retinal artery, and choroidal folds.
- Differential diagnosis
  - The differential diagnosis includes orbital fracture, orbital foreign body, orbital cellulitis, ruptured globe, and carotid-cavernous sinus fistula.
- Evaluation
  - Examination should include assessment of the visual acuity, pupillary reactions, eye movements, IOP, and dilated ophthalmoscopy.
  - CT is useful in localizing the area of hemorrhage for possible drainage.
- Management
  - Drainage of an orbital hemorrhage is not necessary unless vision is threatened by compression of the optic nerve or globe.
  - Urgent decompression should ensue in cases of visual loss. Lateral canthotomy and cantholysis will suffice in most cases; however, surgical wounds should be opened and explored and bleeding points cauterized.
  - Highly elevated IOP (>40 mm Hg) can often be treated successfully with intravenous acetazolamide or mannitol and topical glaucoma drops such as timolol. Anterior chamber paracentesis is contraindicated in this setting.
  - Orbitotomy and bony orbital decompression is seldom necessary.
- Prognosis
  - With prompt recognition and appropriate medical and surgical intervention, the prognosis for visual preservation is very good.

Dysthyroid Ophthalmopathy

- Definition
  - A thyroid-related autoimmune inflammatory orbital disorder
  - Frequently bilateral, the underlying cause remains unknown.
  - Dysthyroid ophthalmology (DO) is also referred to as TRO.
- Epidemiology
  - More common in women than in men, peak incidence rates in fifth and seventh decades, median age at diagnosis was 43 years.
- Etiology
  - Autoimmune reaction resulting in volume expansion of orbital soft tissues
- Signs/symptoms
  - Bulging eyes
  - Ocular irritation
  - Pain
  - Photophobia
  - Decreased vision
  - Diplopia
- Diagnostic criteria
  - Lid retraction and one of the following:
    - Thyroid dysfunction
    - Exophthalmos
    - Optic nerve dysfunction
    - EOM involvement (restrictive myopathy or enlarged muscles seen on imaging)
  - When lid retraction is absent, the diagnosis is made as follows:
    - Thyroid dysfunction and one of the following:
      - Exophthalmos
      - Optic nerve dysfunction
      - EOM involvement
- Differential diagnosis
  - Orbital cellulitis
  - Idiopathic orbital inflammation
  - Orbital tumors
  - Vascular abnormality (arteriovenous fistula, varix)
  - Cranial nerve palsy
  - Parinaud's syndrome
  - Associated systemic disease
    - Myasthenia gravis
    - Thyroid dermopathy
- Evaluation
  - History
    - Systemic symptoms of thyroid disease
    - Ocular symptoms
  - Ocular exam
    - Assess for lid retraction (Figure 5-30)
    - Exposure keratopathy (fluorescein staining)
    - Optic nerve compression (pupils, color vision)
    - Exophthalmometry
    - IOP increased in upgaze versus primary
    - Ocular motility
    - Forced duction testing
  - CT scans of orbits (axial and coronal views) for diagnostic or preoperative purposes (Figure 5-31). Fusiform enlargement of EOM that spares the tendons, increased orbital fat, proptosis, and apical crowding of the optic nerve may be seen. EOM involvement occurs in the following order: inferior rectus (IR), medial rectus (MR), superior rectus (SR), lateral rectus (LR), obliques.

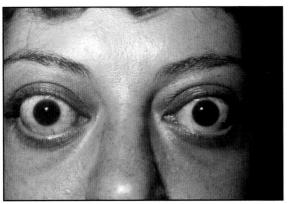

Figure 5-30. Dysthyroid ophthalmopathy. (Reprinted with permission from Leal AG, Rodriguez PM. *The Atlas of Ophthalmology.* Thorofare, NJ: SLACK Incorporated; 2002.)

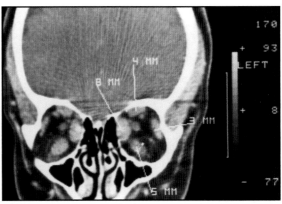

Figure 5-31. CT scans of orbits. (Reprinted with permission from Leal AG, Rodriguez PM. *The Atlas of Ophthalmology.* Thorofare, NJ: SLACK Incorporated; 2002.)

- o Thyroid function tests (T3, T4, TSH): 90% are hyperthyroid, 6% euthyroid, 1% primary hypothyroidism, 3% Hashimoto's thyroiditis. Temporal relationship of DO and hyperthyroidism: 20% diagnosed concurrently, 60% of DO occurred within 1 year of onset of thyroid disease. In patients with DO and no history of thyroid dysfunction, the risk of developing thyroid disease was about 25% within 1 year and 50% within 5 years.
  - o Visual field testing if optic neuropathy is suspected
- Management
  - o Endocrine evaluation for systemic thyroid abnormality
  - o Most patients respond to supportive care (ocular lubricants, prismatic correction to correct diplopia).
  - o Systemic steroids or possibly orbital radiotherapy should be considered if orbital edema and chemosis are severe.
  - o Staged surgical intervention
    - Orbital decompression, followed by strabismus surgery, followed by eyelid surgery (retraction repair)
    - Aside from urgent orbital decompression for compressive optic neuropathy, surgical therapy is not undertaken until the disease is in its stable phase. Operating while the disease is progressing or regressing may lead to under- or overcorrection.
    - Indications for graded orbital decompression: compressive optic neuropathy; exposure keratopathy; spontaneous globe prolapse; disfigurement; orbital pressure/pain; orbital congestion; glaucoma secondary to DO.
  - o Progressive compressive optic neuropathy requires timely intervention.
  - o Systemic steroids may be beneficial, although usually only temporarily.
  - o Definitive treatment consists of orbital decompression, possibly orbital irradiation, or immunosuppressive therapy.
- Prognosis
  - o The inflammatory phase (marked by worsening) may last up to 18 months (Figure 5-32).
  - o The regression phase shows gradual spontaneous improvement over a 1- to 3-year period.
  - o Complete regression typically does not occur.
  - o Following regression is a period of stability.
  - o Most patients do well when appropriate medical and surgical intervention is rendered in a timely fashion.

Orbital Tumors in Adults

- Etiology
  - o Metastatic tumors are more common than primary orbital tumors with breast cancer being the most common metastasis in women and lung cancer in men.
  - o Cavernous hemangioma is the most common primary benign orbital tumor in adults, and lymphoma is the most common malignant tumor in adults.

Figure 5-32. Patient with DO in the inflammatory phase of the disease with conjunctival injection and asymmetrical lid retraction

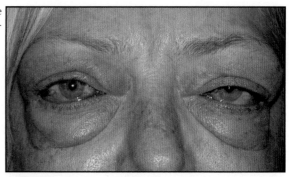

- Signs/symptoms
  - ○ Orbital tumors of significant size produce either proptosis or globe displacement in the direction opposite the tumor mass.
  - ○ Tumors within the EOM cone often limit orbital retropulsion on globe ballottement.
  - ○ Large but slowly growing orbital tumors that do not compress vital structures may cause little or no vision loss or diplopia.
  - ○ In the orbital apex, however, even small tumors may present with vision loss, diplopia, or relative afferent papillary defect, but little proptosis or globe displacement.
- Evaluation
  - ○ CT and/or MRI indicate the location of the orbit lesion (eg, LG or optic nerve) and its appearance (eg, well-circumscribed, infiltrative, cystic, or associated bony erosion)—vital information for diagnosis and surgical planning.
    - ▪ Well-circumscribed lesions tend to be benign, although malignant degeneration is sometimes possible. Cavernous hemangioma, hemangiopericytoma, schwannoma, neurofibroma, fibrous histiocytoma, and solitary fibrous tumor of the orbit are typically well-circumscribed intraconal lesions. Hemangiopericytomas mimic cavernous hemangioma but have a more guarded prognosis. Schwannoma is a common peripheral nerve tumor that may show internal heterogeneity on scanning. When treatment is required for well-circumscribed lesions, complete excision is recommended.
    - ▪ Infiltrative lesions include metastases, lymphoma, orbital inflammatory syndrome (OIS), and lymphangioma.
      - □ Orbital lymphoma (non-Hodgkin B cell) often presents with a conjunctival fornix "salmon patch" mass. Lymphoma often shows "putty like" moulding around orbital structures on neuroimaging and tends to follow an indolent but slowly progressive course.
      - □ In contrast, patients with OIS tend to have abrupt-onset severe pain, without paranasal sinus involvement. Myositis of the EOMs and dacryoadenitis are variants of OIS.
      - □ Lymphangiomas (combined venous-lymphatic malformations) may enlarge with upper respiratory tract infection and often cause sudden hemorrhage of dark subconjunctival or subcutaneous blood. Usually, lymphangiomas bleed in childhood. Lymphangiomas may show cystic fluid levels and occasionally intracranial lesions (Figures 5-33 and 5-34).
      - □ Infiltrative lesions usually cannot be completely excised without significant morbidity. If lymphoma or metastasis is suspected, incisional biopsy or fine-needle aspiration biopsy can be performed in conjunction with a systemic work-up to see if radiation or chemotherapy is appropriate. OIS usually improves dramatically after a day or two of prednisone at doses of 60 mg or greater, but requires several months of gradually tapering systemic steroids to prevent recrudescence. Lymphangioma may be observed, treated with steroids, or partially excised depending on the associated symptoms.
    - ▪ The common cystic lesions of the orbit are dermoid cysts, conjunctival cysts, hematic cysts (post-trauma), sinus mucocele (due to impaired drainage of the sinuses), and lymphangioma.
    - ▪ LG tumors may cause inferonasal globe displacement and ptosis. LG masses are more frequently inflammatory or lymphoid tumors rather than epithelial. Of the epithelial LG tumors, adenoid cystic carcinoma (ACC) is the most common malignant lesion, and PA is the

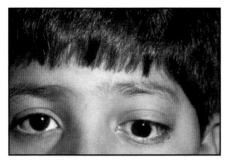

Figure 5-33. Lymphangioma. Lymphangiomas (combined venous-lymphatic malformations) may enlarge with upper respiratory tract infection. (Reprinted with permission from Leal AG, Rodriguez PM. *The Atlas of Ophthalmology.* Thorofare, NJ: SLACK Incorporated; 2002.)

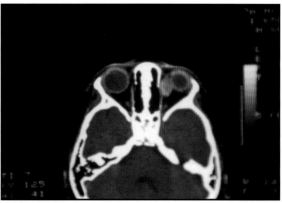

Figure 5-34. Lymphangioma. Lymphangiomas may show cystic fluid levels. (Reprinted with permission from Leal AG, Rodriguez PM. *The Atlas of Ophthalmology.* Thorofare, NJ: SLACK Incorporated; 2002.)

most common benign lesion. ACC tends to present over several months, often with pain from perineural spread and with bony erosion. ACC has a very poor prognosis. PA is a pseudoencapsulated, painless, slowly growing lesion that may scallop the orbital bone but not erode it. PA has a good prognosis when completely excised.

- The most common optic nerve tumors are optic nerve sheath meningioma (ONSM) and OG. ONSM usually occur in adults, especially women. Imaging characteristically shows axial "tram-tracking" and a coronal "target sign." Surgical excision of ONSM usually causes ipsilateral blindness. ONSM can be radiated if there is loss of acuity or visual field. ONSM that spreads intracranially is rarely, if ever, fatal but can be excised. OG usually presents in children, is frequently associated with neurofibromatosis, and on neuroimaging shows fusiform enlargement and, classically, sagittal kinking (Figure 5-35). If OG is not spreading intracranially, it can be observed with serial imaging. OG presentation in adults is an uncommon but highly aggressive lesion with a dismal prognosis for survival.

Proptosis in Childhood

- Definition
  - Proptosis is the protrusion of the eyeball from the surrounding orbital bones.
- Etiology
  - In children, a variety of acute and chronic conditions including infections, inflammation, congenital anomalies, and neoplasms may lead to proptosis.
- Signs/symptoms
  - Redness, pain, foreign body sensation, photophobia, tearing, double vision, or decreased vision
  - Prominent eye(s), failure to completely close eyelids, eyelid retraction, eyelid swelling, chemosis, limited eye movements, or resistance to retropulsion.
- Differential diagnosis
  - Infectious/inflammatory
    - Orbital cellulitis
    - Idiopathic orbital pseudotumor or orbital inflammatory syndrome
    - Thyroid eye disease
    - Sinus mucocele
  - Congenital
    - Dermoid cyst
    - Encephalocele
    - Teratoma
    - Craniosynostosis disorders
    - Infantile glaucoma

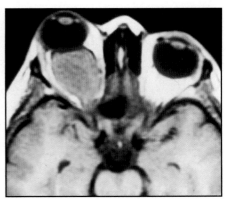

Figure 5-35. Optic nerve glioma. On neuroimaging shows fusiform enlargement and, classically, sagittal kinking. (Reprinted with permission from Leal AG, Rodriguez PM. *The Atlas of Ophthalmology.* Thorofare, NJ: SLACK Incorporated; 2002.)

- ○ Neoplasms
  - ▪ Capillary hemangioma
  - ▪ Lymphangioma
  - ▪ Rhabdomyosarcoma
  - ▪ Metastatic neuroblastoma
  - ▪ Leukemic infiltration
  - ▪ OG
  - ▪ Fibrous dysplasia
  - ▪ Eosinophilic granuloma
  - ▪ Burkitt lymphoma
- • Evaluation
  - ○ History is used to evaluate onset and duration (acute or chronic), age of onset, associated pain, and periocular or systemic symptoms.
  - ○ Ocular exam includes visual acuity, color vision, pupils, IOP, motility, and exophthalmometry. Palpation of the orbital rim is performed to check for masses and check for resistance to retropulsion.
  - ○ Orbital CT scan with axial and coronal views or MRI is helpful.
  - ○ Orbital ultrasound may be useful for a cystic or vascular lesion.
- • Management
  - ○ Treatment depends upon the final diagnosis.
  - ○ Treatment may be designed to reduce the degree of proptosis when there is risk of corneal exposure or optic neuropathy.
  - ○ Intralesional steroids may be used for capillary hemangiomas, oral steroids for idiopathic pseudotumor, antithyroid medication for thyroid eye disease, broad-spectrum antibiotics for orbital cellulitis, and radiation or chemotherapy agents for orbital tumors.
  - ○ Surgery may be necessary in cases of optic nerve compromise or significant corneal exposure not responsive to medical therapy or for tissue diagnosis. Reconstruction of the orbit may be needed for cases of congenital anomalies.
- • Prognosis
  - ○ Benign proliferative and developmental causes of proptosis can usually be satisfactorily treated with medical and surgical therapy.
  - ○ Capillary hemangiomas often spontaneously regress over several years or involute with the use of steroids.
  - ○ Complete excision of dermoid cysts is curative.
  - ○ Orbital reconstruction in congenital malformations such as craniosynostosis can reduce proptosis and corneal exposure.
  - ○ Antibiotic coverage is initiated for orbital cellulites, sometimes with surgical decompression of orbital abscesses.
  - ○ Steroids or other anti-inflammatory agents are useful for idiopathic orbital pseudotumor and other inflammatory disorders and vasculitides.

o Malignant orbital neoplasms in childhood include rhabdomyosarcoma, retinoblastoma, leukemic and lymphomatous infiltrates, and metastatic tumors. Treatment success is determined by the type of tumor, size, grade, and presence of metastasis.

Lacrimal Gland Masses

- Definition
  - o Any lesion causing enlargement of the LG
- Etiology
  - o Infectious, inflammatory, lymphoproliferative tumors and epithelial neoplasms
- Signs/symptoms
  - o LG masses present as fullness or swelling in the superotemporal orbit, often with a characteristic S-shape to the eyelid due to lateral ptosis.
  - o Patients may also develop proptosis and downward globe displacement and diplopia.
  - o Larger tumors may indent the eye, causing choroidal folds and blurred vision.
- Differential diagnosis
  - o Infectious dacryoadenitis
    - ■ Etiology
      - □ The most common organism is *Staphylococcus aureus*, but *Neisseria gonorrhea* and *Streptococcal* species have also been implicated. Viral etiologies include mumps, Epstein-Barr virus, and herpes zoster, and influenza presents with a swollen tender lid and may have a palpable mass due to LG enlargement.
    - ■ Signs/symptoms
      - □ The patient may have a history of preceding upper respiratory illness if the etiology is viral.
      - □ Patients with bacterial dacryoadenitis present with fever, preauricular lymphadenopathy, superotemporal conjunctival injection and chemosis, and an elevated white blood cell count.
    - ■ Evaluation
      - □ The diagnosis is typically made with the clinical exam.
      - □ CT scan will typically show enlargement of the LG with enhancement when contrast material is used.
    - ■ Treatment
      - □ Based on the etiology with broad-spectrum oral antibiotics for a mild bacterial dacryoadenitis and intravenous antibiotics for moderate to severe disease
      - □ Treatment with cool compresses and acetaminophen is appropriate when the etiology is viral.
  - o Orbital inflammation
    - ■ Etiology
      - □ OIS may be nonspecific (orbital pseudotumor) or specific due to an underlying systemic disorder.
    - ■ Signs/symptoms
      - □ Often involves the LG
      - □ Patients present with acute pain and swelling.
      - □ With severe inflammation, restriction of ocular motility and proptosis may develop.
      - □ Bilateral disease is more common with underlying systemic disorders and in children.
    - ■ Differential diagnosis
      - □ Disorders that may be associated with dacryoadenitis include sarcoidosis, Wegener's granulomatosis, tuberculosis, syphilis, and Sjögren's syndrome.
    - ■ Evaluation
      - □ A complete ocular exam looking for uveitis should be performed.
      - □ Laboratory testing and rheumatology referral may be necessary for management of the underlying systemic disorders.
      - □ LG biopsy should be performed for diagnostic purposes (eg, noncaseating granulomas of sarcoid) and to rule out an underlying malignancy such as lymphoma (see next section).

- Treatment
  - Treatment is directed at the specific disorder.
  - If the pathology shows a nonspecific inflammation, treatment with systemic steroids is indicated.
- Lymphoproliferative disorders
  - Etiology
    - Range from benign lymphoid hyperplasia to malignant lymphomas
    - Most of the malignant lymphomas are non-Hodgkins variety and are typically low-grade proliferations of small, monoclonal B cell lymphocytes.
  - Signs/symptoms
    - Account for 50% of all LG neoplasms
    - Commonly present with painless enlargement of the gland, but may present with mild inflammatory signs as an orbital pseudotumor
  - Investigations
    - CT and MRI show a diffuse to moderately well-defined mass.
  - Evaluation
    - The diagnosis is made by LG biopsy.
    - Following the diagnosis, patients need a systemic workup including abdominal and chest CT scans and bone marrow biopsy to rule out systemic involvement.
  - Treatment
    - Treatment of isolated orbital involvement includes external beam radiotherapy at 2500 to 3000 cGy.
- Epithelial neoplasms of the LG
  - Etiology
    - Rare with 50% malignant and 50% benign
    - The most common benign epithelial neoplasm is PA (benign mixed tumor).
  - Signs/symptoms
    - Patients present with slowly progressive, painless proptosis and downward and nasal displacement of the eye (Figure 5-36).
  - Evaluation
    - CT or MRI scans (Figure 5-37) show a well-circumscribed nodular mass in the anterior superiolateral extraconal space.
    - There may be remodeling of the adjacent bone without frank destruction.
  - Treatment/prognosis
    - PAs should be excised completely.
    - This leads to a 99% cure rate.
    - Incomplete excision may be associated with a 30% rate of recurrence.
    - Recurrent growths carry a 10% risk of malignant degeneration.
- ACC
  - Signs/symptoms
    - Most common malignant epithelial neoplasm of the LG commonly seen in the fourth decade but may occur at any age
    - Patients present with relatively rapid (months) proptosis and downward and nasal displacement of the eye.
    - Numbness and pain may occur secondary to perineural invasion.
  - Evaluation
    - CT scans demonstrate a heterogeneous density in the superotemporal orbit with bone destruction.
    - The diagnosis is typically made with an incisional biopsy.
  - Treatment
    - Management of these tumors remains controversial.
    - Most authorities recommend an en-bloc excision with wide margins including bone (orbitectomy).
    - Adjunctive radiotherapy and chemotherapy may also be employed.
  - Prognosis
    - Even with radical treatment, the survival remains poor with a 5-year mortality rate of 60%.

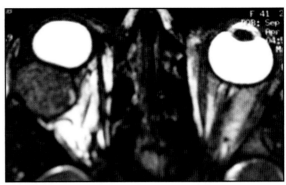

Figure 5-36. Inferonasal proptosis due to pleomorphic adenoma.   **Figure 5-37.** MRI scan of well-defined pleomorphic adenoma.

Enucleation, Evisceration, and Ocular Prosthetic Eyes

- Definitions
  - o Enucleation is the removal of the entire eyeball.
  - o Evisceration is the removal of the intraocular contents, usually along with the cornea, while leaving the white sclera behind.
- Indications
  - o Removal of an eye may be advised in the face of irreparable trauma, intractable pain, severe intraocular infection, certain tumors, or for cosmetic improvement of a disfigured eye.
  - o Pain may arise from refractory glaucoma, phthisis, intraocular inflammation, or corneal decompensation.
  - o Both enucleation and evisceration are effective in controlling pain in these eyes, although the postoperative pain may last somewhat longer after evisceration than enucleation.
- Surgical procedures
  - o The choice of procedure depends on the condition being treated as well as the surgeon's and patient's preferences.
  - o Most surgeons believe that evisceration gives a better final result than enucleation because there is less orbital disruption.
  - o The motility is often better and the risk of enophthalmos is less following evisceration.
  - o However, theoretically, there is an increased risk of sympathetic ophthalmia (SO) following evisceration. SO is a severe granulomatous inflammatory condition that can result in bilateral panuveitis or even blindness. Fortunately, this is a rare and often treatable event.
  - o Evisceration is contraindicated where there is known or suspected intraocular tumor because complete tumor removal cannot be assured. Enucleation is the procedure of choice in this setting.
  - o Evisceration may also be difficult if the eye is phthisical, if infection has damaged the sclera, or if there has been extensive ocular surgery or trauma.
- Ocular implants
  - o Removal of the eye results in a volume deficit that is only partially corrected by placement of an ocular implant.
  - o In order to achieve the greatest natural movement, most surgeons will suture the EOMs to the implant itself or to a wrapping around the implant.
  - o Smooth spherical implants are typically made of silicone or polymethylmethacrylate.
  - o Porous spherical implants are made of coralline, mammalian, or synthetic hydroxyapatite, bone, or high-density porous polyethylene. Fibrous ingrowth into porous implants may reduce the risk of implant extrusion, and a motility peg can be placed in a porous implant to couple with a depression on the back of the prosthesis to improve motility.
  - o Quasi-integrated implants are typically polymethylmethacrylate and have knobs on the anterior surface so that once implanted, the protruding knobs create enough contours in the overlying conjunctiva to couple with the prosthesis.
  - o An autologous dermis-fat graft will provide adequate volume replacement with good motility; however, this requires a second surgical site and the fat may resorb unpredictably.

- Prosthesis fitting and fabrication
  - Several weeks after surgery, a custom-made prosthesis is fashioned by the ocularist.
  - The ocular prosthesis is like a large painted contact lens.
  - An impression is taken of the socket, and a positive mold of the socket surface is made from that.
  - The prosthesis is usually made of polymethylmethacrylate and created so that it fits the contours of the socket precisely, thus affording the greatest comfort and motility.
  - The sclera, iris, pupil, vessels, and cornea are created to match the other eye and give the prosthesis a natural appearance.
  - Care and maintenance of the prosthesis through regular cleaning by the patient and periodic polishing by the ocularist will prolong the life of the prosthesis and maintain the health of the socket.
- Summary
  - Loss of an eye can be a devastating psychological hurdle in a patient's life.
  - A compassionate persona, careful surgery, appropriate implant selection, and collaboration with a skilled ocularist are critical to achieving the most natural appearance possible afterward and facilitating the patient's adjustment to the psychological trauma of organ loss.

Postsurgical Anophthalmic Socket

- Anophthalmic socket syndrome
  - Definition
    - Removal of the eyeball alters the structural and functional relationships within the orbit.
  - Signs/symptoms
    - Anophthalmic orbit syndrome
      - Upper lid ptosis
      - Lower lid laxity
      - Enophthalmos
      - Superior sulcus depression
    - Implant migration, exposure, or extrusion can further complicate the picture.
    - Conjunctival contraction can make it impossible to retain the prosthesis.
    - Meticulous surgical technique will reduce the risk of these problems developing in the first place; however, once they occur, it is important to address these issues to allow patients to comfortably wear their prostheses and to maintain the health of the socket.
  - Treatment
    - Collaboration with a skilled ocularist is invaluable in the management of these problems.
    - Upper lid ptosis may occur from loss of orbital support of the upper lid or from dehiscence or detachment of the levator aponeurosis. In mild cases, building up the superior pole of the prosthesis will lift the lid. This may also fill a mildly depressed superior sulcus. In severe cases, traditional ptosis surgery will correct the upper lid position.
    - The prosthesis is supported mainly by the lower lid. Over time, the canthal tendons can stretch, thus allowing the prosthesis to drop. Horizontal tightening of the lower lid will create needed support for the prosthesis.
    - The prosthesis may look enophthalmic or "sunken in" compared to the normal eye. Volume deficit in the socket may be related to scarring or contraction within the socket, placement of an inadequately sized orbital implant, or a small prosthesis. The prosthesis can only be enlarged to a small degree. If it is enlarged too much, it will be too heavy and will appear to bulge. Placement of a subperiosteal orbital implant, exchanging the ocular implant for a larger one, or placing a dermis-fat graft will all add volume to the orbit. Subperiosteal orbital floor implants also push the orbital contents superiorly and help fill the deep superior sulcus.
    - Exposure of the orbital implant may arise from tension in the tissue overlying an oversized implant or by a poorly fitting prosthesis putting pressure on the tissue. Porous implants have a rough surface, which may contribute to breakdown of the overlying tissue. Small dehiscences can be repaired with a patch graft. Larger dehiscences, recurrent dehiscences, or dehiscences in the presence of an infected implant require implant removal and replacement with a new implant or dermis-fat graft.

- Deep fornices behind the lids are necessary to allow retention of the prosthesis. Contraction of the conjunctival fornices can occur after trauma, chronic inflammation, a poorly fitting prosthesis, or multiple surgeries. This is not only uncomfortable, but also makes it difficult to retain the prosthesis. Grafting mucus membrane, amniotic membrane, or other allograft material into the fornices may be necessary to create enough room to hold the prosthesis.
- o Prognosis
  - Careful enucleation or evisceration surgery with proper implant selection, meticulous closure, and appropriate consultation with the ocularist can avoid many late complications.

Lacrimal System

Evaluation of the Lacrimal System

- Clinical evaluation
  - o Epiphora may result from anatomical obstruction of the nasolacrimal passages or from nonobstructive factors such as tear film instability, primary or reflex hypersecretion, aberrant regeneration, eyelid malposition, or lacrimal pump insufficiency.
  - o Slit-lamp examination
    - The ocular surface should be examined for irritating phenomena or surface keratopathy that may interfere with tear film stability as well as cause reflex tearing.
  - o Staining
    - Fluorescein and rose bengal staining help evaluate for surface keratopathy and dry eyes.
    - A fluorescein paper strip is moistened with saline or water and touched to the palpebral conjunctiva, and the dye spreads over the cornea with several blinks. Using the cobalt blue filter on the slit lamp, areas of abnormal epithelium manifest as bright green areas of staining.
    - A 1% rose bengal solution, applied in the same fashion, may stain the conjunctiva and cornea in a characteristic pattern suggestive of dry eyes or other infectious or inflammatory etiology.
  - o Tear break up time (TBUT)
    - The TBUT is measured immediately after instillation of fluorescein using a broad beam of light and the blue filter.
    - The time it takes from fluorescein instillation to the appearance of the first random dry spot on the corneal surface constitutes the TBUT (<10 seconds considered abnormal).
  - o Tear meniscus level
    - The tear meniscus level should be evaluated prior to any eye drops or eyelid manipulation.
    - The tear meniscus level, or the height from the lid margin to the top of the meniscus along the globe surface, is measured at the slit lamp with a narrow, straight, vertical beam at 0.2 or 1.0 mm.
    - The tear meniscus measures 0.2 mm in unobstructed systems.
    - An elevated tear lake is often a sign of lacrimal outflow obstruction.
    - Measuring the tear meniscus level, on average 0.6 mm in obstructed systems, or the ratio between 2 sides may be useful indicators of nasolacrimal obstruction.
  - o Schirmer's test
    - A Schirmer's test may measure decreased basal or reflex tear production.
    - Topical anesthetic is placed on the eye, and the inferior fornix is dried with a cotton-tipped applicator.
    - A filter strip is placed in the inferior fornix at the junction of the middle and lateral thirds of the lower eyelid to minimize corneal irritation.
    - After 5 minutes, the test strips are removed and measured, with less than 5 mm of wetting suggestive of aqueous tear deficiency.
    - Levels between 5 and 10 mm are equivocal. The Schirmer's test using topical anesthetic measures the basal tear production; if no anesthetic is used, both basal and reflex tear production can be assessed, with less than 10 mm of wetting after 5 minutes suggestive of aqueous tear deficiency.

○ Eyelid position
  ▪ Both eyelids positioned against the globe and punctal apposition to the tear meniscus allow capillary attraction to draw tears into the canaliculi.
  ▪ Margin abnormalities such as entropion, trichiasis, distichiasis, and blepharitis may irritate the ocular surface and cause reflex tearing.
  ▪ Lagophthalmos and eyelid laxity, with or without frank ectropion, result in lacrimal pump insufficiency.
○ Medial and lateral canthal tendon laxity
  ▪ Normally, the tone of medial canthal tendon does not allow the punctum to be pulled laterally more than 2 or 3 mm.
  ▪ Lateral displacement of 5 mm or more, such that the punctum reaches the nasal limbus, would be abnormal (Figure 5-38).
  ▪ Likewise, the lateral canthus should not be lax enough to be pulled medially over to the limbus.
  ▪ A rounded lateral canthal angle or canthal dystopia indicate attenuation of the lateral canthal tendon.
  ▪ The eyelid distraction test and snap back test are performed by pulling the lower eyelid anteriorly with a finger.
  ▪ The eyelid should not be easily distracted more than 6 mm from the cornea.
  ▪ When released, the eyelid should return sharply to its former apposition against the globe. Failure to do so (poor snap back) indicates tarsal attenuation or canthal tendon laxity.
○ Punctal position
  ▪ Causes such as eyelid laxity, inferior retractor disinsertion, cicatricial shortening of the anterior lamella causing medial ectropion or trauma may interfere with the apposition of the puncta to the tear lake.
  ▪ Folds of redundant conjunctiva (conjunctivochalasis) or an enlarged caruncle or plica semilunaris overlying the puncta may cause mechanical obstruction to drainage.
○ Lacrimal probing and irrigation
  ▪ Tests that evaluate anatomic patency include dacryocystography, CT, nasal endoscopy, and probing and irrigation.
  ▪ A cotton-tipped applicator soaked in local anesthetic (proparacaine) is placed on the punctum for several minutes.
  ▪ The stenotic punctum is dilated with a lacrimal dilator, followed by insertion of a small Bowman probe perpendicular to the eyelid for 2 mm into the ampulla, then horizontally toward the medial canthus in a direction parallel to the eyelid margin.
  ▪ Lateral horizontal traction on the eyelid while inserting the probe is necessary to avoid kinking the canaliculus and creating a false passage.
  ▪ Probing helps determine the degree and location of any obstruction present.
  ▪ Lacrimal irrigation can be performed after the probe is removed, in which a lacrimal irrigation cannula on a small syringe is passed into the canaliculus.
  ▪ Saline or water is injected through the system, with partial or complete obstruction manifested by increased resistance to irrigation, lacrimal sac swelling, or reflux of saline from either punctum.
  ▪ Free-flowing irrigation into the nose may indicate patency of the distal system.
○ Dacryocystography
  ▪ A radiopaque dye is injected into the excretory system, and radiographs taken of the dye transit through the passages.
  ▪ Dacryocystography may be helpful to define the presence and location of an anatomic obstruction from a mass.
○ Fluorescein dye disappearance test
  ▪ Functional rather than anatomic obstruction may be determined under normal physiologic conditions without injections using physiologic tests, such as the fluorescein dye disappearance, Jones dye test, and dacryoscintigraphy.
  ▪ In the dye disappearance test, particularly helpful in unilateral outflow obstruction, 2% fluorescein is placed in both conjunctival fornices and the tear film observed using the blue filter. Asymmetrical clearance of the dye from the tear meniscus at 5 minutes suggests relative obstruction on that side.

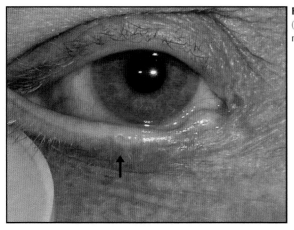

Figure 5-38. With horizontal traction, the inferior punctum (arrow) has been displaced past the pupil, indicating extreme medial canthal tendon laxity.

- ○ Jones dye test
  - ▪ The primary Jones dye test (Jones I) is subsequently performed by placing a cotton pledget at the nasolacrimal duct ostium in the inferior meatus at 5 minutes to evaluate for presence of fluorescein.
  - ▪ In the Jones II dye test, saline is injected through the lacrimal system to evaluate for fluorescein in the irrigating fluid within the nose.
  - ▪ Abnormal results occur frequently, thus limiting the clinical utility of the Jones tests.
- ○ Nasal endoscopy
  - ▪ A complete evaluation of the nasolacrimal system may include nasal examination to evaluate for any abnormalities (deviated septum, obstructed nasolacrimal duct ostium from a membrane, turbinate, polyp, congested nasal mucosa, or mass) that may contribute to the clinical problem.

Disorders of the Lacrimal System

Congenital Lacrimal Obstruction

- See Chapter 10

Adult Epiphora

- Definition
  - ○ Epiphora is spillage of tears onto the cheek and may result from overproduction of tears, a predisposing lower lid contour, failure of tear gathering by the lacrimal puncta, or inadequate clearance through the drainage passages (lacrimal canaliculi, sac, and nasolacrimal duct).
  - ○ Epiphora tends to be worse outdoors, when cold or wind triggers lacrimation, and better in warm, dry environments where there is greater evaporation from the tear lake.
- Etiology
  - ○ Lacrimation is often due to trigeminal nerve stimulation from the ocular, nasal, or oral surface.
  - ○ Stimulation of the ocular surface, especially the cornea, can cause profuse watering and may be seen with corneal foreign bodies or abrasions, corneal erosions, recurrent herpes keratitis, most viral conjunctivitides (such as adenoviral), and early bacterial conjunctivitis before purulence occurs.
  - ○ Corneal inflammation, as with the marginal immune response due to staphylococcal antigens (Figure 5-39) and intraocular inflammation (uveitis), is commonly associated with a red eye and light-induced lacrimation and epiphora.
  - ○ External allergens, such as pollens, dust mites, molds, and animal furs, or chemical irritants can trigger lacrimation from the allergic response in ocular and nasal mucosa. The excessive tear production in hay fever is compounded by poor tear drainage due to chronic nasal congestion.

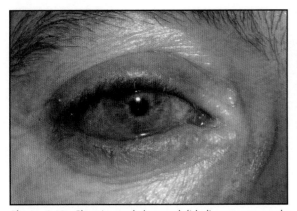

Figure 5-39. Chronic staphylococcal lid disease commonly causes epiphora due to keratitis and reflex lacrimation.

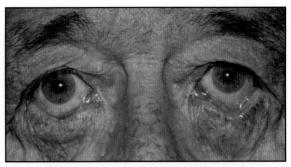

Figure 5-40. With aging of the lower eyelid, the low-point moves towards the outer one-third, impairing tear clearance and encouraging spillage, and eventually marked laxity allows lower lid ectropion with watering due to reflex lacrimation, central tear spillage, and punctal ectropion.

- o Watering eyes may occur from severe oral stimulation by very hot or spicy foods, but "Crocodile tears" (where lacrimation occurs in response to the sight or eating of food) is due to salivary secretomotor fibers passing to the LG in a misdirected reinnervation of the facial nerve, typically after Bell's palsy.
- o Most lower eyelids have a gentle downward slant from the outer canthus toward the inner, this slope (together with the slight medial shift of the lids during the blink cycle) encouraging a medial shift of tears from the LG toward the drainage puncta. The lowest point on the youthful lid margin is often at the junction of the inner one-third and outer two-thirds, but with time it shifts laterally (due to the horizontal laxity of aging tissues and gravity)—this shift both impairs the medial passage of tears and forms a low point for lateral tear spillage.
- Differential diagnosis
  - o Lower lid ectropion (Figure 5-40)
    - Commonly associated with epiphora due to the easy spillage of tears, loss of punctal apposition in the tear lake, and reflex tearing from drying of the exposed tarsal conjunctiva
    - Even with obstructed tear drainage, correction of lower lid ectropion will often lead to a major reduction in epiphora and, where there is no actual ectropion, central or lateral spillage of tears (rather than inner canthal spill) should suggest an abnormality of lower lid contour, such lower lid abnormalities being readily addressed with an enhanced lateral canthal sling procedure.
    - Loss of lower lid movement and tone (as with facial nerve palsy) impairs the medial movement of tears, results in tear retention on the atonic and "sagging" lower lid margin, and impairs the canalicular pump that acts during eyelid closure; for these reasons, it is extremely difficult to completely correct ocular watering due to facial nerve palsy.
  - o Punctal or canalicular blockage
    - May be a congenital anomaly or more commonly it is due to scarring ocular surface disease (such as mucus membrane pemphigoid, SJS, or drug-induced scarring), chemical or physical injury (typically medial lid avulsion or laceration), after viral infections (especially primary Herpes simplex), retained canalicular plugs, with invasive skin tumors such as BCa and with certain systemic chemotherapies (particularly 5-fluorouracil and docetaxel [Taxotere])
    - Canalicular and lid lacerations should usually be repaired with silicone stenting.
    - Skin tumors are treated as necessary, with lacrimal repair a few years later when shown to be recurrence-free.
    - The other conditions may be treated by canaliculodacryocystorhinostomy or dacryocystorhinostomy (DCR) combined with retrograde canaliculostomy or placement of a Jones glass canalicular bypass tube (as a primary or secondary procedure).
  - o Primary acquired nasolacrimal duct obstruction
    - Common cause of adult epiphora due to fibrosis from chronic inflammation, the diameter of the nasolacrimal duct decreases with age

- As fluid collects within the lacrimal sac, a palpable and variable swelling (or mucocoele) may occur beneath the medial canthal tendon, and, on occasion, the mucocoele will develop bacterial infection with secondary facial cellulitis.
- Dacryocystitis requires systemic antibiotic therapy, and a blocked nasolacrimal duct is very effectively treated by DCR, in which the lacrimal sac is opened widely into the lateral nasal wall, under general or local anesthesia. Although the sac can be drained to the nose with endonasal surgery, a wide and complete opening of the system is possible only with the external approach.
  - Secondary obstruction of the lacrimal sac or nasolacrimal duct
    - Trauma (especially the duct in midfacial fractures), stones (just a protein/bacterial coagulum; not calcified), or tumors (either intrinsic to the system or invading the duct from the surrounding maxillary or ethmoid sinus)
    - Lacrimal sac tumors tend to be firmer than the (slightly fluctuant) mucocoele and, whereas tumors may extend above the medial canthal tendon and displace the globe, lacrimal sac mucocoeles never do so.
    - With suspected tumor, dacryocystography and CT scan should be performed before incisional biopsy; if tumor is confirmed, the definitive treatment may involve excision, radiotherapy, or chemotherapy.

Dacryocystitis

- Definition and etiology
  - Inflammation of the lacrimal sac, usually associated with an infection and nasolacrimal duct obstruction
  - Bacteria are the most frequent cause of dacryocystitis, but fungi can also cause dacryocystitis.
  - Dacryoliths, or lacrimal stones, can also block lacrimal outflow and precipitate dacryocystitis. They are generally composed of shed epithelial cells, amorphous debris, and lipids.
- Signs/symptoms
  - Patients with acute dacryocystitis often have pain in the area of the lacrimal fossa and a history of prior ipsilateral epiphora.
  - Patients with chronic dacryocystitis will generally not report pain.
  - With dacryoliths, there may be intermittent epiphora due to a ball-valve effect of the stone in the sac producing episodic obstruction.
  - Edema and erythema inferior to the medial canthal tendon is frequently seen in acute dacryocystitis (Figure 5-41).
  - Often, there is tenderness-to-palpation over the lacrimal sac.
  - Chronic dacryocystitis produces dilation of the lacrimal sac, and, with gentle pressure to the lacrimal sac, a mucoid reflux exudes from the puncta.
- Differential diagnosis
  - Orbital cellulitis may mimic dacryocystitis but it is not typically focally tender over the lacrimal sac.
  - The same is true for severe conjunctivitis associated with periocular erythema or patients with marked blepharitis.
  - A chalazion or hordeolum over the medial aspect of the lower lid may mimic dacryocystitis but will not have antecedent epiphora.
  - Tumors of the nasolacrimal sac typically present with a mass superior to the medial canthal tendon, and patients may not report symptoms of lacrimal obstruction.
- Evaluation
  - No laboratory or imaging studies are routinely ordered in most patients with dacryocystitis.
  - In an immunocompromised host or with severe dacryocystitis, aspiration of the lacrimal sac can be performed for culture and antibiotic sensitivity.
  - A complete blood count may also be indicated in such circumstances. Imaging studies should be performed when there is a suspicion of tumor or sinus disease or a history of trauma.
- Management
  - For acute dacryocystitis, initial treatment is warm compresses and systemic antibiotics.

Figure 5-41. Note the distended nasolacrimal sac, diffuse erythema, crusted debris on the eyelid margin, and high tear lake in this patient with acute dacryocystitis. Fluorescein solution has been placed on the eye to demonstrate delayed tear drainage.

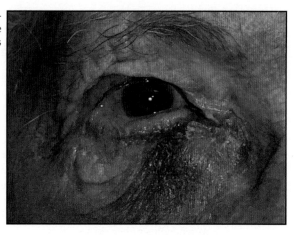

- ○ DCR is generally necessary to restore patency of the lacrimal tract after the initial infection has resolved.
- ○ Chronic dacryocystitis also frequently requires surgical intervention to correct epiphora and treat lacrimal sac distention.
- Prognosis
  - ○ With timely antibiotics and surgical care, dacryocystitis is usually treated successfully.

Canalicular Obstruction and Canaliculitis

- Definition
  - ○ Canalicular obstructions can be divided into nonsuppurative (obstructive) and suppurative (canaliculitis).
- Etiology
  - ○ Canalicular obstruction may be caused by viral infections (herpes simplex and zoster), trachoma, ocular pemphigoid and SJS, radiation, thermal and chemical burns, and glaucoma medications (phospholine iodide or epinephrine). Other causes include systemic chemotherapy (fluorouracil or docetaxel), rare tumors, iatrogenic damage during probing or surgery, postmenopause, and idiopathic.
  - ○ Canaliculitis is often caused by *Actinomycetes israelii*, an anaerobic, gram-positive branching filamentous bacterium normally found in the mouth. Other causes include *Aspergillus fumigatus*, *Candida albicans*, *Fusobacterium neucleatum*, *Nocardia*, and *Rhinosporidiosis*.
- Signs/symptoms
  - ○ Canalicular obstruction
    - ▪ Patients with canalicular obstruction will have tearing (ie, epiphora) that may be intermittent or constant.
    - ▪ Crusting along the medial or lateral canthi and eyelashes can occur.
    - ▪ Canalicular obstruction manifests as increased tear film, conjunctivitis, and possibly punctual occlusion.
  - ○ Canaliculitis
    - ▪ Discharge and conjunctivitis
      - ▫ Punctum is usually pouting with a whitish discharge coming from the punctum that can be milked with pressure on the canaliculus.
      - ▫ There is often inflammation of the eyelid overlying the horizontal canaliculus.
      - ▫ Rarely, there is an underlying dacryocystitis.
- Differential diagnosis
  - ○ Any condition that may mimic tearing or conjunctival infection should be considered when evaluating for canalicular disease (eg, allergic conjunctivitis, dry eye syndrome, blepharitis, eyelid or punctual ectropion, prior lid and facial surgery, corneal abrasion or exposure, corneal infections, FES, lacrimal mucocele, and lid tumors).
- Evaluation
  - ○ Tests of tear secretion (Schirmer's testing) can rule out reflex epiphora due to dry eye syndrome.
  - ○ Fluorescein testing can rule out corneal and conjunctival diseases.

- o Slit-lamp biomicroscopy can measure the tear film, which should usually be at least 0.3 mm.
- o Dye disappearance tests, including Jones I and II, can localize the obstruction.
- o Lacrimal probing and irrigation definitively indicates location of the canalicular blockage.
- Management
  - o Surgical treatment of canalicular obstruction depends on whether one or both are involved and on the precise size and location of the blockage.
  - o Treatments include canalicular intubation, balloon catheter dilatation, canalicular membranectomy with radiosurgery or laser, caniculodacryocystorhinostomy, DCR, and conjunctivodacryocystorhinostomy (Jones bypass tube).
  - o Canaliculitis can be treated with antibiotic drops, but often requires surgical canaliculotomy or punctal dilation with curettage of stones.
- Prognosis
  - o Success rates vary from 40% to 90%.
    - The longer the length of the canalicular obstruction and the more medial its location, the more difficult the surgery and the lower the success rates.
    - Canaliculitis generally responds to canaliculotomy or punctal dilation with removal of any canalicular stones, but may recur.

Lacrimal Duct Disorders Associated With Systemic Disease

- Etiology (Tables 5-4 and 5-5)
  - o Endogenous
    - Wegener's granulomatosis
      - □ Autoimmune disorder that causes inflammation of the blood vessels in the upper respiratory tract, lungs, and kidneys
      - □ Bullen and colleagues reported that 10 of 140 cases of this condition had nasolacrimal duct obstruction
      - □ Nasolacrimal duct involvement is usually associated with advanced nasal disease
    - SJS
      - □ May cause punctal and canalicular obstruction, although nasolacrimal duct obstruction secondary to SJS, although rare, is also possible.
    - Sarcoidosis, cicatricial pemphigoid
  - o Exogenous
    - Iatrogenic stenosis and fibrosis
      - □ Ophthalmic medications may be the most common cause of iatrogenic punctal or canalicular scarring.
      - □ Radiation, systemic chemotherapy, and bone marrow transplantation can cause lacrimal duct obstruction.
      - □ External radiation therapy can incite sufficient inflammation to close the lacrimal drainage passages.
      - □ Brachytherapy for ocular tumors can also cause radiation injury of the lacrimal drainage. The effect of external radiation on the nasolacrimal duct, as an innocent bystander, is dose-dependent.
      - □ Burns and colleagues reported nasolacrimal duct obstruction as a result of I(131) therapy for thyroid carcinoma. Obstructed areas included the nasolacrimal duct, common canaliculus, and the upper and lower canaliculus.
      - □ Systemic chemotherapy with fluorouracil is also known to be associated with occlusion of the puncta or canaliculi.
    - Docetaxel (Taxotere)
      - □ Chemotherapy agent in the group of drugs known as taxanes and is widely used in the treatment of malignancies, such as breast, lung, and prostate cancers
      - □ Esmaeli and colleagues concluded that canalicular and nasolacrimal duct obstruction is a common side effect of docetaxel therapy and recommended early silicone intubation in symptomatic patients to prevent further closure of the lacrimal drainage apparatus and to avoid more invasive lacrimal surgery.
    - Primary tumors of the lacrimal drainage system
      - □ Relatively uncommon and metastatic carcinomas are extremely rare
      - □ Secondary neoplasms are commonly caused by eyelid cancer, BCa in particular.

TABLE 5-4. INFLAMMATORY CONDITIONS CAUSING LACRIMAL DRAINAGE DISORDERS

Endogenous	Wegener's granulomatosis Sarcoidosis Cicatricial pemphigoid SJS (erythema multiforme) Kawasaki's disease (mucocutaneous lymph nose syndrome) Crohn's disease
Exogenous	Radiation therapy Fluorouracil (systemic) Docetaxel (Taxotere) Graft versus host diseases Allergy

Adapted from Bartley GB. Acquired lacrimal drainage obstruction: an etiologic classification system, and a review of the literature. *Ophthal Plast Reconstr Surg.* 1993;9(1):11-26.

TABLE 5-5. OTHER SYSTEMIC CAUSES OF LACRIMAL DRAINAGE DISORDERS

Neoplastic	Lymphoma Leukemia
Infectious	Herpes simplex Infectious mononucleosis (Epstein-Barr Virus)

Adapted from Bartley GB. Acquired lacrimal drainage obstruction: an etiologic classification system, and a review of the literature. Part 3. *Ophthal Plast Reconstr Surg.* 1993;9(1):11-26.

- ◻ Other causes are lymphogenic or leukemic in nature.
- ◻ Metastasis to the lacrimal drainage system can come from breast cancer, prostate cancer, or melanoma.

Lacrimal Outflow Surgery

- Punctoplasty
  - ○ Indications
    - ▪ Tearing due to punctal stenosis
  - ○ Description
    - ▪ The punctum is dilated and then opened using a 1-, 2-, or 3-snip punctoplasty.
    - ▪ The first snip is cut perpendicular to the internal elastic lamina of the punctum.
    - ▪ The second snip is extended from the base of the first snip, parallel to the eyelid margin and through the canaliculus.
    - ▪ The third snip amputates the tissue between the second snip and the punctal orifice.
    - ▪ The procedure may be terminated at any snip according to the surgeon's preference.
    - ▪ There are several commercially available devices for punctoplasty though none are widely accepted in practice.
  - ○ Complications
    - ▪ Bleeding, re-stenosis of the punctum, or infection
- Nasolacrimal duct probing
  - ○ Indications
    - ▪ Congenital nasolacrimal duct obstruction (Figure 5-42)
  - ○ Description
    - ▪ A blunt, semiflexible probe is inserted into the punctum through the vertical canaliculus, horizontal canaliculus, and into the lacrimal sac.

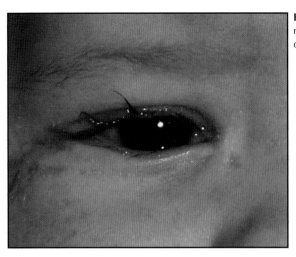

Figure 5-42. Note the crusted debris in the eyelid margin and mucoid discharge in this child with a congenital nasolacrimal duct obstruction.

- The probe is then rotated 90 degrees vertically and passed through the nasolacrimal duct, through the valve of Hasner, and into the inferior nasal meatus.
- Successful passage of the probe is confirmed visually or with a second instrument in the nose.
- The lacrimal system may then be irrigated to confirm patency of the tract.
- Sometimes, infracture of the inferior turbinate will also aid tear drainage.
- Children under 6 months of age may be probed in the office if they can be sufficiently restrained.
- Children over 6 months of age usually require a brief general anesthetic.
  - Complications
    - Unsuccessful surgery and creation of a false lacrimal tract. Nasolacrimal duct probing in adults has a low rate of success.
- Silicone lacrimal intubation
  - Indications
    - Nasolacrimal duct obstruction refractory to simple probing and irrigation
  - Description
    - The nasal mucosa is decongested with oxymetazoline and silicone tubes that have been swedged to blunt lacrimal probes are passed through the inferior and superior canaliculi and nasolacrimal duct similar to nasolacrimal probing.
    - The tubes are tied intranasally to themselves and secured to the lateral nasal wall to be left in place for several weeks.
  - Complications
    - Tube extrusion, failure to improve the occlusion, and infection
    - Tubes will occasionally cause a medially based corneal abrasion
- Balloon dacryoplasty (DCP)
  - Indications
    - Incomplete nasolacrimal duct obstruction
  - Description
    - A balloon catheter is inserted through the lacrimal tract in a manner similar to lacrimal probing and then taken through multiple inflation/deflation cycles, dilating the entire nasolacrimal duct.
    - Performed in an outpatient surgical or office setting, DCP may be combined with silicone intubation.
    - Nasal endoscopy enables identification of intranasal pathology that may contribute to epiphora and firmly establishes successful placement of the catheter.
- DCR
  - Indications
    - Complete nasolacrimal duct obstruction or incomplete nasolacrimal obstruction refractory to other treatments

- o Description
  - This procedure may be performed externally or intranasally and creates a new passage between the nasolacrimal sac and the middle meatus, bypassing the nasolacrimal duct.
  - In the external approach, an incision is made near the anterior lacrimal crest.
  - An osteotomy is made in the medial wall of the lacrimal fossa, and an opening into the middle meatus is made.
  - The lacrimal sac is opened, and a silicone tube is usually passed through both canaliculi, through the lacrimal sac and into the middle meatus.
  - Silicone tubes are thought to help maintain patency of the new tract during healing.
  - In the transnasal approach, the lacrimal sac is opened into the middle meatus either with a balloon or by removing bone transnasally.
  - Silicone tubes are generally placed through both canaliculi to ensure patency of the tract.
- o Complications
  - Infection, CSF leak, meningitis, bleeding (which may be consequential in very young patients), scarring, and failure to improve the obstruction may occur.
- o Prognosis
  - The external approach is generally thought to have a 90% success rate. The success rate may be slightly lower with transnasal techniques.
- Conjunctivodacryocystorhinostomy (CDCR)
  - o Indications
    - Canalicular occlusion, failed DCR
  - o Description
    - □ CDCR involves the creation of a tract through the medial canthus at the level of the caruncle.
    - □ The tract extends through the area of the lacrimal sac and exits into the middle meatus.
    - □ A glass bypass tube is placed in the tract to maintain patency.
    - □ The intranasal tip of the tube should drain well and not be blocked by the turbinates or the nasal septum.
  - o Complications
    - Tube migration into the nose, loss of the tube, bleeding, and ocular irritation from the top of the tube may occur.
  - o Prognosis
    - Success rates are variable, and CDCR is generally considered the "last option" to relieve epiphora.
- Lacrimal outflow occlusion (Punctal occlusion)
  - o Indications
    - Dry eye and for enhancement of therapeutic effect of topical ophthalmic medications
  - o Description
    - A test obstruction with a dissolvable collagen plug is generally undertaken as a trial measure. Such plugs are placed in the horizontal canaliculus and generally dissolve within 2 weeks.
    - Permanent (but theoretically reversible) occlusion can be achieved through use of punctal plugs typically made of silicone. Punctal occlusion devices can be divided into 2 main categories: those that are collared and sit on the punctum and those that are designed to lodge invisibly in the horizontal canaliculus.
    - Collared plugs may be removed in a retrograde fashion, pulling them back out of the punctum the same way they were installed.
    - Noncollared plugs (those meant to reside in the horizontal canaliculus) are theoretically removed by lacrimal irrigation, but noncollared plugs may be associated with an increased rate of irreversible canalicular obstruction.
    - Cautery can be used to stenose the punctal orifice. Cautery occlusion of the puncta can be performed quite simply (or reversed, when necessary) in the office.
  - o Complications
    - Symptomatic epiphora, failure to improve dry eye symptoms, and irreversible occlusion may occur.

Cosmetic Oculoplastic Surgery

Botulinum Toxin

- Definition
  - First identified as a powerful neuromuscular toxin associated with botulism poisoning, BTX was adapted for medical use by Dr. Alan Scott.
  - BTX received FDA clearance in 1989 for the treatment of blepharospasm, hemifacial spasm, and strabismus.
  - In 2002, Allergan (Irvine, CA) received FDA clearance for the use of this agent to smooth corrugator and procerus furrows.
  - Since that time, the use of BTX has increased dramatically.
  - It is now used for facial rejuvenation, headaches, hyperhidrosis, etc.
- Procedure
  - Botulinum toxin A (BOTOX, Allergan) is manufactured as a powder (100 units/vial) and must be diluted before use.
  - Practitioner preference determines the volume of dilution. This author prefers to add 2.5 cc of nonpreserved saline, providing for a solution that contains 4 units BOTOX/0.1 cc.
  - After the administration of a topical anesthetic cream, this solution is injected into the desired facial muscles to elicit a relaxation of dynamic wrinkles (Figure 5-43).
  - The most commonly treated muscles are the procerus, frontalis, orbicularis oculi, orbicularis oris, nasalis, platysma, levator labii superioris alaeque nasi, and mentalis.
  - In general, the relaxant effect takes several days and up to 2 weeks to take effect and lasts up to 3 to 4 months.
- Complications
  - Systemic side effects of BOTOX use are rare in the doses that are recommended.
  - However, postinjection headache (perhaps from frontalis contraction) and bruising may occur
  - As with all procedures, the avoidance of anticoagulation medication and herbs prior to injection (aspirin, Coumadin, Plavix, garlic, gingko, ginger, ginseng, etc) will reduce the risk of postinjection bruising.
  - The use of postinjection ice compresses is recommended as well.
  - If the toxin is injected within the orbital rim, ptosis may occur. This is treatable with Iopidine eye drops. Patients may be reassured that the ptosis will disappear over time.
- Muscles treated with BOTOX and initial doses
  - Frontalis—2 to 4 units/injection
  - Corrugators—4 to 5 units/injection
  - Procerus—4 to 5 units/injection
  - Nasalis—2 to 4 units/injection
  - Orbicularis oculi—2-5 units/injection
  - Orbicularis oris (lipstick lines)—1 to 2 units/injection
  - Popply chin or mental crease—1 to 3 units/injection
  - Marionette lines (depressor labii inferioris)—1 to 2 units/injection
  - Platysma—2 to 3 units/injection

Restylane and Other Fillers

- Definition
  - Unlike BOTOX, which is most useful for the treatment of dynamic wrinkles, fillers are most useful for the treatment of wrinkles at rest.
  - Fillers attempt to replace the skin's cutaneous collagen, fat, and hyaluronic substrate diminished by the aging process.
  - These fillers are manufactured in a multitude of forms, each attempting to optimize longevity, antigenicity, flow, and fill characteristics (Table 5-6).
- Complications
  - With most of these therapies, an expected side effect would be erythema, induration, and some bruising in the immediate postinjection period.

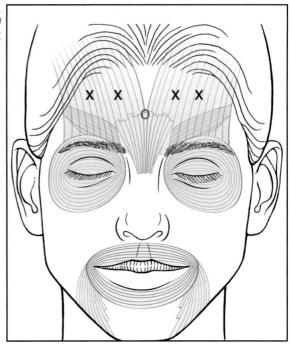

Figure 5-43. Botulinum toxin forehead injection sites. (Reprinted with permission from Lipham WJ. *Cosmetic and Clinical Applications of Botulinum Toxin.* Thorofare, NJ: SLACK Incorporated; 2004.)

- ○ Granuloma formation and a rare abscess may occur.
- ○ There are reported cases of local necrosis and sloughing from injection leading to vascular occlusion and even blindness.

Ablative Laser Skin Resurfacing

- Definition
  - ○ Aging, sun exposure, smoking, and hereditary predisposition all contribute to facial wrinkles and loss of skin tone.
  - ○ The underlying mechanism is breakdown of the dermal collagen and elastin fibers.
  - ○ Blepharoplasty and face lifts may reduce skin laxity by removing excess tissue, but they do not correct the underlying loss of elasticity and structural integrity.
  - ○ Furthermore, these procedures do not correct skin dyschromia.
  - ○ Laser resurfacing is a procedure that both removes sun-damaged epithelium and stimulates new collagen to restore some of the skin's lost elasticity.
- Procedure
  - ○ The principle behind ablative laser resurfacing is selective photothermolysis.
  - ○ Ablative lasers use wavelengths of light that are absorbed by water. The laser energy is absorbed by water in the cells and the cells are vaporized.
  - ○ Every cell in the path of the laser is affected.
  - ○ By carefully controlling the spot size, duration of the pulse, and fluence, or amount of energy delivered in a given area, the depth of penetration can be precisely controlled.
  - ○ Short, high-energy pulse can ablate thin tissue layers with only 20 to 70 μm of residual thermal injury.
  - ○ The lasers used for ablative resurfacing are CO_2 with a wavelength of 10,600 nm and erbium with a wavelength of 2940 nm. Both lasers emit in the infrared light spectrum and are highly absorbed by water. CO_2 lasers penetrate deeper than erbium lasers, but also generate more thermal injury.
    - ▪ The advantage of the CO_2 lasers is that they coagulate the small vessels in the dermis so there is no bleeding during the procedure. Erbium lasers do not have the same coagulative properties, so as ablation is carried deeper, small vessels within the dermis tend to bleed.

TABLE 5-6. WIDELY AVAILABLE FILLERS IN THE UNITED STATES, WITH KEY DIFFERENTIATING FEATURES

CLASS	BRAND NAME	COMMENTS	DURATION
Bovine collagen	Zyderm, Zyplast	Requires skin test (3% incidence allergy), lidocaine in syringe	Lasts 3 to 5 months; rarely used
	Artecoll	Requires skin test	Incorporates PMMA microspheres in a bovine collagen substrate (not FDA approved) Inamed
Human collagen	Cosmoderm, Cosmoplast	No skin test required Lidocaine in syringe	Lasts 2 to 6 months Manufactured from cell culture of human foreskin Inamed
Hyaluronic acid (HA—polysaccharide, identical across species, no skin test required)	Restylane (Medicis Aesthetics Inc. Scottsdale, Arizona)	Bacterial fermentation (20 mg HA/cc)	Lasts 6 to 8 months
	Hylaform-Hylan B gel	Avian derived (rooster comb)	Lasts 3 to 4 months Inamed
	Captique	Bacterial fermentation (5 mg HA/cc)	Lasts 4 to 6 months Inamed
Long lasting—no skin test required	Sculptra	Poly-L-lactic acid (40 to 63 μm in a carboxymethylcellulose gel)	FDA approved for HIV lipoatrophy, lasts 18 to 24+ months
	Radiesse (Radiance)	Calcium hydroxyapatite in polysaccharide gel	FDA approved for use in larynx and bladder, lasts 3 to 5 years
Permanent	Silicone-Adatosil, Silikon	No skin testing	FDA approved for ophthalmic use; use in skin off-label
	Fat	Autogenous, requires second site for extraction; large supply	May require repeat injection of frozen fat to sustain fill as a percentage of graft does not survive

- The disadvantage of the CO_2 laser is that they have more thermal effect in a deeper area of thermal damage; re-epithelialization is slower and redness persists longer after CO_2 laser ablation. Some lasers combine CO_2 and erbium wavelengths or use dual erbium crystals to give more coagulation; with such lasers, the ablative and coagulative properties can be adjusted for any individual situation. Computer-controlled scanners deliver the energy to the tissue in a precise and homogenous pattern.
- Erbium lasers are effective for fine lines and modest laxity, while CO_2 lasers are also effective in treating significant laxity and deeper creases. The parameters of either laser, however, can be modified to be used at either end of the spectrum.
  - Postoperatively, the de-epithelialized skin is kept moist, often with a petrolatum-based ointment, until re-epithelialization is completed over 5 to 10 days. Patients are often treated with oral antibiotics and antiviral medication during the re-epithelialization phase. Once the epithelium has regenerated, the delicate new skin must be protected from the sun for several months.
- Complications
  - Scarring, hyperpigmentation, hypopigmentation, and infection may occur.

Microdermabrasion, Chemical Peels, and Cosmeceuticals

- Introduction/definition
  - Stimulate epidermal and dermal rejuvenation and promote new collagen production
  - Work by disrupting and eventually removing the stratum corneum, which induces regeneration and thickening of the epidermis and dermis
  - Inflammatory responses to skin disruption appear to stimulate new collagen production and improve skin elasticity, as well as stimulate dermal fibroblast proliferation and extracellular matrix production.
  - The end result is thickening of the epidermis and dermis with improved skin appearance and wrinkle reduction.
- Microdermabrasion
  - Physical disruption of the epithelium is created by bombarding the skin surface with a steady stream of microparticles composed of sodium chloride or aluminum oxide crystals.
  - The flow rate of the particles and the numbers of passes applied to a treated area are varied to create the desired individual effect.
  - Removal of superficial epithelium stimulates collagen formation, invigorates epithelial cell maturation, promotes proliferation of the germinal layer, and reduces rete ridges.
  - Microdermabrasion can also improve the appearance of surgical or acne scars, photoaging, rhytids, striae, and melasma.
  - The endpoint of the procedure is removal of the superficial epithelium.
  - Postprocedural care includes daily cleansing of the treated area, mild moisturizing cream, and the application of sunscreen before going outdoors.
- Chemical peels
  - Popular, effective, and have a predictable down time related to the depth of the peel
  - Quite varied and include "lunchtime" procedures, which improve wrinkles, acne scarring, solar keratosis, and benign pigmented lesions
  - Remove the skin layers down to varying depths and concomitantly remove superficial lesions and improve overall skin texture and tone
  - There are 3 categories of chemical peels, which are classified according to effectiveness and depth of penetration.
    - So called "light peels" typically use mild exfoliants such as alpha hydroxyacids found in natural fruits and botanicals. The alpha hydroxyacids exfoliate only the superficial epidermis so recovery often only involves 30 minutes or so of erythema. They improve sun-damaged skin, reduce pore size, and improve fine rhytids. Multiple treatments separated by 2 to 3 weeks are optimal.
    - "Medium depth" peels commonly use more powerful exfoliants such as TCA, and recovery consists of several days of scaling and sloughing of the epidermis. These peels diminish medium wrinkles and some precancerous lesions.
    - The deep chemical peel is performed using phenol (C_6H_6O). Epithelial recovery from this peel is intense. There is oozing of the skin for up to 2 weeks, and redness lasts several months. Results are dramatic although there may be significant skin depigmentation. Severe skin complications may arise from improper application. Furthermore, phenol can also cause cardiac rhythm complications as it is absorbed through the skin, so EKG monitoring and hydration precautions must be taken.
- Topical skin agents
  - Hydroquinone
    - Acts as a bleaching cream by reducing the amount of melanin produced in the skin
    - Reduced melanin production results in diminished skin pigmentation.
    - Hydroquinone in lotion or gel form is applied to the pigmented area nightly before bedtime and is used for a few months or until significant improvement in discoloration is achieved.
  - Tretinoin
    - Increases maturation and regeneration of skin cells, which are exfoliated and replaced
  - The process acts to reduce acne breakouts, improve fine lines, and improve skin texture.

Face Lift, Forehead Rejuvenation, and Neck

- Rejuvenation
  - o Definition
    - From Greek *rhytis*, which means wrinkle; facial aging changes that result in wrinkles and soft tissue descent
    - These wrinkles may be seen at rest (static) or with facial expression (dynamic).
  - o Etiology
    - Facial rhytids are a result of natural (intrinsic) and acquired (extrinsic) factors that result in soft tissue elasticity and volume loss with resultant deflation, as well as gravitational effects resulting in descent.
    - Additional bony and cartilaginous volume loss can accentuate the clinical features of aging.
  - o Symptoms
    - With forehead and brow descent, patients often complain of gradual onset of superior (especially temporal) visual field loss, eyestrain, and headaches from chronic brow.
    - Additionally, patients complain of a fatigued or depressed appearance that does not fit their mood.
  - o Signs
    - Vertical descent of the foreheads, cheeks, and jowls toward the midline: receding hairline; forehead horizontal rhytids; brow ptosis; dermatochalasis; midface descent lengthens the lower eyelid-cheek junction below the inferior orbital rim, creating a "V-pattern" of infra-orbital descent; eyelid laxity with lateral canthal tendon laxity; herniated orbital fat (steatoblepharon); prominent nasolabial and nasojugal folds; jowling; platysmal descent/banding; neck lipomatosis
  - o Differential diagnosis
    - Cranial nerve VII palsy, post-traumatic bony and/or soft tissue facial changes, cicatricial soft tissue changes
  - o Evaluation
    - Systemic evaluation—current and past medications (especially Accutane [isotrentinoin] use); medical and surgical history
    - Social history (tobacco history, sun exposure)
    - Thorough consultation (patient desires, realistic expectations, maturity level, compliance level, risks and benefits of surgery)
    - Complete documentation of stigmata of facial aging changes
    - External photographs (frontal, lateral, oblique views)
    - Facial nerve evaluation (cranial nerve VII)
  - o Management
    - No treatment is necessary unless significant visual field changes are present.
    - Forehead rejuvenation
      - □ Via browlifting (endoscopic [Figure 5-44], coronal, pretrichial, midforehead, direct, transblepharoplasty), with blepharoplasty, chemodenervation of row depressors (with BTX), tissue fillers for furrows, cutaneous skin resurfacing (chemical peels, abalative and nonablative lasers/radiofrequency/pulsed light)
    - Midface rejuvenation
      - □ Tissue fillers, chemodenervation, lower eyelid blepharoplasty; surgical midface elevation (subperiosteal, subcutaneous), bony augmentation (orbital rim/cheek/malar implants), cutaneous skin resurfacing
    - Lower facial rejuvenation
      - □ Tissue fillers, chemodenervation, traditional facial rhytidectomy surgery (subcutaneous, subcutaneous musculoaponeurotic system [SMAS] plication/imbrication/deep plane technique), chin augmentation, cutaneous skin resurfacing
    - Neck rejuvenation
      - □ Liposuction, platysmal plication
  - o Prognosis
    - Cosmetic surgery is associated with high patient satisfaction.
    - The patient must understand that while surgical intervention reverses many stigmata of facial aging, any intervention does not stop the aging process, which will continue.
    - Thus, intervention is temporary and may need augmentation at some future date.

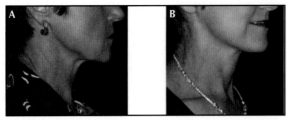

Figure 5-44. (A) Preoperative and (B) 15-month postoperative lateral views of a patient who underwent an endoscopic browlift, deep plane facial rhytidectomy, and platysmal plication for facial aging changes.

Thanks to the following coauthors for their generous contributions and collaboration, without which this chapter would not have been possible: Kathleen Archer, Chaitanya V. Aysola, Cat Nguyen Burkat, Michael A. Burnstine, William Pai-Dei Chen, Raymond S. Douglas, Vikram D. Durairaj, Melanie H. Erb, Christopher D. Gelston, James W. Gigantelli, Tyrone Glover, Andrew R. Harrison, Morris Hartstein, David E.E. Holck, Don O. Kikkawa, Bobby S. Korn, Bradley N. Lemke, Geva Mannor, Michael McCracken, Michael E. Migliori, Yasaman Mohadjer, Manuel O. Palmero, BCK Patel, Julian D. Perry, Karim G. Punja, Geoffrey E. Rose, Stuart R. Seiff, and Rona Z. Silkis, David Weinberg, W. Abraham White, William L. White, and Orin M. Zwick.

Suggested Readings

Bartley GB, Fatourechi V, Kadrmas EF, et al. Clinical features of Graves' ophthalmopathy in an incidence cohort. *Am J Ophthalmol*. 1996;121:284–290.

Culbertson WW, Ostler HB. The floppy eyelid syndrome. *Am J Ophthalmol*. 1981;92:568–575.

Gilden DH. Clinical practice. Bell's palsy. *N Engl J Med*. 2004;351:1323–1331.

Gossman MD, Berlin AJ. Management of acute adnexal trauma. In: Stewart WB, ed. *Surgery of the Eyelid, Orbit & Lacrimal System*. San Francisco, CA: American Academy of Ophthalmology Monograph; 1993:170–196.

Grove AS, McCord CD. Acute orbital trauma: diagnosis and management. In: McCord CD, Tanenbaum MT, ed. *Oculoplastic Surgery*. 2nd ed. New York, NY: Raven Press; 1987:129–154.

Hurwitz JJ. *The Lacrimal System*. Philadelphia, PA: Lippincott-Raven; 1996.

Kennerdell J. *Practical Diagnosis and Management of Orbital Diseases*. Boston, MA: Butterworth-Heinemann, 2001.

Rootman J, ed. *Diseases of the Orbit: A Multidisciplinary Approach*. Philadelphia, PA: Lippincott Williams & Wilkins; 2003.

Saunders DH, Flanagan JC. Disorders of the lids. In: Nelson LB, Calhoun JH, Harley RD, eds. *Pediatric Ophthalmology*, 3rd ed. Philadelphia, PA: W.B. Saunders; 1991:334–354.

Small RG, Sabates NR, Burrows D. The measurement and definition of ptosis. *Ophthal Plast Reconstr Surg*. 1989;5(3):171–175.

Stegman SJ, Tromovitch TA, Glogau RG. *Cosmetic Dermatologic Surgery*. St Louis, MO: Mosby-Yearbook; 1990.

Questions

1. How would you repair left upper eyelid involutional ptosis in a 75 year old with good LF?
   a. Frontalis sling
   b. Upper eyelid blepharoplasty
   c. **Levator advancement**
   d. Botulinum toxin

2. Which, if any, of the following conditions is NOT associated with lacrimal drainage disorders?
   a. Wegener's granulomatosis
   b. Sarcoidosis
   c. Docetaxel (Taxotere)
   d. Graft versus host diseases
   e. **All of the above are associated**

3. What is the innervation of Müller's muscle?
   a. Cranial nerve II
   b. Cranial nerve III
   c. **Sympathetic nervous system**
   d. Parasympathetic nervous system

4. Which of the following "Ps" is not included in the evaluation of the orbit?
   a. Proptosis
   b. Pain
   c. **Pigment**
   d. Pulsation
   e. Progression

5. Which of the following is not associated with preseptal cellulitis?
   a. Eyelid edema
   b. Eyelid erythema
   c. Superficial skin break
   d. **Proptosis**
   e. Tenderness on palpation

6. Immediately after entering into the punctum, tears flow into which of the following:
   a. Lacrimal sac
   b. **Canaliculus**
   c. Lacrimal duct
   d. Common canaliculus

7. What is the most common malignancy to affect the LG?
   a. **Lymphoma**
   b. Squamous cell carcinoma
   c. Adenoid cystic carcinoma
   d. Pleomorphic adenoma

8. Which of the following is false regarding essential blepharospasm?
   a. Oromandibular dystonia occurring with blepharospasm is called Meige's syndrome.
   b. Inability to open the eyes is called apraxia of eyelid opening.
   c. EMG studies may show abnormalitie.s
   d. **Antiseizure medications such as carbamazepine have a high rate of success.**

9. Xanthelasma palpebrarum may be associated with multiple disorders, but most commonly may be an indicator of increased
   a. Blood sugar levels
   b. **Serum cholesterol**
   c. Blood pressure
   d. Serum calcium

10. What is the most common cause of unilateral or bilateral proptosis in an adult?
    a. Orbital metastasis
    b. **Graves ophthalmopathy**
    c. Giant cell arteritis
    d. Orbital helminthic infection

Cornea and Anterior Segment

Julie H. Tsai, MD, and Edward J. Holland, MD

Outline

Probst LE, Tsai JH.
Ophthalmology: Clinical and Surgical Principles (pp. 199–262).
© 2012 SLACK Incorporated

i. Cicatricial Pemphigoid (Mucous Membrane Pemphigoid)
ii. Stevens-Johnson Syndrome
iii. Phlyctenular Keratoconjunctivitis
iv. Staphylococcal Marginal Keratitis
v. Mooren's Ulcer
6. Trauma
  a. Blunt/Penetrating Injuries
	b. Thermal Injuries
	c. Chemical Injuries
	7. Complications Related to Contact Lens Use
	8. Corneal Surgery
	  a. Lamellar Keratoplasty
	  b. Corneal Transplantation
	  c. New Techniques in Endothelial Kerato-plasty

Diseases of the Conjunctiva

Conjunctivitis

- Inflammation of the conjunctiva
  - Infectious or noninfectious
  - Chronic (greater than 4 weeks) or acute
  - Often associated with keratitis

Acute Infectious Conjunctivitis

Bacterial Conjunctivitis

- Etiology
  - *Staphylococcus aureus*
  - *Streptococcus pneumoniae*
  - *Haemophilus* species
  - *Moraxella catarrhalis*
  - *Neiserria gonorrhoeae*
    - Hyperacute
    - May cause corneal perforation
    - Important cause of neonatal conjunctivitis
- Signs/symptoms
  - Conjunctival injection
  - Papillary reaction of conjunctiva
  - Purulent discharge
- Treatment
  - Broad-spectrum topical antibiotic shortens course of disease
    - Second-, third-, and fourth-generation fluoroquinolones
    - Trimethoprim-polymyxin B
    - Sulfacetamide
    - Erythromycin

Viral Conjunctivitis

- Etiology
  - Adenovirus (most common)
    - Epidemic keratoconjunctivitis
    - Subtypes 8 and 19
    - Pharyngoconjunctival fever
    - Subtypes 3 and 7
  - Herpes simplex virus (see keratitis section on p. 234)
  - Other viral etiologies
    - Varicella zoster
    - Influenza
    - Mumps
    - Rubeola
    - Mononucleosis

- Signs/symptoms
  - Serous discharge
  - Eyelid edema
  - Possible pseudomembranes
  - Pre-auricular lymphadenopathy
  - Corneal subepithelial infiltrates
- Treatment
  - Generally self-limited
  - Prevention of transmission

Chronic Infectious Conjunctivitis

Molluscum Contagiosum
- Umbilicated lesions usually on eyelid margin
- Treatment
  - Often self-limited
  - Various topical medications
  - Curettage

Chlamydia
- Sexually transmitted
- Follicles on inferior palpebral conjunctiva
- Preauricular node
- Treatment is oral tetracycline.

Allergic Conjunctivitis
- Signs/symptoms
  - Itching
  - Bilateral
  - Inflammation
  - Usually chronic, recurrent
  - Tearing
  - Stinging
- Classification

Seasonal
- Most common
- Type 1 hypersensitivity reaction
  - Interaction of allergen with mast cell IgE receptors
  - Histamine released from mast cells results in majority of symptoms.
- Mostly in spring and fall
- Due to airborne allergens
  - Pollen
- Perennial type usually milder
  - Usually household allergens
    - Dust mites
    - Dander

Vernal Keratoconjunctivitis
- Mostly males younger than 20 years of age
- Usually spring and fall
- Intensely itchy
- Thick ropy discharge
- Types 1 and 4 allergic reaction
  - Both mast cell and lymphocyte mediated reaction
  - Tissue infiltrated by lymphocytes, plasma cells, and eosinophils
  - Large number of cells accumulate, creating nodules of tissue (giant papillae)

- o May be primarily palpebral or limbal in location
  - Palpebral form mostly affects upper tarsal plate.
  - Limbal form has jelly-like gray bumps with vascular core usually greatest at superior limbus.
    - □ A white center may form in the bump.
      - • Filled with eosinophils and epithelioid cells
      - • Called Horner-Trantas dot
- o Corneal epithelial defects can occur.
  - Called a shield ulcer

Giant Papillary Conjunctivitis

- Similar findings to vernal conjunctivitis due to foreign body
  - o Mostly with contact lens use
  - o Also prosthesis, suture, etc

Atopic Keratoconjunctivitis

- More common in teens and adults
- Includes types 1 and 4 allergic reaction
- Inferior palpebral conjunctiva frequently involved
- Not seasonal
- Associated with history of atopy and tendency for hypersensitivity reactions
- Asthma, atopic dermatitis, eczema
- Conjunctival scarring, corneal vascularization, cataracts common
  - o Treatment
    - Mast cell stabilizer/antihistamine combination
    - Mild topical steroid especially to start with vernal and atopic disease
    - Artificial tears may be helpful adjunct.
      - □ Dilutes allergic mediators and lubricates
    - Systemic antihistamines in some cases
      - □ These may also make eye drier and concentrate mediators.
      - □ Helpful to use artificial tears simultaneously
    - Topical nonsteroidal anti-inflammatory drugs (NSAIDs)
    - Topical antihistamine

Episcleritis

- Relatively benign condition, usually self-limited and involving the episclera (outer layer) of the eye
  - o Etiology
    - Majority idiopathic; some may have associated systemic disorder, most commonly rheumatoid arthritis or vasculitis
  - o Histology
    - Nongranulomatous inflammation of the episcleral tissue with dilation of the vasculature, with infiltration of lymphocytes and plasma cells in the surrounding tissues
  - o Signs/symptoms
    - Lid edema
    - Chemosis
    - Conjunctival injection (either diffuse or sectoral)
    - "Violaceous hue" in natural sunlight
- Differential diagnosis
  - Conjunctivitis (especially viral)
  - Phlyctenulosis (confusion with nodular episcleritis)
  - Scleritis
  - o Evaluation
    - Engorgement of the episcleral vessels can be visualized at the slit lamp, and delineation is achieved using the red-free filter.
    - Topical phenylephrine 2.5% can also blanch the conjunctival vasculature so that the deeper structures can be better visualized.
      - □ Topical phenylephrine 10% will blanch the conjunctival and episcleral vessels, allowing for delineation of episcleritis versus scleritis.

- o Management
    - ▪ Laboratory evaluation including rheumatoid factor (RF), antinuclear antibody (ANA), erythrocyte sedimentation rate (ESR), complete blood count (CBC), and treponemal testing may help to determine the cause of episcleritis.
    - ▪ Treatment is generally directed at the underlying etiology, though the natural course of the disease is such that treatment is not generally necessary.
        - ▫ Topical NSAIDs may be helpful. Topical corticosteroids may play a role in persistent cases, though systemic NSAIDs may be of more benefit.

Scleritis

- • Etiology
    - o Generally due to changes in the immune response that cause local damage to tissue and blood vessels. Often associated with systemic autoimmune disorders. Occasionally can be secondary to local infectious etiologies (ie, *Pseudomonas*).
    - o Classification
        - ▪ Often broken down into anterior and posterior scleritis, with diffuse, nodular, or necrotizing (with or without inflammation) types.
    - o Signs/symptoms
        - ▪ Marked pain, described as "boring" or aching. Dilated, tortuous sclera vessels can be noted upon biomicroscopy, with or without sclera edema.
        - ▪ Anterior scleritis
            - ▫ Involving the anterior portion of the sclera. May be diffuse in nature or present in the following manner:
                - • Nodular scleritis
                    - o Presents with a firm, immobile, and tender nodule
                    - o Can be small or large with a broad base
                    - o Often associated with systemic disease
                - • Necrotizing anterior scleritis with inflammation
                    - o The most severe form with potential for visual loss
                    - o Patients complain of extreme discomfort, and examination reveals avascular areas of sclera with surrounding edema and congestion.
                - • Necrotizing scleritis without inflammation (scleromalacia perforans)
                    - o May present with minimal symptoms including blurry vision or discoloration of the sclera
                - • Posterior scleritis
                    - o Often difficult to diagnose
                        - ▫ May be confused with other posterior segment diseases
                    - o Pain with eye movement, vision loss, chemosis, proptosis, lid edema, or ophthalmoplegia may result.
                    - o Other findings may include optic disc edema, optic neuritis, choroidal thickening, and choroidal folds.
    - o Differential diagnosis
        - ▪ Episcleritis, Mooren's ulcer, and peripheral ulcerative keratitis may be mistaken for scleritis; however, a detailed history and clinical examination will be able to distinguish these clinical entities from scleritis.
    - o Evaluation
        - ▪ Laboratory testing, including RF, ANA, ESR, CBC, antineutrophil cytoplasmic antibodies (ANCA), human leukocyte antigen (HLA) typing, and infectious serologies are most commonly obtained to determine the systemic associations and to direct therapy.
    - o Management
        - ▪ Systemic therapy with oral NSAIDs is the first-line treatment.
            - ▫ Usually effective at controlling pain and reducing inflammation. However, in necrotizing cases with underlying systemic associations, systemic immunosuppression may be required to manage and prevent complications.

Diseases of the Cornea

Developmental Abnormalities

- Corneal size and shape
  - The normal newborn cornea measures 10 mm in horizontal diameter; in the adult, the normal cornea measures 12 mm in horizontal diameter.
  - The horizontal diameter always exceeds the vertical diameter by approximately 1 mm due to prominent scleral encroachment in the superior and inferior limbus.
  - The cornea reaches adult size by 2 years of age.

Congenital Corneal Opacities

- Definition
  - Hereditary, developmental, or infectious etiologies that result in opacity of the cornea noted in the newborn (Table 6-1)
- Etiologies
  - Best summarized by the following STUMPED classification/mnemonic:
    - S—Sclerocornea
      - Scleralization of peripheral cornea (Figure 6-1), or of the entire cornea, secondary to mesodermal dysgenesis (error likely during seventh week of gestation)
      - Sporadic (can be autosomal dominant or recessive)
      - Nonprogressive, usually bilateral, may be asymmetric
      - Appears smooth, white, and vascular, not inflamed
      - Differential diagnosis
        - Arcus juvenilis, interstitial keratitis, Peters' anomaly, microcornea
      - Management
        - Penetrating keratoplasty in order to obtain useful vision if condition is bilateral
    - T—Tears in Descemet's membrane
      - Congenital glaucoma
        - Most important in differential diagnosis of congenital corneal clouding as delayed diagnosis can result in irreversible visual loss (Figure 6-2)
        - Mutations found in the CYP1B1 gene on chromosome 2p21
        - Signs/symptoms
          - Epiphora, photophobia, blepharospasm (classic triad); increased corneal diameter; diffuse corneal haziness (may precede breaks in Descemet's membrane in early disease); buphthalmos due to increased elasticity of infant cornea and sclera
        - Tears due to thinner Descemet's membrane in infants ($\sim$3 to 4 μm); appear as either single or multiple glassy parallel ridges on the posterior cornea either peripherally or in the visual axis (random distribution)
        - Management
          - Surgical (ie, goniotomy, trabeculotomy)
      - Birth trauma
        - Usually due to forceps injury (blunt trauma) (Figure 6-3), also seen with other soft tissue injuries (orbital/lid edema, ecchymosis)
        - Seen centrally, and in vertical or oblique pattern; acute elevation of intraocular pressure (IOP) (due to compression of globe from forceps) leads to distension of the globe and subsequent tears in Descemet's membrane
        - New endothelium resurfaces the area of the break.
        - Signs/symptoms
          - Diffuse central clouding, stromal and epithelial edema, high residual corneal astigmatism (steep axis parallels rupture lines)
        - Management
          - Amblyopia therapy, rigid gas permeable lenses for correction of astigmatism; surgical later in life if cornea decompensates

TABLE 6-1. CONGENITAL CORNEAL CONDITIONS

CONDITION	DESCRIPTION	PATHOGENESIS	CLINICAL FINDINGS	MANAGEMENT	PROGNOSIS
Megalocornea	Rare condition, corneal enlargement not associated with congenital glaucoma; histologically normal cornea (normal thickness, endothelial cell count, clarity) measuring 13.0 to 16.5 mm in diameter; keratometrically may be steeper (not always evident on keratometry)	May be arrested buphthalmos and exaggerated growth of the cornea in relation to the rest of the eye; may be associated with abnormal collagen production	May be associated with cataract, ectopia lentis, arcus lipoids, CCD, microcoria, goniodysgenesis; X-linked recessive; likely located in the Xq21.3–q22 region	Rule out congenital glaucoma	Nonprogressive
Microcornea	Fairly common, normal thickness cornea, horizontal diameter less than 10 mm (9 mm in newborns); anterior microphthalmos if whole anterior segment is small; distinct from nanophthalmos	Unknown; may be related to arrest of growth during fetal development; arrest of cornea development in fifth month	Hyperopia; higher incidence of ACG; associated PFV, cataract, anterior segment dysgenesis, ON hypoplasia; systemic associations include myotonic dystrophy, FAS, Ehlers-Danlos, achondroplasia; transmitted as AR or AD (more common), with equal sex predilection	Treatment of hyperopia and concurrent pathology	Excellent if isolated finding; otherwise dependent upon severity of associated conditions
Cornea plana	Flat cornea with a radius of curvature <43 D, with readings commonly in 20 to 30 D range; corneal curvature same as adjacent sclera is pathognomonic	Similar to sclerocornea; second wave of neural crest fails to form the limbal anlage and differentiates into tissue resembling sclera instead of corneal stroma (absence of limbus associated with failure of the corneal curve to develop)	Associated with sclerocornea or microcornea/ Systemic associations include cataract, anterior/posterior colobomas, Ehlers-Danlos; marked hyperopia, ACG due to morphologically shallow AC; recessive (most severe) and dominant forms exist; sporadic cases linked to chromosome 12q21.	Neutralize refractive errors; treat glaucoma; PK if central clarity is lost (note increased risk of graft rejection/post-PK glaucoma)	Dependent on severity of associated ocular disorders

CCD = Congenital corneal dystrophy; ACG = Angle closure glaucoma; PFV = Persistent fetal vasculature; ON = Optic nerve; FAS = Fetal alcohol syndrome; AD = Autosomal dominant; AR = Autosomal recessive; AC = Anterior chamber; PK = Penetrating keratoplasty

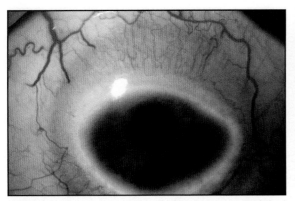

Figure 6-1. Peripheral sclerocornea. (This figure was published in *Cornea*. 2nd ed. Krachmer JH, Mannis MJ, Holland EJ, eds. Copyright Elsevier [2005].)

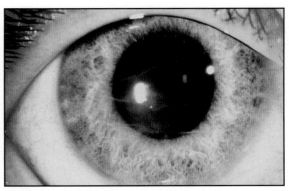

Figure 6-2. Haab's striae. Note the horizontal orientation of the tears in Descemet's membrane. (This figure was published in *Cornea*. 2nd ed. Krachmer JH, Mannis MJ, Holland EJ, eds. Copyright Elsevier [2005].)

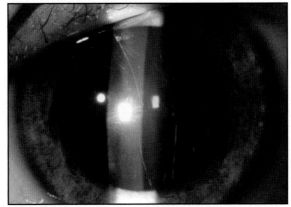

Figure 6-3. Forceps injury resulting in tears in Descemet's membrane. Note the vertical orientation of the tears. (This figure was published in *Cornea*. 2nd ed. Krachmer JH, Mannis MJ, Holland EJ, eds. Copyright Elsevier [2005].)

- U—Ulceration
  - □ Rarely present at birth
  - □ Etiologies
    - Viral (herpes simplex virus [HSV]), congenital rubella), bacterial (*Neisseria gonorrhoeae*, chlamydia), neurotrophic (familial dysautonomia)
  - □ Signs/symptoms
    - Epithelial defect, dendritic ulcer, lid edema with or without skin vesicles, conjunctival injection, transient stromal opacity, chemosis, watery or serosanguinous discharge, peripheral corneal infiltrates, perforation (*N. gonorrhoeae*, if untreated or infection occurs in utero)
  - □ Management
    - Intravenous acyclovir for neonatal HSV keratoconjunctivitis (prevent dissemination), trifluorothymidine (Viroptic) 5 to 9 times daily for epithelial disease. Vidarabine (Vira-A) is difficult to obtain in some areas of the country but may also be used. Topical erythromycin (prophylaxis) for *N. gonorrhoeae*, systemic erythromycin for systemic chlamydial infection, IV penicillin G or IV cefotaxime for systemic *N. gonorrhoeae* infection, fortified gentamycin/tobramycin for *Pseudomonas*.

TABLE 6-2. MUCOPOLYSACCHARIDOSES: CLINICAL FEATURES

Type	Inheritance Pattern	Clinical Findings	Syndrome	Other Systemic Abnormalities	Diagnostic Tests
I-H: Hurler	Autosomal recessive, severe corneal clouding in childhood	Diffuse punctuate stromal opacities not affecting epithelium or endothelium	Mental retardation, large head; abnormal-appearing face; neurological defects	Enlarged abdomen; hepatosplenomegaly; chest enlargement; cardiac defects	Laboratory confirmation: peripheral leukocyte levels of α-1-iduronidase
VI: Mariteaux-Lamy	Autosomal recessive, severe corneal clouding in childhood	Narrow angle glaucoma	Mild facial abnormalities; multiple skeletal changes; genu valgum;	Optic neuropathy; hydrocephalus	
I-S: Scheie	Autosomal recessive; corneal opacification at birth which progresses to visual loss by second decade	Thickened/edematous corneal (periphery > central), ± glaucoma	Claw hand deformities, bony changes in feet	Aortic valve abnormalities	
V: Morquio	Autosomal recessive; corneal opacities after 10 years old	Dwarfism, aortic valvular disease	Joint laxity		
II: Hunter	X-linked recessive; co-congenital corneal opacity	Milder phenotypes with corneal opacity later in life	Heart defects; deafness	Clinically similar to Hurler's syndrome	
III: Sanfilippo	Autosomal recessive, rare corneal opacification				

Adapted from Rezende RA et al. Congenital corneal opacities. In: Krachmer JH, Mannis MJ, Holland EJ, Eds. *Cornea*. 2nd ed. St. Louis, MO: Elsevier-Mosby; 2005:311–338.

- M—Metabolic
  - Mucopolysaccharidoses (Table 6-2)
    - Presents differently, depending on the specific enzyme deficiency; corneal clouding (Figure 6-4), pigmentary retinal findings, and optic atrophy are common to all disorders
    - Heparin and keratin sulfate (glycosaminoglycans) accumulate in cells and extracellular matrix of the cornea, and heparin sulfate accumulates in the retina and central nervous system.
    - Diagnosis
      - Increased urinary excretion of glycosaminoglycans

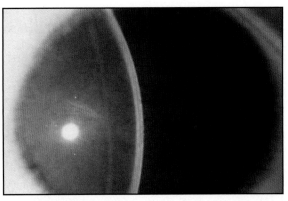

Figure 6-4. Corneal haze secondary to mucopolysaccharidosis. (This figure was published in *Cornea*. 2nd ed. Krachmer JH, Mannis MJ, Holland EJ, eds. Copyright Elsevier [2005].)

- Mucolipidoses (Table 6-3)
  - Autosomal recessive with neuraminidase deficiency with abnormal accumulation of sphingolipids, glucolipids, acid mucopolysaccharides
  - Corneal opacities commonly present at birth only MLS II and IV
- Cystinosis
  - Rare autosomal recessive metabolic disorder due to a defect in cystine transport. Biochemically, there is an abnormally high intracellular content of free cystine, which is deposited as crystals in various tissues including the eye (Figure 6-5)
  - Aberrant gene mapped to chromosome 17p
  - Corneal and conjunctival needle-like crystals are seen by age 1, starting centrally and progressing peripherally to involve the entire cornea.
  - Signs/symptoms
    - Irritation, pain, photophobia, erosions
  - Systemic manifestations
    - Renal failure, hypothyroidism, pancreatic endocrine insufficiency, myopathy, neurologic defects
- Tyrosinemia
  - Only Type II (Richner-Hanhart syndrome) is associated with corneal opacity.
  - Characterized by triad of dendritiform keratitis, hyperkeratotic lesions of the palms and soles, and mental retardation
  - Can be distinguished from HSV keratitis by morphologic presentation, bilateral presentation, lack of response to antiviral therapy, and associated systemic findings
  - Restriction of phenylalanine and tyrosine can reverse ocular abnormalities.
- Fabry's disease
  - X-linked recessive sphingolipidosis due to a lack of α-galactosidase A, mapped to chromosome Xq22
  - Multisystem disorder (genitourinary, nervous, musculoskeletal, and cardiovascular systems), characterized by angiokeratomatous skin lesions
  - Corneal opacities in 90% (corneal verticillata), conjunctival vascular changes in 65%, retinal vessel tortuosity in 55%, and cataract in 50%
- P—Posterior corneal disorders
  - Peters' anomaly
    - Most common congenital opacity requiring penetrating keratoplasty; 80% bilateral; most often sporadic, though autosomal dominant and recessive inheritance patterns have been noted
    - Characterized by central corneal opacity (Figure 6-6) with corresponding defects in posterior stroma, Descemet's membrane, and endothelium
    - Synechiae may extend from the iris collarette to the edge of the defect either in thin bands or in broad sheets forming iridocorneal adhesions.

TABLE 6-3. MUCOLIPIDOSES

MUCOLIPIDOSIS	*MLS I*	*MLS II (I-CELL DISEASE)*	*MLS III (PSEUDOHURLER)*	*MLS IV*
Systemic findings	Hepatospleno-megaly; hernia; mental retardation (moderate)	Mental retarda-tion (severe); skin/gingival thickening; skel-etal deformities; hepatomegaly	Musculoskeletal abnormalities; small stature, mental retardation (moderate); gargoyle-like facies	Profound psychomotor retardation
Corneal findings	Fine epithelial and stromal opacification (rare)	Mild corneal haze, megalocornea	Fine corneal opaci-ties (not affecting acuity)	Epithelial irregu-larities; recurrent erosions; most severe corneal clouding of all mucolipidosis
Ocular findings	Cherry-red spot, tortuous retinal and conjunctival vessels; spotlike cataract; strabismus	Retinal degenera-tion; cortical cat-aracts; glaucoma; optic atrophy	Retinal and optic nerve abnormalities	Cataract; retinal degeneration; optic atrophy

Adapted from Rezende RA et al. Congenital corneal opacities. In: Krachmer JH, Mannis MJ, Holland EJ, Eds. *Cornea*. 2nd ed. St. Louis, MO: Elsevier-Mosby; 2005:311–338.

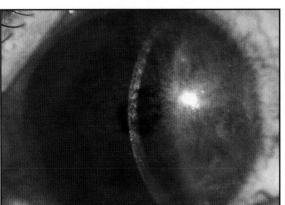

Figure 6-5. Crystalline deposits in the cornea from cystinosis. (This figure was published in *Cornea*. 2nd ed. Krachmer JH, Mannis MJ, Holland EJ, eds. Copyright Elsevier [2005].)

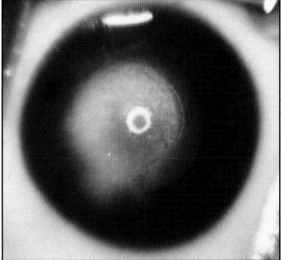

Figure 6-6. Central corneal opacity in an infant with Peters' anomaly. (This figure was published in *Cornea*. 2nd ed. Krachmer JH, Mannis MJ, Holland EJ, eds. Copyright Elsevier [2005].)

- Lens abnormalities including cataract and central corneolenticular adhesions are common.
- Success rate of penetrating keratoplasty is up to 65%, with glaucoma as the most common postoperative complication.
  □ Axenfeld-Reiger syndrome (Table 6-4)
    - Initially categorized into an anterior segment cleavage disorder
    - Bilateral, congenital hereditary disorders involving anterior segment structures

TABLE 6-4. COMPONENTS OF AXENFELD-REIGER SYNDROME

Component	Angle Abnormalities	Iris Abnormalities	Systemic Associations	Glaucoma
Posterior embryotoxin	Posterior embryotoxin easily visualized on gonioscopy	None	None	None
Axenfeld anomaly	(+) Posterior embryotoxin (+) Abnormal iris processes; normal angle appearance ± High iris insertion	None	None	(+) Risk
Reiger anomaly	(+) Posterior embryotoxin (+) Abnormal iris processes; normal angle appearance ± High iris insertion	(+) Iris hypoplasia (thin stroma with easy visualization of iris sphincter); (+) corectopia	None	(+) Risk
Reiger syndrome	(+) Posterior embryotoxin (+) Abnormal iris processes; normal angle appearance ± High iris insertion	(+) Iris hypoplasia; (+) corectopia	Maxillary hypoplasia, midface flattening; hypertelorism; telecanthus; broad flat nasal bridge; microdontia; hypospadias; mental retardation; empty sella syndrome	(+) Risk

- Posterior embryotoxin (anterior displacement of Schwalbe's line; found in 15% of normal population), prominent iris processes (discrete bands to broad sheets covering several clock hours of the angle); iris hypoplasia and corectopia; secondary glaucoma in 50%
- Mapped to chromosome 4q, 13q
  - Posterior keratoconus (Figure 6-7)
    - Uncommon, discrete local conical internal protrusion of the posterior corneal curvature, associated with stromal thinning and variable haze; noninflammatory
    - Well-circumscribed lesion, may be central or eccentric; most commonly sporadic, unilateral, and nonprogressive
    - Amblyopia, refractive errors, or astigmatism may occur, though vision is usually acceptable and penetrating keratoplasty usually not necessary.
- E—Endothelial dystrophy (Figure 6-8)
  - Congenital hereditary endothelial dystrophy (CHED)
    - Diffuse corneal edema and thickening of Descemet's membrane, bilateral
    - Appearance may be blue-gray color to total opacification.
    - Type I (autosomal recessive) is present at birth, nonprogressive, with nystagmus.
    - Type II (autosomal dominant) appears within the first 2 years of life, is slowly progressive, and is associated with pain, tearing, photophobia, and familial findings of posterior polymorphous dystrophy (PPMD) changes.
  - PPMD
    - Autosomal dominant with variable expression; bilateral; nonprogressive and mostly asymptomatic

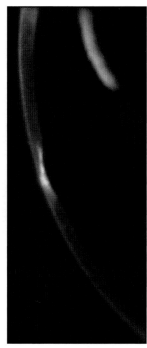

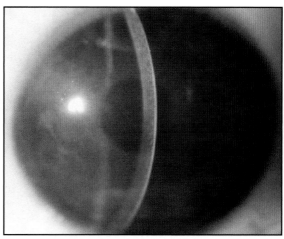

Figure 6-8. Corneal edema and haze secondary to CHED. (This figure was published in *Cornea*. 2nd ed. Krachmer JH, Mannis MJ, Holland EJ, eds. Copyright Elsevier [2005].)

Figure 6-7. Localized, well-circumscribed area of posterior keratoconus. (This figure was published in *Cornea*. 2nd ed. Krachmer JH, Mannis MJ, Holland EJ, eds. Copyright Elsevier [2005].)

- Thickening of Descemet's membrane with irregular or warty appearance; associated with grouped vesicles or bands, discrete gray lesions, or broad bands with scalloped edges ("snail tracks")
- Penetrating keratoplasty may not be necessary unless in severe cases of completely opacified corneas.
- D—Dermoid
  - Solid, benign congenital tumors (Figure 6-9) that arise at the inferotemporal corneoscleral junction. Classified as choristomas (contains cellular components not normally present in the limbal area: hair follicles, sebaceous and sweat glands, muscle, cartilage, teeth)
  - Can range from 2 to 15 mm in diameter, exhibiting little or no growth
  - Associated with Goldenhar's syndrome in one-third of cases (epibulbar dermoids, preauricular appendages, and pretragal fistulas/tags)
  - May induce high astigmatic error; correction of refractive error and patching may be necessary for prevention of amblyopia
  - Evaluation
    - Extensive ophthalmic, birth, and developmental history; detailed clinical examination with focus on external examination, cornea, gonioscopic examination of the angle, and tonometry. May require examination under anesthesia for full evaluation.
  - Differential diagnosis
    - Sclerocornea; tears in Descemet's membrane; microbial, viral, or neurotrophic ulcers; metabolic disorders; posterior corneal defects; endothelial dystrophies; dermoids

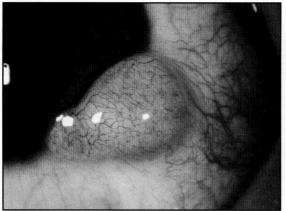

Figure 6-9. Congenital dermoid straddling the limbus. (This figure was published in *Cornea*. 2nd ed. Krachmer JH, Mannis MJ, Holland EJ, eds. Copyright Elsevier [2005].)

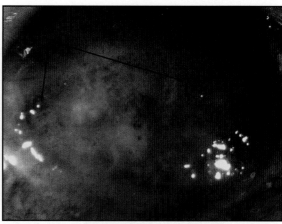

Figure 6-10. Spheroidal degeneration. (This figure was published in *Cornea*. 2nd ed. Krachmer JH, Mannis MJ, Holland EJ, eds. Copyright Elsevier [2005].)

- □ Management
  - • Correction of any baseline refractive error. If amblyopia is present, patching or occlusion therapy may be required. Treatment of elevated IOP and penetrating keratoplasty may be required. Surgical excision of the dermoid should be considered if the affected area involves the visual axis or if there is significant astigmatism induced by the mass that is unable to be treated with spectacle correction.

Corneal Depositions

Superficial

- Verticillata
  - ○ Linear opacities within the corneal epithelium that appear whorl-like in pattern
  - ○ Primarily seen in the inferior cornea, the opacities are not elevated and vary somewhat in color.
  - ○ Most commonly seen in Fabry's disease (X-linked lysosomal storage disease; findings in both heterozygote females and homozygous males), but also found in patients taking systemic medications such as amiodarone, chlorpromazine, chloroquine, and indomethacin
- Iron
  - ○ Yellow-brown lines in the epithelium can be both normal and pathologic. Iron from the tear film often deposits in regions where pooling of tears is common (areas with irregular topography).
  - ○ Types of lines include the following:
    - ▪ Interpalpebral (Hudson-Stahli)
    - ▪ Anterior to head of pterygium (Stocker)
    - ▪ At head of a filtering bleb (Ferry)
    - ▪ At the base of the cone in keratoconus (Fleischer)
    - ▪ At the head of sutures in corneal grafts (Mannis)
- Spheroidal degeneration (Figure 6-10)
  - ○ Golden-yellow globular deposits in Bowman's layer usually restricted to the interpalpebral area.
  - ○ May be primary (bilateral) or secondary (adjacent to areas of corneal scarring or vascularization)
- Adrenochrome (epinephrine) deposits
  - ○ Rarely seen on the cornea, these brown-black deposits occur in patients on chronic epinephrine therapy for glaucoma.
- Band keratopathy
  - ○ Calcium is deposited within the epithelial basement membrane, Bowman's layer, and anterior stroma.
  - ○ Mostly found in the interpalpebral area, it is often described as having a "Swiss cheese" appearance, with the holes often occurring where corneal nerves penetrate Bowman's layer.
  - ○ It is often found secondary to hypercalcemia or in cases of chronic inflammation.

- Fluoroquinolone deposits
  - Chalky white precipitate within the area of an epithelial defect, usually caused by ciprofloxacin and norfloxacin
- Gout (urate deposits)
  - Often seen in the superficial cornea, the urate appears as fine, yellow scintillating crystals in the interpalpebral area.
  - May become confluent and resemble pigmented band keratopathy
- Tyrosinemia (Richner-Hanhart)
  - Opacities are branching, linear, and seen bilaterally.
  - Do not stain with fluorescein, though they often have an appearance similar to dendrites seen in HSV keratitis.

Stromal

- Blood staining
  - Most commonly occurs in the presence of a hyphema and elevated IOP
  - Initially, small yellow granules are noted within the posterior stroma. At this stage, surgical evacuation of the hyphema is advocated if possible.
  - The deposits become rust-colored in the presence of persistent hyphema.
  - The opacity can involve the entire cornea and can take several years to clear, beginning at the limbus.
- Bilirubin
  - Elevated levels lead to staining in the peripheral cornea that is found throughout the stroma, though more prominently in the posterior stroma.
  - It is almost always associated with conjunctival bilirubin staining and is found in cases of advanced liver disease (ie, hepatitis, cirrhosis) or biliary obstruction.
- Siderosis
  - Deposition of iron within intraocular structures; may be associated with the presence of a foreign body or systemic iron overload (ie, hemochromatosis)
- Lipid deposition
  - Most commonly seen as arcus senilis, lipid deposition is most common in the peripheral cornea.
  - Initially deposited in the superior and inferior margins, it often becomes more circumferential.
  - The deposits are a hazy-white circumferential band separated from the limbus by a lucid interval.
  - Primary lipid degeneration is seen as an exaggeration of arcus senilis and is not associated with an elevated lipid profile.
  - Secondary lipid deposition is seen in areas of corneal neovascularization. Adjacent areas of trauma, interstitial keratitis, and corneal ulceration are often present. The lipid deposition in these cases appears more fine and crystalline.
- Immunologic crystalline deposition
  - Often seen in systemic diseases that result in excessive immunoglobulin production
  - Primary amyloidosis, multiple myeloma, waldenstrom's macroglobulinemia, lymphoma, cryoglobulinemia, and benign monoclonal gammopathy
  - The crystals are often the initial signs of the disease.
- Cystinosis
  - Crystals are often deposited in the anterior peripheral stroma and with time involve the entire corneal surface.
  - Severe photophobia and recurrent erosions are often seen.
- Copper (Kaiser-Fleischer)
  - Deposition in the deep stroma, associated with Wilson's disease
  - The deposition is seen in 95% of patients with the liver disorder.
  - The deposition is seen at Schwalbe's line initially prior to progression centrally.
- Gold (chrysiasis)
  - More commonly seen in the era where oral or intramuscular gold therapy was used for rheumatoid arthritis
  - Yellow-brown granules at the level of Descemet's membrane have a metallic sheen but are not visually symptomatic.

- Cornea farinata
  - o Multiple tan or white opacities allocated in the posterior stroma, often bilateral
- Argyrosis
  - o Deposition of silver within the eye, mostly seen as a diffuse, slate-gray discoloration of Descemet's membrane

Dystrophies, Ectasias, Degenerations

Anterior Dystrophies

- Primary, inherited corneal diseases presenting early in life; not associated with systemic disease or pre-existing corneal pathology; usually bilateral, symmetric, and progressive
- Anterior basement membrane
  - o Also known as epithelial basement membrane dystrophy (EBMD), Map-Dot-Fingerprint dystrophy, or Cogan's microcystic dystrophy
  - o Most common anterior corneal dystrophy, seen in 50% of patients with recurrent corneal erosions
  - o Of patients with EBMD, 10% will have corneal erosions.
  - o Etiology
    - Irregularity and redundancy of the epithelial basement membrane within the epithelium itself, sometimes arranged in sheets extending into the substance of the epithelium (Figure 6-11)
    - Abnormal basal epithelial cells with microcysts and abnormal hemidesmosomes are seen.
    - Concentration of changes in the visual axis can cause irregular astigmatism and blurring of vision.
  - o Inheritance
    - Autosomal dominant
  - o Signs/symptoms
    - Spontaneous recurrent corneal erosions and blurred vision, pain, tearing
  - o Evaluation
    - Clinical history of trauma and careful examination for the presence of microcysts or areas of aberrant basement membrane both in the affected eye and the fellow eye.
    - Best seen with tangential illumination, retroillumination, and sclerotic scatter
  - o Management
    - Patching and lubricating ointments at bedtime as initial therapy
    - Severe erosions due to either trauma or EBMD can be treated with anterior stromal puncture (for lesions outside of the visual axis) or superficial keratectomy, with or without adjunct excimer phototherapeutic keratectomy (PTK) (advocated for lesions within the visual axis).
  - o Prognosis
    - Lubrication with ointment alone is effective in the great majority of erosions.
    - Anterior stromal puncture is effective in 80%.
- Gelatinous drop-like dystrophy
  - o Subepithelial, central mulberry-like opacity composed of amyloid without an inflammatory component
  - o Destruction of Bowman's membrane is seen histopathologically.
  - o Findings may be a variant of primary localized amyloidosis.
  - o Inheritance pattern is thought to be autosomal recessive.
  - o Signs and symptoms include decreased vision, photophobia, and tearing.
  - o Management includes either lamellar or penetrating keratoplasty.
  - o Recurrences are common.
- Meesman's dystrophy (Figure 6-12)
  - o Bilateral, symmetric epithelial dystrophy, inherited in autosomal dominant pattern
  - o Etiology
    - Mutation in keratin (K3 or K12)
    - Thickened epithelium and basement membrane are seen
    - Microcysts are filled with an electron-dense, peripheral anterior synechiae (PAS) positive material ("peculiar substance")

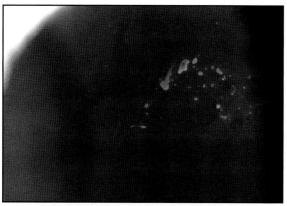

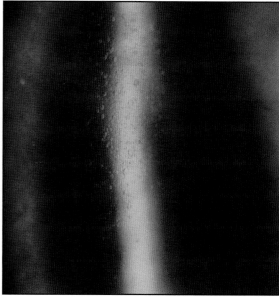

Figures 6-11. EBMD. Note the differing presentations. Microcysts are associated with faint "map" lines in areas of irregular epithelium. (This figure was published in *Cornea*. 2nd ed. Krachmer JH, Mannis MJ, Holland EJ, eds. Copyright Elsevier [2005].)

Figure 6-12. Meesman's dystrophy. Note the intraepithelial cysts noted on retroillumination. (This figure was published in *Cornea*. 2nd ed. Krachmer JH, Mannis MJ, Holland EJ, eds. Copyright Elsevier [2005].)

- o Inheritance
    - ▪ Autosomal dominant
- o Signs/symptoms
    - ▪ Occasionally, pain, recurrent erosions (rare), intraepithelial microcysts, or vesicles visible only at the slit lamp present in the visual axis and midperiphery.
    - ▪ Microcysts are most numerous in the interpalpebral area.
- o Evaluation
    - ▪ Careful clinical history (lack of recurrent erosions)
- o Management
    - ▪ Recurrent erosion is not common; therefore, superficial keratectomy and lamellar corneal transplantation are not appropriate.
- o Prognosis
    - ▪ Vision is usually good in the first few years of life and may diminish if the cysts increase in number and cause irregularity of the epithelium.
- • Corneal dystrophy of Bowman's layer (Figure 6-13)
    - o Subepithelial opacification and scarring of Bowman's membrane
    - o Type I (Reis-Bückler) is considered a superficial variant of granular dystrophy, while type II has been called Thiel-Behnke dystrophy and has the classic "honeycomb" appearance.
    - o Etiology
        - ▪ Fibrocellular scar tissue in a "sawtooth" configuration replaces the area of Bowman's membrane and basement membrane.
        - ▪ Type I
            - □ Rod-shaped bodies and Masson-positive band-like subepithelial deposits similar to those seen in granular dystrophy
        - ▪ Type II
            - □ Curly fibers in the region of Bowman's membrane
    - o Inheritance
        - ▪ Both types are autosomal dominant, mapped to chromosome 5q, with mutations seen in the βig-h3 gene, which is responsible for formation of keratoepithelin.

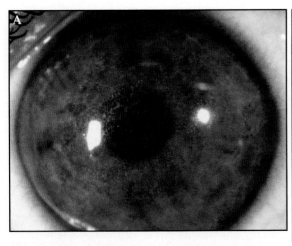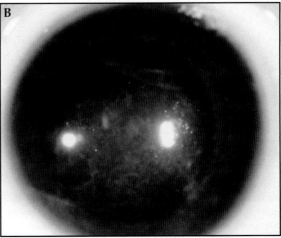

Figure 6-13A. Corneal dystrophy of Bowman's membrane. (A)Type I, or Reis-Bückler's dystrophy. (B) Type II, or Thiel-Behnke honeycomb dystrophy. (This figure was published in *Cornea*. 2nd ed. Krachmer JH, Mannis MJ, Holland EJ, eds. Copyright Elsevier [2005].)

- o Signs/symptoms
    - Recurrent erosions in first or second decade, with onset of visual loss earlier for Type I than Type II
    - Superficial geographic or honeycomb areas of reticular opacification are seen most often in the central cornea.
- o Evaluation
    - Clinical history with emphasis on onset of visual loss, family history, and biomicroscopy
- o Management
    - Lamellar or penetrating keratoplasty
- o Prognosis
    - Good, however, there is a high rate of recurrence in the corneal graft

Stromal Dystrophies

Avellino Dystrophy

- Findings are a combination of granular and lattice with discrete granular-like opacities.
- Three clinical signs characterize the dystrophy (Figure 6-14):
    - o Anterior stromal discrete gray-white granular deposits
    - o Mid to posterior stromal lattice lesions
    - o Anterior stromal haze
- Granular deposits occur first, followed by lattice lines and eventually stromal haze in late disease.
- Etiology
    - o Composed of hyaline and amyloid; stains with Congo red and Masson's trichrome
    - o Mapped to chromosome 5q with mutation seen in the βig-h3 gene similar to that seen in lattice dystrophy, though different from those seen in granular and corneal dystrophy of Bowman's layer
- Inheritance
    - o Autosomal dominant
- Signs/symptoms
    - o Foreign-body sensation, pain, photophobia, recurrent erosions
- Differential diagnosis
    - o Lattice dystrophy, granular dystrophy
- Evaluation
    - o Careful clinical history to determine pattern of inheritance

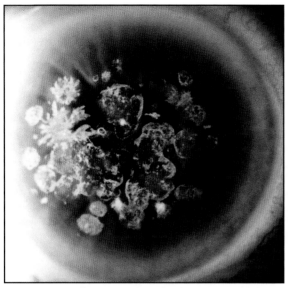

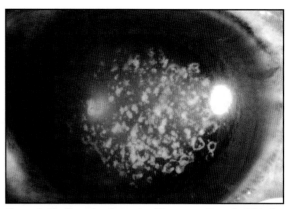

Figure 6-15. Granular dystrophy (Groenouw Type I). (This figure was published in *Cornea*. 2nd ed. Krachmer JH, Mannis MJ, Holland EJ, eds. Copyright Elsevier [2005].)

Figure 6-14. Avellino dystrophy. (This figure was published in *Cornea*. 2nd ed. Krachmer JH, Mannis MJ, Holland EJ, eds. Copyright Elsevier [2005].)

- Management
  - Lubricants, patching, therapeutic contact lenses, or PTK for recurrent erosions and superficial lesions
  - Lamellar or penetrating keratoplasty, if necessary
- Prognosis
  - Good, though recurrence is common

Granular Dystrophy (Groenouw Type I)

- Most common stromal dystrophy; exhibits central, discrete white breadcrumb-like opacities with clear intervening stroma and periphery (Figure 6-15)
- Stroma may become hazy ("ground glass" appearance) with late disease.
- Type I
  - Corresponds to Groenouw Type I dystrophy
- Type II
  - Presents with later onset, usually in the second decade and with fewer, larger ring-shaped granular deposits in the anterior stroma. These lesions are found in progressively deeper layers of the stroma with increasing age.
- Type III
  - More superficial, presents with erosions in infancy, and is clinically indistinguishable from corneal dystrophy of Bowman's layer Type I (Reis-Bückler)
- Etiology
  - Eosinophilic rod or trapezoidal-shaped deposits composed of hyaline; stains with Masson's trichrome
- Inheritance
  - Autosomal dominant, mapped to chromosome 5q and mutations in keratoepithelin gene (β transforming growth factor-induced gene, or βig-h3)
- Signs/symptoms
  - Decreased vision late in the course of the disease, no discomfort
- Differential diagnosis
  - Corneal dystrophy of Bowman's layer (Type I)
  - Avellino dystrophy

- Evaluation
  - Elicit family history
  - Biomicroscopy with use of retroillumination or oblique illumination to highlight stromal opacification
  - Fluorescein staining may show areas of rapid tear film break up.
- Management
  - Recurrent erosions should be managed with therapeutic contact lenses and lubrication.
  - If vision is markedly affected, superficial keratectomy or PTK may be considered for superficial lesions.
  - Lamellar keratoplasty can also be considered for lesions located deeper in the stroma.
  - Penetrating keratoplasty is uncommon prior to the fifth decade.
- Prognosis
  - Recurrence is common, and lesions are often different from those noted in primary disease.
  - Clinically, they are diffuse subepithelial lesions coming from the periphery.

Lattice Dystrophy (Biber-Haab-Dimmer)
- Bilateral, primary localized corneal amyloidosis
- Opacities are shaped like branching lines and dots with associated central haze (Figure 6-16).
- Lesions are often refractile and are associated with cloudy intervening stroma, which has a "ground glass" appearance.
- Etiology
  - Composed of amyloid, stains with Congo red, and exhibits "apple-green" birefringence
- Inheritance
  - Autosomal dominant, mapped to chromosome 5q, with mutations in keratoepithelin gene (β transforming growth factor-induced gene, or βig-h3) and gelsolin gene (on chromosome 9)
  - Type I
    - Branching stromal lattice lesions with subepithelial opacities and anterior stromal haze
  - Type II (Meretoja's syndrome, familial amyloid polyneuropathy type IV)
    - Systemic amyloidosis associated with corneal changes, usually later in onset and a more favorable visual outcome. Recurrent erosions are rare, and lesions involve peripheral cornea with relative sparing of the central stroma.
  - Type III
    - Late onset of visual symptoms, lack of recurrent erosions, and opacities thicker than those seen in Types I and II
- Signs/symptoms
  - Decreased vision, recurrent erosions, and decreased sensitivity of the central cornea
- Differential diagnosis
  - Avellino dystrophy
- Evaluation
  - Careful history to elicit systemic amyloidosis, clinical examination using retroillumination and direct illumination to highlight lattice lines and dots
- Management
  - Dependent on the patient's symptoms; recurrent erosions can be treated with patching, hypertonic agents, lubricants, or therapeutic contact lenses.
  - PTK can also be used to treat erosions and superficial lesions.
  - Lamellar or penetrating keratoplasty can be performed for optical rehabilitation.
- Prognosis
  - Good, though frequent recurrences occur (greater than granular or macular dystrophy)

Macular Dystrophy (Groenouw Type II)
- Focal, irregular whitish-gray spots associated with diffuse haze
- Extends to limbus. Least common of stromal dystrophies and most severe (Figure 6-17)
- Etiology
  - Abnormal glycosaminoglycans deposited both intra- and extracellularly, stains with Alcian blue.
  - Multiple irregular, dense, white-to-gray nodules cause irregularity of the epithelial surface.
- Inheritance
  - Autosomal recessive, genes as yet unidentified

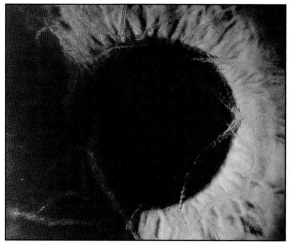

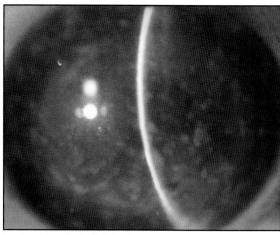

Figure 6-16. Lattice dystrophy. Note the appearance of the lattice lines shown in tangential illumination on the left and retroillumination on the right. (This figure was published in *Cornea*. 2nd ed. Krachmer JH, Mannis MJ, Holland EJ, eds. Copyright Elsevier [2005].)

Figure 6-17. Macular dystrophy (Groenouw Type II). The lesions extend to the limbus. (This figure was published in *Cornea*. 2nd ed. Krachmer JH, Mannis MJ, Holland EJ, eds. Copyright Elsevier [2005].)

- Signs/symptoms
  - o Recurrent erosions, decreased vision early on with fine superficial clouding of the central stroma to involvement of the entire thickness of the cornea by the third decade
- Differential diagnosis
  - o Granular dystrophy
- Evaluation
  - o Careful family history to determine recessive inheritance pattern
  - o Clinical examination using indirect illumination to visualize opacities, and examination of the peripheral cornea to determine extent of stromal involvement
- Management
  - o Reduction of photophobia using tinted lenses, treatment of recurrent erosions using therapeutic contact lenses and lubricants, PTK and lamellar keratoplasty for early disease, and penetrating keratoplasty
- Prognosis
  - o Good. Recurrences do occur in both lamellar and penetrating keratoplasties and initially affect the peripheral donor stroma.

Central Cloudy Dystrophy (of Francois)

- Appears as small, indistinct cloudy areas in the central and paracentral posterior stroma with intervening clear cracks (similar to crocodile shagreen)
- Etiology
  - o Currently unknown
- Inheritance
  - o Autosomal dominant
- Symptoms
  - o Usually asymptomatic
- Differential diagnosis
  - o Crocodile shagreen, especially if there is a lack of autosomal dominant inheritance pattern; corneal edema; posterior amorphous corneal dystrophy
- Management
  - o No treatment is necessary.
- Prognosis
  - o Good. Nonprogressive.

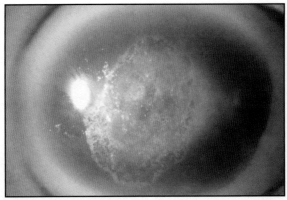

Figure 6-18. Schnyder's central crystalline dystrophy. (This figure was published in *Cornea*. 2nd ed. Krachmer JH, Mannis MJ, Holland EJ, eds. Copyright Elsevier [2005].)

Central Crystalline (Schnyder's) Dystrophy

- Bilateral gray disc-like lesions noted centrally, as well as fine needle-like polychromatic crystals, accompanied by stromal haze (Figure 6-18)
- Associated with dense arcus
- Composed of cholesterol and neutral fats; stains with Oil-red-O
- Etiology
  - Associated with hyperlipidemia
- Inheritance
  - Autosomal dominant, very rare, mapped to chromosome 1p
- Signs/symptoms
  - Usually asymptomatic, though corneal sensation can decrease over the area of the lesions
- Differential diagnosis
  - Bietti's crystalline dystrophy
  - Cystinosis
  - Dysproteinemias
- Management
  - Hypercholesterolemia is strongly associated with the disease; therefore, investigation of systemic hyperlipidemia should be conducted. Lamellar or penetrating grafts can be used if visual acuity decreases.
- Prognosis
  - Good, though cholesterol crystals may recur in transplants

Congenital Hereditary Stromal Dystrophy

- Bilateral congenital opacification not related to abnormal endothelial cell function
- Lesions are superficial, central, and feathery in appearance.
- Etiology
  - Alternating layers of abnormal collagen lamellae
- Inheritance
  - Autosomal dominant
- Signs/symptoms
  - Amblyopia, esotropia, nystagmus
  - No evidence of recurrent erosions, edema, or decreased corneal sensation
- Differential diagnosis
  - CHED, congenital glaucoma, posterior polymorphic dystrophy
- Evaluation
  - Careful clinical history and examination; pachymetry, tonometry
- Management
  - Penetrating keratoplasty at an early age to maintain useful vision, as well as amblyopia therapy
- Prognosis
  - Good. The disease is nonprogressive and does not recur in corneal grafts.

Fleck Dystrophy

- Bilateral, asymmetric disorder exhibiting subtle, grayish white specks that extend to the limbus, sparing Bowman's layer
- Etiology
  - Abnormal glycosaminoglycans (stain with Alcian blue, colloidal irons) and lipid deposits (Oil-red-O or Sudan Black)
- Inheritance
  - Autosomal dominant
- Signs/symptoms
  - Can be unilateral, asymmetric, usually asymptomatic
- Differential diagnosis
  - Macular dystrophy
- Evaluation
  - Careful history and examination to determine if associated conditions (keratoconus, atopic disease, central cloudy dystrophy, limbal dermoid, and pseudoxanthoma elasticum) are present
- Management
  - Treatment is not necessary.
- Prognosis
  - Nonprogressive

Pre-Descemet's Dystrophy

- Focal, fine linear or punctate dots located in the posterior stroma
- Often bilateral, symmetric, and seen after the third decade
- May appear in diffuse, central, or ring shapes, sparing the central and peripheral cornea
- Includes punctiform and polychromatic pre-Descemet's dominant dystrophy (more uniform deep stromal lesions/filaments that extend to the limbus) and systemic associations, such as X-linked recessive ichthyosis
- Etiology
  - Likely a degenerative, age-related process with findings of membrane-bound vacuoles and fibrillogranular material associated with phospholipid and neutral fat deposition
- Inheritance
  - No definitive pattern
- Signs/symptoms
  - Visual acuity spared
- Differential diagnosis
  - Polymorphic amyloid degeneration, corneal farinata, PPMD
- Evaluation
  - Careful clinical history and examination to rule out associated systemic disorders
- Management
  - None necessary
- Prognosis
  - Good

Posterior Dystrophies

Congenital Hereditary Endothelial Dystrophy

- Bilateral, noninflammatory edematous, cloudy corneas at birth due to endothelial dysfunction. Opacification extends to the limbus without clear zones.
- Etiology
  - Primary dysfunction of endothelial cells, likely in the late prenatal period as evidenced by abnormal posterior nonbanded Descemet's membrane
- Inheritance
  - Autosomal recessive more common than autosomal dominant; rare, mapped to chromosome 20p
- Signs/symptoms
  - The following 2 types exist:

- Autosomal recessive form (early presentation at birth or soon thereafter with dense corneal opacification, nonprogressive), which is relatively asymptomatic and associated with nystagmus
- Autosomal dominant form (slowly progressive clouding develops during first and second years of life) with photophobia and tearing
- Differential diagnosis
  - Congenital glaucoma
  - Forceps injury
  - Congenital infections
  - Congenital hereditary stromal dystrophy (CHSD)
  - Metabolic disorders
  - Early onset PPMD
- Evaluation
  - CHED is a diagnosis of exclusion.
  - Careful clinical history and examination are required to rule out other etiologies.
  - Tonometry, pachymetry, and examination under anesthesia may be required.
- Management
  - Penetrating keratoplasty
- Prognosis
  - Mixed. Some studies show graft survival may be greater in patients with "delayed onset" of corneal edema.

Fuchs' Endothelial Dystrophy

- Bilateral stromal and epithelial edema in elderly patients
- Etiology
  - Exact mechanism is multifactorial.
  - Endothelial cell density decreases with age, and research has shown a decrease in anti-apoptotic genes in Fuchs' corneas.
- Inheritance
  - Autosomal dominant, with late onset and slow progression
  - Females develop corneal guttae 2.5 times more often than males and progress to corneal edema 5.7 times more often than males.
- Signs/symptoms
  - Decreased visual acuity, usually worse in the morning/upon awakening
  - Presence of corneal guttae (seen as dark spots on direct illumination and highlighted in retroillumination) can be noted (Figure 6-19).
  - Progressive development of guttae produces a beaten bronze appearance consistent with increased pigmentation.
  - Stromal edema may present as fine vertical wrinkles or striae in Descemet's membrane.
  - Microcystic edema may follow and coalesce into bullae.
  - Progressive edema results in "ground glass" opacification of the central cornea.
  - Avascular subepithelial fibrosis/scarring between the epithelium and Bowman's membrane occurs in the end stages.
- Differential diagnosis
  - Guttae are found in interstitial keratitis, macular dystrophy, PPMD after trauma/inflammation/infection.
  - Chandler's syndrome (beaten bronze appearance of endothelium)
  - Aphakic/pseudophakic corneal edema
  - CHED
  - PPMD
  - Iridocorneal endothelial (ICE) syndrome
- Evaluation
  - Detailed history outlining temporal aspect of visual loss and history of intraocular surgery, clinical examination with emphasis on pachymetry and tonometry
  - Specular microscopy may be helpful in following endothelial cell loss.

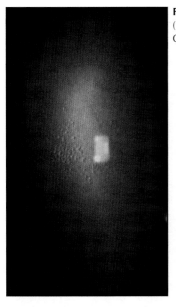

Figure 6-19. Corneal guttae seen in retroillumination in a patient with Fuchs' dystrophy. (This figure was published in *Cornea*. 2nd ed. Krachmer JH, Mannis MJ, Holland EJ, eds. Copyright Elsevier [2005].)

- Management
  - Topical hypertonic saline solutions in the initial phases, with or without corneal dehydration using a blow-dryer; reduction of IOP
  - Therapeutic contact lenses to prevent erosions from epithelial bullae
  - Penetrating keratoplasty
  - Lamellar endothelial keratoplasty
- Prognosis
  - Good. Corneal graft clarity has been noted to be 80% to 90% (with follow up between 2 and 5 years).

Posterior Polymorphous Dystrophy

- Bilateral, asymmetric disease usually occurring during the second and third decades of life.
- Abnormalities lie at the level of Descemet's membrane and endothelium.
- The following 3 clinical patterns exist:
  - Vesicular lesions appear in almost all patients and are considered the hallmark of the disease (Figure 6-20).
  - Band-like lesions often appear in the inferior paracentral cornea.
  - Diffuse opacity may be small or large, seen with haze in the posterior stroma. Corneal edema is uncommon but can range from mild to severe cases, including bullous keratopathy.
- Etiology
  - Thickened Descemet's membrane is seen with focal areas of bilayered endothelial cells or irregular patches of large endothelial cells.
  - The endothelial cells have been shown to exhibit epithelial cell characteristics (presence of microvilli, positive staining for keratin, multilayered, lacking tight junctions seen in endothelium, with cell polarity, and manifesting proliferative tendencies).
- Inheritance
  - Autosomal dominant, variable expressivity
- Signs/symptoms
  - Generally asymptomatic, rarely progressive/debilitating
  - IOP may be elevated.
  - Peripheral anterior synechiae may be seen (either fine strands or broad, shiny areas).
  - Areas of iris atrophy and corectopia may also be present.
- Differential diagnosis
  - ICE syndrome

Figure 6-20. PPMD. (A) "Snail tracks" and (B) vesicles seen on specular microscopy. (This figure was published in *Cornea*. 2nd ed. Krachmer JH, Mannis MJ, Holland EJ, eds. Copyright Elsevier [2005].)

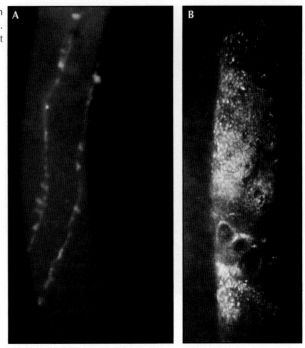

- Evaluation
  - Careful clinical history and examination with emphasis on tonometry, pachymetry, and gonioscopy
- Management
  - Observation in most cases; penetrating keratoplasty in severe cases
- Prognosis
  - Correlated with the presence of PAS and elevated IOP
  - Disease recurrence has been noted in corneal grafts.

Noninflammatory Ectasias

- Keratoconus
  - Bilateral, noninflammatory progressive thinning and protrusion of the cornea into a conical shape
  - Usually affects the central portion, with the apex of the cone centered slightly below the visual axis
  - No specific gender or racial predominance
  - Onset is typically noted at puberty, associated with irregular astigmatism and steep curvatures noted on keratometry.
  - Typically, progression is noted over a period of 10 to 20 years and gradually stops.
  - Etiology
    - Undetermined
    - Biochemical assays have shown up-regulation of proteolytic enzymes, as well as cytokine-induced apoptosis.
    - Only 6% of cases have a positive family history.
  - Signs/symptoms
    - Decreased visual acuity
    - Irregular astigmatism
    - Steep keratometric readings
    - Iron ring (Fleischer's ring)
    - Vogt's striae
    - Corneal edema/opacity (hydrops)
    - Corneal scar

- Differential diagnosis
    - Pellucid marginal degeneration
    - Keratoglobus
- Evaluation
    - Clinical history and examination with emphasis on biomicroscopy, keratometry, topography, pachymetry
    - Rule out the following associated systemic disorders:
        - Atopy
        - Down syndrome
        - Ehlers-Danlos
        - Osteogenesis imperfecta
        - Mitral valve prolapsed
        - Chronic eye rubbing
- Management
    - Spectacle correction and rigid gas permeable contact lenses early in the course of the disease
    - Penetrating keratoplasty once the patient becomes contact lens intolerant
    - Advances in intrastromal ring segments have allowed for temporary stabilization in cases that otherwise would have failed contact lens management and required penetrating keratoplasty.
    - There is currently a clinical trial underway to determine if collagen cross-linking may be beneficial in preventing progression of the disease.
- Prognosis
    - Good. Rarely recurs following penetrating keratoplasty.
- Pellucid marginal degeneration
    - Bilateral peripheral corneal ectasia, with a band of thinning 1 to 2 mm in width usually located in the inferior cornea (from 4 to 8 o'clock position)
    - Maximal corneal protrusion typically superior to the area of thinning, and the area of protrusion is of normal thickness
    - Can occur with keratoconus in the same eye
    - No racial or gender predilection
    - Etiology
        - Changes in collagen (fibrous long-strand collagen) periodicity within the stroma of the cornea
    - Signs/symptoms
        - Blurring of vision starting between the second and fifth decades (due to irregular astigmatism)
    - Differential diagnosis
        - Keratoconus
        - Keratoglobus
        - Terrien's marginal degeneration
        - Mooren's ulcer
        - Idiopathic furrow degeneration
    - Evaluation
        - Careful biomicroscopy
        - Videokeratography
        - Keratometry
        - Pachymetry
    - Management
        - Rigid gas permeable (RGP) lenses (large diameter)
        - Combination lens design of RGP center with soft hydrophilic skirt
        - Large-diameter or eccentric penetrating keratoplasty
        - Crescentic lamellar keratoplasty
        - Crescentic or wedge excision
    - Prognosis
        - Good

- Keratoglobus
  - Bilateral, noninflammatory, ectatic disorder
  - Entire cornea becomes thinned and has a globular shape (keratometry readings 60 to 70 D).
  - Cornea is normal in size, clear, within 20% to 30% of normal corneal thickness.
  - Etiology
    - Absent or fragmented Bowman's layer
    - Thinned stroma with normal lamellar orientation
    - Thinned Descemet's membrane
    - Normal endothelium
    - Breaks in Descemet's membrane heal over weeks to months
  - Signs/symptoms
    - Decrease in visual acuity
    - Corneal edema/opacity (with breaks in Descemet's membrane)
  - Differential diagnosis
    - Keratoconus
    - Pellucid marginal degeneration
    - Megalocornea
    - Buphthalmos
  - Evaluation
    - Clinical examination with emphasis on keratometry/topography, tonometry, pachymetry
  - Management
    - Treatment of associated myopia to prevent amblyopia
    - Protective eyewear for increased risk of corneal rupture with trauma to eye or head
    - Associated with Ehlers-Danlos disorder
    - Lamellar or penetrating keratoplasty only if absolutely necessary
  - Prognosis
    - Guarded, especially in settings of ruptured globe (secondary to complications from surgical repair of thin cornea and sclera)
- Posterior keratoconus
  - Uncommon, localized internal protrusion of the posterior corneal curvature
  - Associated with stromal thinning and variable haze
  - May be central or eccentric
  - Most commonly sporadic, unilateral, noninflammatory, and nonprogressive
  - Etiology
    - Indeterminate. May be a variant of the anomalies of mesodermal dysgenesis
  - Signs/symptoms
    - Decrease in visual acuity
    - Stromal scarring
    - Amblyopia
    - Paracentral or central area of excavation in the posterior cornea
  - Differential diagnosis
    - Keratoconus
    - Keratoglobus
    - Pellucid marginal degeneration
  - Evaluation
    - Biomicroscopy
    - Keratometry
    - Pachymetry
  - Management
    - Treatment of amblyopia
    - Correction of refractive error
    - Penetrating keratoplasty not usually necessary
  - Prognosis
    - Good

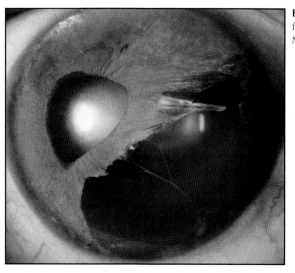

Figure 6-21. ICE syndrome. Note the area of iris atrophy. (This figure was published in *Cornea*. 2nd ed. Krachmer JH, Mannis MJ, Holland EJ, eds. Copyright Elsevier [2005].)

- Iridocorneal endothelial syndrome
  - Unilateral, nonhereditary abnormality of the corneal endothelium associated with a spectrum of disease processes
  - Slowly progressive, and complications often include corneal edema, iris irregularity, and secondary angle-closure glaucoma
  - Components include essential iris atrophy (Figure 6-21), Chandler's syndrome, and Iris Nevus (Cogan-Reese) syndrome.
  - Etiology
    - Undetermined
    - Abnormal corneal endothelium produces abnormal basement membrane that extends beyond Schwalbe's line, over the anterior chamber angle, and onto the surface of the iris.
    - Contraction of the membrane draws the iris to the periphery, stretching the opposite iris quadrant and resulting in corectopia and atrophy of the iris stroma.
    - Iris nodules seen in late disease are actually areas of normal iris stroma that protrude through the membrane-lined iris surface.
  - Signs/symptoms
    - Decreased visual acuity with halos around lights due to corneal edema with or without associated increase in IOP
      - Worse in morning (seen in Chandler's syndrome)
    - Beaten metal appearance of corneal endothelium (finer than that seen in Fuchs' dystrophy)
    - Peripheral anterior synechiae
    - Corectopia
    - Iris atrophy
    - Glaucoma (80% to 100%)
  - Differential diagnosis
    - Posterior polymorphic dystrophy
    - Ectopia lentis et papillae
    - Aniridia
  - Evaluation
    - Biomicroscopy
    - Gonioscopy
    - Specular microscopy
    - Confocal microscopy (if corneal edema precludes evaluation with specular microscopy)
  - Management
    - Treatment of elevated IOP; penetrating keratoplasty or glaucoma surgery, if necessary
  - Prognosis
    - Chronic progressive disease with poor prognosis if associated with glaucoma

Corneal/Conjunctival Degenerations

- Definition
  - o Acquired lesions secondary to aging or previous corneal injury/insult
  - o Often unilateral, asymmetric, and without an inheritance pattern
- Arcus senilis
  - o Degenerative change involving lipid deposition in the peripheral cornea, beginning as a gray or cream-colored arc in the inferior cornea, which eventually circumscribes the cornea with a lucent area between the arc and the limbus
  - o Findings are secondary to deposition of extracellular cholesterol, cholesterol esters, and phospholipids.
  - o Often seen with increased age, the appearance of corneal arcus in patients under 40 should prompt evaluation for hyperlipoproteinemia (especially types IIa and IIb) as well as genetic disorders of cholesterol metabolism (ie, lecithin cholesterol acyltransferase [LCAT] deficiency).
- Band keratopathy
  - o Deposition across the interpalpebral area of the cornea at the level of Bowman's layer
  - o Usually begins in the 3 and 9 o'clock positions and appears sharply demarcated from the limbus by a lucent area
  - o Initially gray, the opacity becomes white and chalky with lucent areas corresponding to areas of penetrating corneal nerves.
  - o Lesions are slowly progressive
  - o Etiology (Table 6-5)
    - Usually secondary to
      - □ Hypercalcemic states (hyperparathyroidism, chronic renal failure)
      - □ Chronic uveitis (juvenile rheumatoid arthritis)
  - o Signs/symptoms
    - Early stages are asymptomatic
    - Decreased vision once the band crosses the visual axis
    - Irritation
    - Foreign-body sensation
    - Tearing
    - Photophobia
  - o Management
    - In patients presenting with band keratopathy of unknown etiology, systemic evaluation is warranted.
    - Chelation of calcium using ethylenediaminetetraacetic acid (EDTA) in 0.05 molar concentration or PTK
- Crocodile shagreen
  - o Commonly bilateral mosaic pattern seen in the anterior or posterior cornea
  - o Opacities appear clinically as polygonal gray to white "cracked ice."
  - o Histologically, stroma is thrown into folds at either Bowman's layer or at Descemet's membrane with a sawtooth pattern of irregularly arranged collagen in the areas of opacity.
  - o Often seen as senile change
- Polymorphic amyloid degeneration
  - o Age-related change of the cornea
  - o Usually bilateral, with mild decrease in visual acuity (20/40 or better)
  - o Often seen as refractile, gray-white opacities and lines in the posterior stroma
  - o These deposits are not associated with systemic amyloidosis.
  - o There is associated central cornea thinning that appears as an area of flattening on topography.
  - o Etiology
    - Thick collagenous layer posterior to Descemet's membrane, within thickening of Descemet's itself (up to 14 μm from 4 to 5 μm in normal cornea)
  - o Inheritance
    - Autosomal dominant, occasionally congenital
  - o Signs/symptoms
    - Slight decrease in visual acuity
    - Topographic changes (central cornea flattening)

TABLE 6-5. GENERAL CAUSES OF BAND KERATOPATHY

Hypercalcemic states
• Hyperparathyroidism
• Milk-Alkali syndrome
Chronic ocular inflammation and disease
• Juvenile rheumatoid arthritis
• Chronic uveitis
• Chronic corneal edema, glaucoma
Eyedrops/irritants
Genetic/Inherited disorders
• CHED
• Ichthyosis
• Norrie's disease
• Still's disease
• Tuberous sclerosis
Systemic diseases
• Multiple myeloma
• Sarcoidosis
• Uremia
Idiopathic

- o Differential diagnosis
  - ▪ PPMD
  - ▪ Pre-Descemet's dystrophy
  - ▪ Congenital hereditary stromal or endothelial dystrophies
  - ▪ Interstitial keratitis
  - ▪ Posterior crocodile shagreen
- o Evaluation
  - ▪ Careful clinical history and examination including the following:
    - □ Tonometry
    - □ Gonioscopy
    - □ Pachymetry
- o Management
  - ▪ No treatment necessary
- o Prognosis
  - ▪ Good
- • Furrow degeneration
  - o Rare degeneration seen in the elderly
  - o Peripheral thinning in the avascular zone between the limbal arcades and arcus senilis
  - o Usually the thinning is of no visual significance, and patients are asymptomatic.
  - o No treatment is required.

- Lipid keratopathy
  - Yellow-white subepithelial and stromal infiltration, often with feathery or crystalline appearance
  - Primary forms are rarer, whereas secondary forms are more common and likely due to lipid deposition from chronic inflammation and vascularization. More common in women than in men (70:30).
  - Clinical manifestation of the disease, aside from cosmetic appearance, is decreased vision.
- Spheroidal degeneration
  - Clear to yellow-gold spherules of hyaline-like material are seen in the subepithelium, within Bowman's layer, and/or the superficial stroma.
  - Etiology
    - Ultraviolet radiation and trauma (from sand, dust, wind, drying) are etiologic factors in the development.
  - Signs/symptoms
    - Usually asymptomatic until the disease advances to the point of decreased vision or advanced lesions break through the epithelium causing foreign-body sensation/irritation
  - Management
    - Lamellar or penetrating keratoplasty may be helpful to rehabilitate vision.
- Salzmann's nodular degeneration
  - Degenerative process that follows episodes of keratitis/microtrauma
  - Rarely associated with other noninflammatory conditions (ie, EBMD)
  - Appear as whitish-blue elevated nodular lesions, either single or multiple, adjacent to corneal scarring or corneal pannus and located in the midperiphery (Figure 6-22)
  - Etiology
    - Nodules are dense collagen plaques with hyalinization found between epithelium and Bowman's layer
  - Signs/symptoms
    - Slowly progressive, usually asymptomatic, though epithelial erosions may cause tearing, photophobia, or irritation
    - Nodules in or adjacent to the visual axis can cause decreased vision.
  - Management
    - Treatment includes superficial keratectomy, PTK, and, in severe cases, lamellar or penetrating keratoplasty.
  - Prognosis
    - Good
- White limbal girdle of Vogt
  - Crescentic yellow or white band in the interpalpebral limbus
  - Usually symmetric, occurring at the limbus, nasal more than temporal
  - Separated from the limbus by a narrow lucent area
  - Incidence increases with age, up to 100% in those older than 80 years.
  - The following 2 types exist:
    - Type I
      - Predominantly calcific and separated from the limbus by a lucid interval
    - Type II
      - Predominantly due to elastic changes and not separated from the limbus by a lucid interval
- Terrien's marginal degeneration
  - Rare peripheral inflammatory condition and most common in second to fourth decades and in men more than women (3:1)
  - Typically bilateral, but may be asymmetric
  - Lesions often begin superonasally with fine punctate opacities noted in the anterior stroma and a lucent area adjacent to the limbus.
  - Fine, superficial vascularization extends from the limbal arcades, and a gutter forms between the opacity and limbus.
  - Over time, the stroma progressively thins, the peripheral edge slopes, and the central edge steepens (Figure 6-23).
  - There is no overlying epithelial defect.

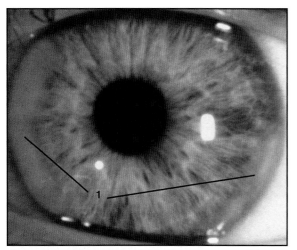

Figure 6-22. Salzmann's nodular degeneration. Nodules are marked by (1). (This figure was published in *Cornea*. 2nd ed. Krachmer JH, Mannis MJ, Holland EJ, eds. Copyright Elsevier [2005].)

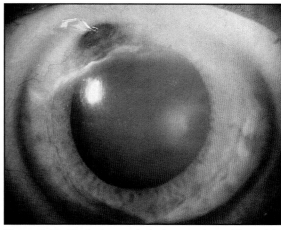

Figure 6-23. Terrien's marginal degeneration with peripheral thinning. (This figure was published in *Cornea*. 2nd ed. Krachmer JH, Mannis MJ, Holland EJ, eds. Copyright Elsevier [2005].)

- ○ A zone of lipid can be seen at the advancing edge of the gutter.
- ○ The lesion may eventually extend circumferentially.
- ○ Etiology
  - Unknown
  - Histologic examination shows fibrillar degeneration of collagen with changes in the epithelium, Bowman's layer, and Descemet's membrane.
- ○ Signs/symptoms
  - Decrease in visual acuity
- ○ Management
  - As a slowly progressive disease, treatment is limited to correction of induced astigmatism.
  - Perforation may occur spontaneously or secondary to trauma in roughly 15% of patients.
  - Eccentric lamellar or penetrating grafts can be used.
- Dellen
  - ○ May occur as age-related changes or secondary to other topographical abnormalities
  - ○ Usually lasting only 24 to 48 hours, they are found most commonly in the peripheral cornea and adjacent to an area of paralimbal elevation.
  - ○ They appear as saucer-like depressions and show thinning of the corneal epithelium, Bowman's layer, and anterior stroma on histologic evaluation.
  - ○ Treatment includes use of lubricants and patching.
- Pingueculae
  - ○ Degeneration of the conjunctiva adjacent to the limbus, most commonly found in the interpalpebral area and in the 3 and 9 o'clock positions
  - ○ Histologically, actinic changes (elastotic degeneration) are seen, likely secondary to damage from ultraviolet radiation.
  - ○ Usually insignificant, they may become inflamed and irritated.
  - ○ Treatment includes topical lubricants, corticosteroids, or NSAIDs.
  - ○ Excision is rarely necessary.
- Pterygium
  - ○ A wing-like mass of fibrovascular tissue that extends from the conjunctiva to the cornea (Figure 6-24)
  - ○ It is highly vascular and often located in the interpalpebral fissure (seen in the 3 and 9 o'clock positions, though more common nasally).
  - ○ The leading edge invades and destroys Bowman's layer
  - ○ There is increased prevalence with age, time spent working outdoors, and increased proximity to the equator.

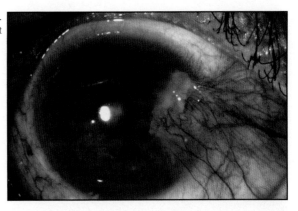

Figure 6-24. Pterygium. (This figure was published in *Cornea*. 2nd ed. Krachmer JH, Mannis MJ, Holland EJ, eds. Copyright Elsevier [2005].)

- o Etiology
  - ▪ Hyperkeratotic, acanthotic, or dysplastic epithelium can be seen with increased goblet cell density and squamous metaplasia.
  - ▪ Elastotic degeneration is seen in the substantia propria.
- o Symptoms/signs
  - ▪ Decrease in visual acuity, irritation, inflammation of pterygium
- o Management
  - ▪ Treatment includes topical lubricants, corticosteroids, and NSAIDs for irritation and inflammation.
  - ▪ Surgical excision is warranted in cases where the head of the pterygium crosses the visual axis or significant regular and irregular astigmatism are induced.
- o Prognosis
  - ▪ Good, depending on technique of removal
  - ▪ Bare sclera excision is associated with high recurrence rates, whereas conjunctival autografts and mitomycin C have been used with low rates of recurrence.
  - ▪ Conjunctival autografts are safe and effective, though technically demanding.
  - ▪ Mitomycin C, though effective, has associated complications, including corneal and scleral ulceration, uveitis, and secondary glaucoma.

Infections

Bacterial

- Most common etiology of infectious keratitis and suppurative corneal ulceration, usually due to
  - o *Staphylococcal* species (*S. aureus, S. epidermidis*)
  - o *Streptococcus* (*S. pneumoniae, S. viridans*)
  - o *Haemophilus* (*H. influenzae, H. aegyptius*)
  - o *Moraxella* (*M. catarrhalis*)
  - o *Pseudomonas* species
  - o *Neisseria* species
  - o *Corynebacterium diptheriae*
  - o Listeria
- Definition
  - o Destruction of corneal epithelium and stroma due to inflammatory reaction from an infectious organism
- Etiology (Table 6-6)
  - o Trauma
  - o Dry eyes
  - o Exposure keratopathy
  - o Bullous keratopathy
  - o Neurotrophic cornea

TABLE 6-6. COMMON ETIOLOGIC AGENTS FOR BACTERIAL KERATITIS

CLASS/ORGANISM	COMMON ISOLATES
Gram positive	
Gram positive cocci	• S. aureus
	• Coagulase negative *staphylococci*
	• *Streptococcus pneumoniae*
	• *Streptococcus viridans*
Gram positive bacilli	• *Corynebacterium* spp.
	• *Propionibacterium* spp.
	• *Mycobacterium* spp.
Gram negative	
Gram negative bacilli	• P. aeruginosa
	• *Serratia marcescens*
	• *Proteus mirabilis*
	• Enteric gram-negative bacilli (other)
Gram negative cocci	• *Neisseria* spp.
Gram negative coccobacilli	• *Haemophilus* spp.
	• *Moraxella* spp.

Adapted from Preferred Practice Patterns: Bacterial keratitis. *American Academy of Ophthalmology.* San Francisco, CA; 2005.

- o Lid abnormalities
- o Contact lens use (identified as the most common risk factor for bacterial keratitis in developed countries)
- o *Pseudomonas* species is the most common isolate in cases of bacterial keratitis and corneal ulceration.
- o Contact lenses with surface protein and mucin deposits are more susceptible to bacterial adhesion
- o Contact lenses may also adversely affect the healthy cornea.
- o Corneal abrasions during insertion
- o Induced corneal changes (epithelial thinning, microcysts, endothelial dysfunction)
- o Tight-lens syndrome (poor lens hydration, inadequate oxygen permeability of the lens, repeated overnight hypoxic stress)
- Signs/symptoms
  - o Usually variable and dependent on the virulence of the microorganism, duration of infection and pre-existing corneal conditions
  - o Pain, photophobia, decreased vision, conjunctival injection, anterior chamber reaction with or without a hypopyon, tearing with or without mucopurulent discharge
  - o Dense suppurative stromal infiltrate with indistinct edges, edema, and white cell infiltration is highly suggestive of bacterial keratitis.
- Differential diagnosis
  - o Viral (herpes simplex, varicella zoster, Epstein-Barr), fungal (yeast and mold), and parasitic (Acanthamoeba) causes of corneal infiltrates, noninfectious causes of corneal infiltrates (associated with contact lens wear; rosacea; atopic keratoconjunctivitis; vasculitic disorders; systemic collagen vascular disorders)

- Evaluation
  - Clinical history
    - History of contact lens wear/abuse
  - Examination
    - Emphasis on biomicroscopy (lid margins, tear film, conjunctival abnormalities, foreign bodies, inflammation of the sclera/cornea, and changes to the corneal surface including but not limited to epithelial defects, keratopathy, stromal infiltration/thinning/perforation)
  - Location
    - Central
    - Peripheral
    - Perineural
  - Other causative factors
  - Laboratory evaluation
    - Gram stain
    - Culture
    - Smear
    - Biopsy specimen
  - Management
    - Medical therapy with appropriate antibiotics
      - Cephalosporins
        - Bactericidal
        - Often used in a fortified form: Cefazolin 15 mg/mL
      - Glycopeptides
        - Bactericidal, with activity against penicillin-resistant staphylococci and primarily active against gram-positive bacteria
        - Compounded in fortified form as Vancomycin (25 to 30 mg/mL)
      - Aminoglycosides
        - Bactericidal, effective against aerobic and facultative gram-negative bacilli
        - Some are active against *P. aeruginosa*, including tobramycin, gentamicin, amikacin, and netilmycin.
        - Fortified tobramycin, at a concentration of 14 mg/mL, is commonly used.
      - Macrolides
        - Bacteriostatic and bactericidal dependent on concentration of the drug
        - Active against *N. gonorrhea*, *N. meningitides*
        - Not indicated for gram-negative bacteria
      - Fluoroquinolones
        - Bactericidal, due to inhibition of bacterial DNA gyrase and topoisomerase IV
        - Effective against most aerobic gram-negative and some gram-positive bacteria
        - Increasing resistance of *P. aeruginosa* and gram-positive organisms, such as *Staphylococcus aureus* and *streptococcus* species, has been noted with the wide use of fluoroquinolone monotherapy.
    - Surgery should be considered if medical therapy fails to eradicate the pathogens or if vision is threatened by infection or decreased by the resultant scar.
  - Prognosis
    - Dependent on the location, duration, and extent of keratitis/corneal ulceration

Viral

- HSV
  - Most common cause of central infectious keratitis with multiple strains of the virus
  - Etiology
    - Primary infection with viral replication in an end organ with subsequent retrograde travel to various ganglia (including trigeminal, cervical, and sympathetic ganglia). Latency is then established.

○ Signs/symptoms
  ▪ Congenital and neonatal ocular HSV
    □ Rare, usually due to HSV-2 due to infection acquired in conjunction with genital herpes in the mother
    □ Note that infection can be acquired from oral lesions, maternal breast lesions, and nosocomial transmission.
    □ Ocular manifestations include periocular skin lesions, keratoconjunctivitis, epithelial keratitis, stromal keratitis, and cataract.
○ Primary ocular HSV
  ▪ HSV affects 60% of the population.
  ▪ Latent infection is the usual course, as only 6% of those infected actually develop clinical manifestations (perioral lesions more common than ocular lesions).
  ▪ Acute follicular conjunctivitis, keratoconjunctivitis, periocular and eyelid skin vesicles, diffuse punctate keratopathy, corneal vesicles, and dendritic lesions can be seen.
○ Recurrent ocular HSV
  ▪ Recurrence occurs at a rate of 18% in the first year per the Herpetic Eye Diseases Study (HEDS).
  ▪ Immune status, sunlight, trauma (surgery), heat, menstruation, other infectious diseases, and emotional stress have all been implicated in the activation of herpetic disease in humans.
  ▪ Usually unilateral
○ Presentation
  ▪ Blepharitis, conjunctivitis, epithelial keratitis (Table 6-7)
  ▪ Dendritic ulcer (Figure 6-25)
    □ A true ulcer with extension through basement membrane
      • Linear, stains positively with fluorescein with swollen, raised epithelial borders compared to neighboring epithelium
      • Swollen margins contain live virus.
      • May have persistent HSV dendritic epitheliopathy for several weeks after the ulcer heals
  ▪ Geographic ulcer (Figure 6-26)
    □ Enlarged dendritic ulcer that has lost the linear configuration
    □ Scalloped margins differentiate this lesion from healing abrasions and neurotrophic keratopathy (smooth margins).
    □ Associated with longer duration of symptoms and time to healing compared to dendritic ulcers
  ▪ Marginal ulcer (Figure 6-27)
    □ Active viral disease with proximity to the limbus accounts for anterior stromal infiltrate underlying the ulcer with adjacent limbal injection.
    □ More symptomatic due to intense inflammation associated with location of lesion
    □ More difficult to treat as the immune response gives the appearance of more intense and longer-lasting disease
  ▪ Stromal keratitis
    □ Accounts for 20% to 48% of recurrent ocular HSV
      • Two types
        ○ Necrotizing stromal keratitis
          □ Due to direct viral invasion of the stroma
          □ Rare
          □ Findings include necrosis, ulceration, and dense infiltration of the stroma with an overlying epithelial defect.
          □ Often refractory to antiviral and anti-inflammatory medications
        ○ Immune stromal keratitis (Figure 6-28)
          □ A result of immune reaction within the stroma
          □ Common chronic recurrent manifestation of HSV, seen in 20% of patients
          □ Likely due to retained viral antigen within the stroma
          □ Overlying epithelium is intact.
          □ Findings include subepithelial haze and scarring.

TABLE 6-7. CLASSIFICATION OF HSV KERATITIS AND COMPARISON OF RECOMMENDED NOMENCLATURE TO COMMON TERMINOLOGY

CLASSIFICATION OF HSV KERATITIS (USING RECOMMENDED NOMENCLATURE)	ALTERNATE TERMS
Infectious epithelial keratitis	
• Cornea vesicles • Dendritic ulcer • Geographic ulcer • Marginal ulcer	Dendrite Herpetic epithelial keratitis Infectious epithelial herpes Limbal keratoconjunctivitis
Neurotrophic keratopathy	
• Punctate epithelial erosions • Neurotrophic ulcer	Trophic ulcer Neurotrophic ulcer Metaherpetic ulcer Indolent ulcer
Necrotizing stromal keratitis	Viral necrotizing keratitis Ulcerating interstitial keratitis
Immune stromal keratitis	Interstitial keratitis Disciform keratitis Herpetic disciform keratitis Herpetic stromal keratitis Stromal keratitis Non-necrotizing stromal keratitis Immune ring Wessely ring Limbal vasculitis
Endotheliitis	
• Disciform • Diffuse • Linear	Disciform keratitis Disciform edema Disciform disease with endotheliitis Central disciform endotheliitis Central endotheliitis Peripheral endotheliitis Keratouveitis

Adapted from Holland EJ, Brilakis HS, Schwartz GS. Herpes simplex keratitis. In: Krachmer JH, Mannis MJ, Holland EJ, Eds. *Cornea*. 2nd ed. Elsevier-Mosby, St. Louis, MO; 2005:1043–1074.

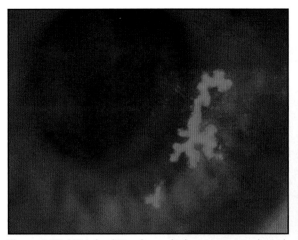

Figure 6-25. HSV dendritic ulcer, which stains positively with fluorescein. (Reprinted with permission from Krachmer JH, Mannis MJ, Holland EJ, Eds. *Cornea*. 2nd ed. St. Louis, MO: Elsevier-Mosby; 2005.)

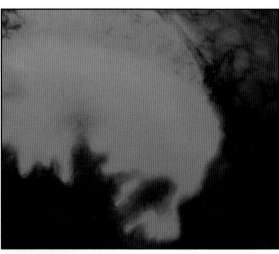

Figure 6-26. HSV geographic ulcer. (Reprinted with permission from Krachmer JH, Mannis MJ, Holland EJ, Eds. *Cornea*. 2nd ed. St. Louis, MO: Elsevier-Mosby; 2005.)

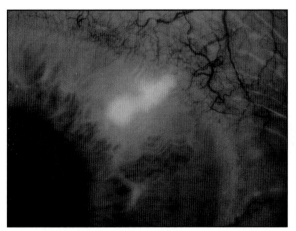

Figure 6-27. Marginal ulcer secondary to HSV. (Reprinted with permission from Krachmer JH, Mannis MJ, Holland EJ, Eds. *Cornea*. 2nd ed. St. Louis, MO: Elsevier-Mosby; 2005.)

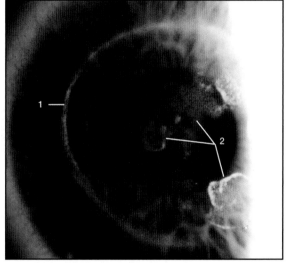

Figure 6-28. HSV immune stromal keratitis. (1) Immune ring and (2) anterior stromal haze and scarring. (Reprinted with permission from Krachmer JH, Mannis MJ, Holland EJ, Eds. *Cornea*. 2nd ed. St. Louis, MO: Elsevier-Mosby; 2005.)

- Endotheliitis
    - Reaction to virus at the level of the endothelium
    - Often seen as diffuse, disciform, or linear and accompanied by stromal edema
    - Keratic precipitates are always present and are associated with the areas of stromal edema (Figure 6-29).
- Differential diagnosis
    - Bacterial keratitis
    - Fungal keratitis
    - Acanthamoeba keratitis
    - HSV
    - Sterile corneal thinning/ulceration
    - Staphylococcal hypersensitivity
    - Sterile corneal infiltrates
    - Topical anesthetic abuse

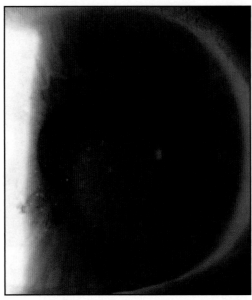

Figure 6-29. Diffuse HSV endotheliitis. Keratic precipitates and stromal edema can be seen. (This figure was published in *Cornea*. 2nd ed. Krachmer JH, Mannis MJ, Holland EJ, eds. Copyright Elsevier [2005].)

- Specifically
  - Dendritic ulcer
    - Healing epithelium
    - Varicella zoster pseudodendrites
  - Geographic ulcer
    - Healing corneal abrasion
    - Neurotrophic keratopathy
  - Marginal ulcer
    - Staphylococcal marginal disease
- Evaluation
  - Clinical history (immune competent or immunocompromised), biomicroscopy with emphasis on evaluation of the epithelium, stroma, and endothelium
  - Corneal sensation, size and depth of ulcer, location and character of ulcer/infiltrate, tonometry, and evaluation of the anterior chamber for cellular reaction
- Management
  - Infectious epithelial keratitis
    - Débridement of the ulcer with sterile cotton-tipped applicator
    - Topical antivirals (Trifluridine 1% drops every 2 hours while awake, Vidarabine 3% ointment 5 times a day as an alternative, gancyclovir ophthalmic gel 0.15%)
    - Cycloplegia and prophylaxis with broad-spectrum antibiotic if treating large geographic ulcers
    - Consider oral antivirals.
  - Neurotrophic keratopathy
    - Discontinuation of all unnecessary topical medications, especially topical antivirals
    - Frequent use of nonpreserved artificial tears
    - Consider broad-spectrum antibiotic if ulceration is large
    - Tarsorrhaphy (tape or surgical)
  - Immune stromal keratitis
    - Topical corticosteroid regimen resulted in significant reduction of stromal inflammation and decrease in the duration of immune stromal keratitis.
    - Oral antiviral therapy for long-term prophylaxis (topical antivirals have long-term side effects of toxic keratoconjunctivitis, allergic conjunctivitis, or punctal stenosis)

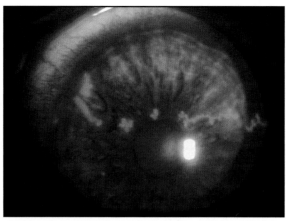

Figure 6-30. VZV keratitis. Note the rounded ends of the dendrites, which do not stain as well with fluorescein as compared to the HSV dendritic ulcer. (This figure was published in *Cornea*. 2nd ed. Krachmer JH, Mannis MJ, Holland EJ, eds. Copyright Elsevier [2005].)

- o Prognosis
  - Visual acuity dependent on location and extent of stromal scarring
- Varicella Zoster virus (VZV)
  - o Primary disease causes a vesicular eruption on the skin of an affected individual.
  - o The diffuse exanthem is usually found on the face and trunk more so than peripheral limbs.
  - o Mucus membrane involvement is rare.
  - o Ophthalmic findings occur externally on the periocular skin, lids, conjunctiva, and cornea as well as on the intraocular structures.
  - o Vesicles on the cornea can lead to scarring and vascularization. Nonspecific papillary conjunctivitis can occur.
  - o Less commonly, dendritic keratitis from active viral growth in the corneal epithelium can occur (Figure 6-30).
  - o Etiology
    - Reactivation of latent VZV from sensory ganglia occurs with increasing age and immunocompromised state.
    - Involvement of the ocular and periocular structures is called Herpes Zoster Ophthalmicus (HZO).
  - o Signs/symptoms
    - Pain, photophobia, discharge, tearing, red eye, and decreased vision may be experienced by patients affected with this infection.
    - Vesicles at the tip of the nose (Hutchinson's sign) are indicative of nasociliary involvement and are also a poor prognostic indicator.
    - Lid edema, hypoesthesia, pain, and pruritis can also be found.
    - Papillary or follicular conjunctivitis, episcleritis, anterior scleritis, or posterior scleritis can occur.
    - Punctate epithelial keratitis, pseudodendrites, anterior stromal infiltrates, and endotheliitis/keratouveitis may occur.
  - o Evaluation
    - Complete ophthalmic history (ie, contact lens use/abuse) and exam with attention to the cornea (ulcer size and depth, corneal sensation, infiltrate location and character, fluorescein and rose bengal staining, area and amount of thinning), tonometry, and anterior chamber examination for evidence of inflammation
  - o Management
    - Supportive therapy with hydration, nonaspirin antipyretics, and careful hygiene to prevent secondary bacterial infection from vesicular skin lesions
    - Antiviral therapy shortens viral shedding duration, accelerates the rate of healing, reduces the severity of acute pain, and reduces the development of ocular complications.

Fungal Keratitis

- One of the most difficult forms of infectious keratitis to diagnose and treat successfully
- Infection is usually due to *Aspergillus, Candida,* or *Fusarium* species.
- *Nocardia* are rare.
- Overall, the incidence of fungal keratitis is low (6% to 20%).
- Etiology
    - Infection after trauma (including contact lenses)
    - Topical medications (ie, corticosteroids and others)
    - Corneal surgery (including LASIK, radial keratotomy, penetrating keratoplasty)
    - Chronic keratitis (HSV, VZV, vernal/allergic conjunctivitis)
- Signs/symptoms
    - Suppuration
    - Conjunctival injection
    - Epithelial defect
    - Anterior chamber reaction
    - Infiltrates with feathery margins, elevated edges, rough texture to the infiltrate, and satellite lesions (Figure 6-31)
    - Often, a deep stromal infiltrate with an overlying intact epithelium may also be found.
- Differential diagnosis
    - Acanthamoeba keratitis
    - Herpes simplex keratitis
    - Sterile corneal thinning/ulceration
    - Staphylococcal hypersensitivity
    - Sterile corneal infiltrates
    - Topical anesthetic abuse
- Evaluation
    - Biomicroscopy
    - Microbiologic evaluation
    - Confocal microscopy
    - Analysis of risk factors for fungal infection
- Management
    - Amphotericin B (0.15%) and natamycin (5%) have been used for treatment for fungal keratitis.
    - Flucytosine 1%, fluconazole 2%, or miconazole 1% can also be added.
    - Note that the duration of treatment can be quite lengthy, and the length of treatment is based on clinical response.
    - Also, the corneal epithelium serves as a barrier to penetration of most topical antifungal agents, and débridement of the corneal epithelium is an essential component of the medical management of fungal keratitis.
    - In severe cases, a therapeutic penetrating keratoplasty can be performed, and an optical keratoplasty can be performed at a later time once the infection is controlled and the integrity of the globe is maintained.
- Prognosis
    - Guarded
    - Success of therapeutic penetrating keratoplasty has been reported as better than medical therapy

Acanthamoeba Keratitis

- Etiology
    - Free-living pathogenic amoeba
- Signs/symptoms
    - Disproportionately severe ocular pain, a paracentral ring infiltrate in the stroma, epithelial haze and irregularity, epithelial ulcers (Figure 6-32), microcysts, punctate epitheliopathy, perineural infiltrates diffuse or nodular scleritis, anterior uveitis, radial keratoneuritis, disciform keratitis, stromal abscess, and resistance to many antimicrobial agents

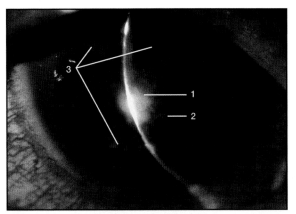

Figure 6-31. Fungal keratitis. (1) Central ulcer, (2) feathery borders of ulcer, (3) satellite lesions. (This figure was published in *Cornea*. 2nd ed. Krachmer JH, Mannis MJ, Holland EJ, eds. Copyright Elsevier [2005].)

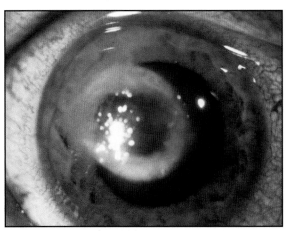

Figure 6-32. Acanthamoeba keratitis. Ring ulcer. (This figure was published in *Cornea*. 2nd ed. Krachmer JH, Mannis MJ, Holland EJ, eds. Copyright Elsevier [2005].)

- Differential diagnosis
  - Herpes simplex keratitis
  - Fungal keratitis
  - Bacterial keratitis
  - Sterile corneal ulceration/thinning
  - Staphylococcal hypersensitivity
  - Anesthetic abuse
- Evaluation
  - Careful history to elicit past and current contact lens use, biomicroscopy with attention to the cornea, sensation, size and location of lesion, laboratory diagnosis (with corneal culture as well as cultured contact lenses and lens cases)
- Management
  - Medical management with topical therapies
    - 0.15% dibrom-propamidine (Brolene ointment)
    - 0.1% propamidine isoethionate (Brolene solution)
    - Polyhexamethylene biguanide (PHMB 0.02%)
  - Penetrating keratoplasty after infection is brought under control and parasites completely eradiated to prevent recurrence in graft.
- Prognosis
  - Early diagnosis yields better visual outcomes.

Interstitial Keratitis

- Definition
  - Vascularization and scarring of corneal stroma due to non-necrotizing inflammation; may be diffuse or sectoral, acute or chronic, and occur with or without edema
- Signs/symptoms
  - Pain, light sensitivity, tearing, decreased visual acuity, peripheral or diffuse stromal haze (Figure 6-33), deep focal stromal vascularization with edema, multifocal or marginal stromal infiltrates, bilateral stromal keratitis, iritis with keratic precipitates, necrotizing stromal keratouveitis, stromal thinning, anterior scleritis (diffuse or nodular), amblyopia if symptoms and signs are congenital
- Differential diagnosis
  - HSV infection
  - VZV infection
  - Hansen's disease
  - Tuberculosis

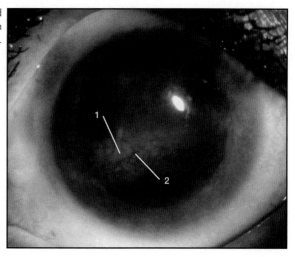

Figure 6-33. Syphilitic interstitial keratitis. (1) Stromal haze and inflammation. (2) Ghost vessels. (This figure was published in *Cornea*. 2nd ed. Krachmer JH, Mannis MJ, Holland EJ, eds. Copyright Elsevier [2005].)

- o Onchocerciasis
- o Human T-lymphotropic virus type I infection
- o Cogan's syndrome
- o Wegener's granulomatosis
- o Sarcoidosis
- o Ectodermal dysplasia
- o Lyme stromal keratitis
- Evaluation
  - o Elicit history of perinatally acquired syphilis, infected sexual contacts, history of syphilis infection, biomicroscopy, tonometry, and indirect ophthalmoscopy
  - o Laboratory evaluation should be conducted to determine infection, including rapid plasma regain (RPR) or Venereal Disease Research Laboratory (VDRL) test as well as fluorescent treponemal antibody absorption (FTA-ABS) or microhemagglutination-Treponema pallidum (MHA-TP) and purified protein derivative (PPD) with anergy panel.
  - o A chest radiograph should be obtained if the patient is PPD positive. Auditory testing should be conducted if there is a high clinical suspicion of Cogan's syndrome.
- Management
  - o Treatment of underlying etiology
    - If acute symptoms are present, if there is evidence for active syphilitic disease, or if serology (ie, RPR, VDRL, FTA-ABS, and MHA-TP) is positive and the patient has not been treated for syphilitic infection, treatment for syphilis is indicated.
    - If the PPD is positive, there is no history of prior treatment for TB, and the patient has active systemic TB infection, a referral to a medical internist is warranted.
    - If Cogan's syndrome is suspected and confirmed by clinical examination and laboratory testing, a referral to an otolaryngologist should be initiated.
    - Penetrating keratoplasty may be considered for old, residual stromal opacification.
- Prognosis
  - o Good. The 10-year corneal graft survival rate is 80%.

Noninfectious Keratitis

Recurrent Erosions

- Definition
  - o Distinct entity characterized by repeated episodes of spontaneous epithelial breakdown
  - o Relatively common and usually due to an abnormality of the adhesion complexes between the epithelium and the basement membrane (secondary to abnormal basement membrane or abnormal deposits of normal basement membrane)
  - o Characterized as primary or secondary, depending on if the defect is intrinsic or acquired

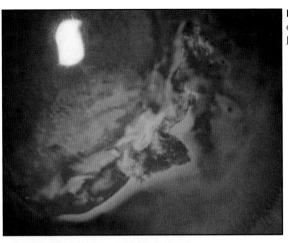

Figure 6-34. Loose epithelium seen in a patient with recurrent erosions. (This figure was published in *Cornea*. 2nd ed. Krachmer JH, Mannis MJ, Holland EJ, eds. Copyright Elsevier [2005].)

- Etiology
  - Primary dystrophies (anterior basement membrane dystrophy)
  - Secondary erosive disorders (mechanical factors, such as lagophthalmos or trauma)
  - Metabolic disorders (diabetes mellitus)
  - Chemical/thermal injury
  - Microbial keratitis
  - Degenerations (band keratopathy, Salzmann's nodular)
- Signs/symptoms
  - Foreign-body sensation upon opening the eye after awakening, which then progresses to extreme pain and photophobia with profuse tearing, corneal abrasions, areas of loose corneal epithelium (Figure 6-34), findings consistent with Map-Dot-Fingerprint dystrophy
- Differential diagnosis
  - Acute trauma
  - Neurotrophic ulcer
  - Infectious keratitis
  - Dry eye
  - Diabetic corneal epitheliopathy
- Evaluation
  - Careful ophthalmic history and exam
    - Use of fluorescein stain may highlight corneal findings.
- Management
  - Superficial keratectomy
    - Débridement with a metal blade or a diamond burr in the affected area. The goal is to remove the abnormal basement membrane by scraping the cornea (without injuring the limbus).
    - Anterior stromal micropuncture
      - Ideal for areas of focal involvement, as can be seen after trauma
    - Excimer laser PTK
      - Modifies the surface structure of the basement membrane and Bowman's layer; often used in conjunction with mechanical débridement for superficial keratectomy
- Prognosis
  - Good. Anterior stromal puncture is effective in 80% of cases.

Filamentary Keratitis

- Definition
  - Filaments are attached to the cornea at their base (Figure 6-35).
  - They are composed of a mucus core, surrounded by degenerated epithelial cells.
  - They may be thin and stringy or short and broad.

Figure 6-35. Filamentary keratitis. The filaments appear as gelatinous lesions seen in on the surface of the cornea. (This figure was published in *Cornea*. 2nd ed. Krachmer JH, Mannis MJ, Holland EJ, eds. Copyright Elsevier [2005].)

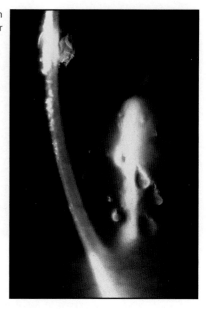

- ○ They are most commonly associated with keratoconjunctivitis sicca, superior limbic keratoconjunctivitis, and neurotrophic keratopathy.
- ○ Filaments are seen in cases of ocular trauma and surgery, including corneal abrasion/erosions, cataract extraction, penetrating keratoplasty, and contact lens overwear.
- Etiology
  - ○ Due to changes in the tear film as well as irregularity of the ocular surface
  - ○ An underlying process damages the basal epithelium, leading to focal areas of basement membrane detachment.
  - ○ The raised epithelium acts as a site of attachment for degenerated cells and mucus.
- Signs/symptoms
  - ○ Decreased visual acuity
  - ○ Pain
  - ○ Mild to severe foreign-body sensation with the following:
    - Epiphora
    - Blepharospasm
    - Photophobia
- Differential diagnosis
  - ○ Epithelial keratitis
- Evaluation
  - ○ Careful biomicroscopy with emphasis on corneal examination
  - ○ Filaments stain with rose bengal and fluorescein, though less brightly with the latter.
- Management
  - ○ Treatment of the underlying disorder, as well as mechanical débridement/removal of the filaments with a jeweler's or tying forceps
  - ○ Aggressive topical lubrication with nonpreserved drops and ointments should be recommended for symptomatic relief.
  - ○ N-acetylcysteine 10% has been used as a mucolytic agent to decrease the viscosity of mucus.
  - ○ The filaments can also be removed carefully with a jeweler's forcep, taking care not to damage the underlying epithelium.
- Prognosis
  - ○ Fair. Treatment is often chronic and can be frustrating for both the patient and physician.

Superficial Punctate Keratitis of Thygeson

- Definition
  - ○ An uncommon epithelial keratopathy with no known association with other ocular or systemic disease

- o Characterized by a coarse punctate epithelial keratitis, the individual evanescent opacities are composed of groups of smaller intraepithelial opacities.
    - o Minimal inflammation accompanies the lesions.
- Etiology
    - o Unknown
- Signs/symptoms
    - o Foreign-body sensation that waves and wanes and is not associated with any conjunctival reaction
    - o Photophobia, tearing, burning, and occasional decrease in visual acuity is also seen.
    - o Epithelial keratitis with discrete oval or round opacities composed of grouped punctate intraepithelial deposits are scattered diffusely across the cornea.
    - o Lesions often change locations, though are more common in the visual axis and central cornea.
- Differential diagnosis
    - o Epithelial keratitis due to staphylococcal blepharitis
    - o Pneumococcal conjunctivitis
    - o Herpes zoster
    - o HSV
    - o Recurrent erosion syndrome
    - o Rosacea
    - o Medicamentosa
- Evaluation
    - o Biomicroscopy with emphasis on corneal examination. There is usually minimal conjunctival inflammation and symptoms are out of proportion with the clinical examination.
- Management
    - o Low-dose topical corticosteroids are commonly used for acute episodes. However, some believe corticosteroids prolong the course of the disease.
- Prognosis
    - o Good. The natural history of the disease is periods of waxing and waning symptoms, with resolution in 2 to 4 years, prior to routine use of steroids.

Neurotrophic Keratitis

- Definition
    - o Degeneration of the corneal epithelium characterized by impaired healing and absence of corneal sensitivity
    - o Persistent epithelial defects can lead to corneal stromal melting and perforation.
    - o The corneal surface is vulnerable to injury, and reflex tearing is reduced.
    - o Healing rates of corneal epithelium also appear to be decreased.
- Etiology
    - o Most common causes for corneal anesthesia are HSV and Herpes zoster infections of the ocular surface.
    - o Iatrogenic injury, tumors, chronic epithelial injury, and systemic disease (ie, diabetes mellitus) all play a role.
    - o Mackie divides the clinical stages of neurotrophic keratitis into the following 3 stages:
        - Stage I
            - □ Includes tear film instability, punctate staining of the corneal epithelium
        - Stage II
            - □ Acute loss of epithelium with a surrounding area of loose epithelium
            - □ The surrounding epithelial cells become hazy, and the edges of the defect become smooth and rolled.
        - Stage III
            - □ Stromal lysis with or without perforation
            - □ These findings ensue in the absence of adequate treatment of Stages I and II and sometimes occur despite appropriate therapy.
- Signs/symptoms
    - o Poor visual acuity
    - o Conjunctival injection

Figure 6-36. Neurotrophic keratopathy. Note the smooth, rolled edges of the ulcer without any accompanying infiltrate in the base. (This figure was published in *Cornea*. 2nd ed. Krachmer JH, Mannis MJ, Holland EJ, eds. Copyright Elsevier [2005].)

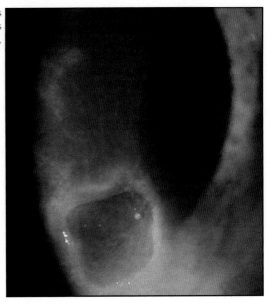

- ○ Hypopyon (rarely)
- ○ Epithelial defect with stromal haze in the base of the defect
- ○ Epithelium at the margins have a smooth, rolled appearance (Figure 6-36).
- Differential diagnosis
  - ○ Infectious corneal ulceration
  - ○ Inflammatory or immune-mediated thinning/ulceration
- Evaluation
  - ○ Biomicroscopy with careful examination of the cornea and area of defect. Corneal sensation is important to document.
- Management
  - ○ Aggressive lubrication with nonpreserved drops or ointments; tarsorrhaphy; lamellar or penetrating keratoplasty
  - ○ Re-evaluate any current ocular therapy that may contribute to corneal anesthesia
- Prognosis
  - ○ Fair

Factitious Keratoconjunctivitis

- Definition
  - ○ Intentionally produced symptoms or physical findings associated with keratitis and corneal ulcers
  - ○ Findings are often patient-induced in order for the individual to assume the role of a sick patient and are believed to have a psychiatric basis.
  - ○ These cases can be differentiated from malingering (evidence of external incentive) and somatoform disorder (including hysteria, conversion disorder, and hypochondriasis).
  - ○ Signs/symptoms
    - ▪ Decreased vision, foreign-body sensation, and marked damage to the cornea, including mechanical injury as well as infectious and inflammatory changes to the cornea
  - ○ Self-induced trauma not associated with an underlying psychopathology include the following:
    - ▪ Mucus fishing syndrome
      - □ Patients present with irritation and inflammation most commonly localized to the nasal and inferior bulbar conjunctiva.
      - □ The findings are often associated with underlying keratoconjunctivitis sicca and overproduction of mucus.

- □ Other associated disorders include allergic conjunctivitis, keratoconjunctivitis, and corneal foreign body.
- □ Upon patient demonstration of the mechanical removal, the source of the irritation will become apparent.
  - ■ Congenital corneal anesthesia
    - □ Usually not associated with repeated self-induced trauma
    - □ This entity should be explored in cases where corneal ulceration fails to heal with standard treatment.
  - ■ Topical anesthetic abuse
    - □ May be the means used by a patient to gain access to the medical system or iatrogenic with occasional cases associated with physician dispensing
    - □ Patients can obtain the anesthetic from a family member or remove the bottles from the examination room.
    - □ Anesthetics are known to inhibit the ability of the corneal epithelium to divide and migrate.
    - □ Initial findings include punctate keratopathy, followed by increased inflammation and conjunctival injection, as well as increased anterior chamber inflammation with keratic precipitates and hypopyon.
    - □ At this point, visual acuity is decreased, as is the corneal clarity within the area of the epithelial defect, and stromal edema and full-thickness stromal infiltration is noted.
    - □ A ring infiltrate is common.
    - □ A high index of suspicion must be maintained in order for the diagnosis to be made.
- • Differential diagnosis
  - o Infectious and inflammatory etiologies producing keratitis, corneal ulceration, and thinning
  - o Trauma (not self-inflicted)
- • Evaluation
  - o Careful history to elicit predisposing factors for infection (such as contact lens wear/abuse, trauma), autoimmune disorders, type of employment, underlying corneal disorder that may induce chronic discomfort and pain, and underlying reason for self-destructive behavior
- • Management
  - o Careful approach is advocated, without harsh accusations and maintaining the patient's confidence.
  - o Treat concomitant infection/inflammation with appropriate medications and obtain psychiatry consultation.

Immune-Mediated Corneal Disorders

Corneal Disease Associated With Rheumatoid Arthritis

- • Definition
  - o Systemic autoimmune disease involving chronic inflammation of unknown etiology
  - o Primarily affects the synovial joints and less frequently the extra-articular tissues such as the eye
  - o Chronic, progressive disease resulting in significant disability and mortality, unless aggressive therapy is initiated
- • Signs/symptoms
  - o Decreased vision
  - o Foreign-body sensation
  - o Conjunctival inflammation
  - o Pain
  - o Chemosis
  - o Proptosis
  - o Exudative retinal detachment

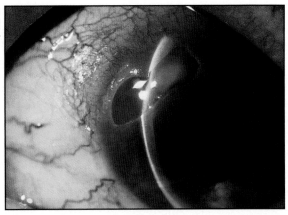

Figure 6-37. Peripheral ulcerative keratitis in a patient with rheumatoid arthritis. (This figure was published in *Cornea*. 2nd ed. Krachmer JH, Mannis MJ, Holland EJ, eds. Copyright Elsevier [2005].)

    o Associated with
- Keratoconjunctivitis sicca (most common)
- Decreased tear meniscus
- Ulcerative keratitis (Figure 6-37)
- Diffuse episcleritis
- Scleritis (anterior, diffuse, nodular, necrotizing, posterior)
- Marginal corneal infiltrates
- Marginal corneal thinning

- Differential diagnosis
  - Other autoimmune disorders such as Wegener's granulomatosis and polyarteritis nodosa
  - Terrien's marginal degeneration
  - Furrow degeneration
  - Drug allergy
  - Phlyctenule
  - Rosacea
  - Mooren's ulcer
  - Herpetic marginal ulceration
  - Zoster keratitis
  - Bacterial or fungal ulcers
- Evaluation
  - History to elicit family history and past medical history, current treatment regimen, and recurrent disease
  - Careful biomicroscopy to determine involvement of the cornea, adjacent conjunctiva, and sclera
  - Laboratory evaluation should include a CBC, RF level, and ANA titers and can be completed in conjunction with a rheumatologic evaluation.
- Management
  - Systemic therapy to slow or reduce the inflammatory process and maintain functional status
  - Use of NSAIDs, corticosteroids, and systemic immunosuppressive medications (including methotrexate, sulfasalazine, cyclosporine, gold, and etanercept [Enbrel]) can be helpful in treating both ocular and systemic symptoms.
  - Rheumatology consultation is recommended.
  - Topical lubrication and low-dose topical steroids for reduction of inflammation can be used to treat keratoconjunctivitis sicca.
  - Topical cyclosporine A may be used as an adjunct.
  - Surgical management may be necessary to maintain the integrity of the globe. Scleral grafting and lamellar corneal grafting have been used as tectonic support.
  - Conjunctival resection may be helpful.
  - Penetrating keratoplasty may be required in cases of corneal perforation from ulceration and inflammation.

Corneal Disease Associated With Nonrheumatoid Collagen-Vascular Disease

- Etiology
  - Destructive and inflammatory disorder involving the connective tissues and vasculature
  - Often presents as keratoconjunctivitis sicca, episcleritis, and scleritis, as well as corneal involvement predominantly caused by changes in tear film stability and eyelid changes
  - Keratitis may occur in the absence of scleritis or may be part of sclerokeratitis.
  - Associated with Wegener's granulomatosis, polyarteritis nodosa, Behçet's disease, systemic sclerosis, mixed connective tissue disease, polymyositis, and dermatomyositis
- Signs/symptoms
  - Decreased visual acuity (dependent on degree of corneal involvement)
  - Foreign-body sensation
  - Decreased tear film/meniscus
  - Conjunctival injection
  - Pain
  - Episcleral and scleral vessel engorgement
  - Anterior uveitis
- Evaluation
  - Family history and past medical history as well as careful biomicroscopy
  - Laboratory evaluations should include CBC (check for anemia, leukocytosis), ESR, antineutrophil cytoplasmic antibody, RF, antinuclear antibody.
- Management
  - Topical lubrication for treatment of keratoconjunctivitis sicca
  - Aggressive systemic therapy should be considered for episcleritis, scleritis, and peripheral ulcerative keratitis.
  - Systemic immunomodulatory and immunosuppressive medications should be considered.
  - Rheumatologic consultation should be obtained.

Cicatricial Pemphigoid (Mucus Membrane Pemphigoid)

- Etiology
  - Autoimmune, cicatrizing disease of mucus membranes
  - Often presents to the ophthalmologist with chronic conjunctivitis, usually of insidious onset
  - Natural course of the disease is usually slow but with occasional aggravated periods of intense inflammation.
  - Often bilateral, though involvement is asymmetric
- Signs/symptoms
  - Decrease in visual acuity
  - Foreign-body sensation
  - Tearing
  - Mucus production
  - Conjunctival injection
  - Vascular dilatation
  - Conjunctival thickening
  - Subconjunctival fibrosis of the tarsal conjunctiva
  - Shortening of the fornices (inferior more than superior)
  - Symblepharon
  - Keratinization of the ocular surface (Figure 6-38)
- Evaluation
  - Careful history to elicit medications that can cause similar findings (ie, chronic topical medications for glaucoma), biomicroscopy to determine level of ocular surface inflammation and degree of conjunctival involvement (Table 6-8)
  - Conjunctival biopsy should be obtained for immunofluorescent stains.
  - Linear deposition of immunoglobulins seen in the basement membrane zone (BMZ) are pathognomonic for the disease.

Figure 6-38. Stage IV cicatricial pemphigoid/mucus membrane pemphigoid. Keratinization of the ocular surface is seen, as well as marked symblepharon, trichiasis, and ocular surface inflammation. (This figure was published in *Cornea*. 2nd ed. Krachmer JH, Mannis MJ, Holland EJ, eds. Copyright Elsevier [2005].)

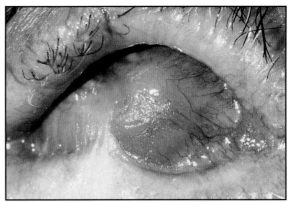

TABLE 6-8. CLASSIFICATION OF OCULAR CICATRICAL PEMPHIGOID/MUCOUS MEMBRANE PEMPHIGOID

GRADE	FINDINGS
I	Subepithelial fibrosis without foreshortening of fornix
II	Subepithelial fibrosis
	Fornix foreshortening
	→ A: 0% to 25%
	→ B: 25% to 50%
	→ C: 50% to 75%
	→ D: 75% to 100%
III	Grade II + Symblepharon
	Degree of horizontal involvement:
	→ A: 0% to 25%
	→ B: 25% to 50%
	→ C: 50% to 75%
	→ D: 75% to 100%
IV	End stage disease, ankyloblepharon and ocular surface keratinization

- Management
  - Aggressive treatment of keratitis sicca, lid hygiene, epilation of trichiatic lashes, treatment of entropion, immunosuppressive therapy for underlying autoimmune process
  - Systemic immunosuppression should be initiated with the assistance of a medical internist, rheumatologist, or immunologist.
- Prognosis
  - Guarded

Stevens-Johnson Syndrome

- Etiology
  - Immune-mediated acute blistering disease involving the skin and mucus membranes
  - Acute phase of ocular disease generally lasts 2 to 3 weeks.

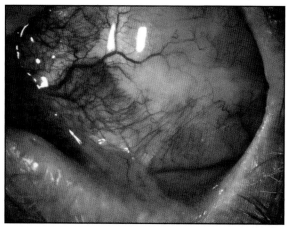

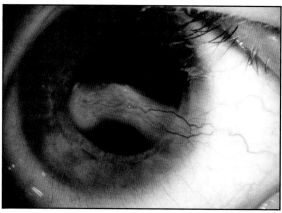

Figure 6-39. Stevens-Johnson syndrome. Marked inflammation is seen on the ocular surface, as well as symblepharon. (This figure was published in *Cornea*. 2nd ed. Krachmer JH, Mannis MJ, Holland EJ, eds. Copyright Elsevier [2005].)

Figure 6-40. Corneal phlyctenule. (This figure was published in *Cornea*. 2nd ed. Krachmer JH, Mannis MJ, Holland EJ, eds. Copyright Elsevier [2005].)

- Signs/symptoms
  - Lid edema and erythema, with crusting/ulceration of the lid margin and conjunctiva
  - Epithelial defects
  - Corneal edema
  - Cicatricial entropion or ectropion
  - Recurrent trichiasis
  - Meibomian gland dysfunction
  - Subepithelial fibrosis
  - Stromal neovascularization (Figure 6-39)
- Differential diagnosis (of chronic SJS)
  - Cicatrizing disorders, including cicatricial pemphigoid, linear IgA disease, atopic keratoconjunctivitis, chemical injury, trachoma, avitaminosis A
- Management
  - Supportive therapy in the acute stages, including lid hygiene, prophylactic topical antibiotics, nonpreserved topical lubricants
  - Surgical treatment of abnormal lid anatomy is important.
  - Symblepharolysis may be necessary.
- Prognosis
  - Dependent on the severity of the disease

Phlyctenular Keratoconjunctivitis

- Definition
  - Localized, noninfectious inflammatory processes of the ocular surface, associated with a form of T-cell mediated hypersensitivity (Figure 6-40)
- Etiology
  - Immune reactions triggered by an antigen. Phlyctenulosis is associated with bacteria (*S. aureus, N. gonorrhea, C. immitis*) and mycobacteria (TB), viruses (HSV), chlamydia fungi, and rosacea dermatitis.
  - *S. aureus* is the most commonly associated etiology in the United States, though tuberculous phlyctenulosis may be more prevalent in other areas of the world.
- Signs/symptoms
  - Pain
  - Photophobia
  - Foreign-body sensation
  - Conjunctival injection
  - Raised, amorphous light pink to gray nodules usually near the limbus, often involving the bulbar conjunctiva.

- o Corneal phlyctenules are whiter and start at the limbus but may migrate to either the cornea or the conjunctiva.
- o Lesions may be solitary or multiple. Staphylococcal blepharitis may be associated.
- Differential diagnosis
  - o Salzmann's corneal nodules
  - o Limbal papillae in vernal keratoconjunctivitis
  - o Inflamed pinguecula
  - o Nodular episcleritis
  - o Infectious corneal ulcers
- Evaluation
  - o Skin testing for tuberculosis and a chest x-ray should be obtained.
  - o Chlamydial infection may be involved in recurrent cases of phlyctenulosis.
  - o Corneal scrapings and cultures should be obtained to rule out bacterial and viral (HSV) etiologies.
- Management
  - o Determined by the underlying cause of the phlyctenulosis
  - o Topical antibiotics should be initiated if there is an overlying epithelial defect.
  - o Topical steroids or a corticosteroid-antibiotic combination is the initial therapy. Treatment for blepharitis and meibomitis should be initiated.
  - o Tuberculosis-associated phlyctenulosis should be treated with topical astringents in addition to topical corticosteroid.
- Prognosis
  - o Good

Staphylococcal Marginal Keratitis

- Etiology
  - o Host antibody response to staphylococcal antigen
- Signs/symptoms
  - o Pain
  - o Photophobia
  - o Foreign-body sensation
  - o Conjunctival injection
  - o Localized peripheral stromal infiltrates that occur most commonly where the eyelid crosses the limbus (2, 4, 8, and 10 o'clock positions)
  - o There is typically a lucid area of cornea separating the infiltrates from the limbus.
  - o The epithelium is initially intact, although with prolonged inflammation, the epithelium breaks down and ulceration/thinning of the underlying stroma can occur.
  - o Increased limbal vascularity may be associated with the areas of stromal infiltrate.
  - o Signs of staphylococcal blepharoconjunctivitis accompany the findings of marginal keratitis.
- Differential diagnosis
  - o HSV marginal keratitis
  - o Mooren's corneal ulcers
  - o Peripheral ulcerative keratitis
  - o Bacterial or fungal ulceration
- Evaluation
  - o Diagnosis is based on clinical findings.
  - o Careful history and clinical examination will reveal associated signs and symptoms of staphylococcal blepharoconjunctivitis.
- Management
  - o In cases of corneal infiltrates without epithelial breakdown, topical corticosteroids may be used in conjunction with an antibiotic or alone.
  - o In cases with epithelial breakdown, a broad-spectrum antibiotic should be used with topical corticosteroids.
  - o If the lesions enlarge and ulceration increases, re-evaluate for an infectious etiology with appropriate microbiologic workup.

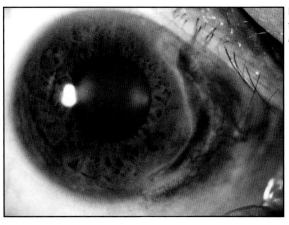

Figure 6-41. Mooren's ulcer with associated inflammation. (This figure was published in *Cornea*. 2nd ed. Krachmer JH, Mannis MJ, Holland EJ, eds. Copyright Elsevier [2005].)

- o Treatment of associated blepharitis with warm compresses, lid hygiene, and topical antibiotic ointment applied to the lids should be initiated along with topical therapy in order to reduce recurrences.
- Prognosis
  - o Good

Mooren's Ulcer

- Definition
  - o Crescent-shaped gray-white infiltrate in the peripheral cornea associated with epithelial breakdown, stromal melting, and chronic, painful peripheral corneal ulceration (Figure 6-41)
  - o Disease progression is associated with spreading of the ulcer peripherally, centrally, and into the sclera (rare).
  - o Corneal re-epithelialization and vascularization is associated with scarring and thinning. Irregular astigmatism may cause a decrease in visual acuity.
  - o The following 2 types exist:
    - ▪ Type I
      - □ Limited, responds well to medical therapy or relatively conservative surgery. Usually unilateral, occurs in older patients, and is not associated with significant pain.
    - ▪ Type II
      - □ Relentless, progressive form that does not respond well to any therapy. Presents at any age but generally occurs in younger patients, frequently shows scleral involvement, is associated with severe pain and hyperemia, is often bilateral, and may progress to corneal perforation.
- Etiology
  - o Likely an autoimmune process
  - o The following 2 groups exist:
    - ▪ Primary
      - □ Can manifest as either Type I or II and is the classic idiopathic variety
    - ▪ Secondary
      - □ Follows a variety of insults to the cornea, including cataract surgery, penetrating keratoplasty, trauma, chemical burns, herpes zoster, syphilis, tuberculosis, and metallic foreign bodies. Often unilateral and behave clinically like Type I.
    - ▪ A small group of patients with aggressive disease progression were found to be seropositive for hepatitis C. Treatment with interferon showed fair to good success when all other therapies and treatment modalities failed.
- Signs/symptoms
  - o Pain
  - o Photophobia
  - o Decreased visual acuity
  - o Epithelial breakdown
  - o Stromal ulceration
  - o Perforation in severe cases

- Differential diagnosis
  - Peripheral ulcerative keratitis
  - Marginal keratitis
  - Terrien's marginal degeneration
  - Furrow degeneration
  - Bacterial ulceration
  - Viral (HSV) marginal keratitis and ulceration
- Evaluation
  - Mooren's ulcer is a diagnosis of exclusion.
  - Bacterial, viral, fungal, and other infectious etiologies need to be ruled out, along with other autoimmune disorders associated with peripheral corneal ulceration.
  - Careful biomicroscopy with emphasis on the corneal examination needs to be conducted to monitor the progress of the ulcer.
- Management
  - Aggressive treatment with topical corticosteroids, with concomitant broad-spectrum antibiotic for prophylaxis against bacterial superinfection
  - If there is no improvement, conjunctival recession is performed adjacent to the ulcer and is recessed to a position 3 to 4 mm posterior to the limbus.
  - Systemic immunosuppressive medications (including cyclophosphamide, prednisone, cyclosporine, methotrexate, mycophenylate mofetil, and azathioprine) may be used with fair to good success.
  - Interferon α-2b may be used in patients with Mooren's ulcer who also are seropositive for hepatitis C.
- Prognosis
  - Dependent on presentation: unilateral disease, bilateral nonsimultaneous disease, or bilateral simultaneous disease
  - Unilateral disease often has the best prognosis, while bilateral simultaneous disease is often the most difficult to treat.

Trauma

- Etiology
  - Corneal tissue destruction due to mechanical, thermal, or chemical (acid or base) injury (Figure 6-42)
  - Alkali causes most severe injury, though strong acids can also cause significant ocular trauma.
- Signs/symptoms
  - Decreased visual acuity
  - Pain
  - Photophobia
  - Tearing
  - Conjunctival injection
  - Ciliary injection
  - Epithelial defects
  - Ischemia of limbus and sclera
  - Corneal edema
  - Opacification of the superficial layers of the cornea
  - Foreign body embedded in the cornea
  - Positive Seidel test
  - Irregular pupil
  - Incarcerated iris
  - Corneal laceration
- Evaluation
  - History is critical in the trauma setting, including details of the traumatic event, as well as surrounding circumstances.

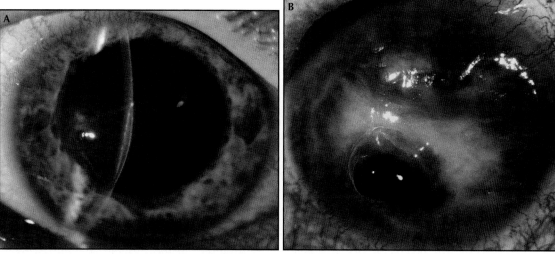

Figure 6-42. Ocular trauma. (A) Partial-thickness laceration with good placement of the corneal flap. (B) Penetrating injury with protrusion of the iris (This figure was published in *Cornea*. 2nd ed. Krachmer JH, Mannis MJ, Holland EJ, eds. Copyright Elsevier [2005].)

○ Careful examination of the external structures surrounding the eye is necessary, taking note of any blunt injury to the lids or lacerations, which may reveal similar injuries to the underlying cornea.

○ Careful biomicroscopy is required in order to fully evaluate the eye and detect occult damage.

• Management

  ○ Epithelial/stromal abrasions

    ▪ Alleviating patient's symptoms

    ▪ Preventing complications

    ▪ Promoting healing of the epithelium

  ○ Cycloplegic agents (cyclopentolate 1%, homatropine 5%, scopolamine 0.25%, or atropine 1%) can be applied twice daily or up to 4 times a day, depending on the size and severity of the epithelial defect.

  ○ Broad-spectrum topical antibiotics should be initiated.

  ○ Consider bandage contact lenses to protect the healing epithelium as well as allow patients to continue to work and perform daily activities.

  ○ Partial-thickness lacerations should be stabilized in order to maintain the tissue in proper anatomic location. Sutures may be necessary to maintain approximation of the injured flap to the stromal bed.

Blunt/Penetrating Injuries

• Ophthalmic emergency

  ○ Careful evaluation of the eye, including external structures, to determine the presence of penetrating injury

  ○ Care must be taken to examine the depth of the anterior chamber and evaluate for the presence of an intraocular foreign body. Once the diagnosis of a penetrating injury has been made, further examination should be completed at the time of surgical repair in the operating room in order to avoid any pressure on the globe and extrusion of intraocular contents.

  ○ Systemic antibiotics should be administered.

  ○ Tetanus toxoid may be administered as needed.

  ○ Obtain any ancillary testing as needed to determine the extent of the injury and to rule out intraocular or intraorbital foreign body.

  ○ Repair of the injury should be scheduled as soon as possible.

Thermal Injuries

- Ophthalmic emergency
  - Determine if the injury is secondary to contact burns or flame burns. Note that flame burns do not often involve the cornea due to the rapid lid closure and insulating quality of the lid. Contact burns are also rare, but happen most frequently in the industrial setting or due to injury from hot curling irons.
  - Treatment involves management of the patients' symptoms for mild cases (ie, associated with curling iron injury). Severe cases require aggressive control of inflammation and prevention of infection with care to manage stromal thinning and symblepharon should they occur.

Chemical Injuries

- Ophthalmic emergency
  - Any prior history of chemical injury (acid or alkali) requires immediate copious irrigation with sterile saline, Ringer's solution, or water.
  - Measure pH both before and after irrigation. Irrigation should be continued until pH is neutralized (7.0). Any precipitate or particulate matter from the chemical should be removed with a sterile cotton swab. The fornices should also be swabbed and inspected.
  - After irrigation is complete, topical lubrication and broad-spectrum antibiotic coverage should be applied.
  - Cycloplegics (cyclopentolate 1%, scopolamine 0.25%, atropine 1%) can be initiated 2 to 4 times a day depending on severity.
  - IOP should be monitored.
  - Prognosis
    - Epithelial abrasions
      - Good
      - Scarring is dependent on degree of injury to Bowman's layer.
    - Partial-thickness lacerations
      - Good
      - Results are dependent on good apposition of injured tissue to stromal bed.
    - Perforating injuries
      - Dependent on the degree of ocular involvement and the number of structures involved
    - Chemical injury
      - Dependent on the degree of injury as well as the strength of the acid or alkali agent involved. Table 6-9 classifies the degree of chemical injury and notes the prognosis based on the initial presentation.

Complications Related to Contact Lens Use

- Symptoms
  - Decreased visual acuity
  - Foreign-body sensation
  - Tearing
  - Photophobia
  - Itching
  - Burning
  - Pain
  - Decreased lens wear time
  - May present with the following:
    - Epithelial defect
    - Hypersensitivity/toxicity to contact lens cleaning solutions
      - Conjunctival injection
      - Punctate staining
      - Once with solutions containing thimerosal
    - Corneal neovascularization
      - Peripheral 1- to 2-mm pannus more common in the superior cornea

TABLE 6-9. CHEMICAL INJURY: HUGHES-ROPER-HALL CLASSIFICATION

GRADE	FINDINGS	PROGNOSIS
I	No limbal ischemia; injury confined to epithelium	Good
II	Stromal haze present (iris details still visible) Limbal ischemia less than one-third	Good
III	Total loss of corneal epithelium Severe stromal haze blurring iris details Ischemia involving one-third to one-half of limbus	Guarded
IV	Severe stromal haze obscuring view of iris or pupil Ischemia involving greater than one-half of limbus Cornea opaque	Poor

Adapted from Kim T, Khosla-Gupta BA. Chemical and thermal injuries to the ocular surface. In: Holland EJ, Mannis MK, Eds. *Ocular Surface Disease: Medical and Surgical Management*. Springer-Verlag: New York, NY; 2002.

- Giant papillary conjunctivitis
  - Irritation from protein deposits
  - Soft contact lens materials and mechanical irritation
  - Seen predominantly on the upper tarsal conjunctiva and associated with thick, ropy mucus discharge
  - Also evident in patients with ocular prostheses or exposed sutures
- Infectious keratitis
  - Infiltrate is noted with an overlying epithelial defect and is often associated with anterior chamber inflammation.
  - Seen more often in extended-wear and soft contact lens wearers. Pseudomonas and Acanthamoeba should be highly suspected.
- Pseudodendritic keratitis
  - Contact lens-induced epitheliopathy
    - Usually seen in the superior cornea
    - Often associated with increased vascularity and sterile infiltrates
    - Application of fluorescein highlights the area of abnormal epithelium.
- Sterile corneal infiltrates
  - Small (1 mm or less) peripheral, multifocal opacities seen, usually with an intact epithelium
- Poor lens fit
  - Associated with increased lid irritation
  - Limbal injection
  - Poor movement of the contact lens with blink (too much or too little movement)
  - Lens edge lift
  - Poor centration of lens
- Evaluation
  - Careful ophthalmic history with emphasis on contact lens wear habits and cleaning habits
  - A full examination with attention to lens fit, palpebral conjunctiva, and cornea should be completed.
  - Evaluation of ocular surface disease, including Schirmer's testing, rose bengal staining, and tear break up time should also be considered.
  - Corneal cultures, contact lens cultures, as well as contact lens cases should be cultured if there is a strong suspicion of infection.
- Management
  - Suspend contact lens use or decrease lens wear time.
  - For hypoxia and neovascularization, consider a lens with higher oxygen permeability.

- o If hypersensitive to lens-care solutions, discontinue lens use and discard lenses until corneal surface is stable.
- o Change the cleaning system and consider a preservative-free regimen or a hydrogen peroxide cleaning regimen.
- o Improve lens fit for poorly fitted contact lenses.
- o Suspend lens wear in patients with sterile corneal infiltrates.
- o Broad-spectrum antibiotics with good gram-negative coverage (ie, fourth generation fluoroquinolones) may be used for empiric therapy of suspected infectious keratitis.
- o Corneal cultures and contact lens/lens case cultures should be obtained to better direct therapy.
- • Prognosis
  - o Good
  - o Infectious keratitis may have good prognosis depending on severity of infection and location of final scar.

Corneal Surgery

Lamellar Keratoplasty

- • Common technique used for optical rehabilitation of the cornea (ie, anterior stromal scarring), as well as an option for tectonic support in markedly thinned recipient beds (cornea or sclera)
- • The theory behind lamellar grafting is to resect only the affected portion of the cornea (usually the anterior portion), leaving behind the patient's own Descemet's membrane and endothelium as a barrier for immunologic rejection.
- • New techniques, such as microkeratome- or femtosecond laser-assisted lamellar keratoplasty, or deep anterior lamellar keratoplasty (DALK), are able to provide better results in visual rehabilitation, with less interface haze and a reduction in endothelial rejection.

Corneal Transplantation

- • Surgical indications
  - o Decreased vision from bullous keratopathy (aphakic and pseudophakic)
  - o Corneal edema (ie, Fuchs' endothelial dystrophy)
  - o Keratoconus
  - o Pellucid marginal degeneration
  - o Stromal dystrophies
  - o Infection
  - o Congenital opacities
  - o Trauma
  - o Stromal dystrophies
  - o Immune-mediated corneal perforation or thinning
  - o Corneal degenerations
  - o A failed previous corneal transplant
- • Preoperative considerations
  - o Any extraocular factors that could compromise the final visual result, including the following:
    - ▪ Malpositioned lids
    - ▪ Poor blink reflex
    - ▪ Trichiasis
    - ▪ Aqueous or mucin deficiency
  - o Also consider intraocular and neurologic abnormalities, including the following:
    - ▪ Neurotrophic keratopathy
    - ▪ Active keratitis or uveitis
    - ▪ Ocular surface inflammation
    - ▪ Pre-existing glaucoma
    - ▪ Retinal pathology (ie, maculopathy, pre-existing retinal disease)
    - ▪ Media opacity (ie, cataract)

- o Poor prognostic factors include the following:
    - Ocular surface disease
    - Active inflammation
    - Stromal inflammation
    - Peripheral corneal thinning
    - Poorly controlled glaucoma
- Intraoperative complications
    - o Choroidal hemorrhage and effusion
    - o Damage to lens or iris with instrumentation
    - o Intraocular hemorrhage from iris or wound
    - o Damage to the donor epithelium during trephination or handling
    - o Iris incarceration in the wound
    - o Vitreous contact with donor epithelium
- Postoperative considerations
    - o Wound leak
    - o Glaucoma
    - o Recurrence of primary disease
    - o Increased astigmatism
    - o Suture abscess
    - o Endophthalmitis
    - o Primary endothelial failure
        - Persistent graft edema from postoperative day 1 without any signs of intraocular inflammation or microbial infection
        - Persistent epithelial defect
            - □ Large nonhealing epithelial defects that continue after 14 days
            - □ Ocular surface disease is a common contributing factor.
            - □ Aggressive treatment with topical lubrication, punctal occlusion, and possibly a lateral tarsorrhaphy may be required.
    - o Transplant rejection
        - Edema and opacification of the corneal graft due to primary donor failure (early)
        - Allograft rejection (usually late, and most often endothelial in origin)
        - Postoperative factors (elevated IOP, neovascularization)
        - Recurrence of primary disease
- Signs/symptoms
    - o Pain
    - o Photophobia
    - o Red eye
    - o Decreased vision
    - o Decreased acuity
    - o Conjunctival injection
    - o Ciliary flush
    - o Corneal edema
    - o Vascularization of the graft
    - o Subepithelial infiltrates
    - o Epithelial rejection line
    - o Endothelial rejection line (Khoudadoust line)
    - o Diffuse keratic precipitates
    - o Anterior chamber inflammation
    - o Possible elevation of IOP
- Differential diagnosis
    - o Herpes simplex keratitis/endotheliitis
    - o Adenoviral keratoconjunctivitis, anterior uveitis
- Evaluation
    - o Complete ophthalmic history and examination with attention to conjunctiva, cornea, suture integrity, anterior chamber, and tonometry

- Management
  - Topical steroid (prednisolone acetate 1% up to hourly dosage in initial phase, then slow taper)
  - Cycloplegia (cyclopentolate 1%, homatropine 5%, atropine 1%, or scopolamine 0.25% 3 times daily)
  - Systemic steroids (oral prednisone 1 mg/kg/day up to 80 mg/day with rapid taper, or Medrol dose-pak) if necessary
  - Sub-Tenon's injection of steroid (triamcinolone; watch for marked steroid response)
  - Topical cyclosporine can be considered, although the effects are not immediate.
  - Acyclovir 400 mg orally 3 times a day for 2 to 3 weeks if HSV is the suspected etiology
  - Treatment of elevated IOP
- Prognosis
  - Good if aggressive therapy is initiated early
  - Poor if there is prior graft failure or penetrating keratoplasty was secondary to previous HSV keratitis, infectious corneal ulcer, chemical injury, or eye disease secondary to autoimmune etiologies (Stevens-Johnson, ocular cicatricial pemphigoid); better if grafts were completed secondary to corneal edema, keratoconus, scar/opacity, or dystrophy
  - Advanced techniques of graft bed preparation (ie, using a "top-hat," "mushroom," or "zigzag" configuration) are in development, and further research may demonstrate the effects on the rate of wound healing and wound stability through use of these surgical approaches.

New Techniques in Endothelial Keratoplasty

- Endothelial lamellar keratoplasty or microkeratome-assisted posterior lamellar keratoplasty (PLK)
  - Large-diameter microkeratome flap of between 160 μm and 230 μm is created and reflected
  - Underlying mid- and posterior stroma is trephinated with a 7.0-mm diameter or smaller trephine.
  - Posterior corneal tissue is removed from the eye, and a same-size or slightly oversized donor is then used to fill the hole.
  - The button is either sutured into place or oversized and secured with an anterior chamber air bubble.
  - Corneal flap is then replaced and sutured into position. Results range from 20/25 to 20/200 with astigmatism levels of 1.25 to 8.0 D.
  - Complications
    - Primary graft failure
    - Epithelial ingrowth flap melt with amputation
    - Frequent wound leaks
  - Advantages
    - Automated lamellar interface
    - Familiar surgical technique with access for anterior segment procedures as necessary (cataract, intraocular lens exchange, vitrectomy, or iridoplasty)
  - Disadvantages
    - Same preoperative and intraoperative requirements of standard PK surgery (the use of surface corneal incisions, sutures, and a significant vertical stromal wound)
- Deep lamellar endothelial keratoplasty (DLEK), PLK, Descemet's stripping endothelial keratoplasty (DSEK), or Descemet's membrane endothelial keratoplasty (DMEK)
  - Endothelial replacement through a limbal incision
  - Partial-thickness stromal dissection is carried out to the limbus (DLEK, PLK).
  - The posterior lamella is trephined or cut with intraocular scissors and the host lenticule removed.
  - The donor lenticule is prepared in similar fashion and is inserted into the recipient, endothelial side down, on a specially designed spatula.
  - In DSEK and DMEK, Descemet's membrane is stripped delicately without compromise of the posterior stroma. Either a surgeon-prepared lenticule or a precut lenticule obtained from an eye bank can be used to replace the diseased endothelial tissue.
  - The lenticule is floated up and apposed to the exposed stromal bed with the introduction of an air bubble in the anterior chamber, and then the bubble is exchanged for balanced salt solution.

o The lenticule is held in position through a mechanism of the endothelial pump, which provides for deturgescence of the overlying stroma.
o Visual acuity results are very good, with one line of vision loss due to interface haze. Astigmatic changes vary up to 1 D of preoperative topography.
o Complications
  ▪ Mainly intraoperative and early postoperative period, with risk of hyphema, dislodged endothelial lenticule
o Advantages
  ▪ Avoidance of corneal surface incisions and sutures
  ▪ Transplantation of the affected tissue, minimal change in corneal topography and astigmatism
  ▪ More predictable corneal stability and power
  ▪ Tectonically stable globe without risk of infection, ulcers, and vascularization of sutures
o Disadvantages
  ▪ Technically difficult
  ▪ Dislocation of endothelial lenticule
  ▪ Final visual acuity may be limited due to coexisting factors or interface haze

Suggested Readings

Auran JD, Starr MB, Jakobiec FA. Acanthamoeba keratitis: a review of the literature. *Cornea.* 1987;6(1):2–26.
Chang RI, Ching SST. Corneal and conjunctival degenerations. In: Krachmer JH, Mannis MJ, Holland EJ, Eds. *Cornea.* 2nd ed. St. Louis, MO: Elsevier-Mosby; 2005:987–1004.
Conners MS, Brasington RD, Padousis JR, Lubiniewski AJ. Corneal disease in rheumatoid arthritis. In: Krachmer JH, Mannis MJ, Holland EJ, Eds. *Cornea.* 2nd ed. St. Louis, MO: Elsevier-Mosby; 2005:1207–1224.
Groos EB Jr. Neurotrophic keratitis. In: Krachmer JH, Mannis MJ, Holland EJ, Eds. *Cornea.* 2nd ed. St. Louis, MO: Elsevier-Mosby; 2005:1189–1196.
Holland EJ, Brilakis HS, Schwartz GS. Herpetic keratitis. In: Krachmer JH, Mannis MJ, Holland EJ, Eds. *Cornea.* 2nd ed. St. Louis, MO: Elsevier-Mosby; 2005:1043–1074.
Hwang AJW, Wichiensin P, Yang M. Bacterial keratitis. In: Krachmer JH, Mannis MJ, Holland EJ, Eds. *Cornea.* 2nd ed. St. Louis, MO: Elsevier-Mosby; 2005:1005–1033.
Jones DB. Diagnosis and management of fungal keratitis. In: Tasman W, Jaeger EA, Eds. *Duane's Clinical Ophthalmology on CD-ROM.* Philadelphia, PA: Lippincott Williams & Wilkins; 2005.
Kenyon KR, Hersh PS, Starck T, Fogel JA. Corneal dysgenesis, dystrophies and degenerations. In: Tasman W, Jaeger EA. *Duane's Clinical Ophthalmology on CD-ROM.* Philadelphia, PA: Lippincott Williams & Wilkins; 2005.
Rezende RA, Cohen EJ, Uchoa UC, et al. Congenital corneal opacities. In: Krachmer JH, Mannis MJ, Holland EJ, Eds. *Cornea.* 2nd ed. St. Louis, MO: Elsevier-Mosby; 2005:311–338.
Rubinfield RS. Recurrent erosion syndromes. In: Krachmer JH, Mannis MJ, Holland EJ. *Cornea.* 2nd ed. St. Louis, MO: Elsevier-Mosby; 2005:1169–1177.
Terry MA. A new approach for endothelial transplantation: deep lamellar endothelial keratoplasty. *Int Ophthalmol Clin.* 2003;43(3):183–193.

Questions

1. All of the following disease processes present with corneal edema *except*
   a. Fuchs' endothelial dystrophy
   b. Pseudophakic bullous keratopathy
   c. CHED
   d. Congenital hereditary stromal dystrophy (CHSD)

2. Management of transplant rejection includes all of the following *except*
   a. Topical corticosteroids
   b. Cycloplegics
   c. Topical antiglaucoma medications
   d. Topical NSAIDs

3. Treatment of sterile corneal infiltrates should include which of the following as a first-line agent?
    a. Artificial tears
    b. Topical corticosteroids
    c. Broad-spectrum oral antibiotic
    d. Topical fluoroquinolones

4. True or **False**: Macular dystrophy is inherited in an autosomal dominant pattern.

5. Which of the following is NOT a finding associated with keratoconus?
    a. Kayser-Fleischer ring
    b. Apical thinning
    c. Acute hydrops
    d. Vogt's striae

6. What finding is associated with PPMD?
    a. Stromal edema
    b. Corneal guttae
    c. Vesicular lesions at the level of the endothelium
    d. Flecks of amyloid in the deep stroma

7. Immune stromal keratitis should be treated with all of the following *except*
    a. Prednisolone acetate
    b. Acyclovir
    c. Trifluridine 1% (Viroptic)
    d. Prednisolone phosphate

8. A 37-year-old man presents to your office with a 2-day history of decreased vision, worsening pain, and red eye after being poked in the eye with a tree branch while out hiking. Clinical examination reveals a dense stromal infiltrate in the paracentral cornea with an overlying defect, as well as several smaller stromal infiltrates scattered around the main lesion. What is the most likely diagnosis?
    a. Traumatic corneal abrasion
    b. Fungal keratitis
    c. Bacterial keratitis
    d. HSV geographic ulcer

9. A 17-year-old girl presents with a 3-month history of worsening vision and increasing problems with her gas-permeable contact lenses. She adheres to her contact lens cleaning regimen religiously and does not sleep in her lenses. Past medical history includes childhood eczema and seasonal allergies. She takes an oral antihistamine and uses Visine (Johnson & Johnson, New Brunswick, NJ) when her eyes feel itchy. Her condition is most likely a result of
    a. Poor fit of the contact lens associated with keratometric changes
    b. Giant papillary conjunctivitis
    c. Protein deposits on the contact lens
    d. Allergy to contact lens solution

10. A cornea transplant is indicated in all of the following conditions *except*
    a. Corneal edema associated with ruptured epithelial bullae
    b. Persistent epithelial defect
    c. Old corneal scarring from syphilitic interstitial keratitis
    d. Corneal perforation from acanthamoeba keratitis

Refractive Surgery

Louis E. Probst, MD

Outline

Probst LE, Tsai JH.
Ophthalmology: Clinical and Surgical Principles (pp. 263–298).
© 2012 SLACK Incorporated

Introduction

Refractive surgery has evolved at a remarkable rate during the past 20 years. Radial keratotomy (RK) was the first refractive procedure to gain widespread acceptance; however, it was quickly replaced by photorefractive keratectomy (PRK) and laser in situ keratomileusis (LASIK) with the advent of the excimer laser. During the past several years, there has been increased interest in phakic intraocular lenses (IOLs) for the correction of high ametropias and accommodative or diffractive IOLs for the correction of cataracts as well as presbyopia. This rapid progress and evolution of technology is likely to continue in this exciting subspecialty of ophthalmology.

Options for Refractive Surgery

There are a variety of procedures available in the armamentarium of the refractive surgeon with different indications for each procedure. The reader should note that the indications for each refractive procedure are rapidly changing as new technologies become available and replace other procedures. For a given refractive error, the refractive procedure is selected by both the surgeon and the patient based on many factors that include the surgeon's experience, tolerance for risk, and goals of the patient.

Food and Drug Administration Studies: Advantages and Challenges

- Aside from the Prospective Evaluation of Radial Keratotomy (PERK) study of RK, there have been no large-scale multicenter trials to evaluate the different techniques and technologies of refractive surgery.
- Refractive procedures involve the use of new devices and therefore require the submission of detailed studies to the Food and Drug Administration (FDA), which are available on the FDA Web site shortly after approval (www.fda.gov).
- The FDA submission criteria require that the data be submitted in a standardized format so the results of different lasers, procedures, and devices can be compared (Table 7-1).
- There are some limitations of the FDA refractive surgery data.
  - Impressive results in an FDA study do not always correlate to excellent results in general practice.
  - FDA studies are generally sponsored by the company seeking FDA approval and are performed by physicians with close relationships with those companies, so at least some degree of bias could be involved.
- FDA studies have been submitted years apart so it is inappropriate to compare the results from one study submitted years before another that used different and probably inferior technology.

Surface Ablation

Photorefractive Keratectomy

- Definition
  - Excimer laser refractive correction is applied to the surface of the corneal stroma after the epithelium has been removed.
- History
  - It was the first refractive procedure to make use of the excimer laser.
- Indications
  - Preferred over LASIK for patients with thin corneas, slightly irregular topography, or in patients with a future risk of eye trauma that could dislodge a LASIK flap, such as military personnel or professional athletes
  - Spherical myopia treatment is up to -6.0 diopters (D) (extended range up to -10.0 D).
  - Astigmatism treatment is up to 3.0 D (extended range 5.0 D).

TABLE 7-1. FOOD AND DRUG ADMINISTRATION STUDIES OF VARIOUS REFRACTIVE TECHNOLOGIES

FDA Data Device	Approval Range	Approval Number	Approval Date	Number of Eyes	>=20/20	>=20/40	0.5 D	1.0 D	Loss 2 Lines BCVA	Loss > 2 Lines BCVA
Conventional Myopic PRK										
Alcon Apex Plus	1 to 6 D myopia, 1 to 4 D astigmatism	P930034/S9	3/11/1998	151	48.3	84.1	49	73.5	n/a	3.4
Alcon LadarVision	1 to 10 D myopia	P970043	11/2/1998	417	69.7	95.9	77.5	92.6	1	0.5
Alcon LadarVision	1 to 10 D myopia w/ 4 D astigmatism	P970043	11/2/1998	177	59.3	93.2	74.3	92	2.1	0
Bausch and Lomb 116	1.5 to 7 D myopia (results 3 to 4 D spherical)	P970056	9/28/1999	33	42.4	81.8	48.5	87.9	0	3
Bausch and Lomb 116	1.5 to 7 D myopia w/ astigmatism (results 3 to 4 D SE)	P970056	9/28/1999	35	45.7	77.5	48.6	80	0	5.7
LaserSight LSX	1 to 6 D myopia	P980008	11/12/1999	265	55.5	87.5	58.5	81.5	n/a	0
Nidek EC5000	0.75 to 7 D myopia	P970053	12/17/1998	441	65.5	94.8	68.6	90.2	2.2	0.3
Nidek EC5000	7 to 13 D myopia	P970053	12/17/1998	145	45.5	80.7	42.8	68.3	2.5	3
Nidek EC5000	1 to 8 D myopia w/4 D astigmatism	P970053/S1	9/29/1999	631	64.3	93.5	62.3	86.1	1.1	0.5

(continued)

TABLE 7-1. FOOD AND DRUG ADMINISTRATION STUDIES OF VARIOUS REFRACTIVE TECHNOLOGIES (CONTINUED)

FDA Data Device	Approval Range	Approval Number	Approval Date	Number of Eyes	>=20/20	>=20/40	0.5 D	1.0 D	Loss 2 Lines BCVA	Loss > 2 Lines BCVA
VISX Star and Star2	0 to 12 D myopia w/ 4 D astigmatism	P930016/S5	3/27/1996	156	50.7	79.5	45.9	70.9	n/a	7.5
Conventional Hyperopic PRK										
VISX Star and Star2	1 to 6 hyperopia	P930016/S7	11/2/1998	158	53.3	96	74.1	90.5	0	1
VISX Star and Star2	0.5 to 5 hyperopia w/ 4 D astigmatism	P930016/S10	10/18/2000	231	50.2	95.4	69.5	91.2	5.1	1.5
Conventional Hyperopic LASIK										
Alcon LadarVision (9 months)	Less than 6 D hyperopia w/ up to 6 D myopia astigmatism	P970043/S7	9/22/2000	66	57.6	95.2	70.2	91.5	5.8	0
Bausch and Lomb 116	1 to 4 D hyperopia w/ 2 D astigmatism	P990027/S4	2/25/2003	233	61.4	94.8	60	86.6	2.1	0.7
VISX S2 and S3	0.5 to 5 D hyperopia w/ 3 D and astigmatism	P930016/S12	4/27/2001	113	54	99.1	70.7	94.7	3.8	0
Wavelight Allegretto	Hyperopia up to 6 D w/ astigmatism up to 5 D	P30008	10/10/2003	212	67.5	95.3	72.3	90.4	n/a	1.5
Conventional Mixed Astigmatism LASIK										
Alcon LadarVision	Hyperopia <6 D w/myopic astigmatism <6 D	P970043/S7	9/22/2000	37	51.4	93.6	82	96	1.9	0

(continued)

TABLE 7-1. FOOD AND DRUG ADMINISTRATION STUDIES OF VARIOUS REFRACTIVE TECHNOLOGIES (CONTINUED)

FDA Data Device	Approval Range	Approval Number	Approval Date	Number of Eyes	>=20/20	>=20/40	0.5 D	1.0 D	Loss 2 Lines BCVA	Loss > 2 Lines BCVA
VISX S2 and S3	Mixed astigmatism up to 6 D (3-month data)	P930016/S14	11/16/2001	115	58.3	98.3	79.1	97.4	0	0.9
Custom Myopic LASIK										
Alcon LadarVision	Myopia to 7 D w/0.5 D astigmatism	P970043/S10	10/18/2002	139	79.9	91.4	74.8	95.7	0	0
Alcon LadarVision	Myopic astigmatism 0.5 to 4 D	P970043/S15	6/29/2004	225	85.8	97.4	80.2	91.8	0	0
Bausch and Lomb 217Z	Myopia to 7 D w/ 3 D astigmatism	P990027/S6	10/10/2003	117	90.1	99.1	71.3	92.4	0	0.4
VISX S4 Wavescan	Myopia to 6 D w/ 3 D astigmatism	P930016/S17	5/23/2003	277	93.9	99.6	90.3	99.3	0	0
Custom Hyperopic LASIK										
VISX S4 Wavescan	Hyperopia up to 3 D and astigmatism up to 2 D	P930016/S17	12/14/2004	131	61.8	95.4	58	88.5	0	0
Conductive Keratoplasty										
Keratec CK	hHperopia from 0.75 to 3.25 D w/ less than 0.75 D astigmatism (16 spots)	P10018	4/11/2002	205	63	96	70	96	4	1
Keratec CK	Presbyopia (16 spots)	P10018/S5	2/6/2004	81	56 (J1)	90 (J3)	82	97	0	2

(continued)

TABLE 7-1. FOOD AND DRUG ADMINISTRATION STUDIES OF VARIOUS REFRACTIVE TECHNOLOGIES (CONTINUED)

FDA Data Device	Approval Range	Approval Number	Approval Date	Number of Eyes	>=20/20	>=20/40	0.5D	1.0D	Loss 2 Lines BCVA	Loss > 2 Lines BCVA
Intacs										
Keravision Intacs	1 to 3 D myopia w/ less than 0.5 D astigmatism	P980031	1/12/1999	442	69	96	68	91	n/a	n/a
Phakic IOL										
Ophtec Verisyse	5 to 20 D of myopia w/ 2.5 D of astigmatism	P30028	2/5/2004	581	33.2	86.7	72	94.5	n/a	0.344234079
Presbyopia										
AMO Array	Cataract—distance	P960028	9/5/1997	400	39	91.5	n/a	n/a	n/a	n/a
AMO Array	Presbyopia—near	P960028	9/5/1997	400	47.5	87.4	n/a	n/a	n/a	n/a
Alcon ReStor	Cataract—distance	P20040	3/21/2005	110	29.2	92.7	n/a	n/a	n/a	n/a
Alcon ReStor	Presbyopia—near	P20040	3/21/2005	110	30.9 (J1)	94.5(J3)	n/a	n/a	n/a	n/a
Eyeonics Crystalens	Cataract—distance	P30002	5/23/2005	368	49.6	91.4	84.5	85.9	7.9	n/a
Eyeonics Crystalens	Presbyopia—near	P3002	5/23/2005	368	14.1 (J1)	89.1 (J3)	84.5	85.9	7.9	n/a

- Technique
  - o Cold balanced salt solution drops are placed on the eye to cool the cornea.
  - o Epithelium is removed from the cornea using alcohol, a rotating brush, scraping with an instrument, or the laser (transepithelial ablation).
  - o Eye tracker and iris registration (IR) is engaged.
  - o Laser ablation is performed.
  - o Mitomycin C 0.02% is applied to the cornea for 10 to 20 seconds if the ablation depth is greater than 70 μm, as this dramatically reduces the risk of haze.
  - o A contact lens is placed on the eye and is removed in 3 to 4 days after re-epithelialization.
  - o Custom wavefront PRK is rapidly becoming the standard of care because of the superior results.
- Results
  - o While the early results of PRK were less impressive, modern technique using custom wavefront ablation and topical mitomycin C when appropriate yields results similar to those of custom LASIK.
  - o PRK is thought to have less risk of inducing keratectasia because it preserves corneal tissue so it is preferred in patients who have any risk factors for ectasia.

Laser Epithelial Keratomileusis

- Hybrid of PRK and LASIK
- Laser epithelial keratomileusis (LASEK) uses an epithelial flap created by exposing the cornea to alcohol.
- Proponents of LASEK believe it reduces the risk of the intraoperative flap complications of LASIK and preserves posterior corneal stroma reducing the risk of ectasia.
- Critics are concerned about the slow visual recovery and the risks of corneal haze.
- The popularity of LASEK has diminished significantly during the past several years.

Epi-LASIK

- Variation of LASEK
- Epithelial flap is created with a modified microkeratome rather than alcohol.
- Proponents state that the flaps created in this manner heal faster, avoid the flap complication risks of LASIK, and the results are comparable to LASIK.
- Others have had less success with this technique, and it has yet to gain widespread acceptance.

Laser In Situ Keratomileusis

- History
  - o LASIK was developed from the flap creation techniques of automated lamellar keratectomy and the excimer surface ablation of PRK.
  - o LASIK quickly replaced RK and PRK as the dominant refractive procedure and remains the mainstay of the refractive surgery armamentarium due to the excellent results, safety, and convenience of the procedure for the patient.
- Indications
  - o For LASIK, the ideal maximum myopia treatment is now -10.0 D (extended range -12.0 D). Other factors that influence the amount of correction include corneal thickness, flap thickness, and curvature of the cornea.
    - A preoperative corneal thickness of at least 480 μm
    - A residual stromal bed after flap creation and laser correction of at least 250 μm
    - A pupil size that is sufficiently covered by the laser ablation
    - The postoperative corneal curvature should not exceed 50 D.
  - o The limit of the hyperopic corrections have been reduced due to regression and night vision disturbances associated with the smaller postoperative hyperopic optical zones noted with corrections over +3.0 D spherical equivalent.

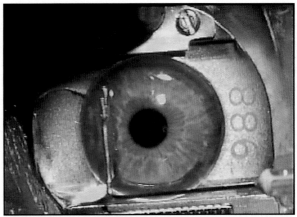

Figure 7-1. LASIK with the Automated Corneal Shaper (ACS) microkeratome. (Reprinted with permission from Probst LE. *LASIK: A Color Atlas and Surgical Synopsis.* Thorofare, NJ: SLACK Incorporated; 2001.)

- Technique
    - o The flap is created with a microkeratome (Figure 7-1) or a femtosecond laser.
    - o The flap is folded back to expose the stromal bed.
    - o The laser ablation is applied to the laser bed.
    - o The flap is replaced.
- Results
    - o The LASIK results have improved dramatically during the past 10 years.
    - o The advent of custom wavefront laser with IR has resulted in more than 90% of eyes achieving 20/20 or better uncorrected visual acuity (UCVA) after the primary procedure (see Table 7-1).

Custom Laser In Situ Keratomileusis and Photorefractive Keratectomy

- Definition
    - o Excimer laser refractive treatment is programmed from a wavefront aberrometry that is used preoperatively to measure the low and higher aberrations of the eye.
    - o Allows the treatment of higher-order aberrations such as spherical aberration, coma, and trefoil as well as spherical and astigmatic refractive errors
- Indications
    - o Greater than 0.4 µm higher-order root mean square (RMS) errors
    - o Greater than 2 D astigmatism
    - o Pupils >6.0 mm
    - o Greater needs for night vision
    - o The results of custom LASIK have been so good that it is now used for virtually all patients.
- Technique
    - o There are several excimer laser systems capable of custom wavefront-driven treatments.
        - ▪ VISX Star S4 CustomVue (Abbott Medical Optics, Santa Ana, Calif.)
        - ▪ Technolas 217Z Zyoptix (Technolas Perfect Vision, Munchen, Germany)
        - ▪ Wavelight Allegretto Wave (Alcon Labs, Fort Worth, Texas)
    - o The aberrometer (Figure 7-2) obtains the wavefront maps (Figure 7-3).
    - o The wavefront map and programming are selected and adjusted.
    - o Laser treatment and the IR data are transferred to the excimer laser by disc or flash drive to guide the laser treatment.
- Results
    - o Greater rate of achieving 20/20 uncorrected vision
    - o Greater rate of achieving better than 20/20 uncorrected vision
    - o Less night vision complaints

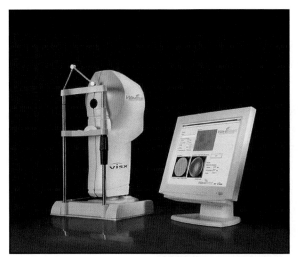

Figure 7-2. VISX WaveScan wavefront system. (Reprinted with permission from Probst LE. *LASIK: A Color Atlas and Surgical Synopsis*. Thorofare, NJ: SLACK Incorporated; 2001.)

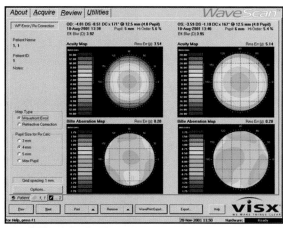

Figure 7-3. VISX WaveScan wavefront capture. (Reprinted with permission from Probst LE. *LASIK: A Color Atlas and Surgical Synopsis*. Thorofare, NJ: SLACK Incorporated; 2001.)

Femtosecond Lasers for Laser In Situ Keratomileusis Flap Creation

- Definition
  - A 1053-wavelength laser is used to produce almost 1 million small microcavitation pulses that create the lamellar stromal flap.
- Indications
  - Produces a more consistently thin flap, so most indicated to preserve posterior stromal tissue with high myopic corrections
  - Patient preference of greater safety profile
- Technique
  - There are several femtosecond lasers available for LASIK flap creation.
    - IntraLase (FS and iFS) (Abbott Medical Optics, Santa Ana, Calif.)
    - Femto LDV (Ziemer Ophthalmic Systems Group, Port, Switzerland)
    - Femtec (20/10 Perfect Vision AG, Heidelberg, Germany)
    - VisuMax (Carl Zeiss Meditec Inc, Dublin, Calif.)
  - Suction ring is placed on the eye and suction engaged.
  - Ring and patient are "docked" under the femtosecond laser.
  - Applanation of the cornea is achieved.
  - The laser treatment is initiated in a raster pattern (Figure 7-4).
  - Early versions required 2 minutes for flap creation while the newer 150-KHz laser creates a flap in approximately 10 seconds.
  - Flap size, depth, and hinge location are completely programmable.
  - Once flap is complete, suction is disengaged.
  - Flap is lifted, and excimer treatment is applied as in microkeratome LASIK.
- Results
  - Slight reduction of induced aberrations, astigmatism, and enhancement rates compared to microkeratome
  - Real advantage is the enhanced safety profile.
  - Vision-threatening flap complications are exceeding rare.

Presbyopic Multifocal Laser In Situ Keratomileusis

- Definition
  - Optical multifocality is produced by laser vision correction for the correction of presbyopia.
- Indications
  - Presbyopia
  - In the future, multifocal ablation could be targeted for the specific needs of the patient.

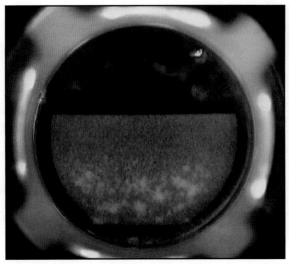

Figure 7-4. The raster pattern of the IntraLase femtosecond laser creating the lamellar flap.

- Technique
  - The LASIK procedure is performed in the standard method with a modified ablation pattern.
  - One area of the cornea is corrected for distance and the other for near.
  - The multifocal ablation profile creates a central area steepened to provide a myopic region for near vision and a peripheral optical zone targeted for emmetropia.
- Results
  - In a study of 12 eyes of 6 patients with a mean preoperative hyperopia of +2.24 D, 90% of eyes achieved an uncorrected vision of 20/40 at distance and near with no eye losing more than one line of best corrected visual acuity (BCVA).
- Complication
  - Moderate night vision disturbances were related by 20% of patients after presbyopic correction

Other Corneal Refractive Procedures

Conductive Keratoplasty

- Approved by the FDA for the treatment of hyperopia and presbyopia
- The thermal corneal burns are applied with a radiofrequency probe down to about 90% of the corneal depth (500 µm).
- The deeper corneal penetration did not prevent the regression associated with all thermal keratoplasty procedures.
- Conductive keratoplasty (CK) is no longer performed by the majority of refractive surgeons; however, it is occasionally used to create "blended vision" in one eye for the correction of presbyopia or for the treatment of iatrogenic hyperopia.

Intracorneal Rings or Intacs

- While the initial intracorneal rings (ICR) FDA studies were promising, the procedure never gained widespread acceptance due to the inability to treat astigmatism, difficulty duplicating the initial FDA results, competition from LASIK, and the high explantation rate.
- Recently, Intacs has been successfully used to treat post-LASIK ectasia or keratoconus.

Radial Keratotomy

- Diamond knife was used to create radial incisions in the cornea.
- It is no longer performed, as other refractive procedures offer a more predictable and stable outcome.

TABLE 7-2. COMPLICATIONS OF LASIK AND PRK

	LASIK	PRK
INTRAOPERATIVE COMPLICATION		
Buttonhole flap (microkeratome)	X	
Thin flap (microkeratome)	X	
Free cap (microkeratome)	X	
Corneal perforation (microkeratome)	X	
Laser complications	X	X
Epithelial defects	X	
Opaque bubble layer (femtosecond laser)	X	
EARLY POSTOPERATIVE COMPLICATION		
Flap striae	X	
Dislodged flap	X	
Infection	X	X
Diffuse lamellar keratitis	X	
Delayed epithelial healing	X	X
LATE POSTOPERATIVE COMPLICATION		
Keratectasia	X	
De-centration	X	X
Night vision disturbances	X	X
Irregular astigmatism	X	X
Central islands	X	X
Dry eyes	X	X
Haze		X
Vitreoretinal complications	X	
Transient light sensitivity (femtosecond laser)	X	

Laser Thermal Keratoplasty

- Peripheral thermal burns were applied to the peripheral cornea for the correction of small degrees of hyperopia.
- It is no longer performed for low hyperopia due to high regression rates.

Complications of Laser In Situ Keratomileusis and Surface Ablation

While some complications, such as those associated with the corneal flap, can only occur after LASIK, other complications, such as infection or de-centered ablations, can occur in either procedure (Table 7-2).

Intraoperative Laser In Situ Keratomileusis Complications

- Intraoperative LASIK complications are often preventable with the appropriate safeguards of the surgical system.

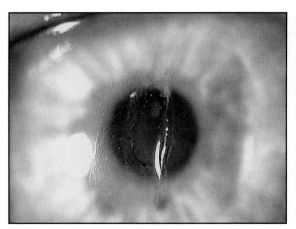

Figure 7-5. Buttonhole half-flap. (Reprinted with permission from Probst LE. *LASIK: A Color Atlas and Surgical Synopsis.* Thorofare, NJ: SLACK Incorporated; 2001.)

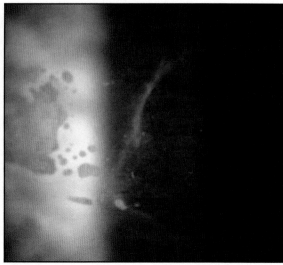

Figure 7-6. Haze around the edge of a buttonhole flap 3 months postoperatively.

- A recent retrospective study evaluated the intraoperative flap complications in 84,771 cases of LASIK with the ACS or the Hansatome. The rate of all flap complications was 0.302%, failures to achieve intraocular pressure in 0.034%, partial flaps in 0.099%, buttonholes in 0.07%, thin or irregular flaps in 0.087%, free flaps in 0.012% of eyes.

Buttonhole and Irregular Flaps

- Etiology
  - Buttonhole flaps occur when the keratectomy has been performed without adequate suction.
- Signs/symptoms
  - The buttonhole flap is evident immediately after the microkeratome has completed the reverse pass.
  - The central aspect of the cornea will appear irregular with a 2- to 3-mm diameter irregular circle in the center representing the buttonhole (Figure 7-5).
  - If the flap is lifted, it will be thin and difficult to manipulate.
  - After 1 month, haze will form around the edges of the buttonhole (Figure 7-6).
- Treatment
  - Performing the laser ablation will result in an irregular astigmatism with central corneal haze.
  - If the buttonhole is identified immediately, the flap should not be lifted.
  - If the flap has been lifted, the flap should be replaced, and then re-floated into position. This can be difficult as the flap is thin and very unstable.
  - The eye is allowed to heal for at least 3 months. LASIK can be performed again using a deeper plate, or PRK can be performed with mitomycin C.
  - Topical steroids are tapered during the healing phase to reduce the risk of haze formation.
- Prevention
  - The keratectomy should never be performed without excellent suction and a perfect blade.

Thin Flaps

- Etiology
  - There is a standard deviation in the average flap thickness of about 25 µm; therefore, the flap thickness can vary considerably, often between 100 and 200 µm.
- Signs/symptoms
  - Flap and the stromal bed may be irregular.
  - Striae are also more prominent with thin LASIK flaps.
  - Once a very thin flap has healed, a hazy area with irregular striae will form in the center of the cornea (Figure 7-7).

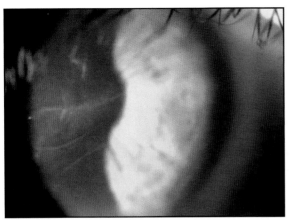

Figure 7-7. Central corneal haze and striae due to a thin flap. (Reprinted with permission from Probst LE. *LASIK: A Color Atlas and Surgical Synopsis*. Thorofare, NJ: SLACK Incorporated; 2001.)

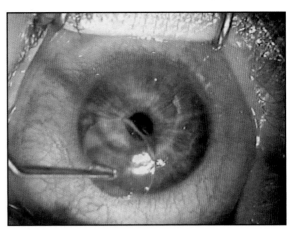

Figure 7-8. Free flap after LASIK using the ACS microkeratome on a cornea with flat K values of 39.0 D at 180 degrees. (Reprinted with permission from Probst LE. *LASIK: A Color Atlas and Surgical Synopsis*. Thorofare, NJ: SLACK Incorporated; 2001.)

- Treatment
  - If the stromal bed is smooth and the flap itself is smooth, LASIK can still be performed with an excellent outcome.
  - If the stromal bed is not smooth or there are perforations or buttonholes of the flap, then performing the laser ablation will result in irregular astigmatism with central corneal haze.
- Prevention
  - The keratectomy should never be performed without excellent suction and a perfect blade.

Free Cap

- Etiology
  - A free cap occurs when the microkeratome does not stop to create a hinge but rather continues across the cornea severing the flap from the bed.
  - Free caps usually occur for 2 reasons:
    - In eyes with very flat preoperative keratometry values, a free cap can occur when using some older microkeratomes.
    - A free cap can also occur if there is a very thin flap due to inadequate pressure.
- Signs/symptoms
  - Free caps are circular and are completely separated from the stromal bed (Figure 7-8).
- Treatment
  - If the stromal bed is irregular, the flap should be replaced and allowed to heal without performing the excimer laser ablation.
  - If the free cap occurred because of low preoperative keratometry readings, the stromal bed may be smooth, and the free cap of normal thickness. In this case, the ablation can be continued with an excellent outcome.
- Prevention
  - In eyes with keratometry readings less than 42 D, it is advisable to use the Hansatome or a larger microkeratome head (9.5) on the Nidek Mk-2000.
  - IntraLase (Abbott Medical Optics, Santa Ana, Calif.) flaps are less dependent on corneal curvature and, therefore, are not associated with free caps.

Corneal Perforation

- Etiology
  - Perforation of the cornea during the keratectomy is the most feared and rare complication of LASIK.
  - Fortunately, it is rare with modern microkeratomes and impossible with the femtosecond laser.

- Signs/symptoms
  - o This complication is obvious during the advancement of the microkeratome as there is a sudden release of a jet of fluid as the cornea is penetrated, followed by a loss of suction with beeping from the suction pump.
  - o Severe ocular damage can result.
- Treatment
  - o The suction should be disengaged immediately.
  - o Removal of the microkeratome reveals the penetration, which could be associated with extruded iris and/or lens material.
  - o Corneal perforation is managed by preserving as much intraocular tissue as possible, suturing the corneal incision to restore the anterior chamber, and immediate referral for further evaluation/surgery that may be required.
  - o An emergency surgical kit that includes a needle driver and sutures should be available in every laser center.
- Prevention
  - o Careful microkeratome assembly is critical for successful LASIK.
  - o Femtosecond lasers for flap creation offer a greater safety profile for flap creation as they have not been associated with corneal perforation.

Laser-Related Complications With Laser In Situ Keratomileusis and Photorefractive Keratectomy

- Etiology
  - o The most avoidable complication is incorrect laser programming.
  - o On rare occasions, the excimer laser will experience a mechanical failure during the procedure.
- Signs/symptoms
  - o There is little to warn of incorrect laser programming during the procedure.
  - o The result will become obvious postoperatively when the patient does not achieve good uncorrected vision.
  - o If there was a transposition error or an astigmatism axis error, the resultant astigmatism may be magnified in a new axis.
- Treatment
  - o Errors in laser programming can be corrected by an enhancement procedure; however, the best strategy is prevention with multiple checks.
  - o If laser failure occurs, the flap should be replaced, and the procedure can be completed later.
- Prevention
  - o It is essential to check and double-check all programming prior to performing LASIK.
  - o IR minimizes programming errors by verifying the patient identity and eye prior to treatment as well as programming the appropriate correction automatically.

Epithelial Defects

- Etiology
  - o Loose epithelium
  - o Excessive use of topical anesthesia
  - o Excessive microkeratome trauma to the epithelium
- Signs/symptoms
  - o Noted immediately after the keratectomy as irregular areas along the epithelial surface of the cornea
  - o The displaced epithelium is usually edematous and gray in appearance (Figure 7-9).
  - o Can be less than 1 mm or as large as the entire corneal flap.
  - o The flap is usually intact and healthy beneath the defect).
  - o Results in a number of highly undesirable complications including prolonged visual recovery, postoperative pain, diffuse lamellar keratitis (DLK), and epithelial ingrowth
- Treatment
  - o If an epithelial defect occurs during the treatment of the first eye, the surgeon should continue with the laser treatment, replace the LASIK flap, and place a bandage contact lens over the eye if the defect is greater than 3 mm in size.

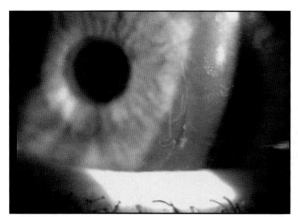

Figure 7-9. Mild peripheral epithelial defect after LASIK. (Reprinted with permission from Probst LE. *LASIK: A Color Atlas and Surgical Synopsis*. Thorofare, NJ: SLACK Incorporated; 2001.)

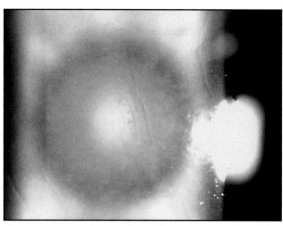

Figure 7-10. Vertical striae due to flap movement after LASIK. (Reprinted with permission from Probst LE. *LASIK: A Color Atlas and Surgical Synopsis*. Thorofare, NJ: SLACK Incorporated; 2001.)

- ○ If the defect is extremely large, it may be elected not to proceed with the treatment of the second eye until the first eye has healed.
- ○ The patient should be followed up for healing of the defect.
- • Prevention
  - ○ Minimal use of topical anesthesia
  - ○ Gentle surgical technique
  - ○ IntraLase has no moving parts on the epithelium during the creation of the flap so it is associated with a lower incidence of epithelial defects.

Early Postoperative Complications

Flap Striae

- • Etiology
  - ○ Misalignment of the corneal flap after flap replacement
  - ○ Movement of the corneal flap during the first postoperative day
  - ○ "Tenting effect" of the corneal flap over the ablated stromal bed
- • Signs/symptoms
  - ○ Striae are oriented horizontally with a nasal hinge and vertically with the superior hinge (Figure 7-10.)
  - ○ Symptoms are related to the severity of the striae (Table 7-3).
  - ○ Displaced flaps will often have oblique striae.
  - ○ Retroillumination of the fixation light and aiming beam through the dilated pupil provides accurate localization of the flap striae and will help identify striae in cases of unexplained reduction of BCVA.
- • Treatment
  - ○ The indications for the treatment of striae include striae that meet the following criteria:
    - ▪ Extend through the visual axis
    - ▪ Cause a decrease in BCVA or diplopia
    - ▪ Induce regular or irregular astigmatism
  - ○ Techniques to remove striae
    - ▪ The stretch and smooth technique (Figures 7-11 and 7-12)
    - ▪ Flap hydration with hypotonic saline
    - ▪ Epithelial débridement
    - ▪ Flap applanation
    - ▪ Phototherapeutic keratectomy
    - ▪ Flap suturing

TABLE 7-3. PROBST CLASSIFICATION OF FLAP STRIAE

GRADE 1 No treatment required	• Fine parallel lines in flap • Difficult to identify • Not in visual axis • No reduction in UCVA or BCVA
GRADE 2 Treatment may be required due to the reduction in the BCVA or the induced astigmatism	• Fine parallel lines in flap • Identification obvious • Extent through visual axis • BCVA reduced to 20/25 to 20/40 • Less than 1 D of induced astigmatism • Patient may complain of diplopia
GRADE 3 Treatment required to restore best-corrected vision and reduce astigmatism, diplopia, and glare	• Large parallel or "basket weave" pattern • Identification obvious • Extend through visual axis • BCVA worse than 20/40 • One or more diopters of induced astigmatism • Patient may complain of blur, diplopia, and glare

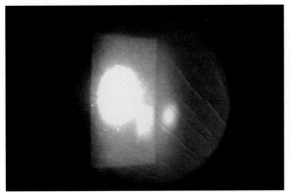

Figure 7-11. Retroilluminated oblique striae. (Reprinted with permission from Probst LE. *LASIK: A Color Atlas and Surgical Synopsis.* Thorofare, NJ: SLACK Incorporated; 2001.)

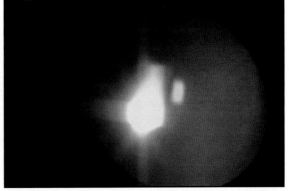

Figure 7-12. Oblique striae from Figure 7-12 are eliminated 24 hours after the "stretch and smooth" technique is used. (Reprinted with permission from Probst LE. *LASIK: A Color Atlas and Surgical Synopsis.* Thorofare, NJ: SLACK Incorporated; 2001.)

- Prevention
  - Intraoperative attention to the repositioning of the flap with minimal manipulation once it has been replaced into the correct position
  - Postoperatively, patients are instructed to avoid rubbing or squeezing the eye.
  - Patients wear eye protection 24 hours a day for the first week to prevent any eye trauma while the flaps are healing.

Dislodged Flap

- Etiology
  - Eye rubbing or squeezing immediately after LASIK (Figure 7-13)
- Signs/symptoms
  - Vision is extremely blurred (<20/200)
  - Severe pain/foreign-body sensation
  - Epithelium can be seen growing over the area of exposed stromal bed.
  - The flap will have obvious striae and folds; however, they may be disguised by the flap edema.
- Treatment
  - Patients with dislodged flaps should be treated as urgently as possible.
  - Flap is unrolled and smoothed out.
  - The stromal side of the flap and the stromal bed must be thoroughly cleaned of all debris, mucus, and epithelium.
  - A bandage contact should be placed on the eye to safeguard a repeat dislodgement of the flap
- Prevention
  - For the first postoperative day, patients are advised to go home and sleep for 4 hours.
  - For the first postoperative week, patients should be warned not to touch or rub their eyes.
  - Patients should be sent home wearing sunglasses and clear eye shields to wear at night.

Infection With Laser In Situ Keratomileusis and Photorefractive Keratectomy

- Etiology
  - The causative organisms vary from gram-positive bacteria to atypical mycobacteria, fungal, and viral pathogens.
  - The infection is usually acquired intraoperatively, but may also be caused by postoperative contamination.
  - While infections are generally unilateral, a bilateral infection after bilateral LASIK has now been reported.
  - Recently, methicillin resistant *staphylococcus aureus* (MRSA) has been identified as the most common cause of postoperative LASIK and PRK infections.
- Signs/symptoms
  - Infections rarely occur after LASIK; however, a recent review of the world literature found that 41 cases have been reported to date.
  - The majority of the bacterial keratitis patients present within 72 hours of the surgery with an acute onset of symptoms.
  - Bacterial infection should be suspected whenever a localized infiltrate is identified either on the surface of the flap or at the flap interface.
  - The infective infiltrate is generally single and localized, about 1 to 2 mm in size, white/gray in color with hazy and indistinct margins. If located on the surface of the cornea, it may be slightly elevated and associated with an epithelial defect.
  - If allowed to progress without treatment, it will slowly increase in size like an early corneal ulcer. Inflammation of the cornea with surrounding interface keratitis, conjunctival injection, and an anterior chamber reaction may all occur if the infection persists.
  - Reactivation of herpes simplex and zoster viral infections has also been reported after LASIK, which present with corneal dendrites in the postoperative period.
  - Fungal infections after LASIK have a delayed onset and have been related to topical prolonged steroid use after LASIK (Figure 7-14).
- Treatment
  - Any suspected corneal infection should be treated immediately.
  - Corneal culture should be obtained.
  - For suspected bacterial infections, hourly topical fluoroquinolones are the obvious first course of treatment followed by specific therapy once the sensitivity data are reported.
  - Topical steroids should be discontinued or reduced.
  - Patients should be followed daily.
- Prevention
  - Prevention of epithelial defects
  - Disposable instruments such as microkeratomes or cannulas ensure the sterility of that step of the procedure.

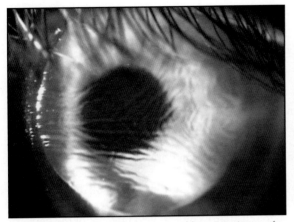

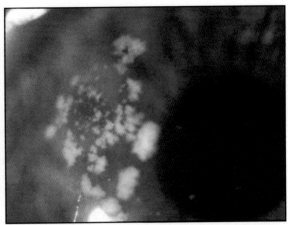

Figure 7-13. Dislodged flap from eye rubbing 20 minutes after LASIK. This flap was refloated without any complications. (Reprinted with permission from Probst LE. *LASIK: A Color Atlas and Surgical Synopsis*. Thorofare, NJ: SLACK Incorporated; 2001.)

Figure 7-14. A case of *Candida albicans* post-LASIK keratitis with a more multifocal appearance and several smaller sized infiltrates with feathery edges. (Reprinted with permission from Probst LE. *LASIK: Advances, Controversies, and Custom*. Thorofare, NJ: SLACK Incorporated; 2004.)

- o IntraLase minimizes the use of reusable instruments.
- o If a patient had a past history of herpes simplex or zoster infection, a prophylactic course of oral antivirals is recommended 1 week prior and 1 week after the LASIK procedure. Doses of acyclovir from 200 to 800 mg 5 times per day have been recommended by various LASIK experts.

Diffuse Lamellar Keratitis (Sands of Sahara)

- Etiology
    - o Probably multiple sources
        - ▪ Bacterial cell wall endotoxins that build up in the wet autoclave reservoirs
        - ▪ Epithelial defects
        - ▪ Ocular trauma
- Signs/symptoms (Figures 7-15 to 7-22)
    - o Begins in the periphery and is confined to the flap interface without extension into the surrounding stroma as white "sand" in the interface.
    - o May present with multiple foci, which are diffusely distributed.
    - o Untreated, this may lead to central inflammation affecting visual acuity secondary to induced hyperopia or irregular astigmatism.
    - o There is no anterior chamber reaction in DLK except in the most advanced cases.
- Treatment
    - o Early identification and intervention are the key steps for successful management of DLK (Table 7-4).
    - o If grades 1 or 2 DLK are identified, the patient should immediately start on a topical steroid every 1 to 2 hours and an antibiotic 4 times daily for prophylaxis against infection.
    - o If grade 3 DLK is identified or grade 2 DLK has not resolved after several days of treatment, the flap should be lifted, and the interface irrigated.
    - o All of these measures aim to prevent the progression to grade 4 DLK with central accumulation of cells, central corneal haze and striae, decreased BCVA, and a hyperopic shift.
        - ▪ Grade 4 DLK also requires urgent flap irrigation along with flap stretching and frequent topical steroids after. While PTK has been suggested as another treatment for DLK, this can cause iatrogenic hyperopia.
    - o Prevention
        - ▪ Minimize epithelial defects
        - ▪ Bacterial endotoxins reduced by cleaning autoclave reservoirs and instruments
        - ▪ Disposable instruments

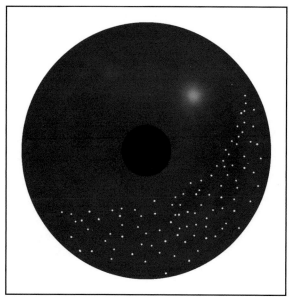

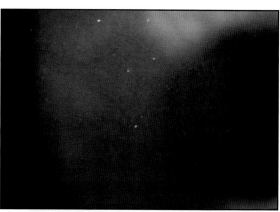

Figure 7-16. Mild sectoral grade 1 DLK. The gray-white interface haze can be seen extending into the superior left region of the pupil. (Reprinted with permission from Probst LE. *LASIK: A Color Atlas and Surgical Synopsis.* Thorofare, NJ: SLACK Incorporated; 2001.)

Figure 7-15. Grade 1 DLK. (Reprinted with permission from Probst LE. *LASIK: A Color Atlas and Surgical Synopsis.* Thorofare, NJ: SLACK Incorporated; 2001.)

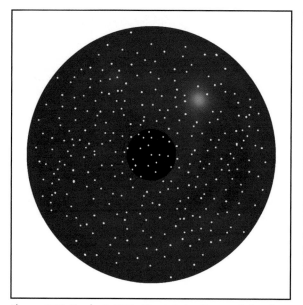

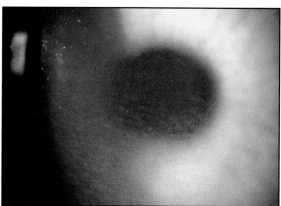

Figure 7-18. Diffuse clumps of inflammatory cells can be seen extending into the papillary region. This patient had myopic LASIK 48 hours previously. (Reprinted with permission from Probst LE. *LASIK: A Color Atlas and Surgical Synopsis.* Thorofare, NJ: SLACK Incorporated; 2001.)

Figure 7-17. Grade 2 DLK. (Reprinted with permission from Probst LE. *LASIK: A Color Atlas and Surgical Synopsis.* Thorofare, NJ: SLACK Incorporated; 2001.)

Late Postoperative Laser In Situ Keratomileusis and Photorefractive Keratectomy Complications

Epithelial Ingrowth

- Etiology
  - Anterior basement membrane dystrophy
  - History of recurrent erosions
  - Postoperative epithelial defects
  - LASIK enhancements

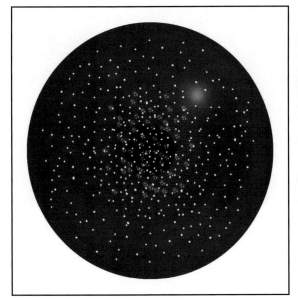

Figure 7-19. Grade 3 DLK. (Reprinted with permission from Probst LE. *LASIK: A Color Atlas and Surgical Synopsis*. Thorofare, NJ: SLACK Incorporated; 2001.)

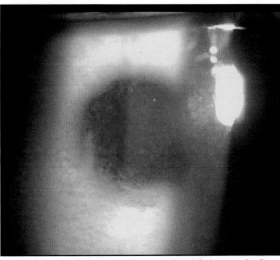

Figure 7-20. Grade 3 LIK. Diffuse, condensed clumps of inflammatory cells in the flap interface. The BCVA was reduced to 20/50. (Reprinted with permission from Probst LE. *LASIK: A Color Atlas and Surgical Synopsis*. Thorofare, NJ: SLACK Incorporated; 2001.)

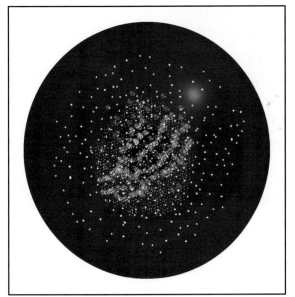

Figure 7-21. Grade 4 DLK. (Reprinted with permission from Probst LE. *LASIK: A Color Atlas and Surgical Synopsis*. Thorofare, NJ: SLACK Incorporated; 2001.)

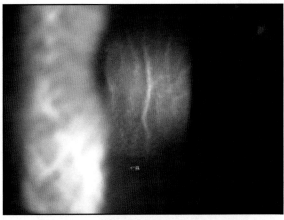

Figure 7-22. Stage 4 DLK. Note the central striae and interface haze. (Reprinted with permission from Probst LE. *LASIK: A Color Atlas and Surgical Synopsis*. Thorofare, NJ: SLACK Incorporated; 2001.)

- Signs/symptoms
  - The patient is usually asymptomatic, and the ingrowth is identified on a scheduled postoperative visit as a faint gray line extending less than 2 mm in from the flap edge.
  - Epithelial ingrowth can be associated with a mild foreign-body sensation that generally indicates an epithelial irregularity along the flap edge associated with the ingrowth.
  - The visual acuity will be unaffected except in the most severe cases when progression occurs into the visual axis.

TABLE 7-4. GRADING OF DIFFUSE LAMELLAR KERATITIS

GRADE 1 DLK

Signs/symptoms	• Focal, white to gray, granular material in the LASIK flap interface 1 to 7 days after LASIK • No other ocular inflammation/anterior chamber reaction • Normal visual acuity
Treatment	• Intensive topical steroids every hour with follow up every 2 to 3 days to ensure complete resolution
Prognosis	• Excellent after topical steroids and 1 week for stabilization

GRADE 2 DLK

Signs/symptoms	• Diffuse, white to gray, granular material under the LASIK flap interface 1 to 7 days after LASIK • No other ocular inflammation/anterior chamber reaction • Normal visual acuity
Treatment	• Interface irrigation has an immediate curative effect • Intensive hourly topical steroids after irrigation • Follow up daily to ensure resolution
Prognosis	• Excellent after interface irrigation, topical steroids and 1 to 2 weeks of stabilization

GRADE 3 DLK

Signs/symptoms	• Diffuse, confluent, white to gray, granular material under the LASIK flap interface 1 to 7 days after LASIK • Slight conjunctival injection • No anterior chamber reaction • Reduced visual acuity
Treatment	• Interface irrigation has an immediate curative effect • Intensive hourly topical steroids after irrigation • Follow up daily to ensure resolution • Repeat irrigation in 1 to 2 days if the inflammation does not resolve • Topical steroid and antibiotics can been placed on the stromal bed to directly address the area of inflammation
Prognosis	• Excellent after interface irrigation, topical steroids, and several weeks of stabilization

(continued)

TABLE 7-4. GRADING OF DIFFUSE LAMELLAR KERATITIS (CONTINUED)

	GRADE 4 DLK
Signs/symptoms	• Diffuse, confluent, white to gray, granular material under the LASIK flap interface 1 to 7 days after LASIK • Inflammation localized to a 2- to 4-mm area of intense central inflammation • Central interface striae in area of inflammation • Slight conjunctival injection • No anterior chamber reaction • Markedly reduced visual acuity
Treatment	• Interface irrigation has an immediate effect • Wipe the stromal bed with Murocel sponges • Topical steroid and antibiotics can be placed on the stromal bed to directly address the area of inflammation • Intensive hourly topical steroids after irrigation • Follow up daily to ensure resolution • Repeat irrigation in 1 to 2 days if the inflammation does not resolve
Prognosis	• Reduced BCVA and irregular astigmatism with residual hyperopia will persist after the resolution of the inflammation due to the residual interface haze and stromal thinning • Persistent interface striae may also reduce the final BCVA

- o Ingrowth is white to gray in color and can be seen to be located beneath the corneal flap with tangential slit-beam illumination.
- o Epithelial ingrowth following LASIK can occur in a number of different patterns, which can be divided into a classification system of grades that assist with identification and treatment (Table 7-5, Figures 7-23 to 7-26).
- Treatment
  - o Indications for treatment of epithelial ingrowth following LASIK include the following:
    - Greater than 2 mm of ingrowth from the flap edge
    - Documented progression, associated flap melting
    - A disturbance of best-corrected vision, which can be attributed to the ingrowth
- Prevention
  - o In cases at risk for epithelial ingrowth, LASIK with IntraLase or PRK should be considered

Undercorrection and Regression

- Etiology
  - o Excessive stromal healing
  - o Epithelial hypertrophy
- Signs/symptoms
  - o The enhancement rate for myopic LASIK can be generally estimated as 1% per diopter of spherical myopic correction and approximately 10% per diopter of astigmatic or hyperopic correction.
  - o Regression of the refractive effect usually occurs several months after LASIK.
  - o Patients may also complain of night glare caused by the residual refractive error.

TABLE 7-5. PROBST/MACHAT EPITHELIAL INGROWTH CLASSIFICATION

GRADE *1* No treatment required	Thin ingrowth, 1 to 2 cells thick, limited to within 2 mm of flap edge, transparent, difficult to detect, well-delineated white line along advancing edge, no associated flap changes, nonprogressive (Figure 7-24)
GRADE *2* Requires nonurgent treatment within 2 to 3 weeks	Thicker ingrowth, discreet cells evident within nest, at least 2 mm from flap edge, individual cells translucent, easily seen on slit lamp, no demarcation line along nest, corneal flap edge rolled or gray, no flap edge melting or erosion, usually progressive (Figure 7-25)
GRADE *3* Urgent treatment required with close follow up, as recurrences are more common due to the altered flap edges	Pronounced ingrowth, several cells thick, greater than 2 mm from flap edge, ingrowth areas opaque, obvious on slit lamp, white geographic areas of necrotic epithelial cells with no demarcation line, corneal flap margins rolled with thickened whitish-gray appearance. Progression results in large areas of flap melting from collagenase release from the necrotic epithelium. Confluent haze develops peripheral to the flap edge as flap pulls away, leaving exposed stromal bed in contact with surface epithelium (Figure 7-26).
GRADE *4*	Melting of the flap edge after prolonged course of epithelial ingrowth (Figure 7-27)

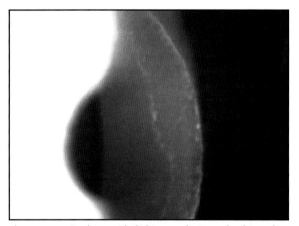

Figure 7-23. Grade 1 epithelial ingrowth. Note the faint white line approximately 1.5 mm central to the LASIK flap edge, which indicates the advancing border of the ingrowth. (Reprinted with permission from Probst LE. *LASIK: A Color Atlas and Surgical Synopsis*. Thorofare, NJ: SLACK Incorporated; 2001.)

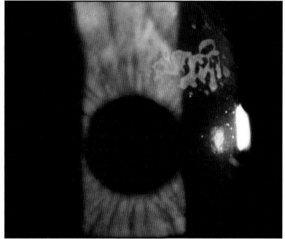

Figure 7-24. Grade 2 epithelial ingrowth. Nests of epithelial cells within 2 mm from the flap edge noted 6 weeks after LASIK. (Reprinted with permission from Probst LE. *LASIK: A Color Atlas and Surgical Synopsis*. Thorofare, NJ: SLACK Incorporated; 2001.)

- Treatment
  - Temporary glasses or fit with disposable contact lens
  - Enhancement once refractive stability is achieved (3 to 12 months)
  - Lifting the original flap for LASIK enhancements has been associated with a high risk of epithelial ingrowth (10% to 20%) when done more than 2 years after the original procedure, so PRK with topical mitomycin is the preferred enhancement technique after this time.

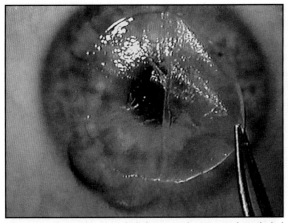

Figure 7-25. Grade 3 epithelial ingrowth. Nests of epithelial cells extend into the visual axis, as shown by retroillumination. (Reprinted with permission from Probst LE. *LASIK: A Color Atlas and Surgical Synopsis*. Thorofare, NJ: SLACK Incorporated; 2001.)

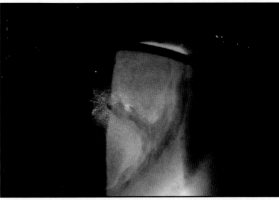

Figure 7-26. Grade 4 epithelial ingrowth with a severe edge melt at the 4 o'clock position of the left eye flap 4 months after LASIK. (Reprinted with permission from Probst LE. *LASIK: A Color Atlas and Surgical Synopsis*. Thorofare, NJ: SLACK Incorporated; 2001.)

Postoperative Keratectasia Following Laser In Situ Keratomileusis

- Etiology
  - o Inadequate posterior stromal thickness
  - o Large myopic corrections and thin preoperative corneas
  - o Preoperative corneal topographic asymmetrical, skewed astigmatism, forme fruste keratoconus, or pellucid marginal degeneration
- Signs/symptoms
  - o Corneal ectasia following LASIK has been recognized as an uncommon complication of LASIK.
  - o Corneal ectasia usually presents from 1 to 12 months after the original LASIK procedure.
  - o Ectasia is usually associated with regression of the refractive effect, loss of uncorrected vision and best corrected vision, and irregular astigmatism.
  - o Topography demonstrates irregular astigmatism often with inferior steepening of the cornea (Figure 7-27).
  - o The Orbscan will demonstrate posterior corneal ectasia on the posterior float map.
- Treatment
  - o Any signs of corneal ectasia on the anterior corneal or posterior cornea should preclude any further LASIK as this could exacerbate the ectasia.
  - o Patients are best treated with hard contact lenses if these can be fit comfortably.
  - o Intacs and CK have been used to help smooth the cornea.
  - o Ultraviolet light and riboflavin (collagen cross-linking) has been used to increase the strength of the cornea in ectasia.
  - o Unfortunately, some of these patients must go on to corneal transplantation in order to restore functional vision.
- Prevention
  - o Patients with keratoconus or other corneal thinning disorders identified on topography should not have LASIK, as LASIK will hasten the onset of keratectasia.
  - o At least 250 µm of posterior stroma should be preserved following LASIK in order to ensure that the risk of long-term corneal ectasia is minimized.

Night Vision Disturbances: Halos and Glare

- Etiology
  - o Large pupils
  - o Small ablation zones
  - o Optical aberrations
  - o Residual refractive errors

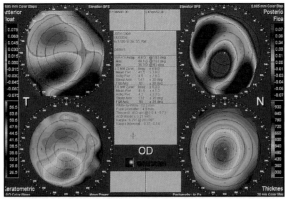

Figure 7-27. Posterior corneal ectasia with irregular astigmatism after LASIK, as demonstrated on Orbscan. The upper right posterior float map demonstrates the increased posterior corneal curvature. The lower left keratometric map appears to indicate the inferior corneal steepening pattern of forme fruste keratoconus. (Reprinted with permission from Probst LE. *LASIK: A Color Atlas and Surgical Synopsis*. Thorofare, NJ: SLACK Incorporated; 2001.)

- Signs/symptoms
  - A study of 236 eyes treated using the Bausch and Lomb 217C laser for mild to moderate myopia found that while mild to moderate glare was reported by 10% more patients at the 6-month follow up, there was no significant increase in marked or severe glare or halos.
  - Halos are the concentric blur circles that surround a point source of light, such as a car headlight, when viewed at night. Halos occur when the optical zone size of the laser treatment is smaller than the mesopic pupil size.
  - Glare is the distortion radiating from light sources at night. Glare occurs because of the optical aberrations of the optical system that are magnified when the pupil dilates at night.
- Treatment
  - Treatment of dry eyes and any residual refractive error or monovision often improve the symptoms.
  - Night driving glasses
  - Turning on the car dome light when driving
  - Alphagan decreases the size of the dilated pupil and is effective in about 75% of eyes.
  - Custom/wavefront LASIK enhancement is particularly effective if there is residual myopia.
- Prevention
  - Pupillometry should be performed in all LASIK patients preoperatively to identify those with pupils larger than 6 mm in dim light. While the risks for night glare are multifactorial, the current most accepted treatment is to adjust the blend zone of the treatment correction to cover the measured pupil size.
  - Custom LASIK has been shown to provide better night vision with fewer night vision disturbances.

Central Islands

- Etiology
  - Large myopic corrections with broad-beam lasers
- Signs/symptoms
  - A central island has been defined as an area of higher refractive power of more than 1.5 D and 2.5 mm or more in diameter or 3 D and 1.5 mm in diameter.
  - Postoperative monocular diplopia, visual distortions, and myopia are the main symptoms associated with central islands.
  - Patients with central islands are difficult to refract and have a disproportionately high degree of residual myopia relative to their UCVA.

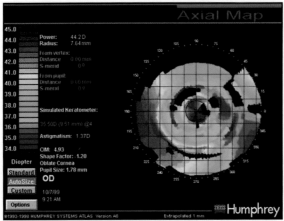

Figure 7-28. Central island noted 1 week following LASIK. (Reprinted with permission from Probst LE. *LASIK: A Color Atlas and Surgical Synopsis*. Thorofare, NJ: SLACK Incorporated; 2001.)

- o A central island cannot be identified on slit-lamp examination, only by topography (Figure 7-28).
- o Unlike central islands observed with PRK, the topographical abnormalities observed with LASIK do not resolve over time.
- o Topographically, a central island appears as a central steepening appearing as red or a lighter shade of blue-green, 2 to 3 mm in diameter, relative to the surrounding area, which is notably a darker green or more typically blue.
- Treatment
  - o Custom wavefront LASIK offers the best option for the treatment of central islands although the results are variable.
- Prevention
  - o Custom LASIK and scanning excimer lasers have effectively eliminated the risk of central islands.

De-Centration

- Etiology
  - o Poor patient fixation
  - o Large angle kappa
  - o Treatment with dilated pupil
- Signs/symptoms
  - o The incidence of de-centrations of 0.5 mm or more has been found to occur in 20.8% of eyes after PRK.
  - o The patient may be noted to have an undercorrection or induced astigmatism. The patient may complain of diplopia and halos at night.
  - o De-centration may produce both a reduction of BCVA secondary to irregular astigmatism and a reduction of UCVA from the associated undercorrection because the maximally treated area is not aligned.
  - o The diagnosis of de-centration is made topographically (Figure 7-29).
- Treatment
  - o Custom wavefront LASIK offers the best option for the treatment of central islands, although the results are variable.
- Prevention
  - o Eye trackers and IR with wavefront LASIK has effectively eliminated the risk of significant de-centrations.

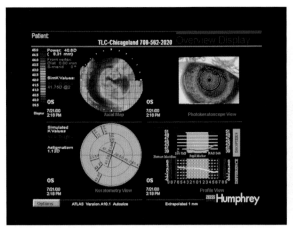

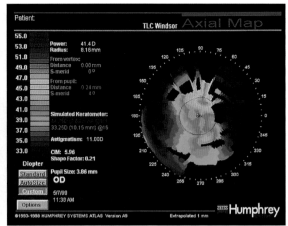

Figure 7-29. Mild to moderate temporally-decentered myopic ablation with some irregular astigmatism on the upper left axial map. The upper right photokeratoscope view demonstrates the nasal fixation with a positive angle kappa. (Reprinted with permission from Probst LE. *LASIK: A Color Atlas and Surgical Synopsis*. Thorofare, NJ: SLACK Incorporated; 2001.)

Figure 7-30. Severe irregular astigmatism demonstrated on topography after LASIK. This patient has had many laser ablations to treat a post-LASIK central island. (Reprinted with permission from Probst LE. *LASIK: A Color Atlas and Surgical Synopsis*. Thorofare, NJ: SLACK Incorporated; 2001.)

Irregular Astigmatism

- Etiology
  - Irregularity of the laser bed or the flap
  - Asymmetrical healing response of the cornea after LASIK
- Signs/symptoms
  - Often associated with other LASIK complications, such as a flap complication, grade 4 sands, flaps striae, or a de-centered ablation
  - Reduced UCVA, blurred vision, diplopia, glare at night, reduced BCVA
  - Topography will demonstrate the areas of asymmetrical elevation or depression of the cornea within the visual axis (Figure 7-30).
  - Hard contact lens over-refraction will improve the BCVA.
- Treatment
  - Flap irregularities such as striae should be treated.
  - Custom wavefront PRK with mitomycin is the best current option.
- Prevention
  - Custom LASIK should minimize the risk of postoperative irregular astigmatism.

Post Laser In Situ Keratomileusis Dry Eyes

- Etiology
  - Caused by the creation of a temporary neurotrophic cornea by severing the corneal nerves during the creation of the LASIK flap
  - During the first year after LASIK, the nerve fiber bundles gradually return, although by 1 year their number remains less than half of that before LASIK.
- Signs/symptoms
  - The post-LASIK dry eye presents immediately after the procedure.
  - The patient experiences the "burning" sensation of the classic dry eye, and the vision is often reduced if a dry eye keratopathy affects the central cornea.
  - Symptoms are resolved temporarily with topical lubrication but may return less than 1 hour after application.
  - Generally, the symptoms resolve over the first postoperative month but can rarely persist for up to 1 year.
  - After hyperopic LASIK, the dry eye can be caused by both the neurotrophic cornea and the reduced tear film of the steeper central cornea. This can cause a central superficial punctate keratitis that dramatically affects both the UCVA and BCVA (Figure 7-31).

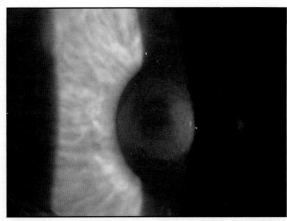

Figure 7-31. Central superficial punctate keratitis after hyperopic LASIK for a +5.50 D correction. This can take months to resolve. (Reprinted with permission from Probst LE. *LASIK: A Color Atlas and Surgical Synopsis*. Thorofare, NJ: SLACK Incorporated; 2001.)

- Treatment
  - The post-LASIK dry eye should be assessed with the same approach used with the classic dry eye patient with Schirmer's testing, staining of the cornea, and blepharitis evaluation.
  - Restasis is a very effective treatment for dry eyes.
  - Punctal plugs are put in the lower and/or upper punctum.
  - Rarely, ointment can be used prior to bed each night. Topical steroids may be useful for treating the inflammatory component of the dry eye as well as any associated eye allergy.
  - Loteprednol etabonate 0.5% is particularly useful as it is not associated with increased risk of cataract or elevated IOP.
  - Environmental controls for dry eyes, including bedroom humidifiers and protective sunglasses, may also be useful for patients who have chronic dry eye problems.
- Prevention
  - During the preoperative process, it is important to identify patients with dry eyes by Schirmer's testing and dye staining of the cornea.
  - Restasis and punctal plugs should be initiated preoperatively to avoid dry eyes postoperatively.

Post Photorefractive Keratectomy Haze

- Etiology
  - Deep excimer laser stromal ablation
  - Excessive stromal healing
  - Ultraviolet (UV) exposure after PRK
- Signs/symptoms
  - Reduced best-corrected vision
  - Myopia and astigmatism
  - White to gray "haze" present on the anterior cornea in a diffuse or reticular pattern (Figure 7-32)
- Treatment
  - Removal of haze
    - Scraping
    - Transepithelial ablation
    - Application of mitomycin
  - Bandage contact lens
- Prevention
  - Mitomycin 0.2% is not applied for 15 seconds after PRK ablations deeper than 70 μm to prevent haze formation in deeper ablations.

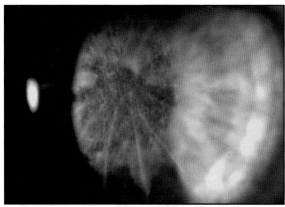

Figure 7-32. A 16-cut radial keratotomy with a small central optic zone treated with PRK and developed dense central haze as a complication of the PRK (occurs in 10% to 20% of RK cases after secondary PRK). (Reprinted with permission from Probst LE. *LASIK: A Color Atlas and Surgical Synopsis.* Thorofare, NJ: SLACK Incorporated; 2001.)

Vitreoretinal Complications After Laser In Situ Keratomileusis

- There has been a theoretical risk of increased risk of retinal detachment after LASIK due to the alteration of anterior retina from the suction ring.
- While the myopic population is already at an increased risk of detachment, no direct cause-effect relationship has been identified. A recent retrospective review of a large number of LASIK cases (38,823) found that the rate of retinal detachment was 0.08%.

Complications Unique to Femtosecond Flap Creation

Opaque Bubble Layer

- Etiology
  - ○ Femtosecond laser produces bubbles as it creates the flap
  - ○ Bubbles collect in the posterior and peripheral stroma
- Signs/symptoms
  - ○ White areas with hazy edges develop during flap creation (Figure 7-33).
  - ○ The white areas range in size from 1 to 8 mm.
  - ○ Can make pupil visualization and eye tracking difficult
  - ○ Can make patient fixation on target difficult
- Treatment
  - ○ Opaque bubble layer (OBL) can usually be wiped away with a Murocel sponge.
  - ○ OBL will absorb in 20 to 30 minutes.
- Prevention
  - ○ OBL is reduced by
    - 60-KHz laser
    - Soft docking with a peripheral meniscus during flap creation
    - Reduced femtosecond laser energy levels
    - Laser maintenance

Gas Breakthrough

- Etiology
  - ○ Gas created from flap creation extends through the anterior stromal under Bowman's layer or epithelium.

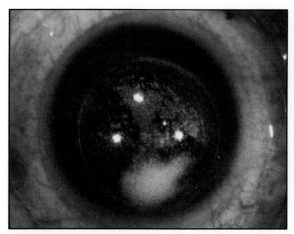

Figure 7-33. The opaque bubble layer can be seen forming in a patchy pattern at the superior portion of the flap.

- Signs/symptoms
  - 1- to 3-mm bubbles can be seen forming underneath the applanation cone during flap creation.
  - Small 1-mm areas of gas breakthrough still allow the flap to be lifted.
  - If bubble is large, flap cannot be lifted as the lamellar plane is incomplete underneath the bubble.
- Treatment
  - Small amounts of gas breakthrough do not affect the lifting of the flap or treatment.
  - If the flap cannot be lifted with a large amount of gas breakthrough, the flap should be replaced and the eye allowed to stabilize for at least 2 weeks.
  - The flap can be re-cut at 40 μm greater depth, or PRK can be performed with mitomycin C.
- Prevention
  - Maintaining a flap depth of 120 μm reduces the risk of gas breakthrough.

Transient Light Sensitivity

- Etiology
  - Higher side cut energy used for flap creation
  - Higher bed energy used for flap creation
- Signs/symptoms
  - Photosensitivity at day and night starting 1 month after IntraLASIK
  - No corneal abnormalities noted on examination
  - Vision acuity unaffected
  - Treatment
  - Topical steroids on a tapering schedule result in resolution.
- Prevention
  - The 60-KHz laser allows lower energy levels to be used for flap creation, which seems to reduce the incidence of transient light sensitivity (TLS).

Intraocular Refractive Procedures

While the corneal refractive procedure offers excellent results, a very low complication rate, and the convenience of bilateral surgery at a laser clinic setting, these procedures are not suitable for all patients. Patients who would benefit from intraocular refractive procedures include those with any of the following:
- Extreme refractive errors
- Corneal abnormalities precluding corneal refractive surgery
- Pre-existing cataracts, making lens replacement surgery more appropriate
- Presbyopia in hyperopic patients who could benefit from a multifocal or accommodating IOL

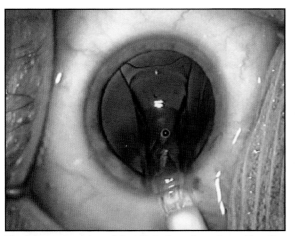

Figure 7-34. Insertion of the ICL is done through a self-sealing 3-mm clear corneal incision. (Reprinted with permission from Hardten DR, Lindstrom RL, Davis AE. *Phakic Intraocular Lenses: Principles and Practice.* Thorofare, NJ: SLACK Incorporated; 2004.)

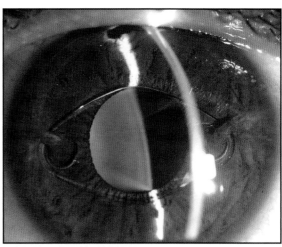

Figure 7-35. Phakic iris fixated lens for hyperopia, 4 years postoperative. The overall width of the lens is 7.25 mm, while the optic is 4.25 mm. (Reprinted with permission from Sher NA. *Surgery for Hyperopia.* Thorofare, NJ: SLACK Incorporated; 2004.)

Phakic Intraocular Lenses

- Definition
  - Phakic IOLs are lens implants that are placed into eye without the removal of the crystalline lens.
    - The Visian phakic IOL, previously the intraocular contact lens (ICL) (STAAR Surgical Company, Monrovia, CA) (Figure 7-34)
    - The Artisan phakic IOL, previously the Worst Iris Claw IOL (Figure 7-35)
    - The Vivarte phakic IOL, previous models known as the Baikoff anterior chamber phakic IOL or Nuvita (Figure 7-36)
- Indications
  - One of the main options for the correction of extreme ametropias
  - Most suitable for prepresbyopic patients because the accommodating crystalline lens is preserved
- Techniques
  - Peripheral iridotomies may be required to prevent postoperative pupillary block.
  - Phakic IOLs can often be inserted under topical anesthesia.
  - Foldable phakic IOLs have allowed insertion through smaller incisions.
  - Delicate surgical technique is required to avoid damage to intraocular structures, such as the corneal endothelium and lens.
  - Toric phakic IOLs allow for the correction of astigmatism and myopia.
  - Hyperopic corrections are more difficult to perform due to the shallow anterior chamber of hyperopic eyes.
- Results
  - Visual results are reasonably good, considering the high amount of refractive error (see Table 7-1).
  - Without the use of toric phakic IOLs, excimer laser correction of residual astigmatism is commonly required as an enhancement procedure.
- Complications
  - Each phakic IOL is associated with its own set of complications (Table 7-6).
  - Phakic IOL surgery is an intraocular procedure, so complications can be more severe.

Refractive Lensectomy

- Definition
  - Refractive lensectomy (RL) is also known as clear lens exchange (CLE).
  - Clear crystalline lens is replaced with an IOL for refractive purposes.

Figure 7-36. Vivarte presbyopic implant. (Reprinted with permission from Hardten DR, Lindstrom RL, Davis AE. *Phakic Intraocular Lenses: Principles and Practice.* Thorofare, NJ: SLACK Incorporated; 2004.)

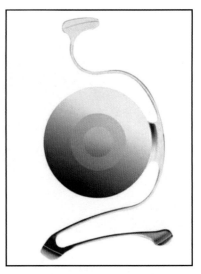

TABLE 7-6. COMPLICATIONS OF PHAKIC INTRAOCULAR LENSES

PHAKIC IOL	MAJOR REPORTED COMPLICATIONS	POTENTIAL COMPLICATIONS
Intraocular contact lens	Cataract (1% to 10%) Pigment dispersion (4%) Pupillary block (4%) Retinal detachment (<1%)	Long-term cataracts Focal closure of anterior chamber angle
Artisan iris-claw phakic IOL	Endothelial cell loss (4 to 5% per year) Chronic anterior chamber flare De-centrations (43%) Retinal detachment (<1%)	Cataract Secondary glaucoma
Nuvita anterior chamber phakic IOL	Endothelial cell loss (1% to 2% per year) Pupillary ovalization (22.6%) Glare/halos (27.8%)	Cataract Focal closure of anterior chamber angle Secondary glaucoma

- Indications
  - Used for the treatment of moderate to extreme hyperopia
  - Usually reserved for presbyopic patients because nature accommodation is lost with removal of the crystalline lens
- Technique
  - Crystalline lens removed and IOL inserted with the same small-incision techniques of cataract surgery
  - RL for high hyperopia has used piggyback IOLs for eyes requiring high corrections; however, high-power foldable IOLs (up to 40.0 D) may make this less necessary in the future.
- Results
  - Excellent at the reduction of the spherical refractive error
  - Often, a secondary enhancement corneal laser procedure is required to completely eliminate any residual sphere and astigmatism.

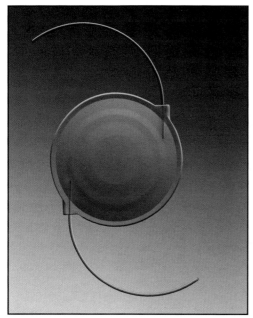

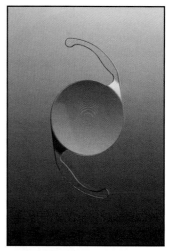

Figure 7-38. The Alcon diffractive-refractive multifocal one-piece acrylic IOL. (Reprinted with permission from Sher NA. *Surgery for Hyperopia.* Thorofare, NJ: SLACK Incorporated; 2004.)

Figure 7-37. The AMO Array Multifocal IOL has a 13-mm overall diameter with a 6-mm silicone optic. It has PMMA haptics (Reprinted with permission from Sher NA. *Surgery for Hyperopia.* Thorofare, NJ: SLACK Incorporated; 2004.)

- Complications
  - Concerns about the increased risk of retinal detachment remain when RL is used for the treatment of high myopia.
  - Other complications are those of cataract surgery.

Multifocal, Accommodating, and Diffractive Intraocular Lenses

- Definition
  - After the removal of the crystalline lens (RL) or a cataract (cataract surgery), a special IOL is implanted that allows for the correction of distance vision as well as presbyopia.
- Types of IOLs
  - ReZoom, previous model was the Array (Abbott Medical Optics [AMO], Santa Ana, Calif) (Figure 7-37)
  - ReStor IOL (Alcon Laboratories, Fort Worth, Texas) (Figure 7-38)
  - Crystalens, previously AT-45 (Eyeonics, Aliso Viejo, Calif.) (Figure 7-39)
  - Tecnis Multifocal IOL (Abbott Medical Optics, Santa Ana, Calif.)
- Indications
  - Presbyopia
  - The presence of a cataract makes this procedure easier to justify as the cataract needs to be treated regardless of the lens inserted.
  - Hyperopes are the ideal candidates, as they will gain both distance and near vision.
- Technique
  - Preoperative counseling is particularly important in these patients as the near and distance results involve compromises.
  - The cataract/clear crystalline lens is removed in the usual manner.
  - The ReZoom and the ReStor are available as foldable IOLs so they can be inserted through a small incision.
  - The Crystalens is not foldable, so it is inserted through a larger incision.

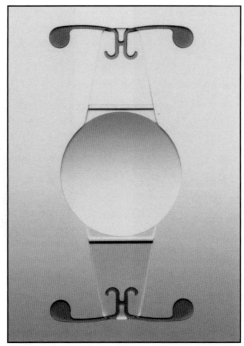

Figure 7-39. The C & C Vision Crystalens. (Reprinted with permission from Sher NA. *Surgery for Hyperopia.* Thorofare, NJ: SLACK Incorporated; 2004.)

- ○ Two different IOL types can be combined to get the best effect.
  - ▪ The IOL for the second eye is based on the patient's satisfaction or visual complaints with the first eye.
  - ▪ A patient with a ReStor lens in the first eye with poor intermediate vision problems would benefit from a ReZoom lens in the second eye to compensate for the deficiencies of the first eye.
- • Results
  - ○ While the results of the presbyopic IOLs are improving, they do not achieve results near those of myopic custom LASIK (see Table 7-1).
- • Complications
  - ○ Same complications as RL
  - ○ Capsular contraction syndrome has been associated with the older version of the Crystalens.
  - ○ Inadequate correction of presbyopia
  - ○ Reduction in the quality of distance vision
  - ○ Night vision disturbances such as glare and halos

Correction of Astigmatism

- • Arcuate keratotomy (AK) and limbal relaxing incisions (LRI) are now limited to use in conjunction with other intraocular procedures (mainly cataract surgery) to partially reduce astigmatism.
- • LASIK, PRK, LASEK, and epi-LASIK are the main methods for the treatment of astigmatism.
- • The limits for the treatment of astigmatism by PRK, LASEK, or LASIK have been expanded by using the cross-cylinder ablation or bitoric ablation technique originally proposed by Vinciguerra and by using custom ablations.
- • Toric pseudophakic and phakic IOLs have recently been introduced for the treatment of astigmatism associated with the lens implantation.

Suggested Readings

Carpel EF, Carlson KH, Shannon S. Folds and striae in laser in situ keratomileusis flaps. *J Refract Surg.* 1999;15(6):687–690.

Colin J, Robinet A. Clear lensectomy and implantation of a low-power posterior chamber intraocular lens for correction of high myopia: a four-year follow-up. *Ophthalmology.* 1997;104(1):73-77; discussion 77–78.

Jacobs JM, Taravella MJ. Incidence of intraoperative flap complications in laser in situ keratomileusis. *J Cataract Refract Surg.* 2002;28(1):23–28.

Kolahdouz-Isfahani AH, Rostamian K, Wallace D, Salz JJ. Clear lens extraction with intraocular lens implantation for hyperopia. *J Refract Surg.* 1999;15(3):316–323.

Linebarger EJ, Hardten DR, Lindstrom RL. Diffuse lamellar keratitis: diagnosis and management. *J Cataract Refract Surg.* 2000;26(7):1072–1077.

Probst LE. *LASIK: Advances, Controversy, and Custom.* Thorofare, NJ: SLACK Incorporated; 2004.

Probst LE. *LASIK Atlas and Surgical Synopsis.* Thorofare, NJ: SLACK Incorporated; 2001.

Probst LE, Machat J. Removal of flap striae following laser in situ keratomileusis. *J Cataract Refract Surg.* 1998;24(2):153–155.

Vinciguerra P, Sborgia M, Epstein D, Azzolini M, MacRae S. Photorefractive keratectomy to correct myopic or hyperopic astigmatism with a cross-cylinder ablation. *J Refract Surg.* 1999;15(2 Suppl):S183–S185.

Wilson SE, Ambrosio R. Laser in situ keratomileusis-induced neurotrophic epitheliopathy. *Am J Ophthalmol.* 2001;132(3):405–406.

Questions

1. Which of the following statements about PRK is false?
   a. PRK involves the removal of the corneal epithelium.
   b. The visual recovery after PRK is slower than LASIK.
   c. Mitomycin C reduces the risk of haze.
   d. PRK is the most popular refractive procedure.

2. Which of the following statements is true about custom wavefront LASIK?
   a. There is greater risk of postoperative night glare.
   b. There is a lower rate of achieving 20/20 uncorrected postoperative vision.
   c. Requires a wavefront aberrometer.
   d. It is not indicated for pupils larger than 6 mm.

3. Which of the following regarding LASIK flap striae is false?
   a. Flap striae can be vertical or horizontal.
   b. Striae can be associated with astigmatism.
   c. Striae often resolve without treatment.
   d. The stretch and smooth technique can be used to remove striae.

4. Which of the following statements regarding DLK is true?
   a. Bacterial endotoxins have not been identified as a cause.
   b. Interface irrigation is not useful.
   c. Grade 4 DLK can result in hyperopia.
   d. The interface inflammation begins in the center of the flap.

5. Epithelial ingrowth has been associated with all the following *except*
   a. Anterior basement membrane dystrophy
   b. Intraoperative epithelial defects
   c. LASIK enhancements
   d. PRK

6. Transient light sensitivity has all of the following characteristics *except*
   a. Femtosecond laser use for flap creation
   b. Normal ocular exam
   c. Light sensitivity immediately after surgery
   d. Treatment with steroid drops

7. Phakic IOLs have been associated with which of the following complications?
   a. Endothelial cell loss
   b. Cataracts
   c. Pupillary block glaucoma
   d. Corneal ectasia

8. All of the following statements about RL are true except
   a. Useful for the treatment of extreme refractive errors
   b. Retinal detachment is not a concern
   c. Piggyback lenses can be required for high hyperopia
   d. Also called "clear lensectomy"

9. Dry eyes after LASIK are associated with all of the following factors *except*
   a. Neurotrophic cornea
   b. Treatment with punctal plugs
   c. Treatment with Restasis
   d. Corneal ectasia

10. Night vision disturbances after LASIK have been associated with which of the following?
   a. Residual refractive errors
   b. Small pupils
   c. Large ablation zones
   d. Low higher-order aberrations

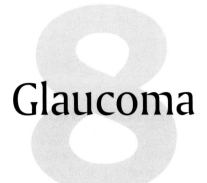

Glaucoma

Catherine M. Birt, MA, MD, FRCS(C) and Khalid Hasanee, MD, FRCS(C)

Outline

Probst LE, Tsai JH.
Ophthalmology: Clinical and Surgical Principles (pp. 299–350).
© 2012 SLACK Incorporated

Introduction

Glaucoma is an optic neuropathy associated with characteristic damage to the optic nerve head (cupping) and the visual field (nerve fiber bundle defects). It is a blinding disease where the peripheral visual field becomes constricted, followed by loss of central visual acuity.

- Glaucoma, if defined with either field or nerve criteria, has a prevalence of 5.6%.
- If defined with both field and nerve criteria, it has a prevalence of 2.4%.
- In the United States, Medicare data demonstrated that 5.3% had a primary open-angle glaucoma (POAG) diagnosis in 1999.
- The appearance of the optic nerve head (ONH) and visual fields is a major factor for a diagnosis of glaucoma.
- An elevated eye pressure is neither necessary nor sufficient to make the diagnosis.
  - In "normal-tension glaucoma," the patient is never found to have a pressure over the normal limits.
  - In "ocular hypertension," the patient has high eye pressures but no signs of optic nerve or visual field damage.
- The level of the intraocular pressure (IOP) is the main risk factor and is important in the monitoring of treatment.
- Gonioscopy is of major importance in the classification of the glaucoma type.
- The extent of damage to the optic nerve and visual field determines the stage of the glaucoma.

Glaucoma Blindness

- Glaucoma is a progressive disease with increased risk of blindness over time
- Studies estimate that 7.5% per year worsen without treatment and 4% per year worsen with treatment.
- Field progression is on average 0.2 decibel (dB)/yr, and stable patients change at 0.1 dB/yr, while progressing patients change at 0.9 dB/yr.
- Patients live (on average) 13 to 15 years from diagnosis to death, so most do not go blind in their lifetime. However, African American patients go blind at a rate of 8% versus 4% for Caucasians.
- Despite low incidence rates, high prevalence means a major burden worldwide. One study looked at 205 untreated patients in a natural experiment, of whom 16% progressed to unilateral blindness in 10 years and 11% progressed to bilateral blindness.

The Basics

Intraocular Pressure

- IOP represents the equilibrium between the rigidity of the cornea and sclera, and the outward pressure of the ocular contents.
- As the vitreous is of fixed volume, the most important variable is the amount of aqueous humor, which varies with respect to production and drainage. In the etiology of glaucoma, however, variation in production is insignificant.
- The pathology of elevated IOP is due to inadequacies of aqueous outflow.
- The normal mean IOP is 15.5 mm Hg, and in the suprachoroidal space, the pressure is approximately 2 mm Hg lower.
- The distribution of IOP is not normal (ie, non-Gaussian) with the curve skewed toward higher pressures.

- Two standard deviations above the mean place 97% of the population below 21 mm Hg, and 2.5 standard deviations above the mean place 99% of the population below 24 mm Hg, hence the derivation of the concept of 21 mm Hg as being the upper limit of "normal" IOP.
- Many factors influence IOP and its measurement. There is a normal diurnal variation of IOP, but a variation of more than 7 mm Hg may be considered significantly abnormal. Much research shows that not only the mean IOP level but also the range within which it varies is of importance to the risk of developing or progressing glaucoma.
  - Increasing age increases IOP due to decreased outflow.
  - Increases in systolic blood pressure also increase IOP slightly.
  - Lying supine increases IOP with dramatic increases seen if the individual lies 30 degrees head down (13 mm Hg more), which is why certain yoga positions can be detrimental to the glaucoma patient.
  - Smoking can increase the IOP.
  - Corticosteroids increase IOP in 25% of the normal population and 90% to 100% of the glaucoma population (see steroid-related glaucoma).

Aqueous Humor

- The volume of the aqueous humor in the anterior segment is 0.25 cc or 250 μL.
- One-quarter of this is in the posterior chamber, and three-quarters is in the anterior chamber.
- The ciliary body (CB) produces 2.5 μL per minute with complete turnover of the aqueous in about 100 minutes (Figure 8-1).
- The CB consists of 70 to 80 ciliary processes, which are fronds of 2 layers of epithelium, pigmented within and nonpigmented superficially. The central core of blood vessels in each frond is surrounded by stroma lying between the blood vessel and the epithelial layers, producing a total surface area of about 6 cm^2.
- Aqueous is produced by the 4×10^6 nonpigmented cells and requires the following 3 prerequisites:
  - An adequate blood supply with sufficient pressure to the CB
  - Ultrafiltration-diffusion down a concentration gradient with hydrostatic pressure added to the driving forces, a process which occurs across capillary walls
  - Active secretion from the sides of the nonpigmented epithelial cells
- The blood supply of the ciliary processes is one area where the blood-ocular barrier is not present. The CB blood supply consists of the following:
  - The long and anterior ciliary arteries leading to the major arterial circle of the iris that also supplies the CB
  - Short radial ciliary artery that produces the capillaries
  - Serum is forced out from the leaky capillary walls and is ultrafiltrated through the stroma
  - The capillaries are thin-walled and fenestrated

Ciliary Body Enzyme Systems

- The active secretion phase of aqueous production requires the following 4 enzymes:
  - Na-K ATPase
  - Carbonic anhydrase
  - Cyclic adenylate monophosphate (cAMP)
  - Chloride secretion
- Na-K ATPase is the most important of these systems.
  - A membrane-bound protein found on the lateral surfaces of the cells
  - Pumps Na$^+$ out of the cells into the intercellular space, producing a hypertonic environment that draws water passively from the ultrafiltrate
- The second major system in aqueous production is carbonic anhydrase, which does the following:
  - Converts CO_2 and H_2O to H$^+$ and HCO_3^-
  - Inhibition of this process with carbonic anhydrase inhibitors alters the ion exchange, as H$^+$ and HCO_3^- are involved in the exchange of Na$^+$ and Cl$^-$ across the basolateral cell membrane of the pigmented ciliary epithelial cells at the stromal side of the bilayer.
  - Na$^+$ and Cl$^-$ move via gap junctions to the nonpigmented cells where they are actively transported into the posterior chamber and water moves passively along this concentration gradient.

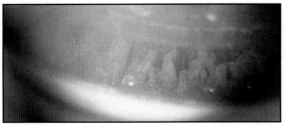

Figure 8-1. Ciliary body.

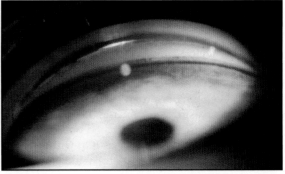

Figure 8-2. Trabecular meshwork.

- cAMP is another enzyme system.
  - ○ Production of cAMP from ATP by adenylate cyclase is stimulated by activation of the α-2 receptors and inhibited by α-2 receptors.
  - ○ Thus, both β-blockers and α-agonists decrease aqueous production by decreasing cAMP levels.
  - ○ The relationship between cAMP and the Na-K ATPase pump is unknown.
- Chloride is the main anion involved in aqueous production but this enzyme system is not amenable to clinical manipulation at this time.

Aqueous Outflow

- Conventional outflow, accounting for approximately 80% to 90% of total outflow, is pressure-dependent and can be increased by the use of miotics. It occurs
  - ○ Through the channels of the trabecular meshwork (TM) (Figure 8-2)
  - ○ Into the canal of Schlemm via pinocytosis and vacuolation of the endothelial cells
  - ○ The site of the major resistance to outflow exists at the juxtacanalicular tissue that lines the canal of Schlemm
  - ○ *Outflow facility* is the term that refers to the ease or difficulty with which the aqueous leaves the eye and is calculated from the following formulas
    - ▪ $C = F/P_o - P_v$
    - ▪ Facility = Flow/(IOP - episcleral venous pressure)
  - ○ The normal value for outflow facility is 0.3 μL/min/mm Hg.
  - ○ In glaucoma, the outflow decreases to about 0.17 μL/min/mm Hg.
  - ○ Pseudofacility refers to the slight drop in production seen with increases in IOP.
- Unconventional or uveoscleral outflow (about 20%) is pressure-independent, decreased by pilocarpine and increased by the use of atropine or prostaglandin agonists, and occurs
  - ○ Through the CB
  - ○ To the suprachoroidal space
  - ○ Then to the choroidal and scleral vessels
  - ○ Through the iris stroma
  - ○ Through the retinal vessels and the optic nerve

Optic Nerve Head

- The optic nerve enters the globe posteriorly and nasal to fixation, about 3 disc diameters away from the fovea.
- It tends to be a vertical oval.
- The exact size and shape is variable.
- It contains about 1 to 1.3 million axons placed around a cup of variable size.
- As the size of the optic nerve increases, so does the cup size.
- A large cup-to-disc (C:D) ratio can be normal in a large nerve and a small C:D ratio can be pathologic in a small nerve.
- The area of the neuroretinal rim is less sensitive to differences in the ONH size.
- Between ±8.00 D of refractive error, there is no relationship between the refractive error, axial length, and ONH size.

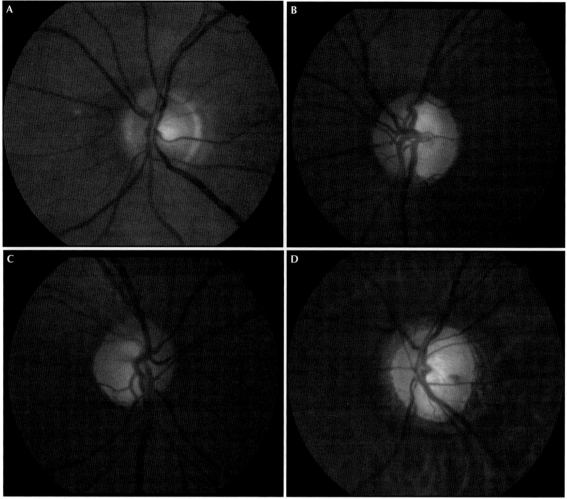

Figure 8-3. (A) Normal optic nerve. (B) Advanced cupping. (C) Optic nerve notch. (D) Optic nerve hemorrhage.

- The size of the disc can be roughly estimated by comparing it to the 5-degree spot in the Welch-Allen direct ophthalmoscope, which subtends about 1.8 mm², approximately the disc size in the phakic eye. This helps to identify the very large and very small disc.
- ONH changes are extremely important in the diagnosis of glaucoma. These changes can be local or diffuse, and local changes may progress to diffuse ones. They may be considered the ends of a spectrum with a large intermingled population. These changes can be seen in the visual field as corresponding paracentral defects that may lead to arcuate or wedge-shaped defects.
    - Local changes include findings such as the following (Figure 8-3):
        - An oval (vertically elongated) cup
        - Thinning of the neuroretinal rim
        - A full rim notch
    - Diffuse changes include the following:
        - Generalized thinning of the neuroretinal rim
        - Increases in the C:D ratio
    - These are seen as constricted isopters on kinetic field testing or changes in the mean deviation (MD) on static perimetry.
- Causative theories
    - There are 2 main theories for the mechanism of glaucomatous optic nerve damage.
        - The mechanical theory suggests that increased pressure interferes with the axoplasmic flow of the nerve fiber layer due to a pressure effect at the lamina cribrosa.
            - This may result in loss of neurotrophic factors that preserve the ganglion cells.

- The vascular theory postulates interference with the autoregulation of the optic nerve blood supply due to the increased IOP leading to ischemia and is considered more important in explaining low-tension glaucoma.
  - □ Autoregulation is the maintenance of a constant blood flow in the face of systemic variations in pressure.
  - □ The retina shows autoregulation, the choroid does not, and the ONH has partial autoregulation.
- Whatever the etiology, factors associated with increased ONH susceptibility to pressure includes the following:
  - □ Polygenic inherited factors associated with a family history
  - □ Age over 40
  - □ Black race
  - □ Female gender
  - □ Prior glaucomatous damage (a weak disc)
  - □ Pressure spikes
  - □ A longer time of pressure exposure
  - □ Prior hemodynamic crises (hypotension)
  - □ High myopia
- Blood supply
  - o The ONH blood supply can be divided into several sections.
    - The superficial nerve fiber layer is supplied from the central retinal artery (CRA) (and occasionally from the choroidal flow via a cilioretinal artery).
    - The prelaminar ONH is supplied from the posterior ciliary arteries via peripapillary and prechoriocapillary vessels.
    - The laminar portion of the nerve is supplied by choroidal circulation via the short posterior ciliary arteries.
    - The postlaminar portion comes from recurrent vessels from the short posterior ciliary arteries to the pial vessels via the pial centripetal vessels and from the centrifugal vessels from the CRA.

Classification

- Glaucoma is not a single disease, but a large number of similar conditions with factors in common. It is usually classified on the basis of the anatomy of the anterior chamber angle as open or closed, and each type has primary and secondary subcategories. Figure 8-4 shows one classification scheme that helps to organize the different diseases that comprise the glaucomas.

Primary Open-Angle Glaucoma

- Epidemiology
  - o Generally, 1% to 2% of the general population is affected, with a 0.4% to 6.6% prevalence in those older than 40 years of age.
  - o The incidence increases with each decade over 40 years of age.
  - o Glaucoma involves about 8% of office visits to an ophthalmologist.
  - o It is one of the leading causes of blindness in North America and is the first in the African American population.
  - o Worldwide, glaucoma is the second or third leading cause of blindness (data vary) with approximately 33 million people affected.
- Risk factors
  - o Elevated IOP
    - The main risk factor
    - The prevalence of the disease increases with higher IOP levels.
    - There is more disease in eyes with a higher IOP.
  - o Age
    - A primary risk factor, with the prevalence of the disease increasing with each decade (see Table 8-1).
    - The prevalence is 3.5 times higher in Caucasians aged 70 or older than in those aged 40 to 49.

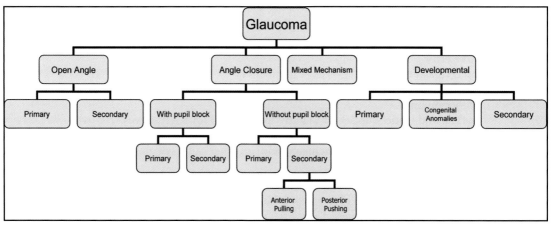

Figure 8-4. Glaucoma classification.

TABLE 8-1. PREVALENCE OF GLAUCOMA BY DECADE OF AGE

40 years	1%
50 years	2%
60 years	4%
70 years	10%
80 years	15%

- The prevalence is 7.4 times higher in African Americans aged 70 or older than in those aged 40 to 49.
  - Race
    - An important risk factor
    - African Americans have a higher incidence of POAG than Caucasians
    - The Baltimore Eye Survey (BES) showed rates of 1.3% in Caucasians and 4.7% in African Americans.
    - The prevalence in Hispanics was 2.1%.
    - Other types of glaucoma are also more commonly seen in certain ethnic groupings. For example, the Inuit have more angle-closure glaucoma (ACG), Scandinavians have more pseudoexfoliation, and normal-tension glaucoma is the most common subtype in Japan.
  - Family history
    - Another risk factor, one that is more important in African Americans (2.5 odds ratio) than in Caucasians (0.97 odds ratio) with parental history of the disease.
    - In the Rotterdam survey, there was a 9.2 times higher lifetime risk of glaucoma in siblings and offspring of glaucoma patients compared to nonglaucomatous individuals.
    - POAG inheritance is considered to be multifactorial with approximately a 1/11 risk for a first-degree relative.
  - Systemic diseases
    - Have been studied for their association with POAG with mixed results
      - For diabetes, the BES showed no age-adjusted risk, and the Blue Mountain Eye Survey (BMES) showed slight increased risk. Overall, 15% of diabetics have glaucoma, and 12% to 21% of glaucoma patients have diabetes.
      - For cardiovascular diseases, the risk is increased with hypertension or migraines. The Rotterdam study showed that having hypertension increased the odds ratio by 2.1, although the BES and Barbados Eye (BDES) studies showed no association.

□ Migraines had no association in the BDES, but the BMES showed a 2.5 increased odds ratio of migraine in POAG patients over 70 years of age than without. The Normal Tension Glaucoma Trial also showed migraine to be a risk factor.

- o Refractive error
  - ▪ Can be relevant to the diagnosis of glaucoma
    - □ Patients with myopia were found by the BMES to have a 2 to 3 times increased risk over nonmyopes.
    - □ The odds ratio was 2.3 for low myopes and 3.3 for a refractive error over -3.0 D.
- Clinical
  - o This is essentially a diagnosis of exclusion with all other causes of glaucoma being ruled out first.
  - o POAG is defined as the following:
    - ▪ A progressive bilateral optic neuropathy
    - ▪ Open angles on gonioscopy
    - ▪ Typical pattern of nerve fiber bundle visual field loss
- Management
  - o The management of POAG is directed at the elevated IOP.
  - o A target IOP is set based on the severity of the disease at the time of diagnosis.
  - o Medical management is the primary form of treatment, generally using the application of topical medications.
  - o Laser trabeculoplasty is often successful but the effects may wear off unpredictably.
  - o The final option is filtration surgery.
  - o Prognosis is generally good with most patients achieving control of their glaucoma with the previously mentioned methods.

Normal-Tension Glaucoma

- Etiology
  - o Nocturnal systemic hypotension
  - o Autoimmune processes
  - o Vasospasm
  - o Hemodynamic crisis (excess blood loss or shock)
  - o Undiagnosed high IOP
- Signs/symptoms
  - o Open angles
  - o Cupping
  - o Visual field defects
  - o IOP less than 22 mm Hg
- Differential diagnosis
  - o Diurnal variation
  - o Intermittent IOP spike (angle closure, glaucomatocyclitic crisis)
  - o Previous high IOP (burned out pigmentary glaucoma, steroid-related glaucoma)
  - o Use of medications that can decrease IOP (β-blockers, digoxin)
  - o Tono-Pen error
  - o Pathology to the optic nerve
    - ▪ Optic nerve compression
    - ▪ Optic disc drusen
    - ▪ Optic nerve coloboma
  - o Systemic disease
    - ▪ Vasculitis
    - ▪ Hypotension
    - ▪ Toxic
- Evaluation
  - o Diurnal pressure monitoring
  - o Visual field testing, which typically demonstrates defects that, compared to POAG, have the following:
    - ▪ Steeper slopes

- Greater depth
- Closer proximity to fixation
- It is important to make sure that any visual field defect is "glaucomatous" in appearance. Any field defect respecting the vertical midline should raise immediate suspicion for an intracranial etiology.
  - A neurologic workup as needed, including neuroimaging
  - A systemic workup as needed (complete blood count [CBC], eosinophil sedimentation rate [ESR], antinuclear antibody [ANA], fluorescent treponemal antibody absorption [FTA-ABS], C-reactive protein, anticardiolipin antibody [ACA], carotid evaluation)
- Management
  - Observation until progression has been determined may be appropriate for some low-risk cases
  - If treatment is required, the same methods as with POAG are used
  - Prognosis more guarded

Secondary Open-Angle Glaucoma

Pigmentary Glaucomas

Pseudoexfoliation

- Etiology
  - Pseudoexfoliation is an age-related systemic disorder of the extracellular matrix, with production and accumulation of fibrillar material in the anterior segment and connective tissue seen throughout the body.
  - Pseudoexfoliation is the most common secondary open-angle glaucoma worldwide.
  - The rates of glaucoma in the setting of pseudoexfoliation vary from 20% to 80%. The IOP tends to be higher than in POAG, and optic nerve and field changes tend to be worse.
  - The presence of pseudoexfoliation carries significant ocular risk. The uninvolved eye may have POAG, and there is also a higher risk of central retinal vein occlusion.
  - Incidence varies, being common in Scandinavia but rare in the Inuit.
  - Incidence increases with age, with 5% of the population over 75 showing signs.
  - Involvement is monocular in 60% of patients.
  - There is a higher prevalence of pseudoexfoliation in the following (in increasing order):
    - Patients older than 50 years
    - Ocular hypertensives
    - Glaucoma patients
    - Glaucoma patients having surgery
    - Glaucoma patients gone blind
  - There is no genetic pattern of inheritance, however,
    - Females outnumber males in pseudoexfoliation syndrome (without glaucomatous neuropathy).
    - Females equal males in the population with pseudoexfoliative glaucoma.
    - There is a higher incidence of the condition in glaucoma populations than normal.
    - There is also an increased incidence of angle closure.
    - Many patients with pseudoexfoliation do not develop glaucoma, but once glaucoma develops, damage is more likely to progress than with POAG.
- Signs/symptoms
  - The pseudoexfoliation material is found throughout anterior chamber, but is most visible on pupil ruff and anterior lens capsule. The classic "target pattern" is due to clearing of the material by iris movement (Figure 8-5).
  - The elevated IOP is due to obstruction of outflow by pigment and/or exfoliation material.
  - Due to this friction, there is loss of pupil ruff pigment and deposition of pigment granules on the iris and in the TM. Small amounts of endothelial pigmentation are also possible.
  - Heavy angle pigmentation is common, and pigment deposited anterior to the meshwork in pseudoexfoliation is known as "Sampaolesi's line" (Figure 8-6).

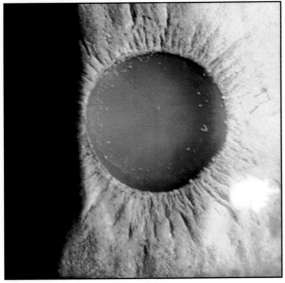

Figure 8-5. Capsule exfoliation (target pattern).

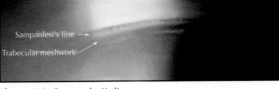

Figure 8-6. Sampaolesi's line.

- o A differential diagnosis for pseudoexfoliation is rarely necessary as the findings are classic but include any other causes of pigment within the anterior segment, such as pigment dispersion syndrome, true exfoliation of the lens capsule, toxic exfoliation, trauma, or tumor.
- Pathology
  - o The pseudoexfoliation deposit is a form of fibrillar basement membrane or elastotic material.
  - o The lens epithelium may contribute to the material, and it is seen as "iron filings" on the lens capsule using light microscopy (Figure 8-7).
  - o The same pseudoexfoliation material is also seen in the iris, conjunctiva, and throughout the body when sought with electron microscopy.
  - o There have been reported systemic associations including transient ischemic attack (TIA), stroke, angina, myocardial infarction, hypertension, retinal vein occlusion, and Alzheimer's disease.
  - o In 2007, a gene was identified for pseudoexfoliation-lysyl oxidase-like 1 (PXE-LOXL1).
    - Thorleifsson and colleagues showed that 2 nonsynonymous single-nucleotide polymorphisms (SNPs) in exon 1 of the LOXL1 gene on chromosome 15q24.1 confer risk for pseudoexfoliation glaucoma.
    - Lysyl oxidase maintains elastic fibers; the product of LOXL1 catalyzes the formation of elastin fibers found to be a major component of the lesions in exfoliation glaucoma (XFG).
    - About 25% of the general population is homozygous for the highest-risk haplotype, and their risk of suffering from XFG is more than 100 times that of individuals carrying only low-risk haplotypes.
    - The population-attributable risk is more than 99%.
- Management
  - o The management of pseudoexfoliative glaucoma is directed at the elevated IOP.
  - o Medical management is the same as for POAG, but typically may be more resistant to topical treatment.
  - o Laser trabeculoplasty is often successful, but the effects may wear off unpredictably.
  - o The final option is filtration surgery, with surgical success generally equal to that of patients with POAG. However, surgery involving the lens in pseudoexfoliative patients has an increased risk of complications including poor pupil dilation, capsule rupture, lens dislocation, and zonular dialysis.

Pigment Dispersion

- Etiology
  - o *Pigment dispersion syndrome* is defined as the presence of pigment dispersion without glaucoma.
  - o Pigmentary glaucoma was originally defined as the presence of pigment dispersion with elevated IOP, with or without the presence of optic nerve or field changes.

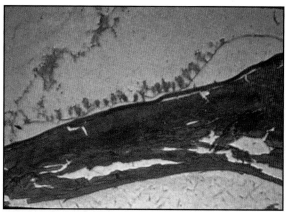

Figure 8-7. Pseudoexfoliation pathology—"iron filings."

- o With the current definition of glaucoma eliminating the reference to elevated IOP, one usually considers pigment dispersion glaucoma to also require changes in the nerve or field.
- o Pigment dispersion is typically seen in the following:
  - A patient with moderate myopia between −1 and -4 D
  - Males are more affected than females with a ratio of 2:1.
  - It is mostly seen in Caucasian patients.
  - The age of onset is younger than is seen with POAG:
    - □ Males are typically affected between the ages of 35 and 45.
    - □ Females are at a slightly later age, between 40 and 50.
- Pathology
  - o There have been several theories regarding the cause of pigment release from the iris.
    - Early theories postulated that an intrinsic iris abnormality, possibly ischemic in nature, was the cause.
    - Later, it was realized that contact between the iris and zonules released pigment in those areas only. It was thought that a lax iris contacted the zonules with mechanical rubbing liberating pigment.
    - The current theory is that of the "reverse pupil block."
      - □ Aqueous is "pumped" into the anterior chamber by the following:
        - Accommodation
        - Eye movement
        - Blinking
        - Exercise
    - A one-way valve exists at the iris-lens interface.
    - This produces a temporary rise in the anterior chamber pressure over the posterior chamber pressure.
    - This results in posterior bowing of the iris that pushes the iris back onto the zonules.
    - Contact between the iris and the zonules releases pigment that accumulates in the TM.
    - Chronic elevation in IOP is due to damage to the trabecular beams and cells from pigment overload over time.
- Signs/symptoms
  - o The findings in pigment dispersion are very typical.
    - Pigment lost from the iris epithelium may end up within the endothelial cells of the cornea in a vertical oval known as the Krukenberg spindle (Figure 8-8A).
    - Retroillumination through the pupil will usually show midperipheral iris transillumination defects, although these may not be visible in patients with a thick iris stroma (Figure 8-8B).
    - Pigment is found throughout the anterior chamber, and pigment deposition is very heavy in the angle.
    - The anterior chamber is generally deep, with posterior iris bowing in the periphery that is more easily seen on gonioscopy.
    - An elevation in IOP is seen in less than half of patients with pigment dispersion.

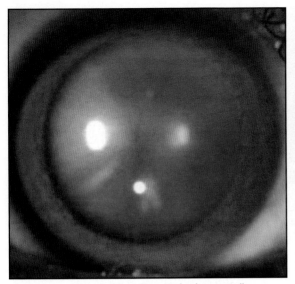

Figure 8-8A. Pigment dispersion—Krukenberg spindle.

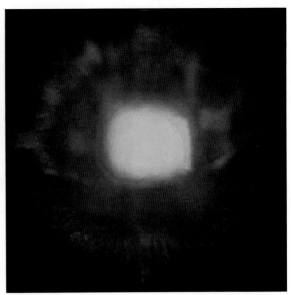

Figure 8-8B. Pigment dispersion—Midperipheral transillumination defects.

- If glaucomatous changes are found, they usually develop within 15 years of presentation.
- Exercise or dilation may liberate pigment from the iris and elevate the IOP in a temporary but possibly severe fashion. A report of blurry vision, halos around lights, and eye pain in a myopic patient, particularly after exercise, should raise the suspicion of a pigment shower and temporary outflow obstruction.
- Differential diagnosis
  - The differential of pigment dispersion covers any other source of pigment within the eye, including uveitic glaucoma, melanoma cell deposition, iris or CB cysts, surgery, trauma, aging changes, and pseudoexfoliation.
- Management
  - Management is intended to prevent further pigment liberation and/or to manage elevations in IOP:
    - Topical miotic agents keep the iris taut but are poorly tolerated, particularly in this younger patient group.
    - Conventional medical management is used to decrease aqueous production and lower IOP once chronic damage has produced chronic IOP elevations.
    - The theory of the reverse pupil block has led to the use of a Neodymium Yttrium-Aluminum-Garnet (Nd:YAG) laser peripheral iridotomy (PI) as a treatment.
      - In theory, this will allow aqueous flow to bypass the valve at the iris/lens interface, decrease the posterior bowing, and halt the release of pigment.
      - Retrospective studies have confirmed the safety of this procedure and that it decreases iris bowing.
      - There is yet no prospective evidence for decreased IOP or slower disease progress.
      - It is used because it is generally safe, although one must watch closely for IOP spikes immediately following the procedure.
    - Laser trabeculoplasty works well, but control may decrease with time.
  - When necessary, filtration surgery is used with success rates similar to age-matched controls.
- Prognosis
  - The condition may "burn out" with time as pigment release decreases. However, permanent meshwork damage may result in permanently elevated IOP.
  - Visual field and optic nerve changes are permanent even if IOP control improves.

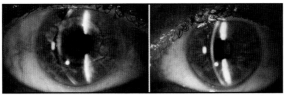

Figure 8-9. Fuchs' heterochromia with anterior IOL in the blue right eye.

Inflammatory Glaucoma

Posner-Schlossman Syndrome

- Etiology
    - Also known as glaucomatocyclitic crisis, this condition consists of recurrent mild anterior uveitis with marked elevation of IOP.
    - The condition usually affects young to middle-aged patients and is rare in those over 80 years of age.
    - The cause is unknown, but there is a possible immune etiology.
- Signs/symptoms
    - Posner-Schlossman syndrome is usually unilateral.
    - Symptoms are usually not dramatic, with mild discomfort, blurred vision, and mild ciliary flush.
    - Hypochromia of the iris may be seen with time.
    - The IOP is usually very high, typically 40 to 80 mm Hg during an attack.
    - The angle is open.
    - The iritis is recurrent and mild, with a trace flare, few cells, small keratic precipitates (KPs), and no posterior synechiae.
    - The average crisis lasts hours to weeks, and the eye appears normal between attacks. During an attack, there is significantly decreased outflow facility and high concentrations of prostaglandin E found in aqueous humor.
- Management
    - Standard medical management is used to decrease the IOP.
    - The iritis responds to anti-inflammatories (steroid or nonsteroidal anti-inflammatory drug [NSAID]). Use of an NSAID may reduce the prostaglandin concentration and lower IOP faster than just aqueous suppression alone.
- Prognosis
    - The condition is self-limited but the significant level of the IOP requires management.

Fuchs' Heterochromic Iridocyclitis

- Etiology
    - Fuchs' usually presents in the third to fourth decades of life and is usually unilateral.
    - The incidence in males is equal to females.
    - Fuch's can be seen in both Caucasians and African Americans.
    - Raised IOP is seen in 13% to 59% of patients, and the incidence increases with time.
    - The disease may be caused by autoantibodies to corneal epithelium, which are found in 90% of cases.
- Signs/symptoms
    - Fuchs' heterochromic iridocyclitis is a chronic iridocyclitis associated with the following:
        - Changes in iris color
        - Cataract formation
        - Possible glaucoma
    - Usually, the iris color changes in the direction of the affected eye being lighter due to loss of iris stroma (Figure 8-9).
    - The clinical course is mild with a chronic anterior chamber reaction (flare and cells) present.
    - In addition to the chronic flare and cells, stellate KPs are seen mostly on the inferior cornea, and Koeppe nodules are also possible.

- o On gonioscopy, fine-angle blood vessels are seen and may bleed during surgery but do not close the angle as ischemic neovascular vessels do.
- o Cataract formation is common, but IOP elevation is not necessarily seen.
- Management
  - o The iritis does not respond to steroids as it is due to chronic incompetence of the blood-ocular barrier.
  - o The management of the IOP involves standard medical and surgical approaches.
  - o Laser trabeculoplasty is less likely to be useful.
- Prognosis
  - o Management of IOP is generally successful.

Steroid-Related Glaucoma

- Etiology
  - o Steroid-related glaucoma is an open-angle glaucoma associated with a marked increase in IOP as a response to topical or systemic steroids.
    - ▪ The major risk factor is pre-existing POAG.
    - ▪ The elevated IOP is due to decreased outflow facility as the steroids induce meshwork genes (GLC1 also known as myocilin or TIGR gene) and the metabolism of proteins in the meshwork is altered.
    - ▪ The highest risk of a response comes from the following:
      - □ Ophthalmic steroid ointments
      - □ Ophthalmic steroid drops
      - □ Periocular/intraocular steroid injections
    - ▪ Local nonophthalmic preparations such as creams used on the face may also be a significant source.
    - ▪ Systemic administration and inhaled or nasal steroids are less likely to cause a pressure rise, but this has been reported.
    - ▪ Endogenous sources of steroid may also affect the IOP but are much more rare. These include conditions such as
      - □ Adrenal hyperplasia
      - □ Adrenal adenoma/carcinoma
      - □ Ectopic adrenal corticotrophic hormone (ACTH) syndrome
- Signs/symptoms
  - o The IOP rise can occur at any time after initiation of steroid treatment, but is most common at 2 to 3 weeks with strong steroids and after months with weaker ones.
  - o The timing and amount of the IOP rise is related to the following:
    - ▪ Drug dose
    - ▪ Frequency
    - ▪ Potency
    - ▪ Patient responsiveness
  - o A topical source is more significant than systemic but they can be additive.
  - o Prednisolone is the most effective, and fluorometholone (FML) is the least effective in causing IOP rise.
  - o The clinical findings resemble POAG, and a prior steroid response can resemble normal-tension glaucoma if nerve and field changes have occurred at a high pressure that has since resolved.
  - o The features of steroid glaucoma are more frequent and more marked in patients with POAG than controls, and patients with angle recession may be more at risk.
  - o A family history of POAG is more common in responders than nonresponders.
- Management
  - o The best management is prevention and a high index of suspicion.
    - ▪ Avoid steroids where possible and use the smallest, briefest possible effective dose.
    - ▪ Use NSAIDs as steroid-sparers if possible.
    - ▪ It is important to establish a baseline IOP before starting therapy and to monitor the IOP carefully during steroid treatment. If a clinically significant IOP rise occurs, the management is to minimize the steroid if possible, and add aqueous suppressant topical therapy if necessary.

- Laser trabeculoplasty is relatively ineffective in steroid-related glaucoma.
- Surgery may be necessary, although this is relatively rare. The outcome of surgery may be affected by the underlying need for steroid, in that uveitic glaucoma can be surgically challenging.
- Prognosis
  - Good if steroid use can be curtailed

Traumatic Glaucoma

Angle-Recession Glaucoma

- Incidence
  - Angle recession is one of the findings that may be seen following anterior segment trauma.
    - True recession is a split between long (outer) and circular (inner) muscle fibers of the CB (Figure 8-10).
      - With angle recession, it is TM scarring that causes outflow obstruction but recession is the "warning sign."
      - The risk of glaucoma is increased if more than 270 degrees of the angle is affected.
      - The prevalence of recession is between 60% and 90% if a hyphema occurred with the trauma.
      - The incidence of glaucoma developing is 2% to 10%, and the contralateral eye also has an increased risk of developing POAG over time, possibly because there is less outflow facility in both eyes, and the trauma results in loss of reserve earlier.
    - An iridodialysis is a tear in the root of the iris.
    - A cyclodialysis is a separation of the CB from the scleral spur.
- Clinical findings
  - The clinical findings are similar to POAG.
    - The anterior chamber is deeper than normal.
    - The angle is wider than normal on gonioscopy.
    - Because the angle changes may be subtle, it is important to do the following:
      - Compare the quadrants within the eye
      - Compare the same quadrants between the 2 eyes, looking for widening
- Management
  - Medical management is usually initiated with aqueous suppression in the early period.
  - Miotics are contraindicated because the angle is dissociated from the scleral spur, and miotics will only serve to decrease uveoscleral outflow. Chronic IOP elevation, however, responds poorly to drops.
  - Laser trabeculoplasty has a low success rate.
  - Surgery or cycloablation is used if necessary.
- Prognosis
  - Variable, depending on the degree of angle damage

Hyphema

- Etiology
  - Hyphema (Figure 8-11), or blood in the anterior chamber, may be caused by the following:
    - Trauma
    - Surgery
    - Rubeosis
    - The risk of IOP elevation may be related to the underlying cause and is more common with a re-bleed than with the primary hyphema.
    - The meshwork becomes blocked by the following:
      - Red blood cells
      - Fibrin
      - Debris
      - There is a possibility of a pupil block with a collar button clot.
    - With a traumatic hyphema, the re-bleed incidence is less than 10%.

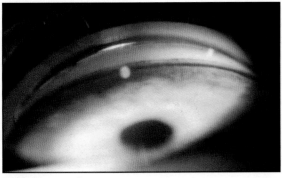

Figure 8-10. Angle recession.

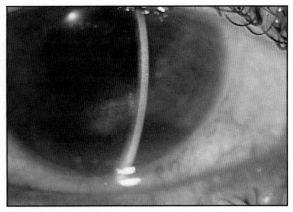

Figure 8-11. Hyphema.

- The glaucoma risk is increased to about 30% with a re-bleed, or in the presence of a total hyphema to between 50% and 100%.
- The incidence is highest in young males.
- Sickle cell patients have a greatly increased risk of IOP rise and central retinal vein occlusion (CRVO), therefore, all African American patients with a hyphema must have their sickle status determined.
- Clinical
    - Blood in the anterior chamber
    - Blood clot in the anterior chamber
    - Elevated IOP
    - Blood staining of the cornea
- Management
    - Initial management includes the following:
        - Aqueous suppression plus hyperosmotics if needed in the acute phase.
        - If the hyphema is not clearing after 7 to 10 days, a surgical washout should be considered, as well as if there is severe pain or corneal blood staining occurring.
        - Corneal blood staining results from a prolonged total hyphema, usually with elevated IOP. The cornea takes up hemoglobin and becomes discolored, and clearing of the stroma may take up to 3 years. Thus, one should consider surgery to clear a total hyphema if
            - It lasts longer than 4 days
            - The IOP is more than 40 to 50 mm Hg (in the setting of a healthy nerve)
            - Patients have sickle cell or POAG
        - A trabeculectomy may control IOP without tugging on the clot, but it is usually possible to remove some or all of the clot and allow the meshwork to begin to clear.

Lens-Related Glaucoma

Phacolytic Glaucoma

- Etiology
    - Phacolytic glaucoma is seen in patients with a mature or hypermature lens that loses lens protein through the capsule (Figure 8-12).
    - Macrophages appear in response to the lens protein.
    - The TM is blocked by the following:
        - Macrophages
        - High molecular weight lens protein
- Signs/symptoms
    - The presentation usually includes the following:
        - Typically a very high IOP, with an acute onset of symptoms that are similar to those seen in angle closure
        - Corneal edema due to the high IOP

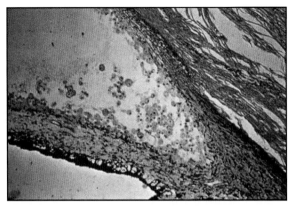

Figure 8-12. Phacolytic glaucoma—Pathology.

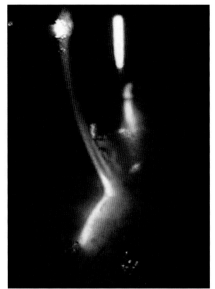

Figure 8-13. Lens-particle glaucoma—High power of fragments in anterior chamber.

- An intense anterior chamber flare due to liberated lens protein
- The anterior chamber cells are macrophages and white chunks, which are actual lens fragments that may also be seen
- The lens is mature or hypermature, and there are white particles seen on the lens capsule, which are macrophages
- Differential diagnosis
  - Differential diagnosis of sudden severe elevations of IOP includes the following:
    - Acute pupil block angle closure
    - Neovascular glaucoma
    - Uveitic glaucoma
    - Traumatic glaucoma
- Management
  - The immediate need is to control the IOP by the following:
    - Medical management including hyperosmotics if necessary
    - It is mandatory to perform a B-scan ultrasound to rule out a posterior mass lesion.
    - Then one may proceed to a semiurgent cataract extraction usually with good results. Theoretically, an intracapsular technique (ICCE) may release less lens protein than an extracapsular technique (ECCE or phacoemulsification), but it is better that the surgeon use the technique with which he or she is most familiar.
- Prognosis
  - Good with lens removal

Lens-Particle Glaucoma

- Etiology
  - Lens-particle glaucoma (Figure 8-13) refers to elevated IOP due to cortical fragments blocking the meshwork, usually following cataract surgery or trauma.
- Signs/symptoms
  - These can be seen as small chunks of white material in the anterior chamber; small fragments may mimic the white blood cells seen in iritis but they are larger.
- Management
  - The condition may respond to medical management if
    - The pressure elevation is mild
    - The amount of lens material is small
    - However, the patient may require surgical removal of the fragments, especially if nucleus material is involved.

Phacoanaphylaxis

- Etiology
  - o Phacoanaphylaxis is a granulomatous uveitic response to liberated lens material.
  - o It may follow surgery or traumatic capsule rupture, with a latent period during which sensitization to lens protein occurs.
- Pathology
  - o The pathology is a zonal granulomatous inflammation surrounding the retained lens material that consists of the following:
    - ▪ Lens material
    - ▪ Polymorphonuclear cells
    - ▪ Epithelioid cells—lymphocytes, mononuclear cells, and giant cells
- Signs/symptoms
  - o The uveitis may be mild or intense, possibly with KP or a hypopyon being seen.
  - o Hypotony is actually more common than elevated IOP.
  - o Posterior synechiae may develop and lead to angle closure.
- Differential diagnosis
  - o Other lens-associated glaucomas
  - o Other granulomatous uveitis, such as sympathetic ophthalmia, or infective endophthalmitis
- Management
  - o The initial medical management requires the following:
    - ▪ Control of the IOP and the inflammation
    - ▪ Surgical removal of all lens material is definitive—a posterior approach may be necessary
- Prognosis
  - o More guarded, aggressive management required

Elevated Episcleral Venous Pressure

- Etiology
  - o Elevated episcleral venous pressure (EVP) results in elevated IOP.
  - o The Goldmann equation is as follows:
    - ▪ $IOP = (F)/(C) + Pv$
      - □ Where
        - • F = aqueous formation
        - • C = outflow facility
        - • Pv = EVP
  - o The IOP increases almost 1:1 with increases in the EVP. The average EVP is 8 to 12 mm Hg, but measurement of the EVP is difficult and not in general clinical use.
  - o Episcleral veins
    - ▪ Lie deep to the conjunctiva
    - ▪ Do not blanch with phenylephrine
    - ▪ Do not move with a cotton-tipped applicator
  - o Causes of elevated EVP include the following:
    - ▪ Venous obstruction such as the following:
      - □ Superior vena cava syndrome
      - □ Thyroid ophthalmopathy
      - □ Retrobulbar tumors
      - □ Congestive heart failure
    - ▪ Arteriovenous abnormalities such as the following:
      - □ Sturge-Weber syndrome (Figure 8-14)
        - • A systemic condition in which ocular involvement with an abnormal plexus of episcleral vessels can result in glaucoma in one-third of cases
      - □ Carotid-cavernous fistula
      - □ Dural-cavernous fistula
      - □ Cavernous sinus thrombosis
      - □ Orbital varix

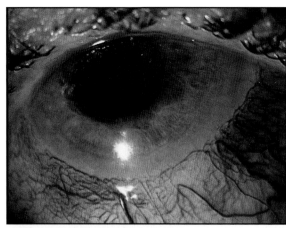

Figure 8-14. Sturge-Weber conjunctiva.

- Signs/symptoms
  - A patient with elevated EVP will present with a chronic red eye that may be either unilateral or bilateral depending on the cause.
    - Findings may include the following:
      - Conjunctival chemosis
      - Proptosis
      - Dilated episcleral veins
      - Limited motility of the extraocular muscles
      - Blood in Schlemm's canal is sometimes seen on gonioscopy
    - There will be some degree of elevated IOP.
    - An ocular bruit can sometimes be auscultated.
  - The etiology of a carotid-cavernous fistula is 75% traumatic and 25% idiopathic.
    - Low-flow fistulas are due to a dural-cavernous connection.
    - High-flow fistulas are due to a carotid-cavernous connection. Head trauma is typically associated with high-flow fistulas.
    - Signs and symptoms can be bilateral, but the fistula is usually unilateral.
    - There may be a bruit audible to the patient as a swooshing sound.
    - The globe may pulsate due to arterialization of the venules that may give strongly pulsing mires on tonometry.
    - Imaging may show an enlarged superior ophthalmic vein or enlarged extraocular muscles.
- Management
  - The work-up of elevated EVP includes the following:
    - A complete ocular, medical, and family history
    - A complete eye exam
    - Neuroimaging such as magnetic resonance imaging (MRI) or magnetic resonance angiogram (MRA) is used to investigate for a tumor or dilated superior ophthalmic vein.
      - If present, a neuroradiological procedure for angiography with possible embolization may be requested.
  - Miotics and prostaglandin agents are less effective than aqueous suppressants for management of elevated IOP.
  - Laser trabeculoplasty is usually ineffective.
  - There is a high risk of choroidal effusions and hemorrhage with trabeculectomy. The surgeon may decide to use prophylactic sclerostomies to decrease this risk.
  - If the underlying cause can be treated, embolization may be curative.
- Prognosis
  - Variable depending on the etiology

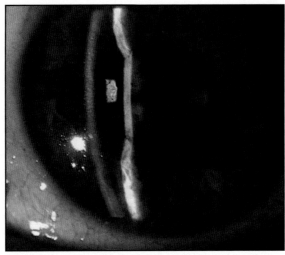

Figure 8-15. Angle closure with iris bombé.

Acute Angle Closure

- Angle-closure patients may be classified in the following ways:
  - ○ Suspects—narrow angles, normal exam otherwise
  - ○ Angle-closure—closed angles, elevated IOP
  - ○ ACG—documented optic nerve and/or visual field changes
- Acute angle closure may be subdivided into the following 2 mechanisms:
  - ○ Primary (with or without pupil block)
  - ○ Secondary (with or without pupil block)

Primary Angle Closure With Pupil Block

- Also known as *acute glaucoma* although the term *glaucoma* should be reserved for situations in which optic nerve and/or visual field changes have been documented
- Etiology
  - ○ Develops when a functional block occurs at the pupil with contact between iris and lens preventing aqueous flow from the posterior to anterior chamber
  - ○ The iris is pushed into an "iris bombé" configuration where the peripheral iris tissue blocks the TM and obstructs aqueous outflow (Figure 8-15).
- Signs/symptoms
  - ○ Signs
    - ▪ Conjunctival hyperemia
    - ▪ Corneal edema
    - ▪ A shallow anterior chamber
    - ▪ Poorly reactive or nonreactive pupil in a mid-dilated position
    - ▪ Closed angle on gonioscopy
    - ▪ Very high IOP (typically over 50 mm Hg)
  - ○ Symptoms
    - ▪ Halos and rainbows around lights, particularly at night or in dark conditions
    - ▪ Blurred central vision
    - ▪ Red eye
    - ▪ Ocular and periocular pain
    - ▪ Nausea and vomiting
- There are variable degrees of primary angle closure on the spectrum of severity and timing.
  - ○ Narrow-angle configuration is characterized with the following:
    - ▪ Narrow angles on gonioscopy
    - ▪ Normal IOP
      - □ No evidence of damage

- Primary ACG has the following:
  - Narrow angles on gonioscopy
  - Signs of disc or field damage (as seen with POAG)
- Acute-angle closure characteristically has the following:
  - High IOP
  - Classic signs and symptoms (below) but not necessarily nerve damage
- Subacute ACG has the following:
  - Mild to nonexistent symptoms
  - Repeated mild attacks may occur
  - IOP may be normal between the attacks, but eventually the patient may have a classic acute attack or develop chronic angle closure secondary to formation of peripheral anterior synechiae (PAS).
- Chronic angle closure is also known as creeping angle closure, where PAS formation occurs and pressure becomes chronically elevated.
  - If this occurs slowly, the IOP may be extremely high (>60 mm Hg) with no symptoms and no corneal edema.
- Mixed mechanism glaucoma is diagnosed
  - After an angle-closure attack where a PI is performed and the angle opens but the IOP remains elevated, indicating a chronic problem with outflow.
  - This may have predated the angle-closure attack.
  - The patient is then managed as an open-angle glaucoma patient.
- Plateau iris configuration/syndrome refers to primary angle closure without pupil block and will be discussed later.

- Angle-closure risk factors
  - Certain risk factors are associated with the possibility of developing angle closure.
    - The most important risk factor is increasing age with concomitant thickening of the lens.
    - Hyperopes have a much higher risk than myopes with 5% to 6% having narrow angles. However, only about 1% have critically narrow angles requiring treatment.
    - In myopes with narrow angles, one should look for spherophakia, or a displaced lens.
    - Racial factors are also important with people of Inuit or Asian race having a higher incidence.
    - Family members may have an increased risk of a narrow angle, but this may not predict an actual ACG attack.
    - Angle closure is more common in women, probably due to a slightly more shallow anterior chamber.
  - Precipitating factors include the following:
    - Dim illumination
    - Emotional stress
    - Medications—most commonly anticholinergics and adrenergic, miotics rarely
    - The position of the iris that most predisposes to angle closure is the mid-dilated position, so anything that dilates the pupil can precipitate an attack.

- Management
  - The first step in management is to acutely lower the IOP.
    - Aqueous suppression is used first.
    - Hyperosmotic agents are the most effective at rapidly drawing water out of the vitreous and lowering the IOP.
    - Pupil constriction is also required to pull the iris out of the angle and open the meshwork (1 to 2 drops of pilocarpine 2% or 4%).
    - If the patient is too nauseated to tolerate the oral glycerol, then intravenous mannitol should be given.
  - The definitive treatment is a laser PI (see the laser section) (Figure 8-16).
    - This opens a channel for aqueous flow between the posterior chamber and the anterior chamber and bypasses the pupil block. The iris bombé relaxes and the angle opens.
    - In rare situations when a laser iridotomy cannot be performed, a surgical iridectomy must be done. However, surgically opening an eye with a high pressure is risky and should be avoided where possible.

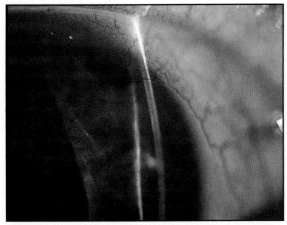

Figure 8-16. Laser peripheral iridotomy.

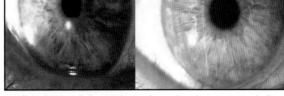

Figure 8-17. Penlight test—(A) deep chamber and (B) shallow anterior chamber.

- Should the PI fail to normalize the IOP, then medical management for chronic (mixed mechanism) glaucoma is instituted.
- Filtration surgery is used when all else fails.
- Other options for treatment of acute glaucoma are less standard, but include the following:
  - Laser gonioplasty
  - Paracentesis
  - Cataract extraction
  - Goniosynechialysis
- Prevention
  - An important component to the management of the acute glaucoma patient is prevention by recognition of the patient at risk by history.
  - In all cases where one eye has had an attack, avoidance of medications with sympathomimetic activity prior to laser is recommended.
  - Chronic pilocarpine treatment should be considered if laser is not possible.
  - It is important to first recognize the narrow angle by examination.
    - Penlight at the bedside (Figure 8-17)
      - Look for a shadow cast on the nasal iris by a prominent central iris bulge.
    - The Von Herrick test at the slit lamp
      - Look at the peripheral anterior chamber depth and if it is less than one-quarter of the peripheral corneal thickness, the angle may be dangerously narrow.
    - Suspicious findings should be confirmed using gonioscopy.
  - A PI to the fellow eye after an acute attack is mandatory, and a prophylactic iridotomy to both eyes is recommended when an angle is potentially occludable, even in the absence of symptoms.
  - Provocative tests are rarely used as they lack sufficient sensitivity or specificity. These include the following:
    - Use of a short acting mydriatic (ie, 0.5% tropicamide)
    - The dark room test, with 60 to 90 minutes awake in the dark
    - The prone position test, with the patient positioned face down for 60 minutes
    - A positive result is considered to be over 8 mm Hg pressure rise with gonioscopic confirmation of closure.

Primary Angle Closure Without Pupil Block (Plateau Iris)

- Also known as plateau iris (Figure 8-18)
- Etiology
  - Classically defined as angle closure in the presence of a patent iridotomy
  - Ultrasound biomicroscopy (UBM) has shown that the ciliary sulcus is closed in these patients, with the peripheral iris held forward by the first ciliary process, so that upon pupillary dilation the iris may crowd into the angle and close the TM to outflow.

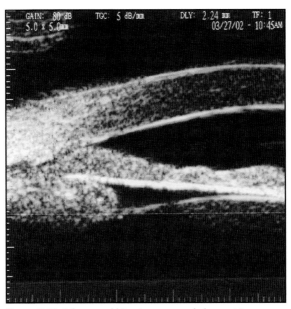

Figure 8-18. Ultrasound biomicroscopy of plateau iris.

- ○ Plateau iris can be separated into the following:
  - ▪ Plateau iris configuration—where the IOP does not rise with dilation
  - ▪ Plateau iris syndrome—where, despite a patent PI, pupillary dilation causes angle closure
    - ▫ Typically, plateau syndrome shows a closed angle with a flat iris (no bombé) and relatively deep central anterior chamber.
- Signs/symptoms
  - ○ Similar to those of primary ACG
- Management
  - ○ The configuration may only need observation.
  - ○ If the syndrome exists
    - ▪ Chronic pilocarpine can be used to prevent full dilation
    - ▪ An iridoplasty may be performed (see the laser treatment section)

Secondary Angle Closure With Pupil Block

- Etiology
  - ○ Posterior synechiae, usually from iritis
  - ○ Miotic induced
  - ○ Intumescent lens
  - ○ Subluxed/dislocated lens
  - ○ Spherophakia
- Signs/symptoms
  - ○ Secondary angle closure with pupil block may present in a fashion similar to primary, but there is some identifiable cause for the pupil block such as
    - ▪ Adhesions from iritis
    - ▪ Intumescent lens
- Management
  - ○ If it is possible to perform a laser iridotomy, it may solve the problem.
  - ○ However, it may be more difficult to produce an adequate and patent iridotomy in an inflamed iris.
  - ○ In this case, pretreatment with the argon laser may be very helpful.

Secondary Angle Closure Without Pupil Block

- Etiology
  - The secondary angle closures without pupil block are divided into those with an anterior pulling or posterior pushing mechanisms.
  - Can be due to anterior pulling or posterior pushing mechanisms that bring the iris tissue into the angle. These include the following:
    - Anterior pulling
      - Neovascular glaucoma
      - Iridiocorneal endothelial syndrome
      - Epithelial downgrowth
      - Penetrating keratoplasty
      - Aniridia
    - Posterior pushing
      - Ciliary block
      - Iris/CB cysts
      - Tumors
      - Suprachoroidal hemorrhage
      - Scleral buckle/intravitreal gas

Neovascular Glaucoma

- Neovascular glaucoma (Figure 8-19) is one of the most important causes of anterior pulling mechanisms.
- Etiology
  - The causes of neovascular glaucoma include anything that will produce ischemia of the posterior segment and liberation of vascular endothelial growth factor (VEGF).
  - The most common of these include the following:
    - Diabetes
    - CRVO with ischemia
    - Carotid insufficiency
    - Various other intraocular and vascular disorders
- Signs/symptoms
  - Rubeosis iridis presents
    - First at the pupil edge and in the angle, or at the edge of an iridotomy—wherever aqueous concentrates
    - It forms a fibrovascular membrane, which grows over the TM and blocks filtration.
    - Later, contraction pulls iris tissue into the angle and closes it irreversibly with PAS.
    - Ectropion uveae at the pupil may be seen due to contraction of the membrane.
    - With a gradual onset of elevated pressure, there may be no symptoms of pain and no corneal edema. Visual function depends on the underlying pathology.
- Management
  - The first line of treatment is
    - Aqueous suppression with
      - β-blockers
      - α-agonists
      - Carbonic anhydrase inhibitors
    - Laser panretinal photocoagulation to ablate the ischemic retina is mandatory.
    - Avoid pilocarpine as the meshwork is blocked, and pilocarpine will decrease uveoscleral outflow.
    - Because there is no pupil block, laser PI is not helpful.
    - If there is potential for useful vision, filtration surgery will usually be necessary.
    - If the eye is nearly blind, then a palliative cycloablative procedure may be preferable (see laser section).
    - Prevention of the disease involves early identification of patients at risk and early and aggressive panretinal photocoagulation prior to angle closure.

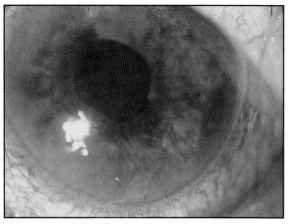

Figure 8-19. Neovascular glaucoma.

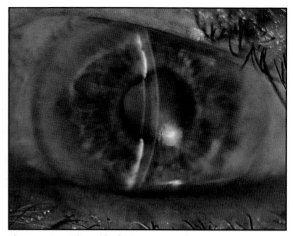

Figure 8-20. Ciliary block/aqueous misdirection.

Ciliary Block Glaucoma

- Ciliary block glaucoma is the most important glaucoma due to a secondary nonpupil block posterior pushing mechanism. It is known by multiple other terms, including
  - Malignant glaucoma
  - Aqueous misdirection
  - Vitreociliary block
  - Ciliolenticular glaucoma
  - Vitreous entrapment/displacement glaucoma
- Etiology
  - The risk of ciliary block is increased in patients who
    - Are hyperopic
    - Have a shallow anterior chamber
    - Are on miotic therapy
    - Have had a high IOP presurgery
  - The condition may be due to
    - Shallow CB detachment
    - CB rotation
    - Ciliovitreal block with aqueous misdirection into the vitreous (Figure 8-20)
  - Postulated mechanisms include
    - Forward movement of vitreous/lens/iris
    - In small eyes, vitreous contacts more of lens and CB, leaving less area for aqueous diffusion.
    - The lens also moves forward, increasing pupil block, and as the IOP increases, less aqueous moves across vitreous face producing a vicious cycle.
    - Smaller eyes have thicker sclera, which reduces trans-scleral fluid movement, increasing the risk.
- Signs/symptoms
  - Ciliary block glaucoma is almost always seen following glaucoma surgery.
    - It typically has a very shallow or flat anterior chamber, both centrally and peripherally (ie, not iris bombé).
    - It typically has elevated IOP.
    - It responds to mydriatic/cycloplegic therapy but not miotic.
- Differential diagnosis
  - Pupillary block
  - Suprachoroidal hemorrhage
  - Serous choroidal detachment
  - Other causes are relatively rare.
    - A suprachoroidal hemorrhage is usually painful and is diagnosed with a B-scan while serous choroidals usually have a low IOP.
    - Anterior serous choroidals can be diagnosed with UBM.

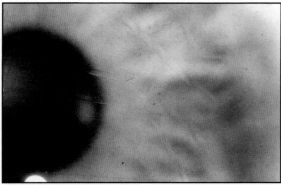

Figure 8-21. Haab's striae.

- Treatment
  - Medical treatment is the first line.
    - Intense cycloplegia, with multiple mydriatics (Tropicamide, Cyclogyl, and Atropine) used every 15 minutes for an hour, then 4 times daily
    - Aqueous suppression and hyperosmotics are used as necessary for IOP control. Medical management has an approximately 50% success rate.
    - If after 5 to 7 days of intense cycloplegia the anterior chamber is not deepening, then further treatment is required.
      - Laser treatment—a YAG hyaloidectomy in an aphakic or pseudophakic patient (see the laser section)
      - Surgical treatment, usually a pars plana vitrectomy and anterior chamber reformation

Developmental Glaucoma

- The types of developmental, or childhood, glaucoma may be categorized according to age of onset.
  - Congenital glaucoma occurs in infants less than 3 months old and may be primary, secondary, or associated with a syndrome.
  - Infantile glaucoma usually occurs between 3 months and 3 years of age.
  - Juvenile glaucoma occurs between 3 and 35 years of age.
- Clinical findings
  - Infants with congenital glaucoma typically present with a triad of
    - Photophobia
    - Epiphora
    - Blepharospasm
  - Children younger than 3 years old may also present with
    - Corneal clouding
    - Associated buphthalmos
    - Enlarged corneas
  - Presentation after 3 years old tends to be asymptomatic with
    - Progressive myopia
    - Insidious visual field loss
  - Classic features of primary congenital glaucoma include the following:
    - IOP >21 mm Hg
    - C:D ratio >0.3
    - Reversible cupping
    - Buphthalmos
    - Enlarged cornea diameter >13 mm
    - Corneal edema with Haab's striae (horizontal Descemet's rupture) (Figure 8-21)
    - Limbal ectasia
    - Zonular stretching leading to lens subluxation

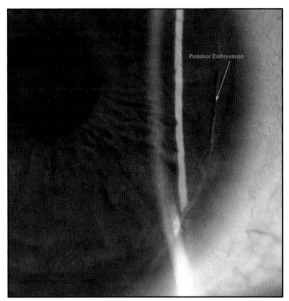

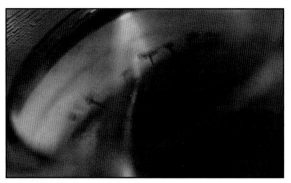

Figure 8-22B. Axenfeld-Reiger syndrome—Iris processes.

Figure 8-22A. Axenfeld-Reiger syndrome—Posterior embryo-toxin.

- Gonioscopy reveals poorly recognized angle structures due to the following:
  - Anterior iris insertion above the scleral spur
  - Thickening of the TM
  - Peripheral iris hypoplasia
  - It was once postulated that "Barkan's membrane" covered the TM. However, no histological evidence has supported this, and it may be due to anterior insertion of the iris causing diminished outflow.
- Ocular features that may be associated with congenital glaucoma include the following:
  - Microcornea
  - Cornea plana
  - Sclerocornea
  - Axenfeld-Reiger syndrome (Figure 8-22A and B)
  - Peters' anomaly
  - Microspherophakia
  - Nanophthalmos
  - Persistent hyperplastic primary vitreous
  - Retinopathy of prematurity
  - Intraocular tumors (retinoblastoma, juvenile xanthogranuloma)
- Systemic syndromes associated with congenital glaucoma include the following:
  - Sturge-Weber syndrome
  - Neurofibromatosis Type 1
  - Marfan's syndrome
  - Weil-Marchesani syndrome
  - Lowe's oculocerebrorenal syndrome
  - Hallerman-Streiff
  - Trisomy 13
  - Stickler's syndrome
  - Mucopolysaccharidosis
- Management
  - Most children require examination under anesthesia for a complete examination.
  - Be aware that certain agents like ketamine and succinylcholine may raise the IOP while general anesthetics (halothane, thiopental, barbiturates, and tranquilizers) may lower IOP.

- A complete exam under anesthesia includes the following
  - IOP measurement (Perkins/Tono-Pen)
  - Portable slit-lamp exam
  - Corneal diameter measurement
  - Gonioscopy
  - Ophthalmoscopy
  - Retinoscopy
- Definitive management is surgical while medications may be used to temporize in the meantime. Surgical options include the following:
  - Goniotomy (ab interno)—Usually performed in cases where the cornea is clear enough to visualize the angle or in children younger than 1.5 years of age.
  - Trabeculotomy (ab externo)—Usually the procedure of choice if goniotomy fails twice, the cornea is hazy, or if the child is older than 1.5 years.
  - Goniotomies and trabeculotomies have approximately a 77% success rate.
  - If both fail, then one can consider a trabeculectomy with mitomycin C, drainage implant, or cycloablation of the CB as a last resort.

Diagnosis of Glaucoma

- The diagnosis of glaucoma is not necessarily easy. One begins with a full ocular history and physical examination. It is important to keep in mind that POAG patients are often asymptomatic. The best corrected visual acuity is taken (and the refraction noted), but the early effect of glaucoma on vision is nothing. The IOP measurement is critical, as higher pressure equals higher risk, but normal pressure does not rule out glaucoma.

Ocular History

- The central portions of the ocular history include the following:
  - Patient demographics such as
    - Age
    - Gender
    - Occupation
    - Race or birthplace
      - Note that self-reporting of race is very inexact
  - Prior ocular history
    - History of ocular trauma
    - Laser treatment
    - Surgery
  - If the patient is using glaucoma drops, record what is currently used as well as what has been tried in the past.
  - Prior medical history
    - Cardiovascular conditions
    - Vasospasm
    - Diabetes
    - Asthma
    - Oral medications used
  - Family history (with particular attention to a known glaucoma diagnosis and in whom)
  - Record of known drug allergies or adverse reactions to both oral and topical medications

Clinical Examination

- Given the asymptomatic nature of much of glaucoma, it is not unreasonable to state that all patients have glaucoma until proven otherwise.
- The clinical examination is used
  - To perform a risk assessment based on IOP and other risk factors
  - To classify the glaucoma (if any) based on gonioscopy and other anterior segment findings
  - To stage the disease based on optic nerve and field changes

Vision

- Best-corrected distance acuity is required for all glaucoma examinations.
- Knowledge of the patient's refractive status is also mandatory, as the glaucoma risks are different for myopes and hyperopes.

Intraocular Pressure

- The IOP should be measured at each visit. IOP is considered to be the major risk factor for the diagnosis of glaucoma, and IOP control has been shown to improve the likelihood of glaucoma progression.
- Applanation tonometry is based on the Imbert-Fick law:
  - $W = Pt \times A$
- Force equals the pressure within sphere x area flattened. This formula was adapted for a central corneal thickness (CCT) of 500 μm, which is slightly less than the ultrasonic average of 540 μm. The area flattened by the prism is 3.06 mm to balance the surface tension of tears.
  - Applanation tonometry errors can include the following:
    - Use of too much fluorescein, giving wide menisci and a falsely high reading
    - Uneven semicircles from poor vertical placement on cornea giving falsely high reading
    - A structurally thick cornea giving a falsely high reading (see pachymetry section)
    - An edematous thick cornea (or loose laser in situ keratomileusis [LASIK] flap) will give a falsely low reading
    - Astigmatism correction is necessary for higher degrees of corneal astigmatism, as there is about 1 mm Hg error per 4 D of astigmatism. This can be minimized by rotating the prism until the red line is aligned to the flatter axis of the astigmatic ellipse. Noncontact tonometry uses a puff of room air to deform the cornea, which is measured optically and is calibrated against Goldmann applanation.
  - The time of the test should be recorded, as diurnal variation is extremely important.
  - Goldmann applanation tonometry is the current gold standard for IOP measurement.
    - Other techniques should be used only when necessary.
  - Target IOP levels are chosen based on optic nerve and visual field parameters.

Gonioscopy

- Gonioscopy is a major part of the clinical examination of the glaucoma patient. However, the anterior chamber angle cannot be directly viewed due to the phenomenon of total internal reflection at the tear film-air interface. Gonioscopy alters the critical angle by changing the tear film-air interface to a cornea-glass one. Several goniolenses are used in clinical practice.
  - The Koeppe goniolens is a direct viewing lens and is used with a binocular viewer and a light source, but the patient must be lying down.
  - Mirror lenses are all indirect viewers, allowing one to see into the opposite quadrant of the angle and can be used at the slit lamp.
    - The 3-mirror Goldmann lens is in common use
    - Indentation lenses such as the Sussman have a small face to allow artificial deepening of the chamber through compression to rule out PAS in narrow-angle situations.
  - Once viewed, the angle must be classified, and several systems exist.
- Scheie classification:
  - Grade I = Wide open (CB visible)
  - Grade II = Scleral spur visible (CB not visible)
  - Grade III = Only anterior TM visible
  - Grade IV = Closed angle (TM not visible)
- Shaffer classification:
  - 0 = Closed angle
  - I = Potentially closable/narrow slit; Schwalbe's line and TM are visible but not scleral spur or deeper structures; a PI is indicated
  - II = A narrow, potentially closable angle; scleral spur may be visible with manipulation, ie, indentation gonioscopy; a PI may be indicated
  - III = The average angle is of this depth; scleral spur and CB easily visible
  - IV = The angle is wider than normal (ie, in an aphake or high myope)

- Spaeth classification (4 elements):
  - First element
    - A = Anterior to TM
    - B = Behind Schwalbe's line or at TM
    - C = At scleral spur
    - D = Deep angle, CB visible
    - E = Extremely deep, large CB band
  - Second element
    - Number that denotes the iridocorneal angle width from 5 to 45 degrees
  - Third element
    - r = regular (flat)
    - s = steep (convex)
    - q = queer (concave)
  - Fourth element
    - Pigmentation of posterior TM (graded 0 [none] to 4 [maximum])
- It is most important to be consistent in the use of any grading system, and one option is to simply record the deepest structure visualized in each quadrant, rather than using an indirect classification system that may be subject to ambiguity (eg, the Scheie and Shaffer classifications record the angle structures in the opposite direction).

Adjunctive Tests

- Imaging techniques
  - Analysis of the nerve fiber layer and the optic nerve has been greatly advanced over the past years by the availability of sophisticated imaging tools. These include scanning laser polarimetry, ocular coherence tomography (OCT), and scanning laser tomography.
- Scanning laser polarimetry—GDx
  - Polarized light is passed through the retinal nerve fiber layer (RNFL), where the microtubules of the tissue produce a shift in phase of the light, with the degree of retardation varying according to the RNFL thickness.
  - The original readings were affected by corneal polarization, but the newer machine incorporates a variable corneal compensation technique.
  - The machine calculates the likelihood of glaucoma and produces a numerical output, but has little ability to detect change over time.
- OCT
  - This machine measures the peripapillary NFL thickness for glaucoma detection and creates a cross-sectional image of the retina (up to 10 μm).
  - A diode mounted on a slit lamp beams infrared light through a fiberoptic Michelson interferometer at both the eye and a reference mirror.
  - The light reflected from the retina is compared to the light from the reference mirror and analyzed. From this, the tissue reflectivity and density can be determined.
  - The overall sensitivity and specificity are fair but there is yet no longitudinal data available. High-resolution OCT may improve the usefulness of this technique.
- Confocal scanning laser tomography—HRT
  - The HRT uses a combination of confocal microscopy and scanning laser ophthalmoscopy, using a 670-nm wavelength
  - Thirty-two to 64 reflectance images at increasing depth are used to build up a topographic analysis of the optic nerve.
  - The technique requires an arbitrary contour line to be placed by the operator on the false color image generated by the computer, and then the optic nerve and NFL parameters are determined by relationship to an arbitrary reference line.
  - The Moorfield's regression analysis gives information about glaucoma status, with the optic nerve being divided into 6 sectors and each compared to a normal database. The sectors are determined as being normal, borderline (outside the 99% confidence interval), or outside normal (less than the 99.9% confidence interval).
  - A progression probability analysis gives information about change from the baseline scan, determined on a pixel-by-pixel basis, whenever there is change present in 3 successive subsequent scans.

Pachymetry

- Pachymetry, or measurement of CCT, has become important in glaucoma care.
  - ○ The original design of the Goldmann applanator was based on an assumption that the average thickness of the central corneal is 500 μm
  - ○ The ultrasonic mean CCT is about 540 μm but was higher at 573 μm in the Ocular Hypertension Treatment Study (OHTS) population (see the OHTS discussion); however, measured CCT actually varies very widely.
  - ○ Racial differences in corneal thickness exist, with African Americans tending to have a thinner cornea than Caucasians.
  - ○ IOP, as measured by applanation, is affected by thicknesses over or under the 500 μm used by Goldmann applanation.
  - ○ Estimates of correction factors for this vary widely.
    - ▪ Ehlers has estimated 7 mm Hg per 100 μm
    - ▪ Whiteman estimated 2 mm Hg per 100 μm
    - ▪ From the OHTS, a CCT less than 545 μm led to a higher risk of progression, while a CCT greater than 588 μm was associated with a lower risk.

Visual Field Testing in Glaucoma

- Visual field (VF) testing is done to determine and quantify any loss of peripheral visual function.
  - ○ Glaucomatous damage usually occurs in the midperiphery and is asymptomatic in the early stages—significant axon loss can occur prior to changes in automated field testing.
  - ○ VF testing by any technique that the clinician is comfortable with is a necessary adjunct to the diagnosis and management of the glaucoma patient.
  - ○ New technology aims to increase the accuracy of VF testing, but results must always be interpreted within the individual clinical situation.
- VF physiology
  - ○ The size of the normal VF extends
    - ▪ 60 degrees superiorly
    - ▪ 75 degrees inferiorly
    - ▪ 100 degrees temporally
    - ▪ 60 degrees nasally
  - ○ Most commercial perimeters test the central 24 or 30 degrees, where damage is most often seen.
  - ○ The retinal NFL has 3 major parts.
    - ▪ The papillomacular bundle, which runs from the fovea to the temporal disc and consists of 65% of the retinal NFL
    - ▪ The superior and inferior nasal radiating fibers
    - ▪ The superior and inferior arcuate fibers, which arc around the papillomacular bundle to converge on the superior and inferior disc. These fibers form the horizontal raphe and are the most susceptible to glaucomatous damage.
- VF technologies
  - ○ The most common technique used in perimetry is white-on-white full-threshold testing, lately modified by Swedish Interactive Threshold Algorithm (SITA) technology. Blue-on-yellow testing and frequency doubling testing are also important options.
- White-on-white full-threshold/SITA
  - ○ The most common perimeter in glaucoma care is the Humphrey Field Analyzer (Figure 8-23)
    - ▪ The Humphrey is usually used with the 24-2 or 30-2 program. A peripheral 30/60 test and central 10-2 can also be used.
    - ▪ The first number refers to the degrees out from fixation tested.
    - ▪ The second number specifies that the test points are offset from the vertical and horizontal meridian.
    - ▪ The test points are
      - □ 6 degrees apart for the 24 and 30 tests
      - □ 12 degrees apart for the 30/60 test
      - □ 2 degrees apart for the 10-2 test

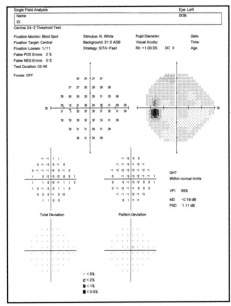

Figure 8-23. Humphrey Visual Field printout.

- Perimetric parameters
  - The standard spot size is referred to as Stimulus III, which subtends 0.43 degrees or 4 mm^2.
  - Occasionally needed is Stimulus V, which subtends 1.72 degrees or 64 mm^2.
  - The dynamic range of the machine extends from 0 dB (10,000 apostilb [asb]) to 40 dB (1 asb).
  - The background illumination is 31.5 asb for Goldmann and Humphrey perimeters.
- Heading
  - The first information on the printout of the Humphrey VF includes the following:
    - The test type (ie, 24-2)
    - The patient's name, age, and birth date
    - The fixation target—central spot versus peripheral diamond
    - The refraction used
    - The pupil diameter (which is important if 2 mm or less)
- Reliability indices
  - Fixation losses are measured and flagged if over 20%.
    - Positive responses when the stimulus was placed in the expected position of the blind spot
    - Movement seen by a gaze tracker
    - Fixation losses may not be real if the blind spot is not where the machine plotted it (ie, due to poor head position)
  - False-positive errors are considered to be a response when no stimulus was given and is flagged if over 33%.
    - False-positive errors are common when the patient is working too fast or is "trigger happy."
    - They will elevate the field, masking a scotoma.
    - The MD will be falsely high.
    - False positives are the most important flag for reliability even if less than 33%.
  - False-negative errors represent no response to a stimulus 9 dB higher than the threshold determined at that point and are flagged if over 33%.
    - False negatives can be due to disease, fatigue, or a "functional" defect.
    - With fatigue, the earlier points will look better, giving a "cloverleaf pattern" to the gray scale.
    - High false negatives seen with disease in Stat Pac strategy may be due to variation within damaged areas of retina; high false-negative rates indicate fatigue more specifically with SITA.

- Gray scale and data plot
  - o The left hand "circle" gives the actual raw data in dB.
  - o The right hand "circle" is a representative "gray scale."
- Probability plots
  - o The circles with numbers are the total deviation plot and the pattern deviation.
  - o Below each of these are the probability plots, which give the probability that each value would occur in a normal age-matched population.
  - o Usually a negative number, the total deviation gives the deviation from the mean normal value of the threshold at that point.
  - o The pattern deviation resets the field with the most normal region adjusted to zero, to eliminate the effect of generalized field depression, such as from cataract.
- Global indices
  - o The global indices represent the overall VF.
    - The MD measures the overall sensitivity of the patient's hill of vision compared to age-matched controls.
      - □ Increased weight is given to points near the fovea.
      - □ Cataracts, other media opacities, small pupils, or poor refraction will give a uniform depression of the VF.
    - The pattern standard deviation (PSD) measures the shape of the hill of vision compared to age-matched controls.
      - □ Localized field defects lead to a high number on the PSD.
    - On Stat Pac printouts, 2 more indices are reported:
      - □ Short-term fluctuation (SF), which tests 10 points twice for consistency
      - □ Corrected pattern standard deviation (CPSD), which corrects the PSD for the effects of SF to eliminate the effect of patient inconsistency
- SITA
  - o SITA is a new program for producing a VF test. It has the same reliability as the older VF thresholding techniques, but takes approximately half the time. Five major techniques are used to decrease test time, including the following:
    - VF modeling
    - An information index to determine endpoints
    - Patient responsive test pacing
    - Post-test recalculation of threshold values
    - Inferential calculations to determine reliability indices rather than specific "catch trials"
  - o To estimate thresholds, SITA uses the following:
    - Bayesian statistics
    - A maximum-likelihood test strategy
    - Probability density functions from normal and glaucoma subjects to generate a frequency of seeing curve
    - Analysis of adjacent points
    - Post-test processing
  - o The model is based on frequency of seeing curves and updates as the test proceeds.
    - It uses all the responses made by the patient during the test, not just the last 2, to calculate the threshold.
    - It is sensitive to typical glaucoma defects.
    - The model uses previously established age-corrected models of normal and glaucomatous VFs, and a probability function is adjusted continuously during the test.
    - The program calculates an "information index" that assesses just how "sure" the threshold estimate is, based on consistency of the patients' responses at each test site and between adjacent sites.
      - □ When consistency is high, the index is reached quickly and testing stops at that location, saving test time.
      - □ The index is reached more quickly in SITA Fast than in SITA Standard, resulting in still shorter test times but with slightly less reliability.

- The program also observes the patient's response time and presents stimuli based on updated response time averages and standard deviations.
  - This allows slow patients more time, but fast responders can go more quickly, saving test time and matching test characteristics to patient needs.
- Postprocessing is the final step.
  - During testing, threshold estimates are made in real time based on the information received so far, and after testing, all the responses are recalculated.
  - Responses that fall outside the calculated response window (either too soon or too late) are considered false and not used for the final threshold estimate.
- Fewer catch trials are needed.
  - False-positive trials are not needed at all, as postprocessing calculates this statistic.
  - Few false-negative trials are required as information from the up and down staircase responses is also used. When done, the 9 dB suprathreshold stimulus is placed within the most normal part of the field to reduce short-term variation found in diseased retina.
  - Fixation losses are calculated by a gaze tracker.
- A 24-2 or 30-2 SITA Standard can be used for almost all clinical situations.
  - SITA Fast is useful when a very short test time is desired.
- The range of normal is tighter so that both SITA Standard and SITA Fast detect milder defects than StatPac full-threshold tests, and the SITA printout includes a Glaucoma Hemifield Test (GHT) analysis.
- Blue-on-yellow testing or short wavelength automated perimetry (SWAP)
  - SWAP is also known as blue-on-yellow perimetry.
    - The background in the Ganzfield bowl is intense yellow, which bleaches the red and green cone pigments, leaving the blue cone system less affected.
    - The stimulus is blue, with a wavelength near the maximum sensitivity wavelength of the blue cones. The green cones respond to the same wavelength but with 15 dB less sensitivity so the blue cones are considered to be "isolated."
    - The blue cone system is "coarse," has a maximum visual acuity of 20/200, and is slow in response; therefore, the stimulus is large (size V) and appears to come on slowly.
      - The subjective effect for the patient is of a large and fuzzy drop that comes and goes slowly.
      - This is very different from achromatic field testing, and the patients should have this explained to them.
    - The low acuity means that the system is less affected by uncorrected refractive error, and refractive error will affect the green cones more than the blue ones, further increasing the isolation of the blue system.
      - Theoretically, yellowing of the ocular media (cataract) can interfere with the test results, but testing and adjusting for this has not proven realistic for clinical use and may not be clinically necessary.
    - SWAP has been reported to show glaucomatous defects earlier than white-on-white perimetry and also to show progression earlier.
    - SITA for SWAP is being developed and may increase the usefulness of the test in selected individuals, as the current test is lengthy.
    - Caveats to be aware of include the following:
      - A significant cataract may depress the field and mask local defects.
      - Test time is 15% longer than standard testing and there is more fatiguing due to the more difficult stimulus.
      - SWAP gray scale is darker than is seen in a standard printout, but the probability plots show the significance compared to the normal population.
      - SWAP range of normal is greater than in standard perimetry, so again one must look at the probability plots.
    - Generally, it is recommended to use SWAP where early detection would be useful in cases of significant glaucoma risk (ie, elevated pressure, anomalous discs, race) but with normal white-on-white perimetry.

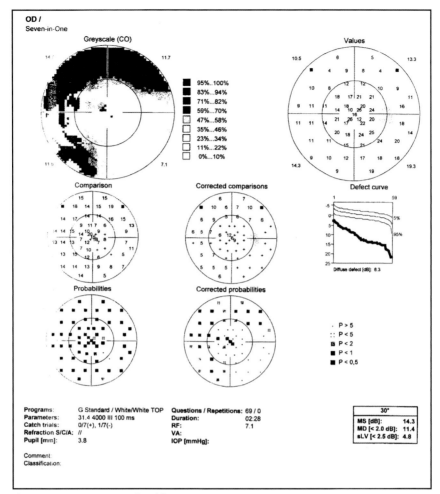

Figure 8-24. Octopus Visual Field printout.

- Octopus Field Analyzer
  - The Octopus Field Analyzer (Figure 8-24) provides most of the same information as is seen with the Humphrey, although with different names. The main parameter provided by the Octopus but not the Humphrey is the Bebie Curve.
    - This shows the deviations for each test point placed in order of rank, from most normal to most abnormal.
    - Expected normal limits are shown.
    - If the curve is normal in shape but depressed downward, it represents a general depression of field.
    - If the curve shows a dip at the right hand side, it suggests a local scotoma.
    - Note that this technique does not differentiate between significant and nonsignificant points (ie, between edge points and a central scotoma).
- Frequency doubling technology (FDT)
  - Frequency doubling perimetry (Figure 8-25) attempts to isolate the magnocellular pathway, thought to be more susceptible to early glaucomatous damage. The test takes advantage of a phenomenon that occurs when large and rapidly flickering bar stimuli are presented in the periphery.
    - The retina produces an illusion whereby twice as many bars are seen as are actually there.
    - In abnormal parts of the retina, the illusion is seen only when the contrast between the bars is higher than is needed by healthy retina.
    - The test can be used for screening, taking about 1.5 minutes, while full-threshold estimation takes 5 to 6 minutes per eye.

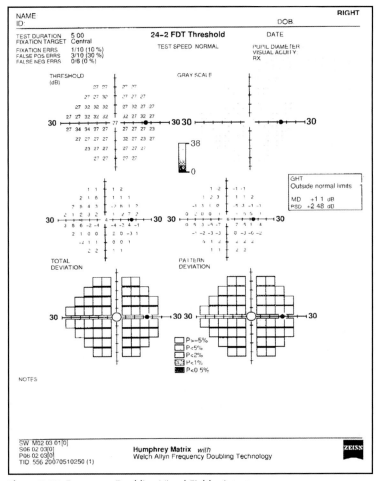

Figure 8-25. Frequency Doubling Visual Field printout.

- The sensitivity and specificity are fairly good, but a strong learning effect is often seen between first and second tests.
- The technique is unaffected by refractive errors of less than 3 D.
- Its usefulness for detection of progression is still unclear.
- The Humphrey Matrix FDT has stimulus patterns similar to SITA (ie, 24-2, 10-2) and includes rapid threshold estimation, fixation monitoring, and better data analysis than the first-generation FDT machines. It is a portable and rapid test and may be useful for screening, but as yet, FDT is not considered a standard technique for diagnosis or monitoring of disease.
- VF analysis
  - Any suggestion of a change in the VF should be confirmed with a second field to rule out patient variability, changes in pupil size, etc. A number of ways to determine an abnormal field exist, including the following:
    - An abnormal glaucoma hemifield test message
    - Three or more nonedge points, 2 of which are at the 5% and 1 at the 1% level on the pattern deviation plot
    - Three PSD points at the 5% level in a local area
    - An abnormal MD with absence of signs of a local defect, indicating a generalized depression
    - It is important to rule out artifacts from
      - The lens rim
      - Lids
      - Retinal disease
      - Fatigue, etc

- ○ The GHT assists in the decision as to whether a defect is significant. The GHT will give 1 of 5 messages:
    - ■ Normal
    - ■ Borderline
    - ■ Outside normal limits
    - ■ General reduction in sensitivity
    - ■ Abnormally high sensitivity
- ○ To look for progression:
    - ■ Find 3 new points at the 5% level
    - ■ A deeper defect of 10 dB worse than baseline
    - ■ An expanded defect with 2 new points 10 dB worse than baseline
    - ■ The Glaucoma Progression Analysis assists in the detection of significant change from baseline.
- Nonspecific VF changes
    - ○ Nonspecific field changes include the following:
        - ■ Baring of the blind spot
        - ■ Generalized constriction, which represents diffuse optic nerve damage
    - ○ Specific glaucomatous changes include ("PANTS")
        - ■ Paracentral defect (isolated) within 10 degrees of fixation
        - ■ Arcuate scotoma arcing from the blind spot
            - □ Also known as a Bjerrum scotoma
        - ■ Nasal step
        - ■ Temporal wedge (temporal island)
        - ■ Sector shape defect
        - ■ The most common presenting field defect is
            - □ An isolated paracentral defect (IPD) and a nasal step, seen in 51% of patients
            - □ About 26% of patients present with an IPD alone.
            - □ About 20% of patients present with a nasal step alone.
            - □ About 3% present with a sector defect only.
        - ■ It is important to remember that up to 50% of axons can be lost before a field defect is seen and that progressive cupping also occurs before field changes are seen.
- Follow up
    - ○ One field is not enough—2 are necessary to establish a baseline:
        - ■ If the first 2 are significantly different, repeat again
        - ■ If the follow-up fields are stable, accept them
        - ■ If follow-up fields show change, repeat
        - ■ The timing of follow-up fields depends on clinical need, but an annual test is recommended for glaucoma patients.
- Treatment
    - ○ Target pressure
        - ■ The concept of setting a target pressure is becoming standard in glaucoma management. Assessment requires the following:
            - □ The presenting IOP
            - □ Optic disc
            - □ VF status
    - ○ A level of treated IOP is then selected. This level may be an absolute figure for the desired pressure or a percent decrease from the maximum level known.
        - ■ Patients may be divided into treatment categories based on evidence from the multicenter trials (Table 8-2).
    - ○ Suspect
        - ■ IOP >22 mm Hg *or*
        - ■ Suspicious disc appearance or asymmetry >0.2 mm Hg *or*
        - ■ Suspicious VF
        - ■ Recommendation:
            - □ IOP <25 mm Hg or 20% from baseline (if treatment recommended)

TABLE 8-2. THE GLAUCOMA STUDIES: TAKE-HOME POINTS

Glaucoma Laser Trial (GLT)	Objective: • To compare efficacy in glaucoma eyes of initial treatment with ALT (laser first [LF]) versus medications first (MF) Conclusions: • Initial laser therapy is safe and effective. • Laser therapy will not guarantee medication not needed. • Laser therapy is a good option for patients noncompliant with medications. • Laser therapy may need to be supplemented with other procedures.
Fluorouracil Filtering Surgery Study (FFSS)	Objective: • Determine whether post-trabeculectomy injections of 5-FU increased the success rate of filtering surgery in high-risk eyes • Examine the safety of 5-FU injections Conclusions: • Use of 5-FU increased the success rate of filtration surgery in high-risk eyes.
Collaborative Initial Glaucoma Treatment Study (CIGTS)	Objective: • Examine long-term outcome of medical therapy versus primary trabeculectomy as initial therapy in newly diagnosed glaucoma patients Conclusions: • Initial medical treatment was as effective as initial surgical treatment. • Initial medical treatment has a better risk-benefit ratio. • Initial medical treatment is reasonable for most patients with mild to moderate disease.
Advanced Glaucoma Intervention Study (AGIS)	Objective: • Compare sequence of laser and surgery in eyes that have failed medical treatment for glaucoma (ALT-Trab-Trab [ATT] versus Trab-ALT-Trab [TAT]) Conclusions: • ALT laser was more successful in African American patients • ATT better in African American patients • TAT better in Caucasian patients • IOP control improved VF stability
Normal Tension Glaucoma Study (NTGS)	Objective: • To determine whether lowering IOP by 30% in NTG patients reduced glaucoma progression Conclusions: • Observational management is satisfactory if fixation is not threatened, but follow up is mandatory. • Untreated patients were more likely to progress.

(continued)

TABLE 8-2. THE GLAUCOMA STUDIES: TAKE-HOME POINTS (CONTINUED)

Normal Tension Glaucoma Study (NTGS) (continued)	• 80% of treated patients were stable versus 40% of untreated patients. • Data were censored if cataract developed. • Damage required confirmatory VF tests (4/5). • Females were twice as likely to progress than males (not significant). • Migraines/vasospasm had 2.58 risk ratio. • Disc heme at presentation had 2.7 risk ratio.
Ocular Hypertension Treatment Study (OHTS)	Objectives: • Determine if lowering IOP prevents VF/ONH progression in ocular hypertensive patients • Determine risk factors for development of glaucoma in ocular hypertensive patients Conclusions: • Lowering IOP by 20% reduced the rate of POAG from 9.5% to 4.4%. • IOP and CCT (thinner) influenced the risk of developing glaucoma. • Age and C:D ratio were also good predictors of POAG development. • Risk was low in the first 5 years, even without treatment. • 90% of untreated patients were stable. • Treatment had little evidence of systemic or ocular risk. • 90% of abnormal fields could not be confirmed with repeat testing.

Early Manifest Glaucoma Trial (EMGT)	Objective:
	• To evaluate the role of immediate IOP lowering versus no or later treatment in patients with newly diagnosed open-angle glaucoma on field loss and nerve changes
	Conclusions:
	• Lowering IOP prevented VF progression.
	• Progression was less with treatment (45% in treated group versus 62% in untreated group).
	• Higher risk associated with certain characteristics:
	  • Higher baseline IOP
	  • Exfoliation
	  • Bilateral disease
	  • Worse mean defect
	  • Older age
	  • Frequent disc hemorrhage during follow up

- o Early glaucoma
  - Definite disc damage but <0.65
  - Definite field defect but not within 10 degrees of fixation
  - Recommendation:
    - □ 20% IOP reduction and/or <21 mm Hg
- o Moderate glaucoma
  - Moderate ONH changes—0.7 < C:D < 0.85
  - Moderate field defect but not within 10 degrees of fixation
  - Recommendation:
    - □ 30% IOP reduction and /or <18 mm Hg
- o Advanced glaucoma
  - Advanced ONH changes—C:D >0.9
  - Field defect within 10 degrees of fixation
  - Recommendation:
    - □ 30% IOP reduction and/or <15 mm Hg

Glaucoma Medications

- Topical medications for chronic use (see Chapter 4) fall into 5 categories:
  - o Prostaglandin agonists
  - o β-blockers
  - o α-agonists
  - o Carbonic anhydrase inhibitors
  - o Parasympathomimetics
- Combination therapy medications used to improve compliance and decrease preservative load generally consist of a β-blocker and 1 of the following:
  - o α-agonist
  - o Carbonic anhydrase inhibitor
  - o Prostaglandin agonist
- Oral agents are more often used for emergency situations.
  - o Oral carbonic anhydrase inhibitor
  - o Oral hyperosmotics
- An intravenous hyperosmotic (mannitol) is also available for emergency use.

Glaucoma Lasers

- Many different laser procedures are done for various indications in glaucoma care.
- The most common laser uses in glaucoma care are the following:
  - o Laser trabeculoplasty
    - Argon laser trabeculoplasty (ALT)
    - Selective laser trabeculoplasty (SLT)
  - o Argon laser
    - Iridoplasty
    - Iridotomy
    - Suture lysis
  - o Nd:YAG laser
    - PI
    - Iris adhesions
    - Hyaloid face
  - o Cyclodestruction

Laser Trabeculoplasty

- Indications
  - o Laser trabeculoplasty is indicated when
    - Drops are ineffective for reaching the set target IOP
    - Poor compliance affects care
    - The physician and patient are trying to avoid surgery

- o ALT
    - The original technique
    - A "hot" laser in which cells die and collagen contracts
- o SLT
    - A new version of laser angle surgery using a frequency-doubled Q-switched YAG laser
    - A fast "cool" laser in which the pigment within meshwork cells absorbs laser energy and kills the cell
- o Early studies suggest both techniques are equally effective, with a 75% to 80% response rate. The indications and techniques are similar.
- Technique
    - o Prelaser
        - An alpha-2 agonist, usually brimonidine, is given 5 to 30 minutes before the laser to provide prophylaxis against a laser-induced IOP rise.
    - o Laser
        - ALT settings
            - □ A Goldmann 3-mirror lens is applied after topical anesthesia.
            - □ Usually, the first treatment is applied to the inferior 180 degrees and the second to the superior 180 degrees.
            - □ The laser energy is adjusted according to the pigmentation of the angle.
            - □ The desired endpoint is
                - Slight blanching of the pigment
                - Formation of a small bubble
                - If a large bubble forms, the energy level should be decreased.
            - □ The typical laser settings are
                - Argon green or blue-green wavelength
                - 50-μm spot size
                - 0.1-second duration
                - 600 to 800 mW
                - 45 to 55 burns placed over 180 degrees
        - SLT settings
            - □ A Goldmann 3-mirror lens is applied after topical anesthesia.
            - □ Usually, the first treatment is applied to the inferior 180 degrees and the second to the superior 180 degrees.
            - □ The laser energy is adjusted according to the pigmentation of the angle.
            - □ The desired endpoint is
                - Formation of a shower of small bubbles, termed *champagne bubbles*
                - If large bubbles form, the energy level should be decreased.
            - □ The typical laser settings are
                - Frequency-doubled 532-nm YAG laser
                - 400-μm spot size
                - 0.000,000,000,3-second duration
                - 0.7 to 1.0 mJ
                - 45 to 55 burns placed over 180 degrees
- Complications
    - o Complications include the following:
        - Development of iritis
        - An IOP spike that may result in central fixation snuff-out
        - The treatment may be ineffective at adequately lowering the IOP

Argon Laser

- Argon laser iridoplasty
    - o Indications
        - In plateau iris configuration or syndrome, the argon laser may be used to shrink the iris stroma and open the angle. This technique uses low power settings.

- o Settings
    - ▪ 200-μm spot size
    - ▪ 0.2-second duration
    - ▪ 200 to 400 mW
    - ▪ Argon green or blue-green wavelength
    - ▪ 10 to 15 burns/quadrant, treating 120 to 180 degrees to start with
- Argon laser iridectomy
    - o Indications
        - ▪ If a YAG laser is not available, if there is a high-risk of bleeding, or in uveitic patients to pre-pare for a subsequent YAG punch-through, the argon may be used to create an iridotomy.
    - o Settings
        - ▪ 200-μm spot size
        - ▪ 0.02 sec
        - ▪ 500+ mW
        - ▪ 50-μm spot
        - ▪ 100+ burns in one location
- Argon laser suture lysis
    - o Indications
        - ▪ Following trabeculectomy, suture lysis may be performed
            - □ When a rise in IOP is detected
            - □ At any time
                - • Commonly after the first postoperative day in surgery without an antimetabolite
                - • One will usually attempt to wait a minimum of 1 week with antimetabolite use.
        - ▪ The effectiveness decreases as time after surgery increases.
    - o Technique
        - ▪ A suture lysis lens is used to compress the conjunctiva and improve the focus on the suture.
        - ▪ It is preferable to cut the suture just where it enters the sclera, so that the short cut end may retract under the sclera.
        - ▪ If the pressure is over 21 mm Hg, only one stitch should be cut, and then the IOP re-checked.
        - ▪ If the pressure is lower and a very low target is desired, it is possible to cut more than one stitch in a single sitting.
    - o Settings
        - ▪ 50-μm spot size
        - ▪ 0.1-second duration
        - ▪ 600 mW
        - ▪ Argon red wavelength

Neodymium Yttrium-Aluminium-Garnet Laser

- Indications
    - o The indications for a laser iridotomy, almost always done with the YAG, are the following:
        - ▪ An angle-closure attack
        - ▪ Production of an iridotomy in the contralateral eye of a patient with an angle-closure attack
        - ▪ Prophylactically in a patient with a potentially occludable angle
        - ▪ In a patient with plateau iris and a possible pupil block component
        - ▪ In pigment dispersion syndrome
        - ▪ To complete an imperforate iridotomy after a trabeculectomy
- Technique
    - o Prelaser
        - ▪ Pilocarpine 1% is instilled to constrict the pupil and put the iris on tension.
        - ▪ An α-2 agonist is used to lower the IOP.
    - o Laser
        - ▪ Some form of iridectomy lens such as the Abraham lens is applied after topical anesthesia is instilled.

- The optimum position for the iridotomy is under discussion; whether placement in the interpalpebral fissure or under the lid is preferable for reduction of the risk of post-treatment glare and diplopia.
- The desired endpoint is visualization of a patent iridotomy and a pigment plume coming forward (or backward).
  - Settings
    - Energy—3 to 8 mJ, depending on the iris and the laser—thicker irides require more energy
    - Burst mode is optional
    - 1064-nm wavelength
- Complications
  - Complications can include the following:
    - Hemorrhage
    - IOP spike
    - A corneal endothelial burn
    - A lens burn
    - A retinal burn
      - The latter 2 are relatively rare
- Other YAG uses
  - The YAG can be used to cut iris free from the ostomy, if it has become plugged after a trabeculectomy.
    - The technique uses a goniolens and similar settings to that of an iridotomy.
  - The YAG can be used to punch through the Descemet's window following nonpenetrating glaucoma surgery to improve filtration.
    - Settings similar to a PI may be used.
  - The YAG can be applied to the anterior hyaloid face to treat aqueous misdirection syndrome in a pseudophakic patient.
    - This uses a similar technique to that of a YAG capsulotomy with maximum defocus.
    - Disruption of the anterior hyaloid may allow aqueous to circulate into the anterior chamber and break the misdirection attack.

Cyclodestruction

- CB ablation can be performed with the following:
  - A contact YAG laser
  - A noncontact YAG laser
  - A diode laser
- The indications are
  - An elevated IOP in a blind painful eye
  - An eye without much pain but with corneal decompensation
  - A sighted nonsurgical candidate
- The aim is to
  - Ablate sufficient CB processes
  - Decrease aqueous inflow to the point that the remaining outflow capacity can normalize the IOP.
- IOP control is achieved in 80% of patients with one or more treatments.
- Loss of vision is reported in about 40% of patients, of which half is due to the underlying disease.
- Technique
  - Prelaser
    - A full retrobulbar block is required as this is a painful procedure.
    - A typical block might consist of 6 to 10 cc of a mixture of 2% xylocaine and 0.5% bupivicaine. Once the eye is anesthetized, the procedure can proceed.
  - Laser
    - The laser is applied to the limbus (10 shots per quadrant).
    - The settings vary between the 1064-nm YAG and the 810-nm diode lasers:
      - Continuous-wave Nd:YAG settings
        - Power: 7 to 8 watts
        - Location: 1 to 2 mm from limbus
        - Number: 40 spots over 360 degrees (sparing the anterior ciliary arteries)

□ Diode settings
- Power: 3 watts
- Location: 1.2 mm from limbus
- Number: 18 spots over 270 degrees
- Time: 1.3 seconds

o Postlaser
- Following the laser, the eye must be patched while blocked.
- Postlaser medications are prescribed at least 4 times daily:
  □ Pred Forte 1%
  □ Atropine 1%
  □ Acular 0.5%
  □ Tylenol #3 as needed for analgesia
- The patient should continue any previously used antiglaucoma medications until the effect of the laser is seen, with follow-up checks at 1 week and 1 month.

- Complications
  o The complications are significant and include the following:
    - Iritis
    - Hemorrhage
    - Pigment dispersion
    - With overtreatment, hypotony and phthisis can be seen.
    - With undertreatment, no effect is achieved.
    - The procedure is usually accompanied by a significant degree of postlaser pain.

Glaucoma Surgery

Trabeculectomy

- The aim of glaucoma surgery is to
  o Lower IOP
  o Reduce or eliminate the need for antiglaucoma medications
  o Preserve vision and field
- The indication for surgery is the inability to reach or maintain the chosen target pressure with a tolerable level of medications and laser.
- The guarded trabeculectomy is the mainstay of filtration surgery.

Phaco-Trabeculectomy

- The phaco-trabeculectomy is a surgical procedure combining phacoemulsification or other cataract extraction techniques with a trabeculectomy. This is done because cataract and glaucoma frequently co-exist in the elderly:
  o The phaco-trabeculectomy is done when there is a visually significant cataract and one or more of the following:
    - An IOP consistently over target
    - Multiple medication use
    - Medication intolerance
    - Advanced VF damage (such as threatened fixation on VF)
    - A fragile optic nerve (over a 0.8 cup)
  o One surgical procedure may
    - Help to alleviate both conditions
    - Provide protection against postoperative IOP spikes
    - Reduce the need for postoperative antiglaucoma medications
    - Protect against risk of postoperative steroid use
  o It is a more demanding and time-consuming procedure with delayed visual recovery compared to cataract extraction alone.
  o There is also the possibility of lower long-term IOP control or the need for more medications than when a filter alone is done.

Nonpenetrating Glaucoma Surgery

- Nonpenetrating glaucoma surgery is aimed at targeting the pathological structures responsible for the increase in IOP without actual penetration into the eye, almost an "extraocular" procedure. Juxtacanalicular TM and the inner wall of Schlemm's canal are removed as they are considered to be the primary site of outflow resistance.
  - Nonpenetrating surgery has been advocated by some to be a safer option than routine trabeculectomy in POAG.
  - This theoretically reduces the risk of intraoperative and postoperative hypotony.
  - A low filtration bleb usually forms after a successful nonpenetrating procedure.
  - It has also been considered a viable surgical alternative in the following:
    - High myopes (who have a higher risk of complications during surgery)
    - Pigmentary glaucoma
    - Pseudoexfoliation
    - Congenital glaucoma
  - Nonpenetrating surgery is more difficult to perform with a steeper learning curve, and the results tend to give a final IOP slightly higher than is usually obtained with an antimetabolite-augmented trabeculectomy.
  - Contraindications to nonpenetrating surgery include the following:
    - Neovascular glaucoma
    - Secondary ACG

Antimetabolite Use

- Antimetabolites are used for filtration surgery when preoperative assessment of risk factors for failure supports the use. These include the following:
  - Mitomycin C (0.2 to 0.5 mg/mL with exposure times varying from 1 to 5 minutes)
  - 5-fluorouracil (5-FU) (50 mg/mL for 5 minutes)
- Risk factors include the following:
  - African American race
  - Uveitic glaucoma
  - Neovascular glaucoma
  - Younger patient age
  - A very low postoperative IOP is desired.
  - Postoperative 5-FU (0.1 cc of 50 mg/mL) is used for incipient bleb failure.

Postoperative Management

- The postoperative care of the filtration patient is as important as the surgical technique itself. Each surgeon has his or her own preferred regimen of medications postoperatively. However, there are some key universal principles. Immediately after surgery, most surgeons use the following:
  - Frequent steroid drops, such as prednisolone every hour, with tapering as the surgery heals
  - Topical antibiotics for 1 to 2 weeks
  - Cycloplegia (Atropine 1% 4 times daily) in phakic patients and in those with shallow anterior chambers
- In the early postoperative period, regular and frequent assessments of the operated eye must be made, including the following:
  - Characteristics of the bleb
  - Anterior chamber depth
  - IOP
- The postoperative IOP must be carefully followed with intervention as necessary if the postoperative IOP remains elevated, including
  - Bleb massage
  - Laser suture lysis

  - o Bleb needling with 5-FU or mitomycin may be necessary if the above options fail or if there is significant scarring postoperatively causing IOP elevation.
- The opposite problem of elevated IOP postoperatively is hypotony. The general management principles are discussed below, but this can usually be attributed to either over-filtration or wound leakage.
- Very avascular blebs caused by excessive mitomycin exposure increase the following risks:
  - o Chronic ocular hypotony (with an IOP less than 5 mm Hg)
  - o Late-onset bleb leak
  - o Blebitis
  - o Endophthalmitis
- In addition to frequent follow up, patients must be cautioned to return for assessment with any symptoms of the mnemonic "RSVP":
  - o Redness
  - o Sensitivity to light
  - o Vision change
  - o Pain

Complications of Filtering Surgery

- Filtration surgery unfortunately includes many potential complications. Many complications have a typical constellation of findings, including those typical of either early or late complications. Neither of the following lists is exhaustive.

Early Complications

- Hypotony and its complications:
  - o Wound leak
  - o Excessive filtration
  - o Cyclodialysis
  - o Iridocyclitis
  - o Retinal detachment
- Flat anterior chamber (Figure 8-26)
- Aqueous misdirection
- Hyphema
- Formation or acceleration of cataract
- Transient increase in IOP
- Choroidal effusion
- Suprachoroidal hemorrhage
- Persistent uveitis
- Infection

Late Complications

- Bleb leakage
- Cataract formation
- Blebitis (Figure 8-27)
- Endophthalmitis
- Symptomatic bleb (dysesthesia)
- Bleb migration
- Failure of filtration

Management of Selected Complications of Filtering Surgery

Wound Leak

- Clinical findings
  - o Shallow or flat anterior chamber

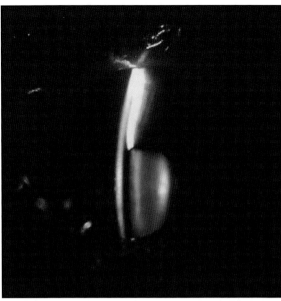

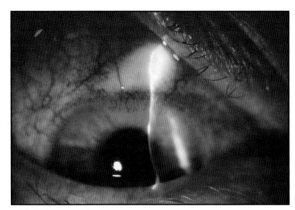

Figure 8-27. Blebitis.

Figure 8-26. Shallow anterior chamber following trabeculectomy.

- o A Seidel positive and poor bleb
- o Low IOP
- Management
  - o Pressure bandage or bandage contact lens
  - o Cycloplegia
  - o Possibly aqueous suppressants
  - o It may be necessary to re-suture the conjunctiva for a large leak

Over Filtration

- Clinical findings
  - o Shallow anterior chamber
  - o A Seidel negative and good bleb
  - o Low IOP
  - o Will often also have a choroidal detachment
- Management
  - o Follow closely, decrease topical steroid dose
  - o Cycloplegia and possibly aqueous suppressants
  - o Reform anterior chamber/drain choroidal detachment if there is lenticulocorneal touch (risk of cataract, corneal edema, PAS) and/or hypotonous maculopathy

Aqueous Misdirection

- Clinical findings
  - o Extremely shallow or flat AC
  - o No bleb and no leak
  - o High IOP (>6 mm Hg)
- Management
  - o Medical
    - Intense cycloplegia (tropicamide, cyclogyl, homatropine, and atropine every 5 minutes for three doses, then 4 times daily), plus mydriatics (phenylephrine)
    - Antiglaucoma medications, including acetazolamide (Diamox) or mannitol if necessary
  - o Laser
    - YAG laser posterior hyaloidotomy through a PI or intraocular lens

- o Surgical
  - Chandler procedure (pars plana tap with 18-gauge needle to break the hyaloid and withdraw liquid vitreous)
  - Pars plana vitrectomy, including removal of the lens if still present

Pupil Block

- Clinical findings
  - o Uneven depth of anterior chamber (shallow peripherally and deep centrally)
  - o Flat bleb and Seidel negative
  - o High IOP
  - o Nonpatent iridectomy
- Management
  - o Complete the iridectomy with the YAG laser

Filtration Failure

- Clinical findings
  - o The anterior chamber is typically deep.
  - o The bleb may be low and inconspicuous or high and encysted with a Tenon's capsule.
  - o The IOP may be any level over the target pressure desired.
- Management
  - o Rule out other causes of high IOP
  - o Digital massage beside the flap for up to 1 week
  - o Argon laser suture lysis from 1 to 3 weeks
  - o Needling with or without 5 FU may be done weeks to months and even years later
  - o YAG laser to ostomy, if iris is blocking it
  - o Medical therapy, if all else fails or if unwilling to proceed for more surgery
    - Further surgery (filtration, shunt, cyclodestruction)

Seton Implants

- Implantation of a glaucoma drainage device, or Seton shunt, is undertaken when a standard trabeculectomy is unlikely to succeed, either based on the underlying disease or in the presence of prior failed attempts (Figure 8-28).
  - o A tube shunts aqueous to a plate on the episcleral surface.
    - A capsule forms around the plate that provides resistance to flow.
    - The final IOP depends on the thickness of the capsule and the surface area of the plate.
    - Many different setons are available, and the choice depends on many factors, including the following:
  - o Ease of implantation
    - Early IOP control
    - Long-term IOP control
  - o Ease of implantation varies
    - With single plates and flexible silicone plates being easier
  - o Early IOP control varies
    - As nonvalved shunts require complete restriction with a suture in the early phase to avoid hypotony until the plate capsule forms
    - Valved implants restrict flow and do not need restriction.
  - o Better long-term IOP control is seen with thinner capsules and larger plates up to a limit, and antifibrotics do not seem to be useful.
  - o Other implants also being used are not traditional tube Setons but include such devices as stents into Schlemm's canal ab interno (the Glaukos iStent), stents replacing a trabeculectomy ostomy (the Optonol Express mini-shunt), and shunts into the suprachoroidal space (the Solx Gold shunt).

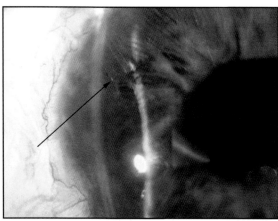

Figure 8-28. Seton tube implant.

- Complications
  - Valved implants reduce but do not eliminate the major early problems, which include the following:
    - Hypotony
    - Flat anterior chambers
    - Possible diplopia is most common with the early Baerveldt designs.

Suggested Readings

Epstein DL. Diagnosis and management of lens-induced glaucoma. *Ophthalmology.* 1982;89:227–230.

Gordon MO, Beiser JA, Heuer DK, et al. The ocular hypertension treatment study. Baseline factors that predict the onset of primary open angle glaucoma. *Arch Ophthalmol.* 2002;120:714–720.

Grosskreutz C, Netland PA. Low-tension glaucoma. *Int Ophthalmol Clin.* 1994;34:173–185.

Janz NK, Wren PA, Lichter PR, et al, and the CIGTS study group. The collaborative initial glaucoma treatment study. *Ophthalmology.* 2001;108:1954–1965.

Kass MA, Heuer DK, Higginbotham EJ, et al. The ocular hypertension treatment study. A randomized trial determines that topical ocular hypotensive medication delays or prevents the onset of primary open-angle glaucoma. *Arch Ophthalmol.* 2002;120:701–713.

Kim YY, Jung HR. Clarifying the nomenclature for primary angle-closure glaucoma. *Surv Ophthalmol.* 1997;42:125–136.

Lichter PR, Musch DC, Gillespie BW, et al, and the CIGTS study group. Interim clinical outcomes in the collaborative initial glaucoma treatment study comparing initial treatment randomized to medications or surgery. *Ophthalmology.* 2001;108:1943–1953.

Migliazzo CV, Shaffer RN, Nykin R, et al. Long-term analysis of pigmentary dispersion syndrome and pigmentary glaucoma. *Ophthalmology.* 1986;93:1528–1536.

Moorthy RS, Mermoud A, Baerveldt G, et al. Glaucoma associated with uveitis. *Surv Ophthalmol.* 1997;41:361–394.

Naumann GO, Schlotzer-Schrehardt U, Kuchie M. Pseudoexfoliation syndrome for the comprehensive ophthalmologist: intraocular and systemic manifestations. *Ophthalmology.* 1998;105:951–968.

Sherwood MB, Midgal CS, Hitchings RA, et al. Initial treatment of glaucoma: surgery or medications. *Surv Ophthalmol.* 1993;37:293–305.

The glaucoma laser trial (GLT) and glaucoma laser trial follow-up study: 7. Results. *Am J Ophthalmol.* 1995;120:718–731.

The fluorouracil filtering surgery study group. Five year follow-up of the fluorouracil filtering study. *Am J Ophthalmol.* 1996;121:349–366.

The collaborative normal-tension study group. Comparison of glaucomatous progression between untreated patients with normal tension glaucoma and patients with therapeutically reduced intraocular pressures. *Am J Ophthalmol.* 1998;126:487–497.

The AGIS investigators. The advanced glaucoma intervention study (AGIS): 4. Comparison of treatment outcomes within race. Seven year results. *Ophthalmology.* 1998;105:1146–1164.

The Glaucoma Laser Trial Research Group: The Glaucoma Laser Trial, II: Results of argon laser trabeculoplasty versus topical medicines. *Ophthalmology.* 1990;97:1403–1413.

Wagner RS. Glaucoma in children. *Pediatr Clin North Am.* 1993;40:855–867.

Questions

1. Which of the following statements about IOP is incorrect?
   a. The mean IOP of a normal population is 15.5 mm Hg.
   b. **The distribution of IOP in a normal population is skewed to the left.**
   c. 99% of the population will have an IOP less than 24 mm Hg.
   d. IOP over 24 mm Hg is not always associated with glaucoma.
   e. Increased IOP is due mostly to decreased outflow facility.

2. Which of the following statements about POAG is correct?
   a. Approximately 5% of the general population is affected by POAG.
   b. Increased C:D ratio is the main risk factor for developing glaucomatous neuropathy.
   c. The prevalence of POAG is greatest in middle age (50 to 70 years).
   d. **POAG is a leading cause of blindness in the African American population.**
   e. Diabetes is highly associated with the risk of developing POAG.

3. Which of the following statements about secondary glaucomas is incorrect?
   a. **Pigment dispersion glaucoma is the commonest secondary OAG worldwide.**
   b. Pseudoexfoliation increases the risk of both open- and closed-angle glaucoma.
   c. Glaucomatocyclitic crisis is a uveitic glaucoma with high pressure and relatively mild symptoms.
   d. The syndrome called Fuchs' heterochromic iridocyclitis includes changes in iris color and cataract formation as well as possible glaucoma.
   e. The risk of angle-recession glaucoma is increased with angle damage over 270 degrees.

4. Which of the following statements about ACG is correct?
   a. A narrow angle configuration can only be diagnosed at the slit lamp.
   b. Acute angle closure will always be associated with nerve and field changes.
   c. Chronic angle closure has the same signs and symptoms as acute angle closure.
   d. Mixed mechanism glaucoma is diagnosed when the patient has known open-angle glaucoma prior to the angle closure.
   e. **Secondary angle closure can be due to formation of posterior synechiae in uveitis.**

5. Which of the following statements about developmental glaucoma is incorrect?
   a. Infants with congenital glaucoma typically present with photophobia, epiphora, and blepharospasm.
   b. Children under 3 years of age may also have corneal clouding and buphthalmos.
   c. **Older children complain of eye pain and blurred vision.**
   d. The corneal diameter is usually over 13 mm.
   e. Haab's striae are typical of congenital glaucoma and represent rupture of Descemet's membrane.

6. Which of the following statements about the diagnosis of glaucoma is correct?
   a. Most patients can be diagnosed with a good history.
   b. The prior ocular history is rarely contributory.
   c. **A positive family history increases the risk of glaucoma.**
   d. Gonioscopy need only be performed when the risk of angle closure is present.
   e. A high level of IOP (>24 mm Hg) is necessary for the diagnosis of POAG.

7. Which of the following statements about optic nerve and nerve fiber layer imaging is incorrect?
   a. Scanning laser polarimetry is affected by corneal and retinal polarization of light.
   b. OCT creates a cross-sectional image of the retina.
   c. Confocal scanning laser tomography uses reflectance to build a topographical image of the nerve.
   d. **OCT shows statistical changes in the RNFL over multiple assessments.**
   e. Confocal scanning laser shows statistical changes in the optic nerve height over multiple assessments.

8. Which of the following statements about the VF testing in glaucoma is correct?
   a. Most glaucoma damage occurs within 10 degrees of fixation.
   b. SITA technology using the Humphrey analyzer is significantly slower than the previous test strategy but more accurate.
   c. Blue-on-yellow testing isolates the blue cone system resulting in earlier detection of field defects.
   d. The Octopus analyzer tests only the central 10 degrees of the VF.
   e. Frequency-doubling perimetry produces a Bebie Curve to aid the analysis of a field defect.

9. Which of the following statements about glaucoma medications is incorrect?
   a. The nonselective β-blockers are contraindicated in patients with chronic obstructive pulmonary disease.
   b. The prostaglandin agonists act by decreasing aqueous production in the CB.
   c. The α-agonists are associated with a characteristic allergic blepharoconjunctivitis in 15% to 20% of patients.
   d. Oral carbonic anhydrase inhibitors have a higher rate of significant side effects than the topical forms.
   e. Poor compliance with prescribed medications is a major source of treatment failure.

10. Which of the following statements about glaucoma lasers and surgery is correct?
    a. Laser trabeculoplasty with either the argon or the selective laser is equally effective.
    b. Laser iridotomy is intended only for patients who have sustained an acute angle-closure attack.
    c. Glaucoma surgery cannot be combined with any other procedures; it needs to be done alone.
    d. Nonpenetrating glaucoma surgery results in a lower IOP than regular surgery with less risk.
    e. Postoperative hypotony is a transient phenomenon with glaucoma surgery and is of no significance.

Lens and Cataract

Irmingard Neuhann, MD; Thomas Neuhann, MD; and Paul Ernest, MD

Outline

Probst LE, Tsai JH.
Ophthalmology: Clinical and Surgical Principles (pp. 351–376).

c. Types of Intraocular Lenses
  i.   Iris Clip (Support)
  ii. Anterior Chamber
  iii. Posterior Chamber
  iv. Multipiece Intraocular Lenses
  v.   Single-Piece Intraocular Lenses
  vi. Plate-Haptic Intraocular Lenses
  vii. Blue-Blocker Intraocular Lenses
  viii. Accommodative Intraocular Lenses
  ix. Multifocal Intraocular Lenses
  x.   Light Adaptive Intraocular Lenses
  xi. Aspheric Intraocular Lenses
d. Insertion Techniques for Intraocular lenses
  i.   Forceps
  ii. Cartridge
14. Complications of Intraocular Lenses
  a. De-Centration
  b. Dysphotopsia
  c. Opacification

Definition of Cataract

- Opacity of crystalline lens
- Can be either primary age-related, congenital, traumatic, or secondary to general condition

Classification of Cataracts by Maturation

Immature

- May show only faint signs of early cataract (eg, yellowing of lens, early cortical spoking)
- Findings may not be clinically evident on physical examination

Mature

- No fundal glow (Figure 9-1)

Intumescent

- Mature cataract swells due to water absorption into the cortex.

Hypermature

- Absorbed water may leak, and lens becomes smaller with wrinkled anterior capsule and sclerotic.

Morgagnian Cataract

- Second type of hypermature cataract formation with completely liquefied cortex allows the nucleus to sink inferiorly (Figure 9-2).

Classification of Cataract by Etiology

Primary Age-Related

- Main form of cataract, which is due to apposition of lens "fibers" with increasing age. May be the following 3 types:

Cortical

- Predominantly cortical 70% (Figure 9-3)

Nuclear

- Predominantly nuclear 25% (Figure 9-4)

Subcapsular

- Predominantly posterior subcapsular 5% (Figure 9-5)
- Rare: Christmas tree cataract. Polychromatic crystals due to cholesterol deposition (Figure 9-6).

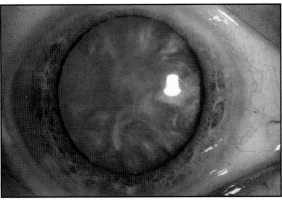

Figure 9-2. Morgagnian cataract.

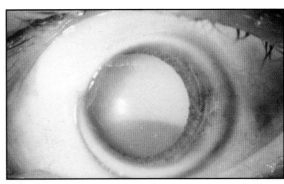

Figure 9-1. Mature cataract.

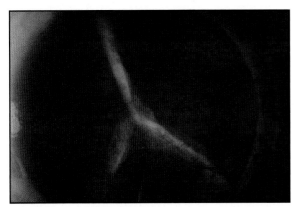

Figure 9-3. Cortical cataract.

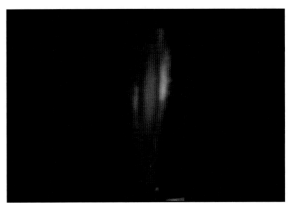

Figure 9-4. Nuclear cataract.

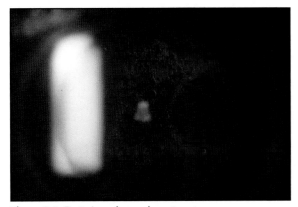

Figure 9-5. Posterior subcapsular cataract.

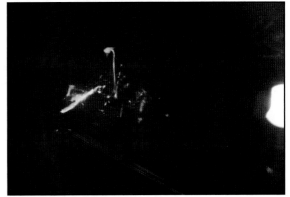

Figure 9-6. Christmas tree cataract.

Secondary

- Some medical conditions cause specific types of cataract and other lens opacities.

Myotonic Cataract

- Associated with myotonic dystrophy. Early stages: dust-like fine and multicolored refractile scattered opacities in the cortex and subcapsular region. May also be known as Christmas tree cataract.

Tetanic Cataract

- Paradoxic calcification of crystalline lens in hypocalcemia

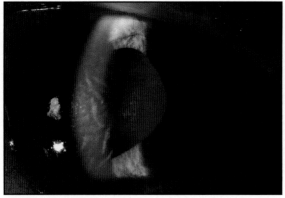

Figure 9-7. Glaukomflecken.

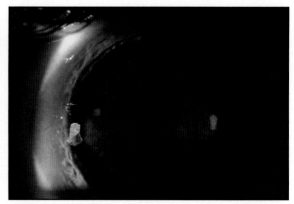

Figure 9-8. Snow flake cataract.

Glaukomflecken

- White patches beneath the anterior capsule after intraocular pressure (IOP) rise due to focal necrosis of lens epithelial cells (Figure 9-7).

Syndermatotic Cataract

- Associated with cutaneous diseases. Anterior or subcapsular bilateral cataract in the third decade of life.

Electric and Lightning Cataract

- Anterior and posterior subcapsular cataracts, dust-like and spoke-shaped opacities

Phenothiazines

- Especially chlorpromazine and thioridazine
- May lead to the deposition of fine yellowish-brown granules under the anterior lens capsule, often asymptomatic

Miotics

- Especially echothiophate, demecarium bromide, di-isopropyl fluorophosphate (DFP)
- Anterior subcapsular vacuoles or more advanced opacities. After discontinuation of drug, these changes may resolve.

Steroids

- Typically axial posterior subcapsular cataract. Regression of early opacities can be observed when the drug is discontinued. Cataract may also progress after withdrawal of steroids.

Amiodarone

- Anterior subcapsular cataract, often asymptomatic

Gold

- Gold therapy of longer than 3 years can be associated with anterior subcapsular cataract formation.

Diabetes

- Characterized by earlier manifestation of cataract with no specific morphology. Snowflake cataract (Figure 9-8) may be seen in young diabetics (multiple spotty cortical opacities as a result of influx of glucose and water into the lens) .

Wilson's Disease and Copper Foreign Body

- Chalcosis lentis. Sunflower cataract due to copper deposition.

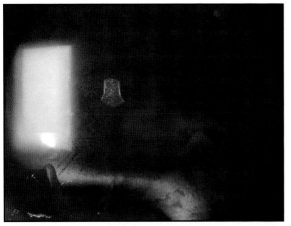

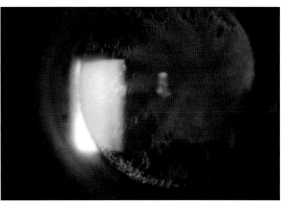

Figure 9-10. Perforation rosette: Posterior subcapsular opacification of crystalline lens due to perforating trauma.

Figure 9-9. Traumatic cataract in anterior subcapsular lens due to blunt trauma (contusion rosette). Note pigment dispersion, iris defect, and concave configuration of lens due to zonular dehiscence caused by trauma.

Nonionizing Radiation

- Infrared—true exfoliation of anterior lens capsule (glassblower's cataract)
- UV—nuclear sclerosis

Ionizing Radiation

- Posterior subcapsular cataract

Traumatic

- Definition
  - Cataract that results from direct trauma to the lens
- Clinical
  - Most commonly presents as a star-shaped opacity in the anterior subcapsular location of the crystalline lens (Figure 9-9), caused by blunt trauma (contusion rosette). The distance of this opacity from the anterior capsule can give a clue as to how long ago the causative trauma lies back in time.
  - Perforating lens trauma may cause a limited opacity with capsular sealing, a posterior "perforation rosette" (Figure 9-10), a rapidly progressing, even intumescent total opacification and/or leakage of some of the lens cortex in the anterior chamber (AC).

Congenital

- Definition
  - Cataract present at birth
- General characteristics
  - Unilateral cases can result from the following:
    - Local dysgenesis
    - Idiopathic 80%
    - Ocular abnormalities 10%:
      - Persistent fetal vasculature (PFV)
      - Anterior segment dysgenesis
      - Tumor
    - Traumatic 10%
    - Masked bilateral cataract
    - Usually not associated with systemic disease
    - Usually sporadic
    - Eye may be microphthalmic

- o Bilateral cases may often be due to the following:
  - ▪ Idiopathic 60%
  - ▪ Inherited 30%—most often autosomal dominant
  - ▪ Prematurity—transient opacities
  - ▪ Intrauterine infections 3%—most often associated with rubella
  - ▪ Genetic, metabolic, systemic 5%
  - ▪ Ocular abnormalities 2%
- Etiology
  - o Metabolic disease
    - ▪ Galactosemia
      - □ Rare, classic oil droplet cataract
      - □ Galactokinase deficiency type may have no other systemic signs and may present late in life.
      - □ Transferase deficiency affects multiple organs.
      - □ Removal of milk prior to 4 months may allow cataracts to be resorbed.
    - ▪ Fabry's disease
    - ▪ Diabetes mellitus
    - ▪ Hypoparathyroidism and pseudohypoparathyroidism
    - ▪ Hypoglycemia
    - ▪ Mannosidosis, sorbitol dehydrogenase deficiency, hyperglycinuria, sialidosis (deficiency of alpha-neuraminidase), Wilson's disease
  - o Chromosomal abnormalities
    - ▪ Down syndrome (trisomy 21)
    - ▪ Patau's syndrome (trisomy 13)
    - ▪ Edwards' syndrome (trisomy 18)
  - o Systemic
    - ▪ Lowe's oculocerebrorenal syndrome
      - □ Frequent association with glaucoma
      - □ X-linked recessive
      - □ Female carriers may have cataract
    - ▪ Myotonic dystrophy
    - ▪ Alport syndrome
    - ▪ Marfan syndrome
  - o Intrauterine infections with cataract
    - ▪ Toxoplasmosis, others (syphilis), rubella, cytomegalovirus, herpes simplex and zoster (TORCH)
- Evaluation
  - o Unilateral
    - ▪ History
      - □ Age of onset, family history, trauma (cannot rule out nonaccidental trauma in children)
    - ▪ Ocular exam
      - □ Associated ocular pathology
    - ▪ Laboratory
      - □ TORCH titers and Venereal Disease Research Laboratory (VDRL) should be obtained.
  - o Bilateral
    - ▪ History
      - □ Family history, age of onset, developmental delays
    - ▪ Pediatric exam
      - □ Genetic evaluation if indicated
    - ▪ Laboratory
      - □ Routine
        - • TORCH
        - • VDRL
        - • Galactosemia screening of urine for reducing substance (post milk feeding)
        - • Fasting blood sugar (hypoglycemia)

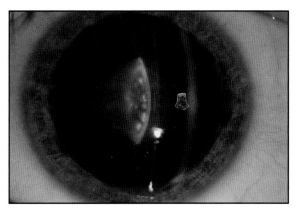

Figure 9-11. Congenital cataract.

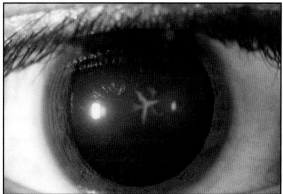

Figure 9-12. Central Y-shaped sutural cataract. (Reprinted with permission from Leal AG, Rodriguez PB. *The Atlas of Ophthalmology*, Thorofare, NJ: SLACK Incorporated; 2002.)

- □ Optional
  - • Red blood cell galactokinase—developmental cataracts
  - • Urine for amino acids—developmental delay glaucoma
  - • Calcium and phosphorus—metabolic

Nuclear Cataract

- Transient problem in development of lens leads to deposition of a powdery looking zone of opaque cells in the center of the lens surrounded by clear zones (Figure 9-11).
- Usually does not affect vision

Lamellar or Zonular Cataract

- Most common congenital cataract, accounting for approximately 50% of the cases
- On the affected layer, small line-shaped opacities that can extend around the edge of the opaque area (so-called "riders") may be present.
- Effect on vision depends on the extent of the opacity.

Sutural Cataract

- Central, Y-shaped, often punctate opacities representing the line of intersection of primary lens fibers that form the anterior and posterior borders of the embryonic nucleus (Figure 9-12)
- Usually have minimal effect on vision

Coronary or Supranuclear Cataract

- Genetically determined opacities that occur during the otherwise normal development of the lens, affecting the deeper cortex or adolescent nucleus
- They increase in number with age but usually do not interfere with vision due to their peripheral position.

Anterior Polar Cataract

- Opacities located at the anterior pole of the lens
- Corneal opacification with anterior polar cataract (Figure 9-13) may be caused by one of the AC cleavage syndromes.

Posterior Polar Cataract

- Opacities are located at the posterior pole of the lens and are caused by the persistence of the posterior hyaloid artery remnant.

Focal Blue Dot Opacities/Punctate Cataract

- Genetically determined small round opacities that are usually scattered throughout the nucleus and deeper layers of the cortex of the lens
- Usually develop during the first 2 decades of life and do not impair vision

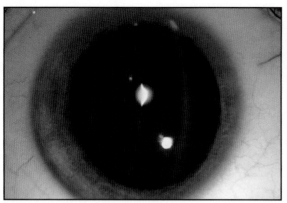

Figure 9-13. Anterior polar cataract.

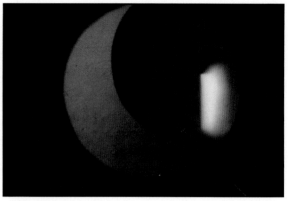

Figure 9-14. Subluxed lens.

Membranous Cataract

- Total or partial absorption of a former congenital cataract allowing the anterior and posterior capsule to fuse together forming a thin membrane, which can be mistaken for congenital aphakia

Other

- Other congenital lens abnormalities include subluxed lens (Figure 9-14) and lens coloboma (Figure 9-15) and may be related to systemic syndromes (ie, Marfan's or homocystinuria) or anterior segment dysgenesis, respectively.

Signs and Symptoms of Cataract

- Decrease in visual acuity/hazy or foggy vision
- Due to irregular birefringence of the light at the lens opacities, the patient may experience glare.
- With nuclear cataracts, the denser inner lens nucleus causes a higher refractive index and may cause myopia and coaxial monocular diplopia.

Differential Diagnosis of Cataract

- Any cause of glare, hazy vision, and myopia should be differentiated from a cataract.
- Corneal problems such as corneal scars or cornea guttata and macular degeneration should be distinguished from cataract symptoms. Hazy vision due to cornea guttata is usually worst in the morning and then ameliorates during the day. Slit-lamp biomicroscopy and endothelial cell count will help confirm the diagnosis.
- In macular degeneration, the patient may also refer to hazy vision. If the symptom is caused by cataract, the patient will confirm that not only the center of vision (faces, when reading) is hazy, but also is the peripheral field of vision. The pinhole vision test will often improve vision considerably with corneal and cataract pathology but will not improve vision with retinal disease.

Treatment of Cataract

- There is no effective treatment of cataract by medication. Those cataracts induced by external agents may be halted in their development and partially reversed with cessation of the causative damage.
- When treatment is indicated, it is by surgical removal of the opacified lens and, whenever possible, replacement by an artificial lens implant.

Indications for Cataract Surgery

- Subjective disturbance of vision
  - ○ Indication for surgery is given if and when the patient feels subjectively bothered by the symptoms caused by the cataract and/or the cataract interferes with visual requirements of occupation or other activities important in daily life, such as driving.

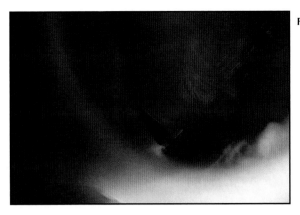

Figure 9-15. Lens and iris coloboma.

- o Commonly, a corrected Snellen acuity of 20/40 vision or worse is considered eligible for cataract surgery although this indication depends on the needs of the patient.
- o Often, the patient's potential visual acuity can be helpful in the decision for surgery (see also Chapter 2, Ocular Examination).
- Mature cataract with potential secondary complications
  - o Patients should not delay surgery if secondary complications from mature cataracts are expected.
- Elevated IOP
  - o After cataract surgery, the IOP may decrease as much as 3 to 5 mm Hg.
  - o This may be a consideration in otherwise equivocal cases.
- Shallow AC
  - o In case of a shallow AC and a lens diameter larger than 5 mm causing acute angle-closure disposition, cataract extraction may be considered, as well as following acute angle closure.

History of Cataract Extraction

- Most ancient techniques employed the principle of dislocating the crystalline lens into the vitreous.
- This was followed by intracapsular (ICCE) and extracapsular (ECCE) techniques with large corneal incisions. ICCE was the standard main technique during the last century until the reintroduction of ECCE in the 1970s.
- In ICCE, the entire lens is removed through a 180-degree corneal limbal incision using a cryoprobe or a capsule forceps.
- In ECCE, only the opaque lens material is removed, leaving the capsular bag in place, enabling intracapsular intraocular lens (IOL) fixation. In planned ECCE, the lens nucleus is expressed, and the cortex is removed via an irrigation/aspiration (I/A) system. Planned ECCE has been replaced by phacoemulsification for modern cataract surgery.

Wound Construction for Cataract Surgery

- There are 3 main access routes to the AC.

Scleral Tunnel

- Advantage
  - o Lowest rate of induced astigmatism because of location farthest from the limbus. Covered by conjunctiva, therefore less endophthalmitis risk.
- Disadvantage
  - o Conjunctival opening/closure needed

Clear Corneal

- Advantage
  - o Aesthetically appealing, rapid recovery, surgically simple (Figure 9-16)

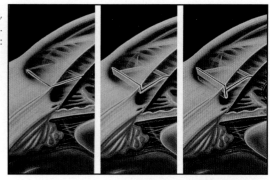

Figure 9-16. Three types of clear corneal incisions (hinge, groove, and single plane). (Reprinted with permission from Wallace RB III. *Refractive Cataract Surgery and Multifocal IOLs.* Thorofare, NJ: SLACK Incorporated; 2001.)

- Disadvantage
  - Astigmatism induction, inner incision closer to corneal center, questionable self-sealing with potentially higher rate of endophthalmitis

Limbal

- Advantage
  - Self-sealing, less astigmatism induction
- Disadvantage
  - Bleeding, potential conjunctival ballooning with irrigation

- Regardless of the location, the tunnel should always be constructed in the following 3 steps:
  - Perpendicular incision until depth of tunnel reached
  - Intrascleral/intracorneal tunnel following curvature of tissue. Ideally, the tunnel is not shorter than its maximum width (square).
  - Perforation of Descemet's membrane with additional step

Lens Removal Techniques

Extracapsular extraction through a small incision by phacoemulsification is today's standard of care. There are other techniques that are or may be the method of choice in selected conditions.

Intracapsular

- Today, only a few indications remain, mainly (very) hard nucleus with weak zonules (eg, in pseudo-exfoliation).

Extracapsular ("Planned")

- Whenever phacoemulsification is not available or is deemed associated with an exaggerated risk (extremely dense nucleus, compromised cornea, lack of surgical expertise for the given case, flat anterior segment, etc) yet preservation of a clear posterior capsule appears desirable and possible, the nucleus in its entirety can be extracted after anterior capsulotomy through an appropriately large incision (Figure 9-17).
- Manual fragmentation (splitting) of the nucleus and softer/smaller nuclei may enable removal through an intermediate-sized incision.

Pars Plana Lensectomy

- This is the method of choice in special situations, such as cataract removal in newborns and infants and soft cataracts (eg, traumatic) with involvement of deeper structures, especially when a vitrectomy is anticipated.

Phacoemulsification

- The main steps of phacoemulsification are as follows:

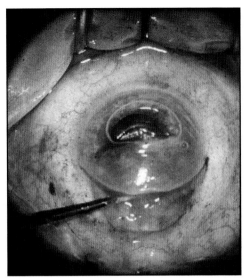

Figure 9-17. Extracapsular cataract surgery utilizes a large limbal incision to express the entire lens nucleus. This technique is rarely used today.

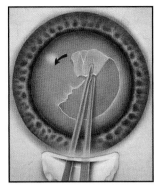

Figure 9-18. Technique of continuous circular capsulorrhexis. (Reprinted with permission from Buratto L, Werner, L, Zanini M, Apple, DJ. *Phacoemulsification: Principles and Techniques*, 2nd ed. Thorofare, NJ: SLACK Incorporated; 2003.)

- o Self-sealing incision at/around limbus (Figure 9-16)
- o (Continuous circular) capsulorrhexis (Figure 9-18)
- o Hydrodissection/optional hydrodelineation (Figures 9-19 and 9-20)
- o Manual mechanical fracturing of nucleus into several segments (grooving and dividing, chopping) (Figures 9-21 and 9-22)
- o Emulsification and aspiration of nucleus fragments (Figure 9-23)
- o I/A of cortical remnants (bimanual, coaxial) (Figure 9-24)
- o Optional capsule polishing
- o IOL implantation, preferably foldable (Figure 9-25)

Special Forms of Cataract Surgery

Congenital Cataract

- Signs/symptoms
  - o Large variation in morphology
  - o Not all cataracts in children affect vision significantly to require extraction.
  - o Poor fixation/nystagmus possible
  - o Amblyopia
  - o Opacified lens is visible particularly after dilation.
- Indications for surgery
  - o The basic principle in evaluating the indication for surgery is weighing the amblyogenic component of the cataract against that caused by the loss of accommodation in case of surgery.
  - o "Rule of thumb": When enough binocularity for at least intermediate quality of stereopsis is preserved, do not operate, especially in younger children.
  - o With visual acuity ≥20/60, stereopsis can be assumed. No surgery and appropriate patching is recommended.
  - o With visual acuity ≤20/200, no stereopsis can be expected; surgery is warranted.
  - o Between 20/200 and 20/80, an individual decision will have to be made, taking additional factors into account (eg, age, compliance expectancy, associated conditions, patch trial).
- Techniques of surgery
  - o Use pars plana lensectomy (PPL) up to approximately 2 years of age. Consider no IOL implantation but preparation for secondary implantation by leaving a small peripheral capsular ring.

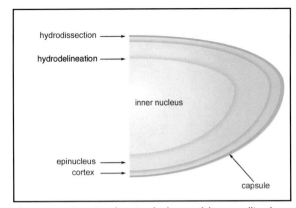

Figure 9-19. Drawing showing the layers of the crystalline lens: capsule cortex, epinucleus, and nucleus. Hydrodissection consents the separation of the epinucleus from the cortex, hydrodelineation is the nucleus from the epinucleus. (Reprinted with permission from Buratto L, Werner, L, Zanini M, Apple, DJ. *Phacoemulsification: Principles and Techniques*, 2nd ed. Thorofare, NJ: SLACK Incorporated; 2003.)

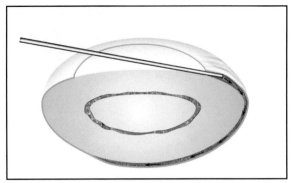

Figure 9-20. Hydrodissection—The cannula enters below the edge of the capsulorrhexis. It proceeds slightly and raises the anterior capsule. The surgeon then injects balanced salt solution, separating the capsule with the cortex from the nucleus. (Reprinted with permission from Buratto L, Werner, L, Zanini M, Apple, DJ. *Phacoemulsification: Principles and Techniques*, 2nd ed. Thorofare, NJ: SLACK Incorporated; 2003.)

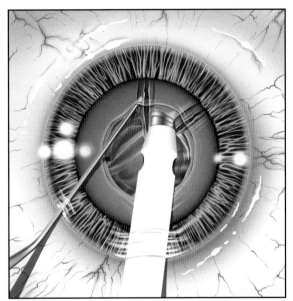

Figure 9-21. Mechanical fracturing of nucleus. (Reprinted with permission from Buratto L, Werner, L, Zanini M, Apple, DJ. *Phacoemulsification: Principles and Techniques*, 2nd ed. Thorofare, NJ: SLACK Incorporated; 2003.)

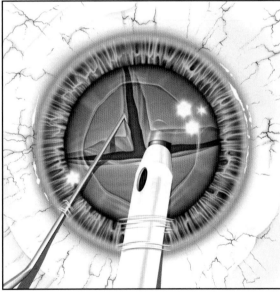

Figure 9-22. Phaco Chop technique after second chop. (Reprinted with permission from Buratto L, Werner, L, Zanini M, Apple, DJ. *Phacoemulsification: Principles and Techniques*, 2nd ed. Thorofare, NJ: SLACK Incorporated; 2003.)

Figure 9-23. Capture of the last piece of nucleus with ultrasound tip. Occlusion, division, and emulsification until the nucleus has been completely removed. (Reprinted with permission from Buratto L, Werner, L, Zanini M, Apple, DJ. *Phacoemulsification: Principles and Techniques*, 2nd ed. Thorofare, NJ: SLACK Incorporated; 2003.)

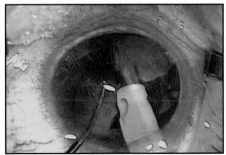

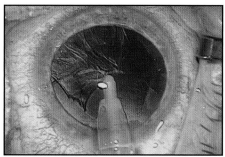

Figure 9-24. The cortex and epinucleus is removed by irrigation/aspiration. (Reprinted with permission from Buratto L, Werner, L, Zanini M, Apple, DJ. *Phacoemulsification: Principles and Techniques*, 2nd ed. Thorofare, NJ: SLACK Incorporated; 2003.)

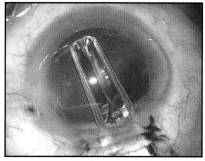

Figure 9-25. The loop is in the bag and lens can slowly be unfolded outside of the bag. (Reprinted with permission from Buratto L, Werner, L, Zanini M, Apple, DJ. *Phacoemulsification: Principles and Techniques*, 2nd ed. Thorofare, NJ: SLACK Incorporated; 2003.)

- ○ With limbal access in older children, use very long scleral tunnels and a paracentesis to obtain watertight closure with soft infantile sclera. Avoid sutures if possible. Consider fibrin glue if necessary.
- ○ With extracapsular extraction, always perform a primary posterior capsulotomy and anterior vitrectomy for maintenance of clear optical axis—the younger the child, the more important this is.
- ○ There is no consensus as to when and with what target refraction to implant an IOL. In doubt, no IOL <2 years with option for secondary implantation.
- • Visual rehabilitation of congenital cataracts
  - ○ Aphakic spectacles
    - ▪ Binocular cases only—would cause aniseikonia in monocular cases
  - ○ Contact lenses
    - ▪ Still most popular choice especially before age 2
    - ▪ Extended-wear lenses (silicone type) most popular
    - ▪ Good choice in monocular cases
    - ▪ Major disadvantages include loss of lenses and cost of lenses.
    - ▪ Infections and corneal ulcers are another concern.
  - ○ IOLs
    - ▪ Increasing in popularity especially after age 2
    - ▪ Studies ongoing from infancy upward
    - ▪ Capsular fixation preferred over sulcus fixation
    - ▪ Posterior capsulorrhexis or vitrectorrhexis essential
    - ▪ Secondary IOLs indicated in those who fail contact lenses
  - ○ Amblyopia treatment
    - ▪ Aphakic patients fit with contact lenses as soon as possible
    - ▪ Patching therapy as soon as possible
- • Prevention
  - ○ Congenital cataracts may be prevented in selected cases by avoiding and treating maternal infection.
- • Prognosis
  - ○ Even with cataract surgery, some degree of amblyopia is common after surgery for congenital cataracts.

Traumatic Cataract

- • Surgical technique
  - ○ Contusion cataracts should essentially be treated like any other adult-acquired cataract with a careful postoperative examination for peripheral retinal trauma damage.

- With perforation of anterior capsule, stabilize AC with viscoelastic, close any perforating wound in the outer wall of the eye, remove all lens matter in a closed system approach, clear anterior capsular situation, consider using vitrector and pupil dilators.
- With perforation of both capsules, proceed as above with a generous, yet controlled anterior vitrectomy.
- Consider implantation of IOL only when clear, controllable situation; in doubt, prefer secondary implantation under controlled circumstances (inflammation, trauma sequels, biometry/target refraction), especially with more significant injury.
- Prevention
  - Eye protection is recommended for high-risk activities and monocular patients.
- Prognosis
  - Generally good if only the lens is involved
  - Otherwise depends on the severity of the associated ocular trauma

Subluxed Lens

- Definition
  - Crystalline lens displaced from normal anatomical location
- Clinical
  - If mild, may be asymptomatic
  - Associated with pseudoexfoliation syndrome due to weak zonules
  - Associated with previous ocular trauma or syndromes (Marfan's, etc)
- Surgical technique
  - Major intraocular maneuvers to preserve a capsule that is too loose to maintain a centered stable position are usually not warranted.
  - Consider PPL in soft cataracts of younger patients (eg, trauma, congenital, Marfan's) or ICCE in older patients with very hard nuclei. Anterior vitrectomy is usually required.
  - A capsular tension ring can be used to stabilize the capsular bag when the subluxated lens is associated with loose zonules.
  - IOL implantation can be achieved with angle fixation, iris clip fixation, or transscleral suture fixation in the ciliary sulcus.
- Prevention
  - Subluxed lens is almost impossible to prevent; however, surgical complications with cataract surgery for a subluxed lens can be minimized with careful technique.
- Prognosis
  - Good with appropriate surgical technique

Complications of Cataract Surgery

Ruptured Posterior Capsule

- Definition
  - Defect in the posterior capsule of the lens that is usually caused during surgery (Figure 9-26)
- Etiology
  - Defect extending into posterior capsule
  - Direct trauma with instruments or implants
  - Defect/weakness in posterior capsule: posterior polar cataract
- Associated complications
  - Loss of nucleus and/or cortex into vitreous
- Clinical
  - Occurs during surgery
  - Associated with postoperative cystoid macular edema
  - Associated with increased risk of retinal detachment
- Prevention
  - Ensure capsulorrhexis is continuous and closed. When lost peripherally, avoid distention. Loose zonules facilitate tear into posterior capsule—consider counterincision 180 degrees away.

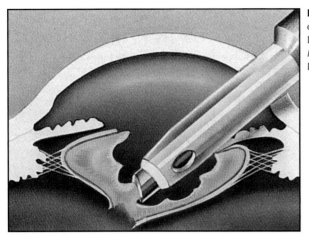

Figure 9-26. Rupture of the posterior capsule with the phacoemulsification tip. (Reprinted with permission from Buratto L, Werner, L, Zanini M, Apple, DJ. *Phacoemulsification: Principles and Techniques*, 2nd ed. Thorofare, NJ: SLACK Incorporated; 2003.)

- o Phacoemulsification tip should remain in the pupillary level, prefer lower flow settings and avoid chamber collapses by adequate setting of parameters of inflow and outflow.
- o I/A tips should be controlled for sharp edges, especially around aspiration port.
- o Posterior polar cataracts should be approached, anticipating a central posterior capsular defect. No partial hydrodissection, tactical use of viscoelastics including dry cortex removal, leaving the posterior polar opacity for removal as the last step.
- Management
  - o Whenever the tear is discovered, it is essential not to allow the chamber to flatten or collapse in order to avoid further extension.
  - o When the tear occurs before complete nucleus removal, it is safest to stabilize the chamber and "freeze" all lens material with profuse use of a dispersive viscoelastic, then remove the nuclear material through the incision, widening it as necessary. A wider incision is much less traumatic than a dropped nucleus or fragment. Then, adequate vitrectomy—preferably bimanual—is mandatory, using the vitrectomy instrument without cutting to remove the cortex.
  - o When loss of the nucleus or a fragment of it is imminent, "posterior assisted levitation" is a helpful maneuver. Through a stab incision of the pars plana, a spatula is introduced to lift the material back into the AC from where it can be removed as previously described.
  - o When all nuclear material is removed at occurrence/detection of tear, bimanual vitrectomy and cortex aspiration can be used.
  - o When the tear does not yet extend too far into the periphery, it can be converted into a posterior capsulorrhexis, which may provide a safe basis for intracapsular lens implantation. Tear edges may also be blunted with the vitreous cutter.
  - o Vitrectomy is required in all but a few exceptional circumstances. When in doubt, vitrectomy should be completed to reduce vitreous traction and vitreous incarceration around the IOL or within the wound.
  - o If nucleus is lost into vitreous beyond where it can safely be retrieved with posterior levitation, management depends on the surgeon's vitreoretinal surgical experience. Without adequate vitreoretinal surgical experience, cortical removal and a limited anterior vitrectomy should be completed. An IOL may be implanted, depending on surgeon skill and other medical and surgical factors. The patient should be promptly referred to a vitreoretinal surgeon for further management.
- Prognosis
  - o Good with appropriate surgical maneuvers
- Prevention
  - o All surgical maneuvers during phacoemulsification aim to preserve the posterior capsule.

Posterior Capsular Opacification

- Definition
  - o Main postoperative complication after extracapsular cataract surgery, occurring in 100% of cases to varying degrees, due to retained lens epithelial cells within capsular bag

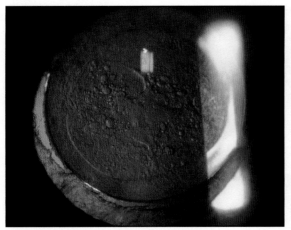

Figure 9-27. Secondary cataract with Elschnig's pearls.

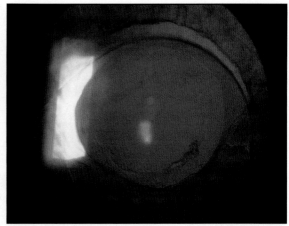

Figure 9-28. Round opening in posterior capsule after treatment with YAG laser.

- Etiology
  - Occurs in 2 basic forms
    - Regeneration (Elschnig's pearls) (Figure 9-27)
    - Fibrotic (fibroblastic metaplasia of lens epithelial cells)
    - Mixed forms of both (most cases)
- Clinical
  - Same symptoms as cataract, with blurred vision occurring months to years after cataract surgery
  - Clinically relevant only when they come close to affecting the visual axis. With modern surgical techniques and implants, there is now an incidence of approximately 10%.
  - A thin membrane of varying degrees of opacity and wrinkles can be seen on slit-lamp examination behind the IOL.
- Prevention
  - Surgery related
    - Hydrodissection-enhanced cortical cleanup
    - In-the-bag fixation of the IOL
    - Capsulorrhexis edge covering the anterior surface of the IOL circularly by approximately 0.5 to 1 mm
  - IOL-related factors
    - Maximal IOL optic—posterior capsule contact
    - Angulated haptic
    - "Adhesive" biomaterial to create a shrink wrap effect
    - Optic geometry with a square, truncated edge
- Treatment
  - Posterior capsulotomy usually with Nd:YAG laser (Figure 9-28)
- Prognosis
  - Excellent after YAG capsulotomy

Endophthalmitis

- Etiology/organisms
  - Usually bacterial contamination during surgery. Enhanced by long surgery time, low postoperative IOP, secondary to wound leak of self-sealing incisions.
  - May be subdivided into the following categories:
    - Early postoperative
      - Peak occurrence on the third postoperative day
      - Usually highly pathogenic gram-positive organisms from the conjunctival sac (eg, streptococcus, staphylococcus)

- Late postoperative
  - Peak occurrence after 2 weeks
  - Usually less pathogenic organisms, such as *Propionibacterium acnes*
- Signs/symptoms
  - Early signs: Increasing signs of postoperative inflammation; pain, ciliary/mixed injection, cells, and flare
  - Late signs: Hypopyon, vitreous infiltration, retinal infiltration, and necrosis
  - Diagnosis is ideally confirmed by proof of organism by AC tap, vitreous tap (highest yield)
- Differential diagnosis
  - Toxic anterior segment syndrome
  - Noninfectious panuveitis
  - Retained crystalline lens material
- Treatment
  - Ophthalmologic emergency
  - Every suspicion to be treated as endophthalmitis unless proven otherwise
  - Immediate AC tap, vitreous tap for culture—do not waste material in nonenriching diagnostics
  - Treatment should follow guidelines as set for in the Endophthalmitis Vitrectomy Study
    - If the vision is hand motion or better, intravitreal injections with vitreous tap is as efficacious as vitrectomy.
    - If the visual acuity is worse than hand motion, vitrectomy is more efficacious.
  - Intravitreal antibiotic injection (eg, vancomycin 1.0 mg in 0.1 mL and ceftazidime 2.25 mg in 0.1 mL)
  - Consider intravitreal steroids
  - Removal of IOL in select cases (eg, *p. acnes* infection)
- Prognosis
  - Variable, depends on severity and speed of treatment
- Prevention
  - Careful technique with cataract surgery
  - Appropriate aseptic technique, application of povidone iodine, use of intracameral antibiotics

Zonular Dialysis

- Definition
  - Absence or loss of the attachment of the lens zonules leading to poor support of the capsular bag/crystalline lens
- Etiology
  - Trauma
  - Pseudoexfoliation
  - Old age
  - Intraoperative iatrogenic trauma
  - Associated with specific disorders (eg, idiopathic, Marfan's syndrome)
- Prevention and management
  - Recognize risk preoperatively
  - Careful and complete hydrodissection
  - Consider dispersive viscoelastic to block vitreous prolapsed.
  - Use capsular suspension hooks.
  - Consider implantation of capsular tension ring as early as practically feasible during lens removal.
  - Do not strip cortex meridionally, but parallel to the dialysis.
  - Avoid chamber collapse to prevent further dialysis and vitreous prolapse.
- Prognosis
  - Excellent with proper surgical approach

Intraocular Lenses

History

- The first IOL was implanted by Sir Harold Ridley in 1949. It was a one-piece polymethylmethacrylate (PMMA) IOL that filled the entire capsular bag. Ridley had observed that pilots from World War I with eye injuries had inert pieces of PMMA glass from plane windscreens in their eyes with little reaction.
- Choyce developed AC angle fixated rigid lenses. Later, many models and variations of this principle were used, but were soon abandoned due to unacceptable complication rates with the models used, the manufacturing quality, and the surgical techniques (ie, ICCE) in general use at that time.
- Binkhorst's iris clip lenses are at the beginning of the modern era of lens implantation.
- Shearing finally developed a posterior chamber IOL, at first for fixation in the ciliary sulcus and then, after the renaissance of extracapsular cataract surgery brought about by the development of phaco-emulsification by Kelman, for fixation in the capsular bag
- Today, all forms of IOLs have been developed further: angle-, iris-, sulcus-, and capsule-fixated lenses are in use to offer a solution for nearly every situation

Materials

Silicone

- All silicone IOLs are high molecular weight polymers of oxygen and silicone (polysiloxanes) that are extensively crosslinked.
- Properties
  - Posterior chamber IOLs
  - Flexible at room temperature
  - Highly hydrophobic
  - High uveal and capsular biocompatibility
  - Stimulate apposition of type IV collagen in the interface between the anterior lens capsule and IOL surface. This results in contraction of the capsulorrhexis rim, thus pulling the posterior lens capsule tightly around the posterior edge and preventing posterior capsular opacification (PCO) formation according to the "no space no cells" theory.
  - Exhibit a much lower threshold for YAG laser damage than other IOL biomaterials

Acrylic

- Acrylic IOLs consist of 3 main groups:
  - Rigid PMMA IOLs
  - Foldable hydrophobic acrylic (hydrogel) IOLs
  - Foldable hydrophilic IOLs
- PMMA is polymer of methylmethacrylate (MMA), which means that it is an acrylic material made from only one type of monomer.
  - Properties
    - Rigid at room temperature
    - Less uveal biocompatibility than silicone or hydrogel IOLs
    - Surface treating of PMMA lenses significantly reduces postoperative inflammation, cell adhesion, and corneal damage
- All hydrophilic acrylic IOLs are water-swollen polymeric gels. The main component is polyhydroxyethylmethacrylate (polyHEMA). The amount of water absorbed expressed as a percentage of weight of the hydrated gel is known as the equilibrium water content, which usually varies between 18% and 38%.
  - Properties
    - Foldable at room temperature
    - High uveal biocompatibility
    - Low damage potential when touching the cornea
    - Lower capsular biocompatibility than other biomaterials
    - Under certain conditions, hydrogels may provoke calcium precipitation on their surface.

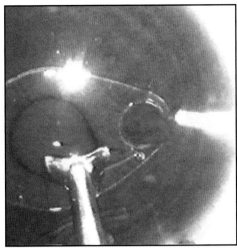

Figure 9-29. Phakic iris claw lens. (Reprinted with permission from Sher NA. *Surgery for Hyperopia.* Thorofare, NJ: SLACK Incorporated; 2004.)

- o The collamer material is a hydrophilic acrylic trademarked by STAAR Surgical. It consists of polyHEMA containing 33% water and 0.2% porcine collagen with an integrated ultraviolet (UV) blocker. IOLs made of this material are foldable.
- Hydrophobic acrylic lenses are made from non-HEMA acrylic compounds.
  - o Properties
    - Foldable at room temperature
    - Lower uveal biocompatibility, especially in uveitic eyes
    - High capsular biocompatibility, provoking less PCO. The low rate of PCO has been attributed in part to the sharp-edge design of the lenses made from this material, but also in part to the adhesive properties of the material itself.

Types of Intraocular Lenses

Iris Clip (Support)

- There are several generations of iris-fixated IOLs (Figure 9-29).
  - o Early iris-fixated IOLs
    - Popular in the 1970s following ICCE but are not used any more due to the high number of complications
    - Made of PMMA
    - The IOL haptics were placed on 2 sides of pupil in the anterior and posterior chamber.
  - o Binkhorst IOL/Worst Medallion IOL
    - Kept in place by a suture (complication: biodegradation of suture and IOL dislocation)
  - o Copland IOL
    - Kept in place by chronic administration of miotics
- Today's iris-fixated IOLs are kept in place by enclavation to the iris
  - o Stay in place with pupillary movement
  - o Originally designed to be placed into the AC
  - o Can also be fixated in PC ("inverse" implantation) in order to respect compartmentalization of eye
  - o Aphakic version is made of PMMA, requires large incision
  - o Also used as phakic implants for high ametropias (also acrylic version available)
  - o Advantages
    - Allow IOL implantation in absence of capsular support
    - Less corneal complications than angle-fixated AC IOL, especially with inverse fixation

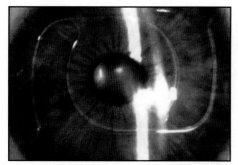

Figure 9-30. ZB 5M implant. It went into production in 1990. (Reprinted with permission from Hardten DR, Lindstrom RL, Davis EA. *Phakic Intraocular Lenses: Principles and Practice.* Thorofare, NJ: SLACK Incorporated; 2004.)

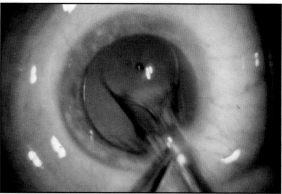

Figure 9-31. Plate lens being inserted. (Reprinted with permission from Buratto L, Werner, L, Zanini M, Apple, DJ. *Phacoemulsification: Principles and Techniques*, 2nd ed. Thorofare, NJ: SLACK Incorporated; 2003.)

      ○ Disadvantages
            ▪ May lead to iris irritation, uveitis
            ▪ Require large incision

Anterior Chamber

- Anterior chamber IOLs (Figure 9-30) are IOLs that are positioned entirely in the AC with their foot plates ideally placed on the ciliary band.
- Early AC-IOLs were introduced in the era of ICCE and displayed several problems due to suboptimal design, which has been altered in newer-generation AC-IOLs.
- Today's AC-IOLs are used for
  - ○ Complicated cataract surgery when there is insufficient support from the bag
  - ○ Phakic IOLs for the correction of high ametropia

Posterior Chamber

- Now the most common location for IOL implantation
- Designed to be positioned within the capsular bag and/or the sulcus
- Posterior chamber IOLs designed for sulcus fixation usually have an overall larger diameter and may have fixation holes for sutures at their haptics.
- Posterior chamber IOLs come in foldable and rigid (ie, PMMA) types. Foldable IOLs are now most commonly used to preserve the small phacoemulsification incision.

Multipiece Intraocular Lenses

- Describes IOLs that have optic and haptics put together secondarily. The optic may be from either material. The haptic material is usually made from a rigid material such as PMMA or prolene.

Single-Piece Intraocular Lenses

- Are manufactured as one piece, meaning that the haptics and the optics are made from the same material or are made from different materials that are covalently bound together

Plate-Haptic Intraocular Lenses

- Foldable IOL at room temperature
- Haptics are solid plates on either side of IOL optic.
- Insertion technique usually involves an injector (Figure 9-31).
- Advantages
  - ○ Low incidence of PCO due to optic/capsular bag contact

- Disadvantages
  - Exact sizing necessary (too large leads to bending of IOL, too small leads to fibrosis)
  - May dislocate in vitreous after YAG laser capsulotomy due to buttonhole effect (recommendation: keep capsular bag opening small)
  - Leads to capsular bag fusion around IOL and makes future explantation difficult

Blue-Blocker Intraocular Lenses

- Several studies have suggested that the yellow discoloration of the crystalline lens might be protective against short-wavelength light and thus prevent macular degeneration.
- On this underlying theory, new "yellow" IOL designs, with an integrated high-frequency blue wavelength filter, were developed.
- There seems to be strong laboratory evidence that the so-called blue-blocking IOLs may prevent light-induced harm to the central retina.
- There are concerns about impaired color vision and circadian rhythm through loss of the blue spectrum.
- Neither the effects nor the concerns have been proven in humans to date.

Accommodative Intraocular Lenses

- Single-optic designs: Based on the anterior shift principle, which means an anterior movement of the IOL optic occurs with accommodative effort. The Crystalens (Bausch and Lomb, Rochester, New York) is an example of this type of IOL.
- Dual-optic lenses: With accommodative effort, a high-power plus lens moves forward while a minus-power posterior optic stays pressed against the posterior capsular bag. In the unaccommodated state, the lenses are closest together.
- Theories to account for the mechanism of these IOLs include constriction of the ciliary body, creating increased vitreous pressure and/or capsule relaxation, permitting the IOL to change its configuration. According to the Helmholtz theory, the loss of accommodation is due to loss of flexibility in the aging, hardening lens. Therefore, research on accommodating IOL designs has included lens refilling using an injectable liquid or flexible polymer.

Multifocal Intraocular Lenses

- Used for the correction of distance acuity and presbyopia
- The multifocal IOLs work on the refractive or diffractive principle, creating separate foci for near and distance vision.
- Truly multifocal IOLs usually have more associated optic phenomena, such as halos, but offer good vision in the intermediate distance.
- Bifocal IOLs may have less associated optic phenomena but only have 2 foci.
- Popular multifocal IOLs
  - ReZoom
  - ReStor
  - Tecnis multifocal

Light Adaptive Intraocular Lenses

- To optimize the achieved refractive correction after cataract surgery, the light-adjustable lens (LAL) has been developed.
- The LAL is a photosensitive silicone IOL whose power can be adjusted noninvasively and cured after implantation using a low-power light source.
- It is composed of a cross-linked silicone polymer matrix with an embedded photosensitive macromer. UV-irradiation to a certain region of the lens will result in polymerization of the macromer and subsequent migration and redistribution of nonpolymerized macromers, which then leads to precise changes in the lens power and thickness.

Figure 9-32. IOL insertion technique with forceps. (Reprinted with permission from Buratto L, Werner, L, Zanini M, Apple, DJ. *Phacoemulsification: Principles and Techniques*, 2nd ed. Thorofare, NJ: SLACK Incorporated; 2003.)

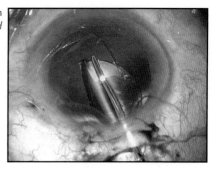

Aspheric Intraocular Lenses

- The cornea has an aspheric anterior curvature, meaning that its radius is greater centrally than peripherally, resulting in negative spherical aberration. In youth, this is balanced by the positive spherical aberration of the crystalline lens, which has a spherical anterior curvature, ie, its radius is smaller centrally than peripherally. Whereas the asphericity of the cornea remains constant throughout life, the positive spherical aberration of the crystalline lens increases in aging eyes. Therefore, the crystalline lens' capacity to neutralize the aberration of the cornea decreases over time, resulting in a loss of contrast sensitivity and mesopic visual quality.
- Aspheric IOLs are designed to increase pseudophakic contrast sensitivity.
- They can feature an aspheric optic, which does not introduce additional spherical aberration into the system.
- They can also be designed with a prolate surface to even (ideally) correct corneal aberration. The optic surface of these IOLs is designed on the basis of theoretical considerations or real measurements.

Insertion Techniques for Intraocular Lenses

Forceps

- Advantage
  - No cartridge necessary, faster (Figure 9-32)
- Disadvantage
  - Incision has to be enlarged to half the IOL optic size, IOL-conjunctiva contact during insertion with possible introduction of bacteria, possible damage of IOL from folding forceps

Cartridge

- Advantage
  - Incision has to be only minimally enlarged if at all; controlled insertion of IOL
- Disadvantage
  - Loading of IOL time consuming; possible cartridge problems may damage IOL or deposit unwanted material on IOL during implantation

Complications of Intraocular Lenses

De-Centration

- Etiology
  - Primarily due to factors directly related to surgery
  - Secondarily related to surgical factors, bag shrinkage, or idiopathic/traumatic factors
- Mechanisms of de-centration
  - IOL is not placed completely within the capsular bag (one haptic or entire sulcus fixation).
  - IOL is displaced within the capsular bag (including anteroposterior tilt).
  - The IOL is displaced within the capsular bag due to loose zonules.
- Predisposing factors are the following:
  - Incomplete or irregular capsulorrhexis

- o Asymmetric shrinkage of the capsular bag due to PCO (enhanced by incomplete or irregular capsulorrhexis)
- o Too small or too large an IOL overall diameter for the capsular bag (for example in highly ametropic eyes)
- o Sulcus fixation of IOL
- o Loose zonules
  - Iatrogenic (zonulolysis during surgery)
  - Idiopathic loose zonules (pseudoexfoliation, myopia)
- Signs/symptoms
  - o Glare/dysphotopsia (see next section)
  - o Loss of best corrected visual acuity
  - o Change in refractive power due to anteroposterior shift
- Management
  - o All factors of PCO prevention will prevent irregular shrinkage of capsular bag.
  - o In cases of irregular capsulorrhexis or discontinuity of capsulorrhexis: Intraoperative or early postoperative IOL—reposition into capsular bag. Recommendation: Place haptics 90 degrees to discontinuity of capsulorrhexis.

Dysphotopsia

- Signs/symptoms
  - o Flare, streaks, halos, and other abnormal visual perception/photic phenomena (shadows)
  - o *Dys*: Refers to directly implied dysfunction secondary to the photic phenomena
  - o *Photopsia*: Subjective sensation of lights, sparks, or colors due to retinal or cerebral disease
  - o Can be positive (light spots) or negative (dark shadows)
  - o Occurs in 20% of pseudophakic patients, but is usually transient and clinically insignificant
- Factors that influence the incidence of dysphotopsia
  - o De-centered or tilted IOL
    - If the IOL margin comes close to the visual axis, light will strike it and may eventually be perceived as reflection.
    - To minimize the effect, the IOL should be centered well in the capsular bag, which is enhanced by a centered capsulorrhexis that is not larger than the IOL optic.
  - o Small optic
    - If the optic is small, the edge of the IOL may scatter light if the pupil becomes larger.
    - Therefore, nowadays, the usual IOLs all have an optic size of at least 5.5 mm.
  - o Edge design of IOL
    - Dysphotopsia problem arose since the introduction of the truncated sharp edge, which is mainly due to internal reflections at the edge in case of an anterior and posterior sharp edge (mainly negative dysphotopsia).
    - To approach this, edge designs that have a sharp posterior edge to minimize PCO but also have a round anterior edge or frosted edge to minimize glare are available.
  - o IOL material
    - The effect of dysphotopsia is larger if the IOL is manufactured from a biomaterial that has a larger refractive index.
    - Some hydrophobic acrylic IOLs tend to have higher refractive indexes than other IOL types.
    - Therefore, in a patient prone to develop dysphotopsia, it is recommended to use an IOL with a low refractive index.
  - o Anterior curvature of the IOL
    - If the anterior curvature of the IOL is flat, the risk for dysphotopsia is higher.
    - Patient factor: Hyperopia, special predisposition of patient
- Treatment
  - o If symptoms are sufficiently symptomatic, the IOL may need to be replaced.
- Prevention
  - o Correct IOL selection and surgical technique
- Prognosis
  - o Generally good, although may require IOL exchange in severe cases

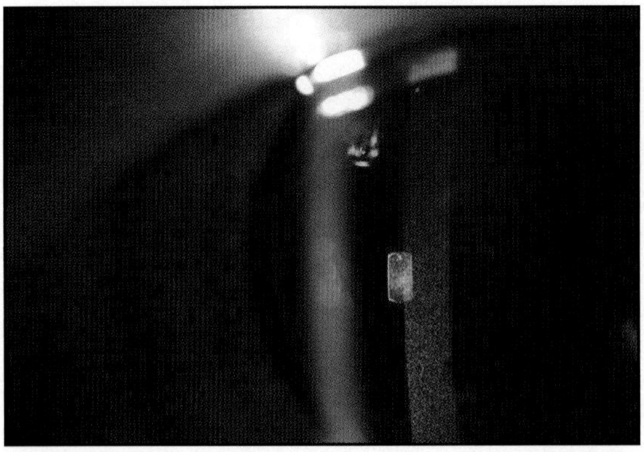

Figure 9-33. IOL opacification due to calcification of IOL optic.

Opacification

- Definition
  - o Loss of transparency of IOL optic
- Signs/symptoms
  - o Vision loss
  - o Glare
  - o Dysphotopsia
- Etiology
  - o Main reason for opacification is calcification of the IOL optic (Figure 9-33).
    - Most reports on calcification of IOL refer to hydrophilic acrylic IOL.
    - All IOL materials have been reported with regard to calcification.
    - May be IOL-related (manufacturing problem) or related to environment (inflammation, complicated surgery).
  - o Hydrophobic acrylic IOL may exhibit "glistenings"
    - Small water-filled vacuoles within IOL material
    - Temperature-dependent
    - Usually not visually significant
  - o Rare causes include uptake of intraoperatively used dyes, systemic medication, material flaws, etc.
- Treatment
  - o Usually only necessary if patient disturbed
  - o Treatment is surgical (IOL exchange).
  - o Do not perform YAG capsulotomy when in doubt, because IOL exchange will become more difficult with open posterior capsule.

Suggested Readings

Buratto L, ed. *Phacoemulsification, Principles and Techniques*. Thorofare, NJ: SLACK Incorporated; 1998.

Chang DF, ed. *Phaco Chop: Mastering Techniques, Optimizing Technology, and Avoiding Complications*. Thorofare, NJ: SLACK Incorporated; 2004.

Ernest P, Tipperman R, Eagle R, et al. Is there a difference in incision healing based on location? *J Cataract Refract Surg*. 1998;24(4):482–486.

Hardten D, Lindstrom RL, Davis E. *Phakic IOLs*. Thorofare, NJ: SLACK Incorporated; 2004.

Jaffe NS, Jaffe MS, Jaffe GF, eds. *Cataract Surgery and Its Complications*. Mosby; 1997.

Wallace B. *Refractive Cataract Surgery and Multifocal IOLs*. Thorofare, NJ: SLACK Incorporated; 2001.

Questions

1. Typical cataract symptoms include
   a. Hazy, foggy vision
   b. Glare
   c. Monocular diplopia
   d. Vision impairment at near more pronounced than for distance
   e. All of the above
   f. a, b, and c

2. Cataract surgery is
   a. Always indicated below 20/40 best-corrected distance vision
   b. Indicated, when individual patient's activities are impaired by typical symptoms
   c. Indicated, when cataract causes or threatens further complications
   d. Will usually worsen pre-existing glaucoma
   e. b and c
   f. a, b, and c
   g. All of the above

3. ICCE is
   a. Obsolete and never indicated today
   b. An option in congenital cataract
   c. Indicated in subluxed hard lenses
   d. Preferred with pseudoexfoliation
   e. Preferred with compromised corneal endothelium

4. Monocular congenital cataract
   a. Should not be operated before age 2
   b. Should be operated when binocularity is (assumed) interrupted
   c. Should be operated regardless of binocularity to prevent amblyopia
   d. Should be operated early to avoid patching for amblyopia treatment
   e. Is usually not an indication for surgery

5. Combine the correct number and letter
   1. Perforation cataract
   2. Contusion (blunt trauma) cataract
   3. Steroid-induced cataract
   4. Diabetic cataract

   a. No specific morphology
   b. Anterior rosette formation
   c. Posterior rosette formation
   d. Posterior subcapsular cataract

   Answer:
   1. **c**
   2. **b**
   3. **d**
   4. **a**

6. Risk factors for posterior capsular rupture in phacoemulsification are
   a. Working near capsule with phaco tip
   b. Posterior polar cataracts
   c. Anterior capsular rim tears
   d. Sharp edges of instruments
   e. a, b, and d
   f. All of the above

7. Anterior chamber angle-fixated IOL lenses
   a. Are obsolete today
   b. Exist only for phakic refractive implantation
   c. Are not used for phakic refractive correction
   d. Are an option in cases of lack of capsular support
   e. Are only used in developing countries

8. Iris-fixated IOL lenses
   a. Are obsolete today
   b. Are today fixated by enclavation of tissue
   c. Must be fixated to the anterior surface of the iris
   d. Are only used for phakic refractive correction
   e. Cannot be used for phakic refractive correction

9. Acrylic IOL lenses
   a. Are hydrophilic
   b. Are hydrophobic
   c. May show late opacifications
   d. Can be foldable
   e. All of the above

10. Dysphotopsia may be caused by
    a. Truncated sharp-edge design of IOL
    b. Decentration of IOL
    c. Bi-/multifocal optics of IOL
    d. High refractive index of IOL material
    e. All of the above

Pediatric Ophthalmology

Robert S. Gold, MD; Louis C. Blumenfeld, MD; and Naval Sondhi, MD

Outline

1. Introduction
2. Examination of the Pediatric Eye
3. Strabismus and Amblyopia
   a. Esodeviations
      i. Infantile Esotropia
      ii. Accommodative Esotropia
      iii. High Accommodative Convergence/ Accommodation Ratio
      iv. Sensory Deprivation Esotropia
      v. Consecutive Esotropia
      vi. Incomitant Esodeviation
   b. Exodeviations
      i. Pseudoexotropia
      ii. Exophoria
      iii. Intermittent Exotropia
      iv. Constant Exotropia
      v. Congenital Exotropia
      vi. Sensory Exotropia
      vii. Consecutive Exotropia
      viii. Exotropic Duane's Syndrome
      ix. Neuromuscular Abnormalities
      x. Dissociated Horizontal Deviation
      xi. Convergence Insufficiency
      xii. Convergence Paralysis
   c. Amblyopia
      i. Strabismic Amblyopia
      ii. Eccentric Fixation
      iii. Anisometropic Amblyopia
      iv. Isometropia (High Bilateral Refractive Errors)
      v. Deprivation Amblyopia
4. Disorders of Ocular Motility
   a. A/V Patterns
   b. Vertical Deviations and Special Strabismus Conditions
      i. Dissociated Vertical Deviation
      ii. Third Nerve Palsy
      iii. Fourth Nerve Paresis (Superior Oblique Palsy)
      iv. Sixth Nerve Palsy
      v. Internuclear Ophthalmoplegia
      vi. Brown's Syndrome
      vii. Inferior Oblique Palsy
      viii. Monocular Elevation Deficiency (Double Elevator Palsy)
      ix. Orbital Floor Fractures
      x. Duane's Syndrome
      xi. Moebius Syndrome
      xii. Myasthenia Gravis
      xiii. Thyroid Eye Disease
      xiv. Congenital Fibrosis Syndrome
5. Nystagmus
   a. Congenital Motor Nystagmus
   b. Latent
   c. Spasmus Nutans
   d. Sensory Nystagmus
   e. Downbeat Nystagmus
   f. Medication
   g. Upbeat Nystagmus
   h. See-Saw Nystagmus
   i. Convergence Retraction Nystagmus
   j. Dissociated Nystagmus
   k. Vestibular
   l. Gaze Evoked
6. Childhood Glaucoma
7. Congenital Disc Anomalies
   a. Optic Disc Hypoplasia

Probst LE, Tsai JH.
Ophthalmology: Clinical and Surgical Principles (pp. 377–418).
© 2012 SLACK Incorporated

b. Morning Glory Disc
c. Optic Disc Coloboma
d. Optic Pit
e. Congenital Tilted Disc Syndrome
f. Myelinated Nerve Fibers
g. Optic Disc in Albinism Papilledema
h. Optic Disc Drusen
8. Leukocoria and Cataracts
    a. Retinoblastoma
    b. Coats' Disease

c. Persistent Fetal Vasculature
d. Cataract
e. Retinopathy of Prematurity
9. Congenital Lacrimal Obstruction
10. Pediatric Red Eye
    a. Kawasaki Syndrome
    b. Stevens-Johnson Syndrome
    c. Neonatal Conjunctivitis
    d. Anterior Uveitis in Children
    e. Juvenile Rheumatoid Arthritis

Introduction

Pediatric ophthalmology involves the evaluation and treatment of the disorders of the eye of children, which include strabismus, amblyopia, retinopathy of prematurity (ROP), as well as a number of other disorders more prevalent in children.

Examination of the Pediatric Eye

- Examination of the pediatric eye involves a specialized approach for the testing of visual acuity (VA), amblyopia, and ocular alignment.
- VA is measured in a manner appropriate for the patient's age.
    - For patients too young to subjectively quantify their VA levels, objective methods are used, such as visual evoked potentials (VEPs).
    - For patients aged 1 to 3 years, subjective methods, such as Allen cards, are often used in addition to objective methods.
    - For patients aged 3 to 5 years, subjective methods, such as Allen cards, tumbling Es, or the letter chart, can be used.
    - For patients older than 5 years, the Snellen alphabet chart can almost always be used.
- Determine stereoacuity using polarized glasses and Randot stereogram.
- Check extraocular movements.
- Measure or estimate the angle of deviation.
    - The easiest method is to evaluate the centration of the corneal light reflex in each eye while the patient fixes on objects at distance or near.
    - Prisms can be used to quantify the deviation.
    - In some cases, performing the alternate cover test is possible.
        - The patient fixes on an object.
        - By alternately covering and uncovering each eye, the examiner can detect a shift in the eye's position with refixation.
        - In esotropia (ET), as an eye is uncovered, it turns out to fixate.
        - In accommodative ET, the angle of deviation is often the same when measured at distance and near fixation (usually 20 to 40 prism diopters [PD]), but it can vary depending on the accommodative convergence/accommodation (AC/A) ratio.
- Measure the AC/A ratio.
    - If the AC/A ratio is high, the deviation measured at near will be significantly greater than that at distance.
    - In true accommodative ET, the AC/A ratio should be normal.
- Perform a complete eye examination.
    - Examine the anterior segment to assess the cornea, anterior chamber, and lens.
    - Examine the fundus with both direct and indirect ophthalmoscopes.
    - Note the appearance of the macula and optic nerve.
- Perform cycloplegic refraction on all children by using the retinoscope and trial lenses.
    - Cycloplegia often can be achieved with Mydriacyl 1% if the patient is younger than 1 year; it is achieved with Cyclogyl 1% if the patient is older than 1 year.

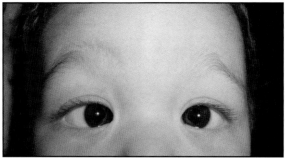

Figure 10-1. Infantile ET of approximately 35 PD in a 6 month old.

Strabismus and Amblyopia

Esodeviations

- Definition
  - Inward deviation of the eye/eyes
- Pseudostrabismus
  - Due to wide flat nasal bridge/prominent epicanthal folds/small interpupillary distance
  - Corneal light reflex test normal (Hirschberg)
  - True crossing may occur on top of false crossing, so follow-up exam may be warranted, especially with positive family history of strabismus and/or amblyopia.

Infantile Esotropia

- Definition
  - Esotropia at birth (congenital) or by 6 months of age
- Signs/symptoms
  - Positive family history may be present
  - Children usually otherwise normal
  - Up to 30% of patients with neurological and developmental problems (cerebral palsy, hydrocephalus)
  - Cross fixation = equal vision
  - Amblyopia can occur if ET with one eye with or without cross fixation
  - Usually >30 PD (Figure 10-1)
  - Vertical deviations become more common over time—usually >1 year of age
  - Dissociated vertical deviation (DVD) and inferior oblique (IO) overreaction common
- Evaluation
  - Usually >30 PD of ET
- Treatment
  - Cycloplegic refraction
    - >+2.50 or 3.00 need optical correction prior to surgery
    - Large deviations will usually not respond to small refractive errors.
  - Surgery
    - After refractive errors and amblyopia treated
    - Repeat measurements before surgery
    - Timing
      - Most advocate age 6 months (maximize binocular fusion potential)
      - Goal is ocular alignment as soon as possible.
      - Surgery by 24 months of age or 12 months from onset of deviation for fusion potential
    - Usual procedure is bilateral medial rectus (MR) recessions or unilateral MR recession/lateral rectus (LR) resection.
- Prognosis
  - Good with early intervention; 70% achieve within 10 PD of orthophoria

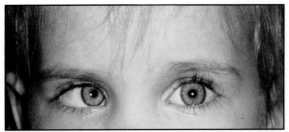

Figure 10-2. Right ET in a 2 year old with an ansiometropic cycloplegic refraction requiring glasses and patching therapy to the left eye.

Accommodative Esotropia

- Definition
  - Esotropia induced by accommodation
- Signs/symptoms
  - Esotropia onset between 6 months and 7 years—most between 18 months and 4 years (Figure 10-2)
  - Intermittent to constant
  - Hereditary
  - Sometimes preceded by trauma or illness
  - Amblyopia common
  - Visual spectrum from diplopia to suppression
  - Types
    - Refractive
    - Hyperopia/insufficient fusion
- Evaluation
  - Angle 20 to 30 PD
  - Hyperopia +2 to 10 (average +4)
- Treatment
  - Glasses (cycloplegic refraction) usually full correction with amblyopia treatment
  - Bifocals if increased ET at near
  - Glasses full-time (cycloplegics for compliance) and surgery for nonaccommodative component (basic) (Figures 10-3 and 10-4)

High Accommodative Convergence/Accommodation Ratio

- Definition
  - Abnormal accommodation convergence
- Signs/symptoms
  - More accommodation required at near, thus ET greater at near
- Treatment
  - Conservative
    - Treat with refraction (most tolerated) with bifocal add (usually +2.50 to +3.00 D)
    - Bifocals can be flat-top style to bisect 1- to 2-mm below pupil border to encourage near use of the bifocal.
    - Progressives can be used, but optical center must be raised 2 to 4 mm to encourage use of the progressive bifocal.
    - Phospholine iodide rarely used due to side effects including iris cysts and susceptibility to muscle relaxants under anesthesia.
  - Surgery
    - Surgery is usually based on residual deviation with glasses in place.
    - Parents must be counseled that patient will need glasses postoperatively and will have crossing without correction postsurgery.

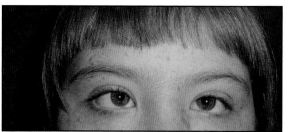

Figure 10-3. A 4-year-old girl with Down syndrome with a right ET.

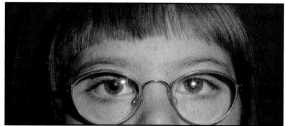

Figure 10-4. Accommodative ET in same patient with a +4.00 sphere cycloplegic refraction OU and orthophoria with glasses in place.

- Prognosis
  - Hyperopia usually increases up to age 4, variably changes from 5 to 7, and usually decreases after age 8.
  - Optical correction titrated after age 7 to have best vision and alignment possible.
  - Bifocal power can also be titrated depending on near measurements but patients often will not outgrow this until the teenage years (50% chance).

Sensory Deprivation Esotropia

- Etiology
  - Cataract
  - Corneal scarring
  - Optic atrophy
  - Retinal image distortion
- Treatment
  - Try to remove or eliminate problem if possible
    - Treat amblyopia if possible
    - Surgery on abnormal eye

Consecutive Esotropia

- Secondary to exotropia (XT) surgery (Figure 10-5)
  - Patients often overcorrected post-XT surgery and usually will resolve if deviation is small.
  - Treat with patching and further surgery if persists or significant angle.
- Slipped or lost LR muscle
  - Demonstrate variable amounts of ET
  - Treatment by exploration for lost muscle

Incomitant Esodeviation

- Definition
  - An incomitant deviation is worsened with gaze into the direction of the paretic muscle.
- Etiology
  - Sixth nerve (abducens) palsy
- Signs/symptoms
  - Uncommon at birth
    - Increased intracranial pressure with birth process
    - Usually spontaneously resolves
  - Older patients
    - Diplopia/head turn toward side of paralysis
    - One-third have intracranial lesions and neurological findings
    - Other etiologies include infections, immunologic, head trauma (Figure 10-6)
- Treatment
  - Occlusion/prisms—usually spontaneously resolves within 3 to 6 months
  - BOTOX into antagonist MR to align eyes and prevent MR contracture

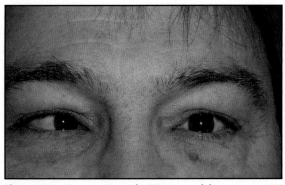

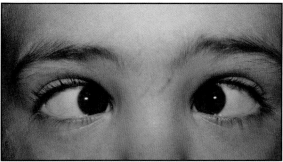

Figure 10-6. A 2 year old with ET secondary to bilateral sixth nerve palsies from closed head trauma.

Figure 10-5. Consecutive right ET in an adult status post-XT surgery.

- ○ Surgery
  - ▪ Wait 3 months minimum—most advocate waiting 6 months or until deviation stabilizes for 3 months
  - ▪ MR recess/LR resect versus transposition versus botulinum injection (BOTOX) + transposition

Exodeviations

Pseudoexotropia

- Positive angle kappa with or without ocular abnormalities (ie, macular dragging from ROP) (Figure 10-7)
- Wide interpupillary distance

Exophoria

- Definition
  - ○ Outward deviation of the eye when fusion is broken
- Signs/Symptoms
  - ○ Controlled by fusion
  - ○ Detected when binocular fusion is interrupted
  - ○ Asthenopic symptoms
- Treatment
  - ○ Observation

Intermittent Exotropia

- Definition
  - ○ Intermittent outward deviation of the eye
- Signs/symptoms
  - ○ Usually occurs before age 5 but can be in much older child
  - ○ Usually seen during fatigue, stress, inattention
  - ○ Usually occurs late in the day with fatigue or when a child is sick or daydreaming
  - ○ Eye closure is common especially with bright lights.
  - ○ Distance deviation more than near
  - ○ IO over action in approximately one-third of patients
  - ○ Categorize XT as good, fair, or poor control
- Classification
  - ○ Basic XT: distance XT and near XT equal
  - ○ Divergence excess XT: distance XT greater than near XT
  - ○ Convergence insufficiency XT: near XT greater than distance XT
- Treatment
  - ○ Nonsurgical
    - ▪ Glasses for significant refractive errors—myopia, astigmatism, hyperopia

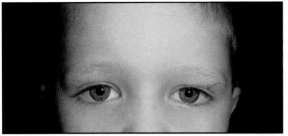

Figure 10-7. Positive angle kappa. Note corneal light reflexes simulating an XT.

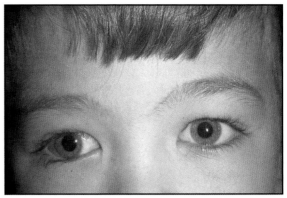

Figure 10-8. A 35-prism-diopter right XT in a 4 year old.

- Minus lenses to stimulate accommodative convergence
- Part-time patching of dominant eye—a passive orthoptic treatment
- Convergence exercises or base-in prism glasses for convergence insufficiency
  - o Surgical
    - Indicated when progression of amount and frequency of the deviation increases despite non-surgical observation and treatments
    - Timing controversial
    - Procedure usually bilateral LR recessions. Unilateral LR recession and MR resection is an alternative especially in basic type XT.
    - Overcorrection desirable postoperatively—if persists, patching with or without prisms. If overcorrection persists and if LR recessions had been previously performed, MR recessions are often advocated.
    - Undercorrections—base-in prisms, patching. If further surgery is needed, MR resections, unilateral or bilateral are recommended depending on amount of deviation.

Constant Exotropia

- Signs/symptoms
  - o More common in older patients with sensory XT or with decompensated intermittent XT (Figure 10-8)
  - o Often see X pattern
- Surgical treatment
  - o Same as intermittent XT surgery with or without oblique surgery

Congenital Exotropia

- Definition
  - o Exotropia before 6 months of age
  - o Large constant angle
  - o Often associated with neurological impairment or craniofacial disorders
- Treatment
  - o Early surgery advocated but late consecutive ET, recurrent XT, and DVD all common

Sensory Exotropia

- Similar to sensory ET

Consecutive Exotropia

- Similar to ET

Exotropic Duane's Syndrome

- Face turn away from affected eye
- Deficient adduction, eyelid narrowing, globe retraction, up and downshoots

Neuromuscular Abnormalities

- Third-nerve palsy
- Internuclear ophthalmoplegia (INO)
- Myasthenia gravis

Dissociated Horizontal Deviation

- Definition
  - Dissociated abduction prominent
- Signs/Symptoms
  - May be confused with intermittent XT
  - DVD and latent nystagmus may coexist with dissociated horizontal deviation (DHD).
- Treatment
  - Treatment usually unilateral or bilateral LR recessions

Convergence Insufficiency

- Definition
  - Poor near point of convergence and near fusional convergence
- Signs/symptoms
  - Asthenopia, blurred vision at near, reading difficulties
  - Usually has an exophoria at near
- Treatment
  - Orthoptic exercises
  - Pencil pushups and other near-point exercises
  - Base-in or myopic reading glasses
  - Rarely MR resections, unilateral or bilateral

Convergence Paralysis

- Definition
  - Normal adduction and accommodation
  - XT and diplopia at near
- Signs/symptoms
  - Usually secondary to an intracranial lesion
  - Acute onset
  - Location of lesion usually corpora quadrigemina, nucleus of cranial nerve III
  - May be associated with Parinaud's syndrome
- Treatment
  - Base-in prisms for diplopia
  - Very difficult to re-establish binocular vision so occlusion often used

Amblyopia

- Definition
  - Decrease of best-corrected vision
  - Amblyopia is unilateral or bilateral
- Etiology
  - It can be caused by strabismus, anisometropia or isometropia, or visual deprivation and is a defect of central vision.
  - Prevalence is 2% to 4% of the population.
- Evaluation
  - Detection of amblyopia is essential at a young age.
  - Screening programs at a primary care physician's office, at school, or in community setting are extremely important opportunities to identify amblyopia at an early stage so it can be treated.
  - Photoscreening is another method of identification that is used most often in large community-based screening programs. Other vision-screening technology is being investigated to further aid in this process including autorefractors.

Strabismic Amblyopia

- Most common form
- Usually, constant tropias with one eye fixation preference

Eccentric Fixation

- Use of a nonfoveal region of the retina to be viewed monocularly by an amblyopic eye

Anisometropic Amblyopia

- Unequal refractive errors with one eye's image being more blurred than the other
- Many patients do not have strabismus, which makes this form of amblyopia more difficult to identify and puts a good deal of the burden on the primary physician to accurately screen these children's vision.

Isometropia (High Bilateral Refractive Errors)

- Usually hyperopia >5 D and myopia >10 D and astigmatism >2 D will cause this problem.

Deprivation Amblyopia

- Usually from a congenital corneal or lenticular opacity
- Can also be caused by occlusion amblyopia from excessive patching or atropine eye drops
- Treatment
  - o Refractive correction
    - Cycloplegic refraction is critical in young children.
    - It has been found that correction of the refractive error (unilateral or bilateral) can aid in VA improvement over several months' time.
  - o Occlusion and penalization
    - Occlusion therapy with patching has been prominent in the ophthalmic literature since the Pediatric Eye Disease Investigator Group (PEDIG) began publishing its protocols and findings in 2001.
    - Many practitioners will now prescribe 6 hours of patching/day and if the patient's vision in the amblyopic eye does not improve significantly, patching is increased to full-time.
    - For mild to moderate amblyopia, 2 hours of patching is initially prescribed and increased accordingly up to 6 hours a day or more if target vision is not achieved.
    - Also, atropine in the sound eye is being used more frequently to treat amblyopia and can increase compliance.
    - Weaning of patching is also important to not have the vision decrease toward the initial treatment level.
    - In addition, while age 9 had been a cutoff age for positive response to amblyopia treatment, children up to age 17 were found to respond to some form of amblyopia therapy to improve vision in their amblyopic eye.
  - o Surgery
    - Consideration of surgery in causes of deprivation, especially lenticular and strabismic issues

Disorders of Ocular Motility

A/V Patterns

- Definition
  - o Eyes adduct in upward gaze and abduct in downward gaze (A pattern) or vice versa (V pattern)
- Etiology
  - o Inferior oblique overaction (IOOA) creates a V pattern.
  - o Superior oblique (SO) overaction creates an A pattern.
- Signs/symptoms
  - o A or V pattern associated with 15% to 25% of all strabismus cases.

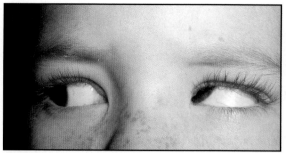

Figure 10-9. Overaction of inferior oblique muscles in a 3 year old with a V pattern ET. Right gaze.

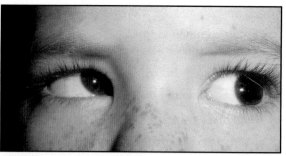

Figure 10-10. Overaction of inferior oblique muscles in a 3 year old with a V pattern ET. Left gaze.

- ○ Oblique muscles
  - ▪ IOOA creates a V pattern (Figures 10-9 and 10-10).
  - ▪ SO overaction creates an A pattern.
  - ▪ Apert or Crouzon syndromes commonly show these strabismic patterns.
- • Management
  - ○ Determine treatment by primary and reading position deviation.
  - ○ Horizontal surgery for primary position independent of oblique surgery
  - ○ Large A or V patterns indicate oblique muscle dysfunction and require oblique muscle surgery
  - ○ If no oblique dysfunction
    - ▪ A pattern—MR to apex, LR to empty space (MALE mnemonic)
    - ▪ V pattern—MR down to apex, LR up

Vertical Deviations and Special Strabismus Conditions

Dissociated Vertical Deviation

- • Definition
  - ○ Upward deviation of one eye, independent of the other eye
- • Signs/symptoms
  - ○ Unknown cause
  - ○ Found in two-thirds of patients with congenital ET
  - ○ Usually bilateral and asymmetrical
  - ○ Can be spontaneous (manifest) or when one eye is occluded (latent)
  - ○ Associated with DHD, latent nystagmus, and horizontal strabismus
  - ○ Observe eye spontaneously and slowly drift up and out when eye is occluded or during periods of inattention
  - ○ Difficult to measure
- Management
  - ○ Observation
  - ○ Patching/optical to change fixation pattern
  - ○ Surgery
    - ▪ Rarely cures problem
    - ▪ Usually needs to be bilateral with IO recessions, anterior transposition versus superior rectus (SR) recessions with or without posterior fixation suture versus inferior rectus (IR) resections

Third Nerve Palsy

- • Anatomy
  - ○ Superior division of nerve innervates SR and levator.
  - ○ Inferior division innervates IR, IO, MR, and parasympathetic fibers to iris sphincter and ciliary muscle.

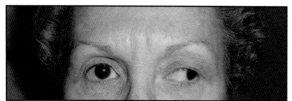

Figure 10-11. A 65-year-old woman with a left third nerve palsy showing fields of gaze. Primary gaze.

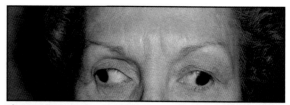

Figure 10-12. A 65-year-old woman with a left third nerve palsy showing fields of gaze. Right gaze.

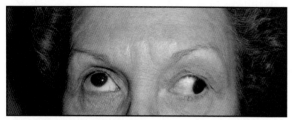

Figure 10-13. A 65-year-old woman with a left third nerve palsy showing fields of gaze. Upgaze.

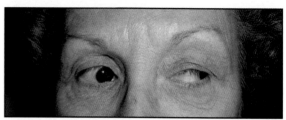

Figure 10-14. A 65-year-old woman with a left third nerve palsy showing fields of gaze. Left gaze.

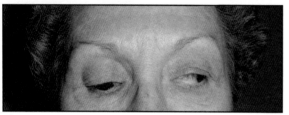

Figure 10-15. A 65-year-old woman with a left third nerve palsy showing fields of gaze. Downgaze.

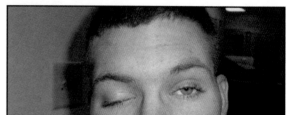

Figure 10-16. Ptosis in a patient with complete third nerve palsy.

- Etiologies
    - Congenital most common in children (40% to 50%)
    - Traumatic
    - Inflammatory
    - Neoplastic
    - Postviral
    - Migraine-related
- Signs/symptoms
    - Eye is typically exotropic and hypotropic with ptosis and sometimes enlarged pupil (Figures 10-11 to 10-16).
    - Amblyopia is common and often requires treatment.
    - May develop aberrant regeneration (misdirection of nerve fibers)
- Treatment
    - Wait 6 to 12 months to allow for any spontaneous improvement
    - Surgical intervention difficult due to large number of muscles involved
    - Goal of surgery is to improve ocular alignment in primary gaze.
    - Often large recession/resection with displacement of tendons upward will allow adequate alignment.
    - SO tenotomy may also be considered for vertical deviation.

Fourth Nerve Paresis (Superior Oblique Palsy)

- Etiology
    - Trochlear nerve
        - Congenital
            - Defect in nucleus or motor portion of IV

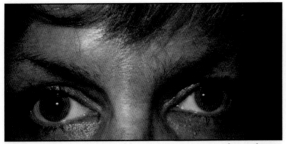

Figure 10-17. A 45-year-old woman status post loss of consciousness from a motor vehicle accident with a left SO (fourth nerve) palsy showing a left hypertropia in primary gaze.

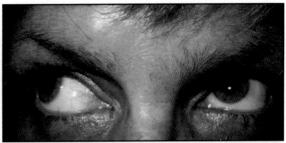

Figure 10-18. Same patient with secondary overaction of the left IO.

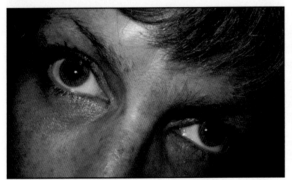

Figure 10-19. Same patient with a left hypertropia in left head tilt during the 3-step test for superior oblique palsies.

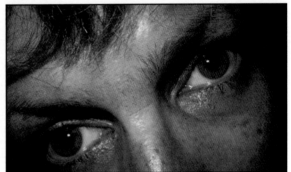

Figure 10-20. Same patient with orthophoria in right head tilt. Current case—left hypertropia in primary gaze > in right gaze and left head tilt = left superior oblique palsy.

- Acquired
  - □ Closed head trauma, central nervous system (CNS) vascular disorders, diabetes, brain tumors
- Signs/symptoms
  - ○ Most common cyclovertical muscle palsy
  - ○ Unilateral or bilateral
  - ○ May be masked bilateral
  - ○ Three-step test—diagnostic hypertropia > opposite gaze and ipsilateral head tilt (Figures 10-17 to 10-20)
  - ○ Abnormal head posturing—head tilt toward opposite side of paresis
  - ○ Amblyopia common in congenital cases, not acquired
- Evaluation
  - ○ Three-step test—diagnostic hypertropia > opposite gaze and ipsilateral head tilt
    - Bilateral
      - □ V pattern ET in downgaze
      - □ Excyclotorsion (>10 degrees diagnostic)
      - □ Head tilt test
        - Right head tilt = Right hypertropia
        - Left head tilt = Left hypertropia
      - □ Bilateral fundus torsion
    - Unilateral
      - □ Little ET in downgaze
      - □ Excyclotorsion < 10 degrees
      - □ SO normal or decreased
    - Measure deviation in all 9 fields of gaze

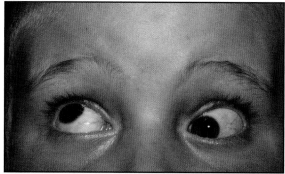

Figure 10-21. Left Brown's syndrome in a 5 year old demonstrating inability to elevate the left eye in adduction.

- Treatment
  - ○ Indicated for abnormal head posture, significant vertical deviation, diplopia
  - ○ Unilateral
    - ▪ IOOA, deviation < 15pd - IO weakening
    - ▪ If deviation is greater than 15, may need to add a second muscle (contralateral IR recession ± adjustable, SO tuck)
    - ▪ No IOOA-contralateral IR resection or ipsilateral SO tuck (side effect of creating Brown's)
  - ○ Bilateral
    - ▪ If bilateral IO overaction, then bilateral IO recession
    - ▪ IR recession, Harada Ito (with significant torsional component), SO tuck

Sixth Nerve Palsy

- See incomitant esodeviations

Internuclear Ophthalmoplegia

- Etiology
  - ○ Disruption of nerve fibers that connect the cranial nerve nuclei that control motility
  - ○ Group of nerve fibers called medial longitudinal fasciculus
- Clinical
  - ○ Causes characteristic ocular motility pattern
    - ▪ Limited adduction ipsilateral eye
    - ▪ Horizontal nystagmus contralateral eye
    - ▪ Normal adduction of both eyes on convergence
  - ○ Unilateral or bilateral
  - ○ Secondary to tumor, cerebrovascular accident, or demyelination
- Treatment
  - ○ If deviation persists, ipsilateral MR resection and contralateral LR recession may be helpful.

Brown's Syndrome

- Also called SO tendon sheath syndrome
- Definition
  - ○ Restriction of elevation in adduction
- Signs/symptoms
  - ○ Bilateral in 10% of cases
  - ○ Often decreased elevation in straight upgaze with divergence (Figure 10-21) that improves with abduction
  - ○ Types
    - ▪ Mild (no hypotropia in primary, no downshoot in adduction)
    - ▪ Moderate (no hypotropia in primary with downshoot)
    - ▪ Severe (hypotropia in primary + downshoot ± chin up head posturing and face turn away from affected eye)

- Congenital
  - Usually constant
  - Felt to be due to a short/inelastic SO muscle/tendon or stenosis of trochlear pulley
- Acquired
  - Constant or intermittent
  - Local trauma to trochlea
  - Systemic inflammatory conditions
  - Prevents free movement through trochlear pulley
  - May have hypotropia with chin up head position
  - Positive forced ductions (FD)
  - V pattern strabismus (helps differentiate from SO overaction pattern)
  - May resolve on own
- Evaluation
  - Positive FD test
    - Restriction of elevation in adduction is diagnostic
    - Increases with retropulsion of globe
- Treatment
  - Observation
  - Treat systemic causes – rheumatoid arthritis, sinusitis
  - Surgery in cases of primary position hypotropia and abnormal head posture
    - SO tenotomy ± ipsilateral IO recession
    - Silicone expander to SO tendon (guarded tenotomy)

Inferior Oblique Palsy

- Rare—unknown etiology
- A pattern (versus V in Brown's syndrome)
- Three-step test
- FDs negative
- SO OA present
- Surgery for abnormal head posturing, vertical deviation in primary gaze, diplopia
  - Ipsilateral SO weakening surgery versus contralateral SR recession

Monocular Elevation Deficiency (Double Elevator Palsy)

- Definition
  - Simultaneous paralysis of the IO and SR of the same eye
- Classification
  - Type 1—Inferior rectus restriction (fibrosis syndrome)
  - Type 2—Double elevator palsy (weak SR and IO)
    - Equal deficit in elevation with eye adducted or abducted
  - Type 3—Combined IR restriction and double elevator palsy
- Signs/symptoms
  - Limitation in elevation in adduction and abduction
  - Hypotropia of involved eye—increases in upgaze
  - Chin up head posturing with fusion in downgaze
  - Amblyopia of involved eye
  - Ptosis versus pseudoptosis of involved eye
  - Marcus Gunn's jaw wink in up to one-third of patients
- Evaluation
  - IR restriction
    - Positive FD in elevation, normal forced generations and saccades
  - Elevator weakness
    - Free FD, reduced forced generations and saccades
  - Combination
    - Positive FD, reduced forced generation and vertical saccades

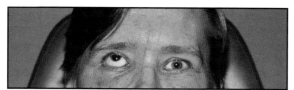

Figure 10-22. Left IR restriction on attempted elevation of both eyes in a patient with a blowout fracture.

- Treatment
  - Surgical intervention if there is a significant hypotropia in primary position or there is a significant chin up head position
  - IR recession if there is significant restriction
  - Horizontal muscle transposition toward the SR (Knapp procedure) if no restriction is present
  - Correction of hypotropia may result in some improvement of apparent ptosis, but additional eyelid surgery may be necessary.

Orbital Floor Fractures

- Etiology
  - Blunt facial trauma (motor vehicle accidents)
  - Fractures of mid face or orbital rim/zygomatic complex (hydraulic effect-blowout fracture)
  - Most frequently related to tethering of the IR muscle with orbital floor fracture
- Signs/symptoms
  - Ecchymosis
  - Diplopia
  - Infraorbital anesthesia
  - Enophthalmos
  - Entrapment of IR, IO, surrounding tissues
  - Hypotropia in primary gaze, increases in upgaze and may decrease (become a hypertropia) in downgaze (combined mechanical restriction and IR paresis/pseudoparesis) (Figure 10-22)
  - Limited horizontal movement, especially abduction, from medial wall fracture, entrapment of MR
- Evaluation
  - Computed tomography (CT) and/or magnetic resonance imaging (MRI) essential for diagnosis and treatment decision making.
  - Complete eye exam essential, especially to rule out ruptured globe
- Treatment
  - Timing of exploration controversial
    - Immediate versus waiting until orbital edema and hematoma subside (5 to 10 days)
    - Entrapment—explore fracture, release IR and surrounding tissues. Early intervention is advised with confirmed entrapment.
    - No entrapment—IR paresis—observe for resolution—muscle surgery after 3 to 6 months if not resolved
  - Surgery—IR resection for partial IR paresis/recess ipsilateral SR
    - Recess contralateral IR ± posterior fixation suture (limits downgaze to equal deficiency in involved eye)
    - Transposition MR/LR to IR for complete IR paresis (inverse Knapp)

Duane's Syndrome

- Etiology
  - Anomalous innervation of the LR by the third cranial nerve with agenesis of the sixth cranial nerve
  - Usually sporadic, but may be familial
  - Usually unilateral, but may be bilateral in up to 20% of cases

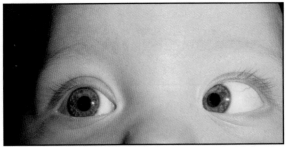

Figure 10-23. Right Duane's syndrome in a 9 month old showing inability to abduct the right eye.

- o Affects females more than males (3:2) and the left side more than the right (3:1)
- o All types show narrowing of palpebral fissure on attempted adduction and widening with attempted abduction due to co-contracture of the horizontal recti.
- Classification
  - o Type 1—Esotropic (Figure 10-23)
    - Abduction deficit > Adduction deficit
  - o Type 2—Exotropic
    - Adduction deficit > Abduction deficit
  - o Type 3
    - Abduction deficit = Adduction deficit
- Signs/symptoms
  - o Frequently may have an upshoot or downshoot of the eye due to a "leash" effect
- Treatment
  - o Treatment may include correction of refractive error, especially if there is a co-existing accommodative ET and treatment of amblyopia when present.
  - o Frequently does not require surgical intervention. Surgery may be performed if there is a significant strabismus in primary position, abnormal head position, or significant upshoot or downshoot. Never resect muscles in Duane's syndrome. Surgery may include recessions, vertical muscle transpositions, and Y-splitting procedures (for upshoots and downshoots).

Moebius Syndrome

- Etiology
  - o Congenital bilateral aplasia of the sixth and seventh cranial nerve nuclei
- Signs/symptoms
  - o Inability to abduct past midline
  - o Masklike faces
  - o May be associated with limb abnormalities and absence of the pectoralis muscle (Poland anomaly)
- Treatment
  - o Bilateral MR recessions or vertical transpositions may be considered for ET.

Myasthenia Gravis

- Definition
  - o Systemic disease of the neuromuscular junction causing muscle weakness
- Signs/symptoms
  - o 90% have ocular involvement
  - o 75% have ocular manifestations on presentation
  - o 20% have ocular involvement only
  - o Increased incidence of other autoimmune diseases
  - o Variability is the hallmark of disease (worsens with fatigue)
  - o May mimic any other type of strabismus
  - o Will also typically have variable asymmetric ptosis

Thyroid Eye Disease

- Signs/symptoms
  - o IR muscle most frequently involved; followed by medial, superior, and lateral in order of decreasing frequency
- Evaluation
  - o Orbital CT or MRI shows muscle enlargement with sparing of muscle tendons.
- Treatment
  - o Prism may be used for diplopia (ground in or Fresnel).
  - o Surgery may be considered if condition is stable for 3 to 6 months and orbital surgery has been completed, if necessary.

Congenital Fibrosis Syndrome

- Etiology
  - o Replacement of some or all of the extraocular muscles with fibrous tissue
- Signs/symptoms
  - o General fibrosis involves all extraocular muscles and levator bilaterally.
    - ▪ Autosomal dominant > autosomal recessive > idiopathic
  - o Unilateral fibrosis may also occur.
  - o Unilateral or bilateral fibrosis of the IR muscle alone may occur
    - ▪ Autosomal dominant inheritance
  - o Vertical retraction syndrome
    - ▪ SR > IR in both eyes
    - ▪ Decreased downgaze
  - o Strabismus fixus—horizontal recti involved, usually medial with severe ET
- Treatment
  - o Surgical correction is difficult.
  - o Recession of tight fibrotic muscles
  - o Surgical goal is good alignment in primary gaze.

Nystagmus

- Definition
  - o Involuntary back-and-forth movement of the eye
- Etiology

Congenital Motor Nystagmus

- Idiopathic
- Periodic alternating nystagmus
  - o Special type of congenital motor nystagmus
    - ▪ Direction of the jerk nystagmus typically changes every 60 to 90 seconds.
    - ▪ There may be a changing head position to compensate for a changing null point.

Latent

- Occurs under monocular conditions
- Both eyes will jerk in the direction of the fixating eye.
- Very commonly associated with congenital ET and DVD

Spasmus Nutans

- Acquired nystagmus between the ages of 3 and 24 months
- High-frequency small amplitude ("shimmering") horizontal nystagmus
- Usually bilateral, but often asymmetric
- Triad of nystagmus, head bobbing, and torticollis

- Benign and self-limited disorder, but
  - o Very similar-appearing nystagmus described associated with chiasmal and suprachiasmal tumors
  - o Recommend neuroimaging when any doubt
- Usually disappears by 3 to 4 years of age

Sensory Nystagmus

- Typically manifests around 3 months of age if vision loss is present at birth
- Associated with other ocular pathology as follows:
  - o Congenital cataract
  - o Congenital glaucoma
  - o Iridocorneal dysgenesis
  - o Aniridia
  - o Retinal dysplasia
  - o Toxoplasmosis
  - o Albinism (oculocutaneous, ocular)
  - o Achromatopsia
  - o Congenital stationary night blindness
  - o Congenital retinoschisis
  - o Retinopathy of prematurity
  - o Retinoblastoma
  - o Retinal dysplasia
  - o Optic nerve hypoplasia
  - o Optic nerve atrophy
- Nystagmus potentially localizing for neurological disease

Downbeat Nystagmus

- Cervicomedullary junction
- Arnold-Chiari malformation
- Multiple sclerosis
- Cerebrovascular accident (CVA)
- Syringomyelia

Medication

- Lithium

Upbeat Nystagmus

- Anterior vermis
- Lower brainstem
- Wernicke's syndrome
- Drug intoxication

See-Saw Nystagmus

- Elevation and incyclotorsion with concurrent depression and excyclotorsion of the fellow eye
  - o Suprasellar lesion
  - o Diencephalic lesion
  - o INO
  - o CVA
  - o Congenital
  - o Traumatic

Convergence Retraction Nystagmus

- Dorsal midbrain
  - Pinealoma
  - Trauma
  - Aquaductal stenosis
  - AV malformations
  - Multiple sclerosis
  - Other associated findings of the dorsal midbrain syndrome
    - Decreased upgaze
    - Light near dissociation of pupil function
    - Impaired convergence

Dissociated Nystagmus

- Different in each eye
- Posterior fossa disease
- INO
- Spasmus nutans

Vestibular

- Often horizontal and rotary
- Associated vertigo, deafness, tinnitus
- End organ disease
- Peripheral nerve (inhibited by fixation)
- Central (not inhibited by fixation)

Gaze Evoked

- May be physiologic if symmetric and fatigues with prolonged eccentric gaze
- Brainstem lesions
- Posterior fossa lesions
- Medications
  - Anticonvulsants

- Classification
  - Direction
    - Horizontal
    - Vertical
    - Oblique
    - Torsional
  - Velocity of movement
    - Pendular
      - Equal velocity in both directions
    - Jerk nystagmus
      - Moves faster in one direction than the other
        - Recorded as the direction of the fast movement (phase)
        - Right jerk nystagmus has greater velocity of eye movement to the right.
  - Frequency
    - Oscillation per unit time
  - Amplitude
    - Degree of movement
  - Monocular or binocular
  - Symmetric or asymmetric

- o Null point
  - Decrease or cessation of nystagmus in certain gaze positions
  - May cause anomalous head position
    - □ Child attempts to bring eyes into a certain gaze to improve his or her vision
  - Typically, this will be in the opposite field of gaze as the direction of a jerk nystagmus.
- Symptoms
  - o Rare
  - o Oscillopsia
    - Sensation that objects are moving back and forth
    - Rarely present unless the nystagmus is acquired after the age of 8
- Evaluation
  - o Vision
    - Near vision
      - □ Normal near vision more likely motor nystagmus
        - More likely benign
      - □ Poor near acuity more likely sensory etiology
      - □ Near VA is often better than distance, due to dampening of nystagmus with convergence
    - Preverbal children can have vision tested with
      - □ Optokinetic drum
        - Response indicates vision of 20/400 or better
        - Preferential looking techniques
  - o Pupils exam
    - Sluggish pupils typically indicate a problem in the anterior visual pathway.
    - Paradoxical
      - □ Initially constrict in response to darkness
      - □ Conditions associated with a paradoxical pupil and nystagmus
        - Congenital stationary night blindness
        - Congenital achromatopsia
        - Leber's congenital amaurosis
        - Best's disease
        - Albinism
        - Retinitis pigmentosa (RP)
  - o Strabismus is often associated with nystagmus.
    - Sensory with poor vision
    - Nystagmus blockage syndrome
      - □ Compensatory strabismus
      - □ Children will dampen their nystagmus by converging their eyes, thus creating an ET.
  - o Anterior segment
    - Any media opacity causing vision loss
      - □ Cataract
    - Iris transillumination defects
      - □ Sign of albinism
  - o Fundus examination
    - Macular hypoplasia
      - □ Albinism
    - Optic nerve hypoplasia or atrophy
    - Retinal disease
      - □ Pigmentary changes
      - □ May still be present with normal fundus
  - o Electroretinogram (ERG)
    - Very helpful in detecting occult retinal disease
  - o MRI
    - Indicated when congenital motor nystagmus is not felt to be the cause and no ocular findings explain the nystagmus
    - Especially necessary when a localizing type of nystagmus is present
    - Rule out a chiasmal or suprachiasmal lesion in suspected Spasmus nutans

- Differential diagnosis
  - Opsoclonus
    - Rapid eye movements in different directions usually with high frequency
    - Not a true nystagmus
    - May be associated with
      - Neuroblastoma
      - Acute cerebellar ataxia
      - Encephalitis
      - Hydrocephalus
  - Voluntary "nystagmus"
    - Horizontal rapid back-and-forth saccades
    - May only be maintained for seconds
    - Functional (hysterical or malingering)
- Treatment
  - Prism therapy
    - May be used to move the position of the image into the null zone with the head straight
    - May also be used to stimulate convergence (base in both eyes) to dampen nystagmus
  - Surgical management
    - Kestenbaum procedure
      - Combined bilateral recessions and resections to move the eyes so that the null point is present with the eyes straight
      - Helpful in eliminating head turns
      - Usually horizontal, but vertical procedures may be used for null point in upgaze or downgaze
    - Large 4 horizontal muscle rectus recessions
      - May decrease the fast phase of the nystagmus
      - Some studies have shown a mild improvement in vision following procedure.
    - Bimedial recessions for nystagmus blockage syndrome
    - Disinsertion/reinsertion of the horizontal recti have also recently been advocated to decrease nystagmus
  - Medications
    - Limited utility
    - Baclofen may be tried with periodic alternating nystagmus

Childhood Glaucoma

- Definition
  - Optic neuropathy secondary to increased intraocular pressure (IOP) subcategorized as
    - Congenital—birth to 3 months
    - Infantile—3 months to 3 years
    - Juvenile—children over 3 years
- Etiology
  - One-third primary
  - One-third secondary to ocular pathology
  - One-third associated with systemic disease
  - Primary
    - Two-thirds bilateral
    - One-third unilateral
    - 85% diagnosed by 1 year
    - Multifactorial inheritance
    - Mutation mapped to chromosomes 1p36 and 2p22–p21
  - Secondary
    - Inflammatory disease
    - Trauma, tumor
    - Medication

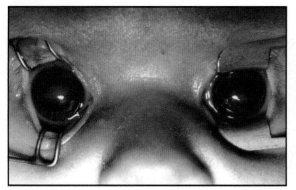

Figure 10-24. Example of congenital cloudy corneas in an infant. Congenital glaucoma must be ruled out as part of the differential diagnosis.

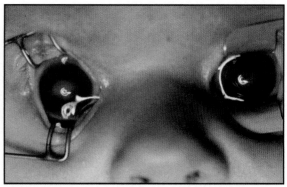

Figure 10-25. Example of congenital cloudy corneas in an infant. Congenital glaucoma must be ruled out as part of the differential diagnosis.

- o Associated systemic disease
    - ▪ Aniridia
    - ▪ Aphakia/pseudophakia
    - ▪ Anterior dysgenesis
    - ▪ Persistent fetal vasculature
    - ▪ Nanophthalmos
    - ▪ Neurofibromatosis
    - ▪ Sturge Weber syndrome
    - ▪ Mucopolysaccharidoses
    - ▪ Marfan's syndrome
    - ▪ Lowe's syndrome
- Mechanism
    - o Decreased aqueous filtration with abnormal angle
- Signs/symptoms
    - o Epiphora
    - o Photophobia
    - o "Cloudy"-appearing eye (Figures 10-24 and 10-25)
    - o Decreased vision
    - o Increased IOP
    - o Corneal edema (Figure 10-26)
    - o Corneal enlargement
        - ▪ Greater than 12 mm at 1 year of age or less
    - o Haab's striae
        - ▪ Breaks in Descemet's membrane usually horizontal or concentric to the limbus
    - o Ocular enlargement (buphthalmos)
    - o Optic nerve cupping
        - ▪ May be partially reversible in young children
- Differential diagnosis
    - o Nasolacrimal duct obstruction
    - o Megalocornea
    - o Congenital hereditary endothelial dystrophy (CHED)
    - o High myopia
    - o Proptosis (simulating ocular enlargement)
    - o Birth trauma (with corneal striae and edema)
    - o Sclerocornea (simulating corneal edema)
    - o Mucopolysaccharidoses
        - ▪ Corneal clouding simulating edema
        - ▪ May also be associated with glaucoma
    - o Generally, with congenital glaucoma, there is severe photophobia that is not present with these other ocular conditions.

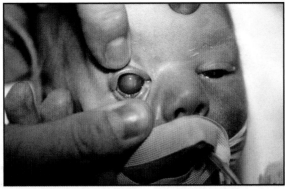

Figure 10-26. Congenital glaucoma in an infant with a cloudy and enlarged cornea.

- Evaluation
  - Complete ocular exam
    - Corneal clarity/size
    - Anterior chamber—gonioscopy when possible
    - IOP
    - Optic disc cupping
    - Refractive error
      - Progressive myopia is a sign of uncontrolled glaucoma in young children.
      - Useful for following glaucoma and also detecting possible cause of amblyopia (anisometropia)
  - Pachymetry (corneal thickness) when possible
    - Thick cornea will record higher than true pressure.
    - Thin cornea will record lower than true pressure.
  - Ultrasonography
    - Measurement of axial length
    - Globe becomes progressively longer with uncontrolled glaucoma.
  - Disc photography when possible
  - Visual fields
    - Reliable fields are difficult to obtain in children under age 10.
  - Optic nerve head analysis in older children when possible
    - Various methods including
      - Optical coherence tomography (OCT)
      - Confocal scanning laser ophthalmoscopy
        - Heidelberg retinal tomograph
      - Scanning laser polarimetry
        - Nerve fiber analyzer, GDx
      - Optic nerve blood flow analysis
        - Color Doppler imaging
        - Laser Doppler flowmetry
  - Examinations under anesthesia may be necessary if child is uncooperative.
    - Anesthetics may alter IOP
      - Lowered by inhalation anesthetics
      - Increased with ketamine
      - IOP should be checked as soon as possible after being placed under anesthesia.
- Treatment
  - Primarily surgical
    - Trabeculotomy
    - Goniotomy
    - Trabeculectomy
    - Glaucoma drainage device
    - Cycloablation

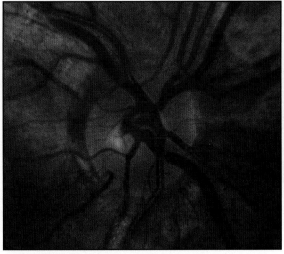

Figure 10-27. Normal optic nerve.

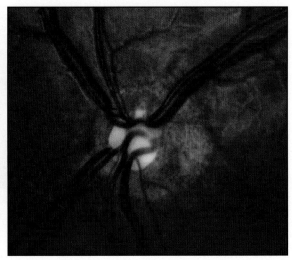

Figure 10-28. Hypoplastic optic nerve.

- o Medical therapy
  - ▪ Temporize while awaiting surgery
  - ▪ Supplement to surgery
  - ▪ Medical therapy alone in very select cases
  - ▪ β-blocker is generally still first line.
    - □ Timolol (timoptic), betalol (betoptic) twice daily
  - ▪ Systemic or topical carbonic anhydrase inhibitor (CAI) is often a helpful addition.
    - □ Diamox 15 mg/kg/day orally
    - □ Dorzolamide (Trusopt) topical 3 times daily
    - □ Timolol/dorzolamide combo (Cosopt) twice daily
      - • Both β-blocker and CAI in one
  - ▪ Prostanoid receptor agonist may be considered once daily.
    - □ Latanoprost (Xalatan)
    - □ Travoprost (Travatan)
  - ▪ Never use brimonidine (Alphagan) in infancy.
    - □ Has been associated with arrhythmia and death
    - □ Alpha-2 adrenergic agonist
- • Amblyopia management
  - o Anisometropic/refractive amblyopia is common.
  - o Check and correct refractive errors frequently.
  - o Treat amblyopia in standard way with occlusion/penalization.

Congenital Optic Disc Anomalies

Optic Nerve Hypoplasia
- • Etiology
  - o Dysplasia of retinal ganglion cells with associated loss of nerve fiber layer
  - o Septo-optic dysplasia (de Morsier syndrome)
    - ▪ Absence of septum pellucidum
    - ▪ Agensis of corpus callosum
    - ▪ Pituitary dwarfism due to growth hormone deficiency
- • Signs/symptoms
  - o Double ring sign (normal optic nerve [Figure 10-27] compared to hypoplastic optic nerve [Figure 10-28])
    - ▪ Histopathology
      - □ Outer ring normal—junction between sclera and lamina cribrosa

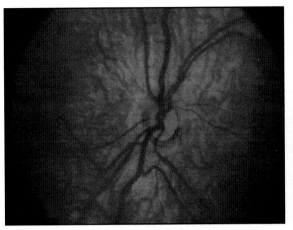

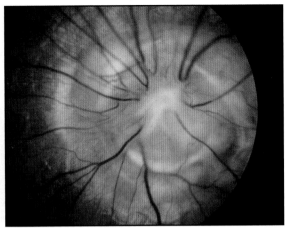

Figure 10-29. Typical appearance of a hypoplastic optic nerve with a characteristic double ring sign.

Figure 10-30. Morning glory disc showing characteristic findings.

- Inner ring abnormal—extension of retina and pigment epithelium over outer portion of lamina cribrosa (Figure 10-29)
  - o Major retinal vessels are tortuous
  - o VA varies from 20/20 to no light perception (NLP)
  - o Nystagmus
  - o Strabismus
  - o Astigmatism
- Treatment
  - o General concepts in management of congenital optic disc anomalies (CODAs)
  - o Bilateral optic disc anomalies generally present in infancy with poor vision and nystagmus.
  - o Unilateral CODAs present during preschool years with sensory ET.
  - o CNS malformations common with CODAs
    - Small discs associated with defects in cerebral hemispheres, pituitary, and midline structures (septum pellucidum, corpus callosum)
    - Large ODs (morning glory) associated with trans-sphenoidal encephalocele.
    - Colobomas are associated with systemic syndromes.
  - o Structural abnormality is associated with decreased vision and amblyopia so occlusion therapy may be warranted.
  - o V- or tongue-shaped zone of infrapapillary retinochoroidal depigmentation in an eye with an anomalous disc is associated with trans-sphenoidal encephalocele.

Morning Glory Disc

- Definition
  - o Peripapillary staphyloma
  - o Excavation of posterior globe that incorporates optic disc (Figure 10-30)
- Signs/Symptoms
  - o Usually unilateral
  - o Usual VA (20/200 or less)
  - o Disc
    - Markedly enlarged
    - Orange or pink color
    - Recessed or elevated within confines of funnel-shaped excavation
    - White tuft of glial tissue centrally
    - Blood vessels appear increased in number and often arise from periphery of disc.
  - o Strong association with myopia, strabismus, and amblyopia (refractive correction warranted)
  - o Serous retinal detachment in 26% to 38% of patients/subretinal neovascularization can occur
  - o More common in females
  - o Rare in African Americans
  - o Associated with trans-sphenoidal basal encephalocele

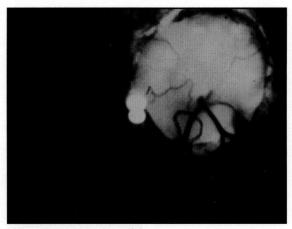

Figure 10-31. Optic disc coloboma.

Optic Disc Coloboma

- Definition
    - Coloboma—Greek for *mutilated*
- Defective closure of embryologic fetal fissure
- Excavated disc, de-centered inferiorly (Figure 10-31)
- Iris and choroidal colobomas often coexist.
- Vision depends on integrity of papulomacular bundle.
- Unilateral = bilateral
- Systemic associations
    - Coloboma of the eye, heart defects, atresia of the choanae, retardation of growth and/or development, genital and/or urinary abnormalities, and ear abnormalities and deafness (CHARGE)
    - Aicardi's syndrome
    - Goldenhar's syndrome
    - Linear sebaceous nevus syndrome

Optic Pit

- Definition
    - Round or oval, gray or yellowish depression in optic disc
- Signs/symptoms
    - Usually temporal (Figures 10-32 and 10-33)
    - Cilioretinal arteries from bottom or margin of pit in 50% of cases
    - Usually unilateral; 15% bilateral
    - Can be a familial (autosomal dominant) form
    - Serous macular detachment in 25% to 75%—usually third or fourth decade
        - Spontaneous reattachment 25%
        - Laser not effective—need vitrectomy/gas/laser treatment
    - Sources of intraretinal fluid
        - Vitreous cavity via the pit
        - Subarachnoid space
        - Blood vessels at base of pit
        - Orbital space surrounding dura
- Differential diagnosis
    - Colobomas
        - Optic pits (OPs) are usually unilateral, sporadic, and unassociated with systemic abnormalities.
        - Colobomas are bilateral as often as unilateral, commonly autosomal dominant, and associated with multisystem disorders.
        - It is rare for OP to coexist with iris or retinochoroidal colobomas.
        - OP usually occur in locations unrelated to the embryonic fissure.

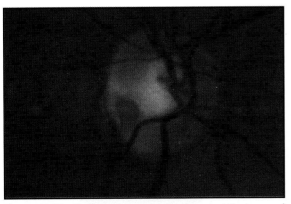

Figure 10-32. Optic nerve pit in its characteristic temporal location.

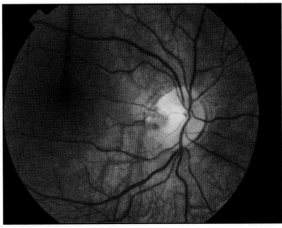

Figure 10-33. Optic nerve pit in its characteristic temporal location.

Congenital Tilted Disc Syndrome

- Nonhereditary, bilateral
- Superotemporal disc elevated and inferonasal disc posteriorly displaced = oval-appearing disc with long axis obliquely oriented
- Situs inversus of retinal vessels
- Inferonasal conus
- Thinning of retinal pigment epithelium and choroid
- Bitemporal visual field defect—incomplete and fails to respect vertical meridian
- Myopia/astigmatism—secondary to posterior ectasia if inferonasal fundus and optic disc
- Rare history of congenital suprasellar tumor, so neuroimaging is recommended
- Tilted discs without retinal ectasia = trans-sphenoidal encephalocele

Myelinated Nerve Fibers

- Affects 1% of eyes—usually unilateral
- Mechanisms
  - o Defect in lamina cribrosa
  - o Fewer axons relative to the size of the scleral canal allows room for myelination to go into eye (Figures 10-34 through 10-36).
  - o Late development of lamina cribrosa
- Can be autosomal dominant
- Rarely due to trauma or optic nerve sheath fenestration
- High association with high myopia/amblyopia

Optic Disc in Albinism Papilledema

- Small disc diameter
- Absence of physiologic cup
- Oval shape with long axis oriented obliquely
- Origin of retinal vessels from temporal aspect of the disc
- Abnormal retinal vessel course (Figures 10-37 and 10-38)

Optic Disc Drusen

- Hyaline or colloid bodies (Figures 10-39 and 10-40)
- Can simulate papilloedema (Figure 10-41)
- Familial drusen autosomal dominant
- Rare in African Americans
- Drusen does not correlate with hyperopia.

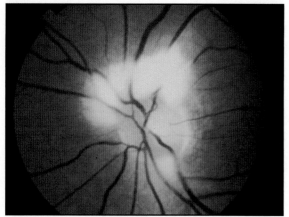

Figure 10-34. Example of myelinated optic nerve fibers.

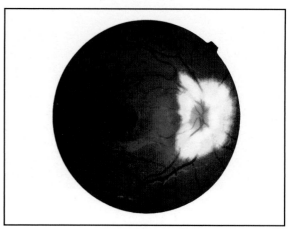

Figure 10-35. Example of myelinated optic nerve fibers.

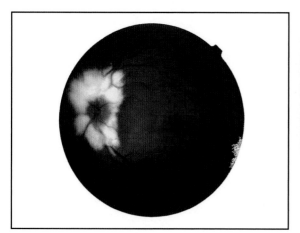

Figure 10-36. Example of myelinated optic nerve fibers.

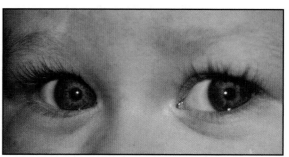

Figure 10-37. An 18 month old with albinitic facial features.

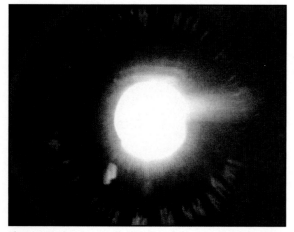

Figure 10-38. Iris transillumination defects typical in patients with albinism.

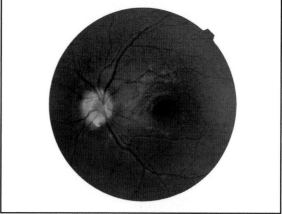

Figure 10-39. Optic nerve head drusen with typical appearance.

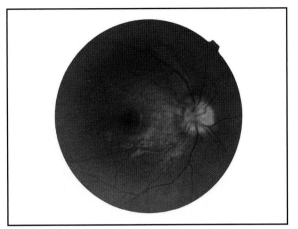

Figure 10-40. Optic nerve head drusen with typical appearance.

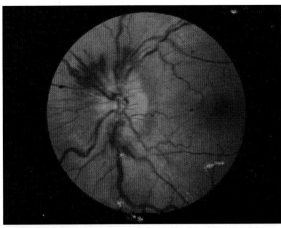

Figure 10-41. Example of true papilledema, which can be confused with optic nerve head drusen.

- Visible disc drusen bilateral two-thirds versus buried drusen bilateral 86%
- Fluorescein angiogram
  - o Autofluorescence in preinjection phase then nodular hyperfluorescence with location of drusen
- Systemic disorders associated with visible disc drusen
  - o RP
  - o Pseudoexfoliation (PXE)
  - o Megalencephaly
  - o Migraines

Leukocoria and Cataracts

- Definition
  - o "White pupil" secondary to multiple ocular disorders
- Differential diagnosis
  - o Retinoblastoma (Figure 10-42)
  - o Persistent hyperplastic primary vitreous (PHPV)
    - Also known as persistent fetal vasculature
  - o Cataract
  - o Toxocariasis
  - o Retinopathy of prematurity
  - o Coats' disease
  - o Uveitis
  - o Endophthalmitis
  - o Coloboma (Figure 10-43)
  - o Hamartoma
  - o Myelinated nerve fiber layer
  - o Pseudoleukocoria
    - Congenital glaucoma
    - Corneal scarring
    - Strabismus
    - Iris irregularities such as flocculi
- Why is leukocoria important?
  - o Retinoblastoma; fatal without treatment.
  - o Early treatment of other disease entities may prevent irreversible blindness.
  - o Most disorders that cause leukocoria are otherwise asymptomatic or the child is too young to communicate vision loss.

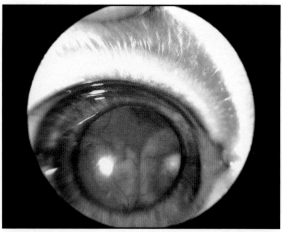

Figure 10-42. Example of leukocoria in a patient with a retino-blastoma.

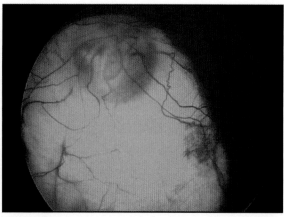

Figure 10-43. Optic nerve and chorioretinal coloboma, which can present with leukocoria.

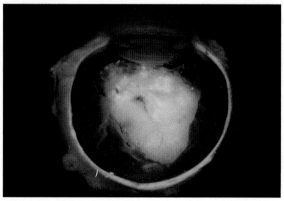

Figure 10-44. Retinoblastoma in an infant presenting with leukocoria.

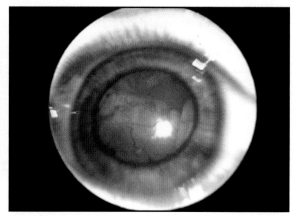

Figure 10-45. Another example of retinoblastoma presenting as leukocoria.

Retinoblastoma

- Etiology
  - All cases considered inherited with the following:
    - Bilateral disease
    - Multifocal unilateral disease
    - Deletion of chromosome 13q14
    - Secondary monocular neoplasms
- Signs/symptoms
  - Leukocoria is most common presenting sign (Figure 10-44).
  - Most common primary intraocular tumor of childhood
  - Remission rate greater than 90%
  - Presenting signs
    - Leukocoria (60%) (Figure 10-45)
    - Strabismus
    - Red eye
  - Is 70% unilateral
- Evaluation
  - Examination of family due to positive family history
- Treatment
  - Shift toward globe- and vision-sparing treatment
  - Large unilateral cases may still require enucleation.

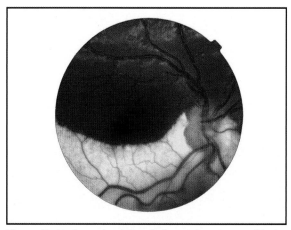

Figure 10-46. Example of Coats' disease in a 5 year old who presented with leukocoria and amblyopia showing the exudative component of the disease process.

- ○ Combined treatments may include the following:
    - ▪ Multiagent chemotherapy
    - ▪ Thermotherapy
    - ▪ Cryotherapy
    - ▪ Laser
    - ▪ Plaque brachytherapy
    - ▪ External beam radiation
    - ▪ Intra-arterial chemotherapy
- Prognosis
    - ○ Almost universally fatal in absence of appropriate treatment

Coats' Disease

- Idiopathic
- Nonhereditary
- Telangectatic and aneurysmal retinal vessels
- Is 80% unilateral
- Is 75% male
- Affects 70% prior to age 10
- Retinal exudate and hemorrhage (Figure 10-46)

Persistent Fetal Vasculature

- PHPV
- Persistence and secondary fibrosis of the primitive hyaloid vascular system
- Have residual stalk of tissue from optic disc to posterior lens
- Eye is frequently small, shallow anterior chamber
- Ciliary processes pulled into center of pupil

Cataract

- See Chapter 9.

Retinopathy of Prematurity

- Definition
    - ○ Abnormal retinal vascular development in premature infants
    - ○ Plus disease—Dilated and tortuous posterior vasculature due to shunting. May also have iris vascular engorgement (Figure 10-47).
    - ○ Rush disease—ROP in Zone 1 with plus disease. High risk of rapid progression.

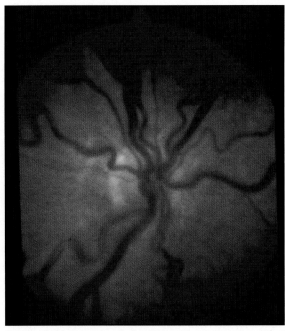

Figure 10-47. Example of plus disease in a premature infant with ROP. Note the significant tortuosity of the retinal vessels.

- Differential diagnoses
  - Other causes of leukocoria such as cataract, retinoblastoma
  - Familial exudative vitreoretinopathy
  - Persistent fetal vasculature
  - Coats' disease
  - Eales disease
- Epidemiology
  - Increased incidence and severity with lower birth weight and gestational age
  - Infants born at less than 750 g have a 90% chance of developing some retinopathy, and 37% develop stage 3 disease (16% threshold).
  - Infants born between 1000 and 1250 g have a 45% chance of some retinopathy; 8% stage 3; 2% threshold.
  - Supplemental oxygen is felt to be a modifying factor in the development of ROP.
- Classification
  - Retinal changes are described by 5 stages according to the International Classification of ROP.
    - Stage 1—Thin demarcation line between vascularized (posterior to line) and avascular (anterior to line) retina
    - Stage 2—Ridge with elevation and thickness develops between vascular avascular retina
    - Stage 3—Fibrovascular proliferation (neovascularization) along ridge
    - Stage 4—Subtotal retinal detachment
      - 4A—Macula attached
      - 4B—Macula detached
    - Stage 5—Total retinal detachment
  - ROP is also described by its location in zones extending circumferentially from the optic disc.
    - Zone 1—Twice the radius from the optic disc to the macula
    - Zone 2—From the border of stage 1 to a radius tangential to the nasal ora serrata
    - Zone 3—The remaining temporal crescent from the border of zone 2 to the temporal ora serrata
- Evaluation
  - <1500 g or less than 30 weeks gestational age
  - Children born at 1500 to 2000 g or 30 to 34 weeks gestational age will be examined if supplemental oxygen is used.

- o Frequency of re-evaluation is dependent on examination findings.
  - Close observation is extremely important.
  - The majority of cases are followed every 1 to 2 weeks.
  - The most severe prethreshold disease may need to be seen more than once weekly.
  - Mild zone 3 disease may be followed every 3 to 4 weeks.
- ROP treatment parameters
  - o Threshold ROP
    - Zone 1 or 2 Stage 3 for 5 contiguous or 8 total clock hours with plus disease
  - o Prethreshold disease
    - Type 1—High-risk prethreshold
      - □ Zone I, any stage with plus disease
      - □ Zone I, stage 3 without plus disease
      - □ Zone II, stage 2 or 3 with plus disease
    - Type 2—Lower risk prethreshold
      - □ Zone I, stage 1 or 2 without plus disease
      - □ Zone II, stage 2 or 3 without plus disease
  - o Treatment in the past has been felt to be indicated once threshold criteria (50% risk of retinal detachment) are met.
  - o More recent studies suggest earlier treatment of high-risk (Type 1) prethreshold may be more appropriate while very close observation of lower-risk (Type 2) prethreshold may be most appropriate.
  - o Treatment is ablation of the avascular retina with argon laser, diode laser (500 μm spot size), or cryotherapy.
  - o Retinal detachment (stage 4 or 5) requires pars plana vitrectomy with or without lensectomy, membrane peel, and scleral buckling.
- Prognosis
  - o Long-term complications of prematurity and ROP
    - Common
      - □ Strabismus
      - □ Myopia
      - □ Anisometropia
      - □ Amblyopia
      - □ Nystagmus
    - Uncommon
      - □ Late-onset retinal detachment due to cicatricial changes and glaucoma (particularly with stage 4 or 5 disease)

Congenital Lacrimal Obstruction

- Definition
  - o Congenital nasolacrimal obstruction is a blockage of the lacrimal outflow tract that is present from birth.
  - o Though the incidence of obstruction may be as high as 50% at birth, clinically significant obstruction is present in only about 5% of infants by 1 month of age.
- Etiology
  - o Membranous obstruction at the level of the valve of Hasner (the opening of the nasolacrimal duct into the inferior meatus) is the most common cause, although the obstruction can be anywhere in the system from the punctal orifice on the eyelid margin to the nasolacrimal duct.
  - o Rarely, obstruction can originate from punctal or canalicular atresia sometimes in association with other congenital anomalies such as cleft palate or amniotic band.
- Signs/symptoms
  - o Incidence varies between 5% and 10% of newborns.
  - o Usually presents by 1 month of age (Figures 10-48 through 10-50)
    - Symptoms of excess tearing and mucus discharge that is often visible with digital pressure on the nasal dorsum and observing the fluid and/or discharge coming out of the inferior puncta (Figures 10-51 through 10-53)

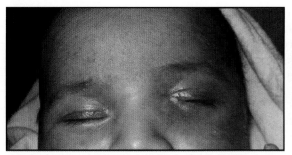

Figure 10-48. A 3 week old with a left tear duct mucocele causing localized swelling and discharge.

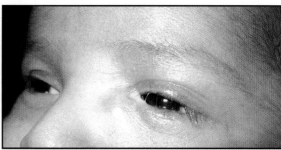

Figure 10-49. Same patient showing elevation of tear duct mucocele.

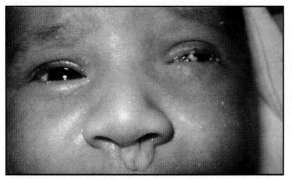

Figure 10-50. Same patient showing discharge from the left nostril and left eye after digital message over the mucocele decompressed the obstruction.

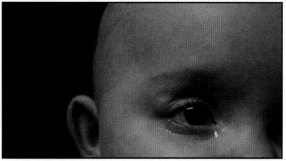

Figure 10-51. A 5 month old with a right tear duct obstruction as well as a dermoid cyst of the right anterior orbit temporally.

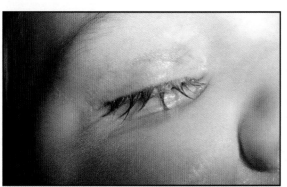

Figure 10-52. Eyelid crusting secondary to a tear duct obstruction in a 7 month old.

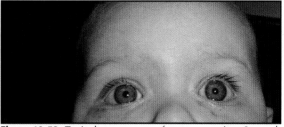

Figure 10-53. Typical appearance of watery eyes in a 9 month old with bilateral tear duct obstructions.

- o Acquired
  - ▪ Etiologies include trauma, sinus disease, granulomatous disease (ie, Wegener's granulomatosis or sarcoidosis).
- o Epiphora (tearing) and discharge are common, often resulting in crusted lashes, periocular erythema, and dermatitis.
- o Patients will exhibit a prolonged dye disappearance test as noted by residual fluorescein in the tear film 5 minutes after instillation in the inferior cul-de-sac (Figure 10-54).
- o Application of pressure over the lacrimal fossa may result in reflux of tears or a mucopurulent discharge from the lacrimal sac.
- o Overt signs of inflammation are often absent.

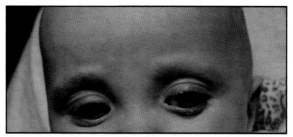

Figure 10-54. Fluorescein dye disappearance test used for diagnostic purposes in the diagnosis of tear duct blockage.

- Differential diagnosis
  - Congenital glaucoma is the most important diagnosis to exclude in an infant with epiphora.
  - Other signs of congenital glaucoma include high IOP, photophobia, corneal haziness or enlargement, and blepharospasm. Infants with congenital glaucoma typically do not have crusted debris in their lashes or mucoid discharge.
  - Occasionally, an infant with conjunctivitis may appear to have lacrimal outflow obstruction.
  - Punctal or canalicular atresia or stenosis
  - Congenital glaucoma
  - Trichiasis, entropion, or ectropion
- Evaluation and management
  - Tear duct obstructions usually resolve with conservative treatment including digital massage in up to 90% of cases by 6 months of age.
  - Conservative measures include broad-spectrum topical antibiotics and Crigler massage of the lacrimal sac, which is done by compressing the pad of a digit lubricated with ophthalmic ointment directly over the nasolacrimal sac in a sweeping downward motion.
  - Although these obstructions can resolve even up to and after 1 year of age, a tear-duct probing procedure can be recommended after 6 months of age depending on the surgeon's and parental preference and the severity of the child's symptoms.
  - A simple probing can be done as an in-office procedure or under general mask or laryngeal mask airway anesthesia, again depending on surgeon and parental preference.
    - The procedure involves dilating the superior puncta and then placing a Bowman probe (usually a 00 or 0) into the superior canalicular system and passing the probe into the common canalicular system and into the bony tear duct and into the nose. Metal-on-metal contact is then established in the nose to confirm a proper passage of the probe. Then, an irrigating cannula is placed into the superior canaliculus and fluorescein-stained saline solution is irrigated into the system and collected in the nose with a suction catheter to confirm patency of the system. Some recommend also probing the inferior system as well as irrigating, particularly if there is an obstruction present at the entrance of the inferior canaliculus to the common canaliculus.
    - The success rate of a simple probing procedure prior to age 2 can be up to 90% successful, depending on various series.
  - Balloon catheter dilation and intubation
    - The balloon catheter device uses a mechanism similar to an angioplasty to dilate the tear duct system after initially probing the system. While it can be used at any age, most use this device to open the tear duct systems in those who have previously failed tear duct surgery or those who are over the age of 2 years during the initial procedure (Figure 10-55).
    - Silicone intubation of the tear duct system can also be used at any age but its use is similar to that for the balloon catheter. The tube serves as a stent to keep the system open and is usually left in place for 6 weeks to 6 months, depending on the series (Figure 10-56).
    - Complications of silicone intubation include dislodging of the tube (10% to 20%), canalicular cheesewiring, corneal abrasion, difficulty of tube placement, postoperative patient monitoring, and possible second general anesthesia for tube removal (Figure 10-57)
    - Another alternative is the placement of a monocanalicular tube (Monoka), which has been found to be both easily inserted and removed but can cause corneal complications (Figure 10-58).

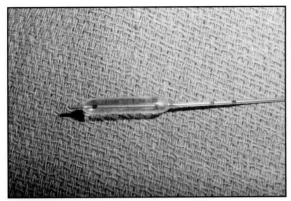

Figure 10-55. Example of the LacriCATH (QUEST Medical Inc., Allen, TX) balloon dilator used in tear duct surgery.

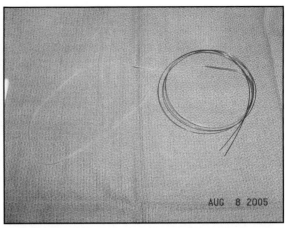

Figure 10-56. Silicone tube used in tear duct surgery.

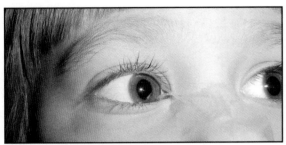

Figure 10-57. Extrusion of silicone tube post tear duct surgery, an example of a common complication of the surgery.

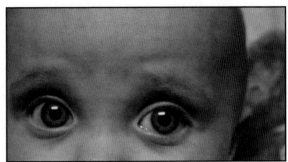

Figure 10-58. Example of the Monoka monocanalicular tear duct tube, an alternative to bicanalicular tubes.

- o Infracturing of the inferior turbinate
    - ▪ This procedure can be performed when there is a significant bony obstruction at the entrance of the tear duct into the nose.
    - ▪ Most surgeons will perform this maneuver during a second tear-duct procedure to enhance a successful surgical result.
    - ▪ It is particularly useful when the entrance is so narrow that there is great difficulty passing the silicone tube and retrieving it in the nose and when it is difficult to place the balloon catheter fully down the tear duct, just below the Valve of Hasner.
    - ▪ A periosteal elevator or hemostat is used to rotate the turbinate to facilitate a larger opening for the tears to flow.
- o Dacryocystorhinostomy (DCR)
    - ▪ DCR rarely needs to be performed today to open tear ducts.
    - ▪ Indicated for multiple probing, intubation, or balloon dilation procedures and is most often performed endoscopically today
- • Prognosis
    - o Congenital nasolacrimal duct obstruction (CNLDO) will resolve spontaneously by 1 year of age with nonsurgical management in as many as 90% of cases.
    - o For symptomatic congenital lacrimal obstruction present at 1 year of age, surgery success rates are as high as 90%. Delayed treatment of CNLDO (after 2 years of age) may be less successful than earlier intervention.

Pediatric Red Eye

- General concepts
    - o Appropriate history will frequently point to the correct diagnosis.
    - o Complete and accurate history is not always possible with children.
    - o Always be prepared for unreported trauma.
    - o Etiologies range from benign to serious.
- Important factors to determine need for immediate exam and a serious etiology are as follows:
    - o Loss of vision
    - o Irregular pupil
    - o Pain
    - o Photophobia
    - o Foreign-body sensation
    - o History of trauma or foreign body
    - o Visible opacity on the cornea
    - o Contact lens wear
    - o Vesicular skin lesions
- Etiology
    - o Pathology of many structures of the eye may give rise to redness of the sclera or conjunctiva including inflammation or irritation of the eyelids, conjunctiva, cornea, or sclera.
    - o Anterior segment diseases causing a red eye that are of particular importance in the pediatric age group include Kawasaki syndrome, Stevens-Johnson syndrome, and neonatal conjunctivitis.

Kawasaki Syndrome

- Also known as mucocutaneous lymph node syndrome
- Diagnosis criteria
    - o Unexplained fever for 5 or more days
    - o At least 4 of the following
        - ▪ Bilateral conjunctival injection
        - ▪ Mucus membrane changes of lips, pharynx, tongue (strawberry tongue)
        - ▪ Erythema of the palms or soles
        - ▪ Rash
        - ▪ Cervical lymphadenopathy
    - o Coronary artery aneurysm is the most serious possible complication
    - o Self-limited anterior uveitis may occur
    - o Usually treated with aspirin
    - o Systemic steroids contraindicated
        - ▪ Increased incidence of coronary artery aneurysm

Stevens-Johnson Syndrome

- Systemic disease affecting skin and mucus membranes
    - o Angiitis leading to bullous lesions
- Has a 5% to 15% mortality rate
- About 50% with ocular involvement
- Associated with the following medications
    - o Sulfonamides
    - o Penicillin
    - o Aspirin
    - o Barbiturates
    - o Isoniazide
    - o Dilantin

Neonatal Conjunctivitis

- Etiology
  - o Neisseria gonorrhoeae
    - Most serious cause
    - Usually present within days, but may take weeks
    - Often severe chemosis and discharge
    - May cause corneal perforation
    - Systemic infection may cause meningitis, sepsis, and arthritis.
    - Treated with systemic penicillin G for susceptible strains or ceftriaxone. Topical irrigation may be helpful.
  - o Chlamydia
    - Most common cause in the United States
    - Usual onset around 1 week of age
    - Frequent association with systemic infection
      - □ Requires systemic treatment
      - □ Treatment of choice is erythromycin 50 mg/kg/day divided 4 times daily for 10 to 14 days.
  - o Herpes simplex
    - Presents around age 2 weeks
    - See above for further discussion of herpetic disease
  - o Chemical conjunctivitis
    - Previously seen frequently in first 24 hours when silver nitrate is used for prophylaxis
- Signs/symptoms
  - o Potentially serious cause of vision loss
  - o First month of life
  - o Dramatically decreased in frequency in industrialized countries
  - o Common problem in developing countries
  - o Usually infectious, obtained by passage through birth canal
  - o May be chemical
  - o Eyelid edema
  - o Conjunctival injection
  - o Chemosis
  - o Papillae
  - o Follicles
  - o Preauricular adenopathy
  - o Ocular discharge
- Differential diagnosis
  - o Nasolacrimal duct obstruction
    - Purulent discharge
    - Lack of conjunctival injection
  - o Subconjunctival hemorrhage
    - Bright red blood under surface of conjunctiva
    - Excellent prognosis without intervention
    - Causes
      - □ Trauma
      - □ Straining (coughing, sneezing, emesis)
      - □ Conjunctival vessel abnormality
      - □ Hypertension (rarely in children)
  - o Telangiectasia
  - o Treatment (see previous)

Anterior Uveitis in Children

- Definition
  - o Inflammation of the anterior uveal tissues
  - o Includes iris (iritis) and ciliary body (iridocylitis)
  - o Breakdown of blood-aqueous barrier allows cells and protein to enter anterior chamber.
  - o See section on uveitis for more complete discussion.
- Etiology
  - o Indeterminate cause in 50% of children
  - o Juvenile rheumatoid arthritis (JRA) is most common cause in children.

Juvenile Rheumatoid Arthritis

- Etiology
  - o Chronic nonsuppurative synovial inflammation
  - o Causes joint effusions and destruction
- Classification
  - o Pauciarticular
    - Up to 4 affected joints
    - 50% of JRA patients
    - Up to 25% develop uveitis
    - Highest risk in young females with early onset (2 to 3 years of age), antinuclear antibody (ANA) positive and rheumatoid factor (RF) negative
  - o Polyarticular
    - More than 4 affected joints
    - 30% of JRA patients
    - 2% to 5% develop uveitis
  - o Systemic (Still disease)
    - Variable number of joints
    - 20% of JRA patients
    - 1% develop uveitis
- Signs/symptoms
  - o Often minimal redness and pain
  - o Regular examinations important because symptoms may be absent
- Evaluation
  - o Examination schedule for diagnosed JRA without documented uveitis
  - o Pauciarticular
    - Onset younger than 7 years of age
      - □ ANA positive
        - Less than 4 years duration, examine every 3 to 4 months
        - Between 4 and 7 years duration, examine every 6 months
        - More than 7 years duration, examine annually
      - □ ANA negative
        - Less than 7 years duration, examine every 6 months
        - More than 7 years duration, examine annually
    - Onset older than 7 years
      - □ ANA positive or negative
        - Less than 4 years duration, examine every 6 months
        - More than 4 years duration, examine annually
  - o Polyarticular
    - Onset younger than 7 years
      - □ ANA positive
        - Less than 4 years duration, examine every 3 to 4 months
        - Between 4 and 7 years duration, examine every 6 months
        - More than 7 years duration, examine annually

□ ANA negative
- Less than 7 years duration, examine every 6 months
- More than 7 years duration, examine annually
■ Onset older than 7 years
□ ANA positive or negative
- Less than 4 years duration, examine every 6 months
- More than 4 years duration, examine annually
o Systemic examination annually regardless of age of onset or duration
- Treatment
  o Nonsteroidal anti-inflammatory drugs (NSAIDs) are used to treat all subtypes of JRA.
  o Aspirin is no longer the drug of first choice because of the increased frequency of gastric toxicity and hepatotoxicity when compared to other NSAID medications.
  o Rarely, systemic corticosteroids are required.

Suggested Readings

Adams A, Lehman TJ. Update on the pathogenesis and treatment of systemic onset juvenile rheumatoid arthritis. *Curr Opin Rheumatol.* 2005;17(5):612.

Early Treatment for Retinopathy of Prematurity Cooperative Group. Revised indications for the treatment of retinopathy of prematurity: results of the early treatment for retinopathy of prematurity randomized trial. *Arch Ophthalmol.* 2003;121(12):1684–1694.

Katowitz JA, Welch MG. Timing of initial probing and irrigation in congenital nasolacrimal duct obstruction. *Ophthalmology.* 1987;94:698–705.

Kittleman WT, Mazow ML. Reoperations in esotropia surgery. *Ann Ophthalmol.* 1986;18(5):174–177.

Kushner BJ. Congenital nasolacrimal system obstruction. *Arch Ophthalmol.* 1982;100:597–600.

Neely DE, Sprunger DT. Nystagmus. *Curr Opin Ophthalmol.* 1999;10(5):320–326.

Pediatric Eye Disease Investigator Group. A randomized trial of atropine vs. patching for treatment of moderate amblyopia in children. *Arch Ophthalmol.* 2002;120:268–278.

Questions

1. Clinical characteristics of accommodative ET include the following:
   a. Usual onset between 18 months and 4 years
   b. Positive family history
   c. Amblyopia is common
   d. All of the above

2. Clinical characteristics of intermittent XT include the following:
   a. Near deviation greater than distance
   b. Onset less than 1 year of age
   c. Eye closure in sunlight
   d. Early surgery essential for binocularity

3. Amblyopia:
   a. Can be unilateral or bilateral
   b. Occurs in 2% to 4% of the population
   c. In unilateral cases, can be treated with patching or atropine eye drops
   d. All of the above

4. Which of the following is true of characteristics of cranial nerve palsies?
   a. Sixth nerve palsies characteristically develop aberrant regeneration
   b. Fourth nerve palsies are the most common cyclovertical palsy
   c. In third nerve palsies, the eye is usually esotropic
   d. All of the above

5. Duane's syndrome:
   a. Is most commonly familial
   b. **Is a "leash" effect causes the upshoot and downshoot**
   c. Does not cause amblyopia
   d. Can be cured by surgery

6. Nystagmus characteristics include which of the following?
   a. With congenital motor nystagmus, a frequent null point develops where the nystagmus dampens for best vision.
   b. The nystagmus and head nodding with spasmus nutans usually disappears by age 4.
   c. Upbeat and downbeat nystagmus are frequently associated with neurological disease.
   d. **All of the above**

7. Differential diagnosis of leukocoria includes which of the following:
   a. Retinoblastoma
   b. PHPV
   c. Cataract
   d. **All of the above**

8. Congenital optic nerve anomalies include which of the following:
   a. Optic nerve hypoplasia does not affect VA
   b. Optic pits are usually bilateral
   c. **Myelinated nerve fibers are frequently associated with high myopia and amblyopia**
   d. Optic disc drusen are associated with normal fluorescein angiograms

9. Retinopathy of prematurity characteristics include which of the following:
   a. Increased incidence with low birth weight and early gestational age infants
   b. Long-term complications include myopia, strabismus, amblyopia, and nystagmus
   c. Rush disease is defined as ROP in Zone I with plus disease and has a high risk of rapid progression
   d. **All of the above**

10. Which of the following is correct about a child with a red eye?
    a. Ophthalmia neonatorum is a self-limiting condition in infants.
    b. Polyarticular JRA is the most common form of the disease to cause uveitis.
    c. **Stevens-Johnson syndrome needs to be considered in children who have been treated with certain antibiotics and antiseizure medications.**
    d. Topical steroids are the first-line treatment for children with allergic conjunctivitis.

Neuro-Ophthalmology

Andrew G. Lee, MD

Outline

Introduction

Neuro-ophthalmology includes a diverse group of conditions that share a common relationship to the nervous system of the eye. Abnormalities of the pupils, paresis of the oculomotor nerves, disorders of the optic disc, and visual field deficiencies are caused by a wide variety of conditions requiring diverse investigations and treatments. A good understanding of the pathophysiology of neuro-ophthalmic disease requires knowledge of the neural anatomical pathways of the eye.

The Pupil

- Definition/anatomy
  - The efferent pupil pathway is composed of a parasympathetic (for constriction) and sympathetic pathway (for dilation).

Probst LE, Tsai JH.
Ophthalmology: Principles and Practice (pp. 419–452)
© 2012 SLACK Incorporated

- The parasympathetic pathway travels with the third cranial nerve.
- Within the peripheral third nerve, the pupil fibers lie within the superior and medial portion of the nerve in the subarachnoid space. In this location, an aneurysm can produce a pupil-involved third nerve palsy.
- The third nerve then travels in the cavernous sinus and enters the orbit as the inferior division to the ciliary ganglion.
- The third nerve fibers synapse within the ciliary ganglion and travel as short ciliary nerves to the iris sphincter.
  - The sympathetic pathway is composed of a 3-neuron arc (ie, central, preganglionic, and postganglionic neuron).
    - The central neuron (first-order neuron) begins in the posterior hypothalamus, descends in reticular formation, and synapses in the intermediolateral gray matter of spinal column at the lower cervical and upper thoracic spine (ciliospinal center of Budge-Waller), level of C8 to T2.
    - The preganglionic (second-order neuron) exits in the ventral roots via the white rami (mainly T1 level) and travels up (without synapse) through the sympathetic paraspinal ganglia to synapse in the superior cervical ganglion (at the level of the mandible).
    - The postganglionic (third-order neuron) then travels with the carotid artery to the cavernous sinus. Within the substance of the cavernous sinus, some fibers join briefly with the sixth nerve and then proceed onto the V1 (ophthalmic branch) nasociliary branch to the iris dilator via the long posterior ciliary nerves.

The Relative Afferent Pupillary Defect

- Definition
  - The relative afferent pupillary defect (RAPD) is a critical assessment of the afferent visual pathway.
- Etiology
  - An RAPD can occur in patients with retinal, optic nerve, or optic tract disease.
  - There is no RAPD from media disease (eg, cataract, corneal disease, refractive error) alone, and there is no RAPD with retrogeniculate disease in adults.
  - A small RAPD may rarely be seen in vitreous hemorrhage or amblyopia but should be considered to be a diagnosis of exclusion.
  - There may not be a RAPD if there is bilateral and symmetric anterior visual pathway involvement (eg, bilateral optic neuropathy) as the finding is relative to the fellow eye. Patients with bilateral and symmetric optic neuropathy thus actually have a bilateral defect in the afferent pupillary despite the lack of a RAPD on exam. Clinically, the bilateral defect in the afferent pathway may manifest as a light-near dissociation of the pupils.
- Signs/symptoms
  - The RAPD correlates roughly with the size and density of the visual field defect but is less tightly correlated with visual acuity.
- Evaluation (Figures 11-1 and 11-2)
  - Testing under low background illumination
  - Patient fixating a distant target to relax accommodation and miosis
  - The examiner should use a bright focused light source (eg, Fenhoff transilluminator).
  - Swing the light briskly and rhythmically from eye to eye.
  - Timing should be consistent with a fast count of about 3 seconds.
  - There should be equal stimulation time to each eye to avoid bleaching one retina asymmetrically.
  - Using a neutral density filter may be useful for grading the RAPD.
- Treatment/prognosis
  - Management depends upon the etiology of the RAPD.

Anisocoria

- Patients with unequal pupil size have anisocoria. If only one pupil is abnormal, then determining which pupil is pathologic is important in localizing the lesion.

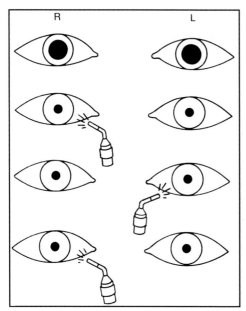

Figure 11-1. Normal response to swinging flashlight test with no change in size of pupils. (Reprinted with permission from Kline LB, Bajandas FJ. *Neuro-Ophthalmology.* 5th ed. Thorofare, NJ: SLACK Incorporated; 2004.)

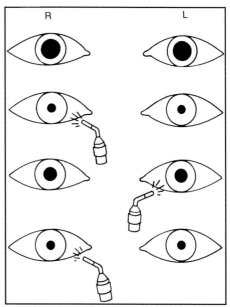

Figure 11-2. Afferent pupillary defect in the left eye using a swinging flashlight test. The pupils constrict when the light is shined in the right eye; however, when the flashlight is swung back to the left eye, both pupils dilate. (Reprinted with permission from Kline LB, Bajandas FJ. *Neuro-Ophthalmology.* 5th ed. Thorofare, NJ: SLACK Incorporated; 2004.)

- The first step in anisocoria is to determine the light reaction in each eye.
  - If the light reaction is abnormal, then the affected pupil is the problem.
  - If the light reaction is normal in each eye, then the anisocoria should be assessed in the light and in the dark.
  - If the anisocoria is greater in the dark, then the differential diagnosis includes the following:
    - Physiologic anisocoria
    - Horner syndrome
    - Sympathetic overaction
  - Physiologic anisocoria is common (about 20% of normals) and is characterized by the following features:
    - Lid position is normal (ie, no ptosis)
    - No dilation lag
    - Variability (pupil size may vary from day to day or even minute to minute)
    - Equal anisocoria in light and dark
    - Usually less than 1 mm of difference in pupil size
  - If there is any doubt, a topical apraclonidine or a topical cocaine test if negative can prove the anisocoria to be physiologic but is usually not necessary clinically. On the other hand, the Horner syndrome (oculosympathetic disruption) has distinctive features compared with physiologic anisocoria.

Horner Syndrome

- Definition
  - Disorder of the sympathetic nervous system causing mild ptosis and miosis as well as other symptoms
- Etiology
  - See Management section

Figure 11-3. External photographs show an anisocoria worse in the (A) dark than the (B) light with associated mild ptosis of right upper eyelid and "upside down" ptosis in a right Horner syndrome.

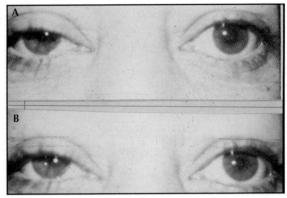

- Signs/symptoms
  - Ptosis (usually <2 mm) due to weak Müller's muscle of upper lid (Figure 11-3)
  - Moderate miosis (smaller pupil)
  - Apparent enophthalmos (due to ptosis and upside-down ptosis)
  - Anhydrosis of the face
  - Dilation lag of pupil
  - Upside-down ptosis (lower lid smooth muscles)
  - Increased amplitude of accommodation
  - Decreased intraocular pressure (IOP) may be present.
  - Lighter iris color may be seen in congenital cases.
- Evaluation
  - Pharmacological assessment
    - Pharmacologic testing may be helpful in confirming the diagnosis of Horner syndrome (versus physiologic anisocoria) and localizing the lesion (pre- versus postganglionic).
    - Topical cocaine inhibits the reuptake of norepinephrine at the neuromuscular junction, and failure of the pupil to dilate is diagnostic of a Horner syndrome. Patients with greater than 0.8 mm of postcocaine testing anisocoria have a Horner syndrome.
    - Topical hydroxyamphetamine (Paredrine 1%) stimulates the release of norepinephrine from the third-order neuron and localizes the lesion after the cocaine test confirms the Horner syndrome. Failure of the pupil to dilate indicates a third-order neuron Horner syndrome, and a greater anisocoria after hydroxyamphetamine compared with predrop test anisocoria indicates a postganglionic lesion. Thus, hydroxyamphetamine testing distinguishes pre- from postganglionic lesions. The hydroxyamphetamine test should be performed 1 or 2 days after the topical cocaine has worn off.
    - Topical iopidine has also been used in Horner syndrome diagnosis and produces a reversing anisocoria.
    - Old photographs should be reviewed to try to establish the duration of the anisocoria if possible.
  - Imaging
    - The oculosympathetic pathway is a 3-neuron arc that includes a central, first-order preganglionic neuron, a second-order preganglionic neuron, and a third-order postganglionic neuron.
    - Central (first-order neuron) Horner syndromes do not typically occur in isolation. Patients with brainstem lesions (eg, tumor, demyelination) or cervical cord lesions typically have other brainstem or spinal cord signs present. Neuroimaging should be directed toward the brainstem and cord to C8-T2 level.
    - Preganglionic (second-order neuron) Horner syndrome involves the high thorax or low cervical cord lesions or the neck. The etiologies include trauma (eg, head and neck injury), head and neck tumors, apical lung tumor (ie, Pancoast tumor, metastatic), lymphadenopathy (neck), or internal carotid artery lesions (eg, dissection). Arm pain may occur in patients with brachial plexopathy. Imaging of the preganglionic Horner syndrome should include hypothalamus to T2 in the chest.

- The postganglionic (third-order neuron) Horner syndrome may be due to headache syndromes (eg, cluster, Raeder's paratrigeminal neuralgia), cavernous sinus lesions, upper neck surgery, cervical lymph nodes or tumor, trauma to orbit/neck, and distal carotid artery lesions (eg, dissecting aneurysm, fibromuscular dysplasia, arteriosclerosis, or thrombosis). Although postganglionic Horner syndromes are usually benign in isolation, imaging of head and upper neck may be necessary, especially in patients suspected of harboring a dissection or cavernous sinus lesion.

- Treatment/prognosis
  - Depends upon the etiology
- Horner syndrome in a child
  - In children, the main consideration is birth trauma.
  - In patients with an acquired Horner syndrome, however, neuroblastoma or other mass lesion of the cervical chain should be considered.
  - Neuroimaging of the cervical sympathetic chain should be considered in all patients without a clear birth trauma or other trauma history or defined etiology.

Poor Light Reaction

- If the light reaction is poor, then the differential diagnosis includes afferent anterior visual pathway disease or efferent pathway disease.
- Patients with severe loss of vision due to retina or optic nerve disease (anterior visual pathway) will have sluggishly reactive or nonreactive pupils. If the visual loss is unilateral or bilateral but asymmetric, then a RAPD will be detected.
- If both eyes are affected, then testing the near reaction will determine if the efferent pathway is intact. If the near reaction is normal, then the patient has light near dissociation of the pupil. This can occur due to severe afferent visual pathway disease, diabetes (autonomic neuropathy), dorsal midbrain syndrome, or the Argyll-Robertson pupils (syphilis).
- If the near reaction is abnormal but tonic, then the patient has the Adie's tonic pupil.

Adie's Tonic Pupil

- Definition
  - Near reaction is abnormal and tonic
- Etiology
  - Although the idiopathic variety is most common (ie, Adie's tonic pupil) the differential diagnosis includes the following:
    - Infectious (eg, syphilis, viruses)
    - Trauma (eg, orbital or ocular)
    - Tumors (eg, orbital, choroidal)
    - Iatrogenic (eg, laser, retrobulbar injection of alcohol, cryotherapy)
    - Diabetes (neuropathic)
    - Giant cell arteritis (GCA) (rare)
    - Inflammation (eg, sarcoid)
    - Infiltrative (eg, amyloid)
    - Dysautonomias (eg, Riley Day, Ross syndromes)
- Signs/symptoms
  - The typical patient with a tonic pupil is a young female (70%) aged 20 to 40 years.
  - Up to 20% of cases are asymptomatic and are detected incidentally.
  - Symptomatic patients may complain about "blurry vision" (accommodative palsy) and difficulty reading, photophobia and glare, ciliary spasm at near (brow ache with near work), or accommodative-induced astigmatism.
  - The incidence of the tonic pupil is estimated at 4.7/100,000, and 10% to 20% are bilateral.
  - The ocular exam shows characteristic slit-lamp findings including sector paresis of the iris sphincter and vermiform movements of the remaining normal iris segments when stimulated by light.
  - The pupil demonstrates a poor constriction to light and a tonic response to near with slow redilation.

- o The pupil is often irregular and dilated but may become miotic over time (ie, "little old Adie's pupil").
  - o It is typically unilateral (90%) at onset, but up to 4% per year become bilateral over time.
  - o There may be regional corneal anesthesia and decreased deep tendon reflexes.
- Evaluation
  - o Cholinergic denervation supersensitivity may be demonstrated with topical low-dose pilocarpine (1/8% to 1/10%).
  - o No further evaluation is needed usually if Adie's tonic pupil syndrome is confirmed clinically or pharmacologically.
  - o Erythrocyte sedimentation rate (ESR) if indicated in elderly patients with a suspicion for GCA but this would be a rare presentation.
  - o Syphilis serology should be considered if the tonic pupil is bilateral and simultaneous.
  - o Other autonomic dysfunction should prompt consideration for the systemic dysautonomic syndromes.
- Differential diagnosis
  - o Iris changes
    - If the pupil light reaction is abnormal but the near reaction is not tonic and the Adie's tonic pupil cannot be confirmed as the cause for the anisocoria, then structural iris changes should be excluded using the slit-lamp biomicroscope (eg, sphincter tears, previous or acute anterior segment inflammation, previous ocular surgery, iris ischemia, angle closure glaucoma, iris atrophy [Figure 11-4], or acute elevated IOP).
  - o Third nerve palsy
    - Patients with anisocoria and a dilated, poorly reactive pupil should be evaluated for an ipsilateral third nerve palsy. Usually, a dilated pupil in isolation is not due to a third nerve palsy, however. Associated motility signs of third nerve palsy (eg, adduction, depression, elevation deficit) or ptosis should suggest the diagnosis. An isolated dilated pupil is more likely to be iris damage, the tonic pupil, or pharmacologic dilation than a third nerve palsy. Pharmacologic testing can differentiate a chronic Adie's tonic pupil (supersensitive to dilute pilocarpine), a third nerve palsy (constricts to pilocarpine 1%), and pharmacologic dilation (does not constrict to pilocarpine 1%). But generally, these entities can be distinguished clinically.
  - o Pharmacological dilation
    - Pharmacologic dilation typically produces a large pupil (often more than 8 to 10 mm) and can be confirmed by a lack of constriction to topical pilocarpine 1%.
    - Purposeful or inadvertent topical or systemic mydriatics (eg, atropine), transdermal scopolamine patches, or exposure to mydriatics in plants (eg, Jimson weed, Belladonna alkaloids) may produce pharmacologic dilation.
    - Patients with pharmacologic dilation typically can be observed for resolution of the mydriasis.
- Treatment/ prognosis
  - o None required

Third Nerve Palsy

- Definition
  - o Paresis of the third cranial nerve
- Etiology
  - o The clinical localization of the third nerve palsy is defined by associated clinical signs.

Nuclear Third Nerve Palsy

- The nuclear third nerve palsy in the midbrain is rare in isolation and is usually associated with other midbrain signs (eg, other cranial neuropathies, ataxia, hemisensory loss, hemiparesis).
- The obligatory nuclear lesions include unilateral third nerve palsy with a contralateral superior rectus palsy and bilateral ptosis or a bilateral third nerve palsy with sparing of both levators (no ptosis).
- Other possible nuclear third nerve lesions include bilateral complete third nerve palsy (eg, basilar artery infarct), a bilateral and symmetric ptosis (single midline nucleus involvement), or isolated weakness of one muscle.

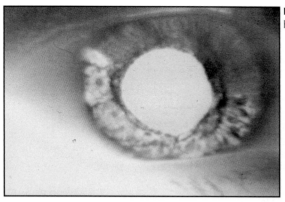

Figure 11-4. Infrared pupillography shows iris atrophy due to prior herpes zoster infection.

- For the same reasons, the following third nerve palsies cannot be nuclear lesions:
  - ○ Complete third nerve palsy with normal contralateral superior rectus function (crossed innervations)
  - ○ Unilateral ptosis alone because both levators are supplied by single caudal subnucleus bilateral innervations
  - ○ Unilateral dilated pupil alone (ie, internal ophthalmoplegia)
  - ○ Isolated unilateral or bilateral medial rectus muscle (3 separate subnuclei and more likely to be an internuclear ophthalmoplegia)
- The etiologies of a nuclear third nerve palsy include ischemia (midbrain), neoplasm, trauma, infection, or rarely demyelination.

Fascicular Third Nerve Palsy

- The fascicular third nerve palsy, like the nuclear palsy, is defined by the "company they keep" (eg, contralateral ataxia, "rubral" tremor, contralateral hemichorea or hemitremor, vertical gaze palsy, contralateral hemiparesis, and face and tongue involvement).
- In the subarachnoid space, the third nerve palsy is particularly important as a sign of possible intracranial aneurysm.
  - ○ The clinical findings for subarachnoid space localization include a pupil-involved third nerve palsy with or without other subarachnoid space signs (signs of subarachnoid hemorrhage present, stiff neck, headache, especially the "worst headache of my life").
  - ○ This presentation should be considered to be a posterior communicating artery aneurysm until proven otherwise (the "rule of the pupil").
  - ○ The etiologies for a subarachnoid space lesion in addition to the posterior communicating aneurysm include basilar artery aneurysm, uncal herniation, basilar meningitis, neoplasm, ischemia, surgical and nonsurgical trauma, and hydrocephalus.
- In the cavernous sinus, the clinical findings usually include other cranial nerves (eg, IV, VI, and V1) or a Horner syndrome. Proptosis may indicate superior orbital fissure or orbital involvement. The etiology for cavernous sinus lesions includes the following:
  - ○ Neoplasm (eg, pituitary tumor, meningioma, metastasis)
  - ○ Infections (eg, mucormycosis, Aspergillus)
  - ○ Vascular lesions (eg, intracavernous aneurysm, fistula, thrombosis)
  - ○ Inflammatory lesions (eg, sarcoid, Tolosa-Hunt syndrome)
  - ○ Trauma
- Orbital third nerve lesions produce orbital clinical signs including proptosis, chemosis, and conjunctival injection. There may be a concomitant orbital optic neuropathy.
- Signs/symptoms
  - ○ Patients with third nerve palsy typically complain of diplopia and/or ptosis.
  - ○ Eye is positioned inferiorly and laterally (down and out).
  - ○ Complete ptosis may act as an occluder and preclude diplopia (Figure 11-5).
  - ○ Other neurological signs and symptoms may also be present depending on the topographical localization of the lesion (see previous).

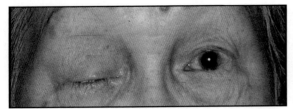

Figure 11-5. External photograph shows complete ptosis of right eye.

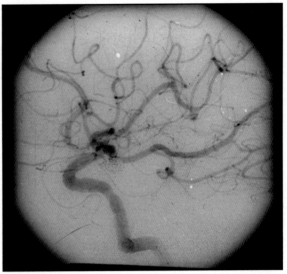

Figure 11-6. Angiogram shows endovascular coil within posterior communicating artery aneurysm.

- Management
  - o Third nerve palsies may be divided into those that are isolated and those that are not isolated.
    - Nonisolated third nerve palsies should undergo neuroimaging with attention to areas suggested topographically by the associated neurologic signs and symptoms
    - Treatment of the underlying etiology of the third nerve palsy may improve the ophthalmoplegia (eg, endovascular coiling of an aneurysm [Figure 11-6]).

Classification of Isolated Third Nerve Palsy

- Isolated third nerve palsies may be classified by degree of internal (ie, pupil function) and external (ie, extraocular muscle function) into complete and incomplete third nerve palsies.
  - o A complete external dysfunction third nerve palsy significantly involves all of the somatic branches (Figure 11-7) of the third nerve (eg, all the extraocular muscles innervated by the third nerve). Third nerve palsies with complete external involvement may be further subdivided into pupil-sparing (normal internal function) and pupil-involved (abnormal internal function) complete third nerve palsies.
  - o An incomplete external dysfunction third nerve palsy does not involve all of the branches of the third nerve (eg superior divisional palsy) or does not involve all of the muscles to a significant degree.
  - o Although severe pain (eg, "worst headache of my life") is suggestive of aneurysm, ischemic palsies may be painful, and the absence of pain does not exclude aneurysm. Aneurysm is less common in children or the elderly but age alone is not a differentiating feature.

Isolated Complete Third Nerve Palsy With Pupil-Sparing

- An isolated third nerve palsy with a normal internal function (normal pupil) but completely palsied extraocular muscles is almost never caused by an aneurysm.
- The isolated, complete, pupil-spared third nerve palsy is most commonly caused by ischemia and can be observed for improvement in a vasculopathic patient.
- Patients with lack of improvement or progression, or a palsy in a nonvasculopathic patient, should probably undergo a neuroimaging study, preferably contrast magnetic resonance imaging (MRI) (Figure 11-8) along the course of the third nerve with magnetic resonance angiography (MRA) or computed tomography angiography (CTA).

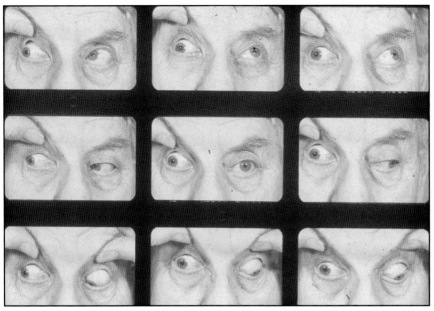

Figure 11-7. Motility photos show adduction, elevation, and depression deficit in the right eye. The right eye is exotropic and hypotropic ("down and out"). Abduction of the right eye is normal. Intorsion of the right eye is intact, suggesting an intact fourth nerve function.

Isolated Incomplete Third Nerve Palsy With No Pupil Involvement

- Patients with an incomplete external (ie, extraocular) muscle involvement but no pupil involvement (eg, divisional palsy) still a require magnetic resonance (MR) scan to rule out a mass lesion and an MRA or CTA to consider aneurysm.
- If the MRI and MRA (or CTA) is normal, cerebral angiography should still be considered to investigate the presence of an aneurysm or a carotid cavernous sinus fistula. MRI and MRA usually disclose an aneurysm causing a third nerve palsy, but cerebral angiography remains the "gold standard" to exclude cerebral aneurysm.
- The combination of an adequately performed and interpreted MRI and MRA or CTA may be up to 98% sensitive in the detection of an aneurysm that will bleed. The decision, however, to solely rely upon the MRI/MRA versus CTA for third nerve palsy remains controversial. Although CTA might be superior to MRA at a particular institution, in general MR is superior to CT scan for the evaluation of nonaneurysmal causes for a third nerve palsy. Thus, from a practical standpoint, an MRI with MRA combination might be easier to obtain than an MRI with CTA combination.
- The risk of the angiography must be weighed against the risk of aneurysm in the individual patient. Patient age, pain, and the quality, reliability, and results of MRI/MRA or CTA should be considered in the decision making. It should be emphasized that pupil sparing is not protective against aneurysm in this setting unlike in the complete pupil-spared third nerve palsy due to vasculopathy.

Isolated Incomplete or Complete External Dysfunction Third Nerve Palsy With Partial or Relative Pupil Sparing (Partial Internal Dysfunction)

- Patients with a partial (internal dysfunction) or "relative" pupil-sparing third nerve palsy should probably undergo MRI and MRA (or CTA) to exclude a compressive lesion.

Isolated Complete or Incomplete External Dysfunction but Pupil-Involved (Internal Dysfunction) Third Nerve Palsy

- Third nerve palsies that produce complete pupilloparesis (ie, complete internal dysfunction) are often due to compressive lesions (including aneurysm).
- The clinical "rule of the pupil" states that an isolated pupil-involved third nerve palsy is due to an aneurysm (usually the posterior communicating artery) until proven otherwise. Thus, patients should undergo MRI and MRA (or CTA). Even if this study is negative, a cerebral angiogram should be strongly considered to exclude aneurysm.

Figure 11-8. MRI shows a right cavernous sinus mass (which proved to be metastatic adenocarcinoma).

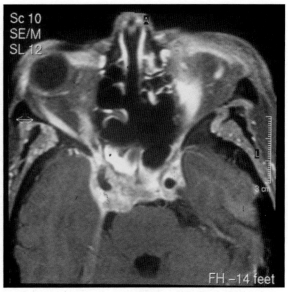

- Catheter angiography should still be considered if risk of aneurysm is higher than risk of angiography. On the other hand, angiography should be deferred if the risk of angiography is higher (eg, stroke risk in elderly or frail individual, renal failure) than the risk of aneurysm (eg, child under 10 years, pupil spared complete, isolated vasculopathic palsy).
- Observation alone initially is appropriate for isolated complete, pupil-spared third nerve palsy in vasculopathic patients.

Fourth Nerve Palsy

- Definition
    - o Paresis of the fourth cranial nerve
- Etiology
    - o The most common causes for a fourth nerve palsy in isolation are congenital, traumatic, ischemic, and idiopathic. Compressive lesions are rare but can occur anywhere along the pathway of the fourth nerve (eg, trochlear schwannoma).
    - o Nonisolated fourth nerve palsies may be ischemic, hemorrhagic, demyelinating, traumatic, or neoplastic.
        - ▪ The clinical signs of a neurologically nonisolated fourth nerve palsy are topographically localizing.
            - ▫ In midbrain (nuclear/fascicular) lesions, the fourth nerve palsy is "defined by the company it keeps," as there are typically other brainstem signs present (eg, hemiparesis, hemisensory loss, other cranial neuropathies, or dorsal midbrain findings).
            - ▫ The subarachnoid space lesions produce stiff neck or other multiple or bilateral cranial neuropathies. The etiologies for midbrain/subarachnoid fourth nerve palsy include traumatic, neoplastic (eg, meningioma, schwannoma, pinealoma), or infectious or inflammatory (eg, meningitis) lesions.
            - ▫ In the cavernous sinus, the fourth nerve palsy is typically not isolated and is usually associated with other intracavernous nerve involvement (ie, III, V, or VI nerve paresis, Horner syndrome). The etiology for the cavernous sinus lesion includes neoplastic (ie, meningioma, pituitary adenoma, metastasis), inflammatory (eg, Tolosa Hunt syndrome), infectious (eg, herpes zoster virus), or vascular (eg, carotid cavernous fistula or thrombosis or carotid cavernous aneurysm) lesions.
            - ▫ In the orbit, other orbital signs are present (eg, proptosis, chemosis, edema), and orbital etiologies include trauma (including surgical), postinflammatory, or orbital neoplasm or orbital inflammatory pseudotumor.

- Symptoms
  - Patients with isolated fourth nerve palsy complain of binocular oblique diplopia.
  - They may assume an anomalous head tilt to avoid diplopia.
  - Some patients have subjective torsion.
  - Acute isolated palsies are typically post-traumatic or ischemic.
  - The isolated and longstanding or congenital palsy typically has a gradual, vague, or early onset. Patients with congenital palsy, however, may decompensate later in life. The patient may have intermittent symptoms of diplopia, suggesting either large fusional amplitudes or variable control of the deviation. Patients may have other localizing neurologic symptoms depending on the location of the lesion (see previous).
  - Chronic, progressive, or nonisolated palsies should be considered to have compressive lesions until proven otherwise.
- Signs
  - The patient with a fourth nerve palsy has an ipsilateral hypertropia that is worse in contralateral gaze and ipsilateral head tilt.
  - Torsion measurement with the double Maddox rod may reveal excyclotorsion (Figure 11-9).
  - The fundus exam may also show objective excyclotorsion (Figure 11-10).
  - The clinical features are summarized in Table 11-1.
  - Ductional measurements may show a slight reduction in the ipsilateral superior oblique muscle function.
  - There may be overaction of the ipsilateral inferior oblique muscle.
  - Over time, in longstanding fourth nerve palsies, the hypertropia may show spread of comitance.
  - Old photographs may disclose a longstanding torticollis or facial asymmetry.
  - Measurement of the fusional amplitudes may suggest a congenital palsy if the vertical amplitudes are very large (>10 to 15 prism diopters) compared with normal values (ie, 3 to 6 prism diopters).
  - A bilateral fourth nerve palsy should be considered in all cases but especially following trauma. There are several clinical features that might suggest a bilateral palsy (see Table 11-2).
- Evaluation
  - The first responsibility of the ophthalmologist in managing a cranial nerve palsy is to document that the palsy is isolated or not.
  - For the nonisolated fourth nerve palsy, the neuroimaging (eg, cranial contrast MRI) should be directed to the topographical localization based upon the associated clinical signs and symptoms (see previous).
  - If the fourth nerve palsy is truly neurologically isolated, then the clinician can consider an etiologic diagnosis based upon the clinical presentation.
  - In the fourth nerve palsy in the vasculopathic patient (eg, diabetes, hypertension, older age), the clinician might elect to follow the patient for improvement over time (eg, 4 to 6 weeks) and control any underlying medical risk factors (eg, blood pressure, blood sugar, blood cholesterol, discontinue smoking). If there is no change in the measurements over time, new neurologic signs develop, or there is progression of the palsy, then a neuroimaging study (preferably a contrast MR scan of the head along the course of the fourth nerve) should be considered (Figure 11-11). If, however, the patient is improved, then no further evaluation may be necessary.
  - For patients with a clearly congenital and isolated fourth nerve palsy (eg, old photographs show longstanding head tilt, patient has been symptomatic for years), no further additional workup may be required.
  - Likewise, for patients with a clearly post-traumatic fourth nerve palsy, no additional workup beyond the original trauma evaluation is necessary. The one caveat, however, is that in cases of minor head trauma out of proportion to the cranial neuropathy, one should consider the possibility of an underlying skull-based tumor, and a contrast MR scan should be performed.
  - In all patients with a painless, pupil-spared, nonproptotic ophthalmoplegia, even a classic fourth nerve palsy, the clinician should consider the diagnosis of myasthenia gravis. Patients with concomitant ptosis, variability, fatigue, or other signs of myasthenia should undergo additional testing (eg, Tensilon testing, antiacetylcholine receptor antibodies, neurology consultation). In addition, one should consider GCA in the differential of diplopia in elderly patients.

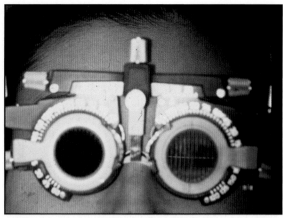

Figure 11-9. Double Maddox rod testing for torsion.

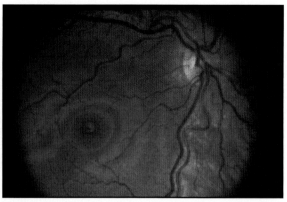

Figure 11-10. Objective torsion seen on fundus exam.

TABLE 11-1. SUMMARY OF FEATURES OF THE FOURTH CRANIAL NERVE PALSY
Three-step test
• Which is the hypertropic eye? (ipsilateral)
• Is the hyperdeviation worse in gaze right or left? (contralateral to the hypertropia)
• Is the deviation worse in head tilt right or left? (ipsilateral to the hypertropia)
Document anomalous head tilt
• Opposite side (70%)
• Same side (3%)
• No tilt (27%)
Chin down or face turn opposite side
Measure torsion with double Maddox rod
• Measure subjective excyclotorsion
• If torsion >10 degrees, consider bilateral palsy
• Check torsion in primary position and downgaze
Document presence of objective torsion on fundus exam

- Management
  - Treatment should be directed at the underlying etiology for the fourth nerve palsy (eg, treatment of tumor).
  - Patients who are anticipated to recover function (eg, vasculopathic) may benefit from short-term patching or prism therapy.
  - Strabismus surgery could be considered for patients with a persistent but symptomatic and stable deviation.
- Prognosis
  - Many patients can be treated symptomatically with prism or surgical therapy.
  - Treatment of the underlying etiology (eg, neoplasm) might alleviate the diplopia.
  - The majority of ischemic fourth nerve palsies resolve spontaneously.
  - Traumatic palsies, depending on the severity of the injury, may also recover without treatment.

TABLE 11-2. FEATURES SUGGESTIVE OF A BILATERAL FOURTH CRANIAL NERVE PALSY

Reversal of hypertropia with gaze positions (alternating hypertropia)
Large >10 degrees excyclotorsion
"V" pattern esotropia (bilateral "overaction" of inferior oblique in upgaze)
No hypertropia or small hypertropia in primary (bilateral hypertropia cancels out)
Marked chin depression
Bilateral underaction of superior oblique muscles on ductions

Sixth Nerve Palsy

- Definition
  - Paresis of the sixth cranial nerve
- Symptoms
  - Patients with a sixth nerve palsy typically complain of binocular horizontal diplopia worse in gaze toward the paretic lateral rectus muscle.
  - Nonisolated sixth nerve palsy may be accompanied by other symptoms depending upon the location of the lesion (eg, headache, other cranial neuropathies, other neurologic symptoms).
- Signs
  - The examination reveals an ipsilateral abduction deficit that might be complete or incomplete
  - There is usually a primary position and incomitant esotropia that is worse on gaze to the paretic lateral rectus muscle (Figure 11-12).
  - A small vertical deviation (less than 2 prism diopters) may also occur in isolated sixth nerve palsy.
  - Other signs may be present depending on the topographical location of the lesion.
- Etiology and clinical syndromes based upon the localization of the sixth nerve palsy
  - Pontine (lower pons) syndromes producing a sixth nerve palsy may involve the nucleus or fascicle.
    - A nuclear sixth nerve lesion produces a horizontal gaze palsy and not an isolated abduction deficit due to involvement of the interneurons of the medial longitudinal fasciculus (MLF). Nuclear sixth nerve palsies are usually associated with other brainstem signs. In the pons, an ipsilateral facial nerve palsy may occur.
    - Likewise, fascicular sixth nerve palsy is defined by involvement of adjacent neurological structures in the pons including the following:
      - Cranial nerves V, VII, and VIII
      - Cerebellar ataxia
      - Central Horner syndrome
      - Contralateral hemiplegia (pyramidal tract)
    - The etiology of nuclear or fascicular lesions in the pons includes ischemic, vascular (eg, bleed, arteriovenous malformation [AVM]), neoplasm (pontine or cerebellar-pontine lesions), and demyelinating disease.
    - In the subarachnoid space, a unilateral or bilateral sixth nerve palsy may be a nonlocalizing sign of any cause of increased intracranial pressure including pseudotumor cerebri, inflammatory (eg, sarcoid) or infectious (syphilis, bacterial, viral) meningitis, subarachnoid bleed, or an intracranial mass lesion.
    - At the level of the petrous apex, the sixth nerve palsy can be associated with other cranial nerve involvement (eg, V, VII, VIII). The etiology of petrous apex involvement includes complicated otitis media/mastoiditis (Gradenigo's syndrome), basilar skull fracture, and neoplasm (eg, nasopharyngeal carcinoma).

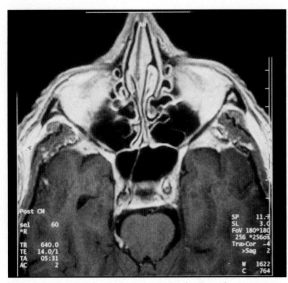

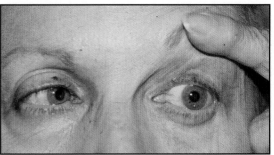

Figure 11-12. Motility photograph shows left abduction deficit with incomitant esotropia on left lateral gaze consistent with a left sixth nerve palsy.

Figure 11-11. Axial postcontrast MRI shows enhancement in intracisternal portion of right fourth nerve consistent with trochlear schwannoma.

- Within the cavernous sinus, the sixth nerve palsy may be associated with other nerve involvement (eg, III, IV, Horner syndrome, or V1 or V2), or it may present in isolation. The etiologies for a cavernous sinus lesion include sellar/parasellar tumors (eg, pituitary adenoma, meningioma), vascular (eg, aneurysm of the internal carotid artery or dissection, cavernous sinus thrombosis or fistula), inflammatory (eg, Tolosa-Hunt syndrome, sarcoid), or infectious.
- Orbital lesions typically are associated with other orbital signs (eg, proptosis, chemosis). The etiology for orbital processes producing a sixth nerve palsy include neoplastic, inflammatory, infectious, and traumatic causes.

- Evaluation
  - The main responsibility of the ophthalmologist in the evaluation of the sixth nerve palsy is to ensure that the palsy is truly neurologically isolated.
  - A bilateral sixth nerve palsy is not isolated. The ophthalmologist should exclude papilledema and a nonlocalizing sixth nerve palsy due to increased intracranial pressure.
  - Myasthenia gravis may mimic a sixth nerve palsy and should be considered in the differential diagnosis.
  - Patients with topographically localizing features should have neuroimaging (preferably cranial contrast MRI along the course of the sixth nerve) directed at the localization.
  - Vasculopathic patients with a neurologically isolated sixth nerve palsy may be observed for improvement over 4 to 6 weeks, although some authors have recommended initial neuroimaging for all ocular motor cranial neuropathies. If observation is selected and the patient improves, then no further evaluation is generally required for the vasculopathic patient beyond diagnosis and treatment of the underlying risk factors (eg, diabetes, hypertension). If, however, the patient worsens, progresses, or develops new neurologic signs/symptoms, then neuroimaging (preferably contrast cranial MRI) and further evaluation may be required.
  - Nonvasculopathic patients probably should undergo at least neuroimaging.
  - Patients with clearly post-traumatic palsies do not generally require additional evaluation outside of that required as part of acute trauma workup. If, however, the sixth nerve palsy occurs in the setting of minor head trauma, consideration for a cranial contrast MRI should be made to exclude skull base tumor (Figure 11-13).
- Differential diagnosis
  - Not every abduction deficit and esotropia is due to a sixth nerve palsy.
  - Table 11-3 lists alternative etiologies that might mimic a sixth nerve palsy and the differentiating features of each entity.

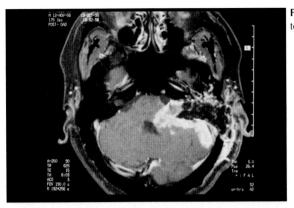

Figure 11-13. Axial postcontrast MRI shows enhancing hyperintense lesion in left cerebellopontine angle.

TABLE 11-3. DIFFERENTIAL DIAGNOSIS FOR AN ABDUCTION DEFICIT AND ESOTROPIA

CONDITION	COMMENT
Convergence spasm	Variable esotropia, variable abduction deficit, miosis during convergence spasm episodes
Duane syndrome I	Lid fissure narrows during adduction and widens during abduction. Usually do not have diplopia but may use an anomalous head position. May have up or downshoot in adduction.
Thyroid ophthalmopathy	Restrictive myopathy involving the medial rectus muscle(s) might produce abduction deficit and esotropia. Proptosis, lid retraction, lid lag, and history of thyroid disease may be helpful.
Childhood strabismus	Typically, no diplopia and longstanding history of comitant esotropia with no abductional deficit.
Myasthenia gravis	May mimic any ocular motor cranial neuropathy including sixth nerve palsy. Look for ptosis, bilateral or multiple muscle involvement, variability, or fatigue.
Restrictive myopathies other than thyroid ophthalmopathy	Medial wall fracture with entrapment of the medial rectus muscle. Mechanical restriction can occur in orbital tumors, orbital pseudotumor, or orbital foreign body (eg, scleral buckle).

- Management
  - Treatment should be directed at the underlying etiology for the sixth nerve palsy (eg, treatment of tumor or pseudotumor cerebri).
  - Patients who are anticipated to recover function may benefit from a short-term patching or prism therapy.
  - Botulinum toxin injection into the medial rectus might produce temporary relief of diplopia and reduce the risk of contracture.
  - Strabismus surgery could be considered for patients with persistent but symptomatic and stable esotropia.
- Prognosis
  - Most ischemic and many traumatic sixth nerve palsies resolve spontaneously over time.
  - The success of the treatment of the underlying etiology determines prognosis for nonisolated palsies.
  - Most patients who remain symptomatic can be treated with patching, prism, or strabismus surgery.

Nystagmus

- Definition
  - Nystagmus is a rhythmic oscillation of the eyes.
  - The eye movement may be unilateral, dissociated, or bilateral.
  - The eye movement can be rotary, horizontal, or vertical or a combination of these movements.
  - The nystagmus should be described in terms of the morphology as jerk (fast phase in one direction, slow phase in the opposite direction) or pendular; conjugate or dissociated, or frankly unilateral; symmetric or asymmetric; vertical, horizontal, or rotary; fast or slow frequency; and small, moderate, or large amplitude.
  - The nystagmus morphology should be described in the primary position as well as the various positions of gaze.
  - Precipitating (eg, head position, gaze position, monocular occlusion) or palliating (null position) features should be documented.
- Etiology
  - The etiology for nystagmus includes nonlocalizing forms of nystagmus (eg, gaze-evoked nystagmus) or localizing forms of nystagmus.
  - Table 11-4 lists some localizing forms of nystagmus.
  - Congenital nystagmus occurs sometime after birth and is associated with specific features listed in Table 11-5.
  - The major role of the ophthalmologist in evaluating congenital nystagmus is the exclusion of sensory visual loss as the cause.
  - Acquired nystagmus is commonly due to drug toxicity or side effect.
  - The localizing forms of nystagmus can result from any lesion in the posterior fossa (eg, demyelinating, neoplastic, toxic, traumatic, ischemic, vascular).
- Symptoms
  - The symptoms of nystagmus are related to the retinal blur induced by the eye movements.
  - This symptom of ocular motion is called oscillopsia.
  - Patients with congenital nystagmus typically do not have oscillopsia, however.
- Signs
  - Nystagmus can be described by its direction (eg, horizontal, vertical, rotary, or combination).
  - In patients with jerk beating nystagmus, the nystagmus is typically named for the fast-phase direction (eg, fast phase down is termed *downbeating nystagmus*).
  - Patients with equal amplitude and frequency in both directions are termed *pendular nystagmus.*
- Differential diagnosis
  - The differential diagnosis of nystagmus depends upon the topographical localization of the findings. Illicit and prescribed drugs (eg, sedatives, antiseizure medications) and exposure to toxins may produce nystagmus and should be considered in every patient. Infectious, inflammatory, ischemic (eg, stroke), demyelinating, toxic, nutritional, and neoplastic etiologies can affect the brainstem, cerebellum, or their connections.
- Evaluation
  - Patients not taking any medications or not exposed to any toxins that can produce nystagmus should probably undergo neuroimaging with attention to the topographical localization of the clinical findings (eg, MRI with contrast).
- Management
  - Some patients with nystagmus have a null point where the nystagmus amplitude and/or frequency are less. Prism therapy or surgical treatment might be able to move the null point into the primary position or relieve an anomalous head position.
  - Botulinum toxin has been used with anecdotal success in selected cases of nystagmus, but obviously the patient will be trading oscillopsia for ophthalmoplegia.
  - Medical therapy has had variable success. Baclofen has been useful in periodic alternating nystagmus. Gabapentin, carbamazepine, scopolamine, valproate, memantine, isoniazid, 4-aminopyridine, clonazepam, and other medications have been used with variable anecdotal success for different forms of nystagmus.
- Prognosis
  - Treatment of the underlying etiology for the nystagmus might resolve the symptoms.

TABLE 11-4. LOCALIZING FORMS OF NYSTAGMUS

Upbeat	Cerebellar vermis or brainstem
Downbeat	Cervicomedullary junction
Rebound	Cerebellum
Periodic alternating nystagmus	Cerebellum
Convergence retraction nystagmus	Dorsal midbrain
See-saw	Parasellar, third ventricular region

TABLE 11-5. FEATURES OF CONGENITAL NYSTAGMUS

Convergence typically dampens the nystagmus, and near vision might be better than distance vision
Oscillopsia is absent
Null point and anomalous head position may be present
Uniplanar movement (stays horizontal in up, down, and horizontal gazes)
May have a latent component

Optic Neuritis

- Definition
    - Optic neuritis is defined as demyelinating or idiopathic inflammation of the optic nerve.
    - Other forms of infectious, inflammatory, or infiltrative optic neuropathy should probably be referred to according to the underlying etiology in order to avoid confusion and miscommunication with other specialists.
- Etiology
    - Multiple sclerosis (demyelinating disease) is the most common association with optic neuritis.
    - Although other etiologies (eg, infectious, inflammatory, and infiltrative disorders) can produce an optic neuropathy, optic neuritis is typically demyelinating or idiopathic.
- Symptoms
    - Patients with optic neuritis are typically young adults (often female) who complain of acute, unilateral loss of vision.
    - There is usually pain with eye movement (90%).
    - There may be a prior history of loss of vision (prior attacks of optic neuritis) or previous or current neurologic deficit (eg, double vision, weakness, numbness, or tingling, or loss of bowel or bladder control).
- Signs
    - The typical clinical features of optic neuritis are acute unilateral loss of visual acuity and visual field (any optic nerve-related field loss but often central loss).
    - An ipsilateral RAPD
    - Dyschromatopsia (often out of proportion to visual acuity loss)
    - A normal (Figure 11-14) optic nerve appearance (most cases are retrobulbar optic neuritis)
    - In some cases, the optic nerve is swollen (ie, papillitis), but in general demyelinating optic neuritis produces only mild hyperemia.
    - The presence of severe optic disc edema, significant hemorrhage, exudate, cotton wool patches, or retinitis or neurosensory detachment suggests alternative etiologies for the optic neuropathy.

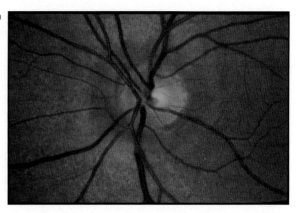

Figure 11-14. Fundus photograph shows normal optic nerve in retrobulbar optic neuritis.

- o The motility, slit-lamp biomicroscopy, and IOP exams are typically normal.
- o Anterior or posterior segment inflammation is uncommon in demyelinating disease and suggests an underlying inflammatory etiology for the optic neuropathy (eg, sarcoid).
- Differential diagnosis
  - o The differential for an acute optic neuropathy includes ischemic, inflammatory, infiltrative, infectious, traumatic, hereditary, and demyelinating disease.
  - o In the Optic Neuritis Treatment Trial (ONTT), laboratory studies and a chest radiograph were performed to evaluate young patients with an acute unilateral optic neuropathy for systemic lupus erythematosus, sarcoid, syphilis, and other etiologies. Although a few patients had positive laboratory testing, none proved to have an underlying infectious or inflammatory disorder causing typical optic neuritis, and the recommendation of the ONTT is that laboratory testing is not necessary for typical cases.
  - o Patients with an atypical presentation, however (see Table 11-6), should be queried about infectious (eg, Lyme, tuberculosis, cat scratch disease, syphilis), inflammatory (eg, sarcoid, autoimmune optic neuropathy, systemic lupus erythematosus), infiltrative (eg, leukemia), or hereditary (eg, Leber's hereditary optic neuropathy) risk factors.
- Evaluation
  - o In the ONTT, typical cases of optic neuritis did not benefit from additional laboratory testing. In patients with atypical presentations, selected and directed laboratory testing may be applicable.
  - o In patients with inflammatory symptoms, signs, or suggestive history, testing for systemic lupus erythematosus (eg, antinuclear antibody), sarcoid (eg, chest imaging, angiotensin converting enzyme), syphilis (eg, serology), tuberculosis (eg, chest imaging, skin testing), Lyme disease (eg, serology for endemic areas), or cat scratch fever (eg, serology) may be indicated.
  - o Lumbar puncture in the ONTT was optional but only showed changes compatible with demyelinating disease in those who had abnormalities.
  - o Cranial MRI was a powerful predictor of demyelinating disease in the ONTT.
  - o Our current imaging recommendation for acute unilateral optic neuropathy is a contrast, fat-suppressed MRI of the brain and orbits (Figure 11-15). In the ONTT, although there were a few compressive lesions detected, the major reason for imaging a typical optic neuritis is to evaluate for demyelinating disease and not to exclude other etiologies. Patients with typical optic neuritis and demyelinating white matter lesions have a significant chance for developing multiple sclerosis (50%) over 5 years. On the other hand, patients with a normal MRI at the time of the optic neuritis have a much lower, but not zero, risk of multiple sclerosis (16%).
- Management
  - o In the ONTT, there were 3 treatment arms: intravenous (IV) steroids followed by an oral taper, oral steroids, or oral placebo.
  - o All 3 treatment groups recovered visual function equally, but IV treatment sped the rate of visual recovery.

TABLE 11-6. TYPICAL AND ATYPICAL FEATURES OF DEMYELINATING OPTIC NEURITIS

	Typical Optic Neuritis	*Atypical Optic Neuritis*
Age	Young patient	Any age, but consider ischemic optic neuropathy in older patient and postviral optic neuritis in children
Gender	Often female	Either gender
Pain with eye movement	Usually present	Beware of severe pain out of proportion to optic neuritis or painless onset
Laterality	Typically unilateral	Consider systemic infectious, inflammatory, or infiltrative etiologies in bilateral and simultaneous cases
RAPD	Present ipsilaterally in unilateral (common) or bilateral but asymmetric cases (uncommon)	Consider alternative etiologies for the unilateral vision loss in the absence of a RAPD (eg, retinal disease, media or refractive, or nonorganic)
Slit-lamp biomicroscopy	Typically no anterior or posterior uveitis	Consider inflammatory etiologies (eg, sarcoid) in the setting of anterior or posterior uveitis
Optic disc appearance	Typically normal optic nerve appearance (retrobulbar) but mild hyperemia in some cases (papillitis)	Consider alternative etiologies in severe optic disc edema, significant hemorrhage, exudate (neuroretinitis), cotton wool patches, or neurosensory retinal detachment
Course	Usually recovers to normal or near normal vision	Lack of recovery suggests an alternative etiology (eg, ischemic, inflammatory)
Treatment response	Intravenous steroid therapy speeds rate of recovery but does not change final visual outcome	Steroid responsiveness or steroid dependency suggests inflammatory (eg, sarcoid, autoimmune optic neuropathy) or rarely infiltrative/neoplastic (eg, lymphoma) etiology

- o Interestingly, oral steroids alone not only did not improve final visual outcome but increased the rate of new attacks. The ONTT concluded that oral steroids in conventional doses should not be prescribed for typical optic neuritis.
- o Additional studies since the ONTT have shown that patients with monophasic neurologic events and MRI studies consistent with demyelination might benefit from immunomodulatory therapy. In one of these studies, the Controlled High Risk Avonex Multiple Sclerosis Prevention Study (CHAMPS) treatment with interferon beta-1a (Avonex) reduced the rate of clinically definite MS after 3 years compared with placebo. Treatment also improved the demyelinating white matter lesions on MRI over time.
- o Other studies have confirmed the utility of other immunomodulatory therapies in monophasic neurologic events including optic neuritis.
- Prognosis
  - o In the ONTT, the majority of patients recovered visual acuity better than 20/40.
  - o The MRI is the most powerful predictor of MS and probably should be considered for prognostic purposes in every patient with optic neuritis.

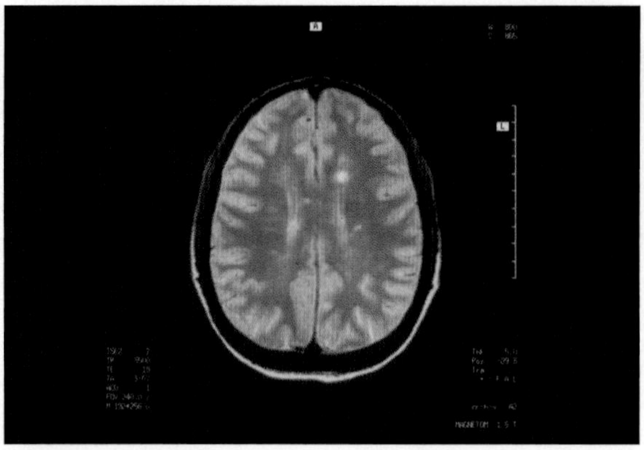

Figure 11-15. Cranial T2-weighted MRI shows multifocal periventricular white matter lesions consistent with demyelinating disease.

Nonarteritic Anterior Ischemic Optic Neuropathy

- Definition
  - Nonarteritic anterior ischemic optic neuropathy (NAION) is an ischemic lesion of the optic nerve head producing visual loss, a RAPD, and optic disc edema in the acute setting.
- Etiology
  - The precise cause of NAION is unknown but several theories have implicated small vessel ischemia, hypotension, and vasculopathic risk factors such as anemia, hypotension, hypertension, diabetes mellitus, hypercholesterolemia, smoking, and atherosclerotic small vessel disease.
  - In addition, obstructive sleep apnea, hyperhomocysteinemia, and other exogenous agents (eg, sildenafil, amiodarone) have also been implicated in the pathogenesis of NAION, but none have proven to be causal, and NAION is likely to be multifactorial. Most patients are older (older than 50 years), but NAION may occur in young patients.
  - Other vascular risk factors may also be contributory including migraine, collagen vascular disease, and vasculitis.
- Symptoms
  - Typically present with acute, unilateral painless, visual loss
  - Patients often notice the visual loss upon awakening.
  - No other neurologic signs or symptoms are typically present.
  - As opposed to arteritic anterior ischemic optic neuropathy (A-AION), NAION is not preceded by transient visual loss (ie, amaurosis fugax).
- Signs
  - There may be a variable loss of visual acuity and/or visual field (often central, arcuate, or altitudinal loss).
  - Decreased color vision may also occur.
  - Most cases are unilateral, but bilateral sequential disease may occur in up to 12% to 14% of cases.
  - Bilateral and simultaneous onset of NAION is atypical, and consideration for alternative etiologies is recommended.
  - A RAPD will be present in unilateral or in bilateral but asymmetric optic neuropathies.
  - In the acute setting, the optic disc will be swollen in a sector or diffuse fashion. The "anterior" in AION requires the presence of optic disc edema at onset (Figure 11-16).
  - Although ischemic optic neuropathy can occur without optic disc edema (ie, posterior ischemic optic neuropathy), alternative etiologies (eg, GCA) should be considered in the acute retrobulbar optic neuropathy.
  - There may be surrounding peripapillary hemorrhages and rarely exudate.
  - Optic atrophy develops after the disc edema phase resolves.
  - There are no other associated neurologic or systemic signs or symptoms.

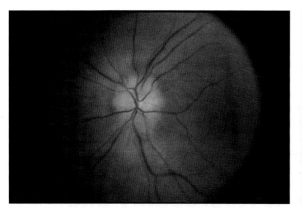

Figure 11-16. Optic disc edema due to NAION.

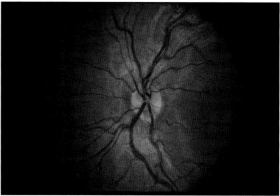

Figure 11-17. Small, crowded, "cupless" disc (the "disc at risk") in the fellow eye of a patient with NAION.

- o A small and crowded optic nerve (ie, "disc at risk") is a presumed predisposing risk factor for NAION and should be searched for in the fellow eye (Figure 11-17). The lack of the "disc at risk" should prompt consideration for alternative etiologies of the optic neuropathy including A-AION.
- Differential diagnosis
  - o The differential diagnosis of optic disc edema is extensive and includes ischemic, inflammatory, infiltrative, demyelinating, toxic, and hereditary optic neuropathies and papilledema.
  - o In most cases, the acute onset of unilateral optic disc edema with visual loss in a vasculopathic patient can be diagnosed clinically as anterior ischemic optic neuropathy.
  - o The presence of anterior or posterior segment inflammation (eg, iritis, vitreitis, retinitis) excludes the diagnosis of NAION.
  - o The major diagnostic consideration in AION is distinguishing arteritic from NAION.
- Evaluation
  - o The diagnosis of NAION is a clinical one, and there is no diagnostic laboratory testing.
  - o Neuroimaging is not necessary for typical NAION. Patients without documented optic disc edema at onset, atypical presentation, or progressive visual loss should be considered for neuroimaging to exclude alternative etiologies (eg, optic nerve sheath meningioma or other compressive lesion).
  - o An ESR and/or C-reactive protein might be useful for patients suspected of having GCA (ie, A-AION). The clinical features that might suggest A-AION include bilateral and simultaneous or rapidly sequential optic disc edema, severe visual acuity loss (eg, light perception or no light perception), pallid edema, or simultaneous retinal (eg, cilioretinal artery occlusion, cotton wool patches) or choroidal circulation ischemia with AION.
  - o Patients with atypical features (eg, anterior or posterior uveitis, bilateral optic disc edema) should undergo appropriate evaluation for alternative etiologies of optic disc edema.
  - o NAION is presumed to be small vessel ischemic disease and is rarely embolic in origin. Therefore, carotid Doppler studies and cardiac echocardiography are not indicated in typical NAION. Evaluation for and treatment of any underlying vasculopathic risk factors, however, is reasonable.
- Management
  - o Although there have been several proposed treatments (eg, corticosteroids, levodopa) for NAION, none have proven effective.
  - o Surgical decompression of the optic nerve was shown in a clinical trial (ie, the Ischemic Optic Neuropathy Decompression Trial) to be ineffective and probably harmful for NAION.
  - o Patients with NAION should be evaluated and treated for any underlying vasculopathic risk factors.
  - o Precipitants of nocturnal hypotension (eg, overaggressive treatment of hypertension, nocturnal use of agents causing hypotension such as antihypertensives, alcohol, or sleeping aids) might be avoided but is unproven.

o Aspirin use has not been proven to prevent contralateral involvement but might be helpful in patients who have other underlying vasculopathic risk factors.

- Prognosis
  - o Most patients with NAION experience acute loss of vision that remains static over time.
  - o A small percentage of patients may have progression in the first few weeks, and a significant minority of patients may improve a few lines.
  - o Patients with NAION should be re-evaluated to ensure that the optic disc edema resolves.
  - o Most cases develop optic atrophy once the disc swelling resolves.
  - o A neuroimaging study (ie, MRI of the head and orbit with gadolinium and fat suppression) should be considered in patients with progressive visual loss or persistent optic disc edema.

Arteritic Ischemic Optic Neuropathy and Giant Cell Arteritis

- Definition
  - o A-AION is an ischemic lesion of the optic nerve due to GCA that presents with optic disc edema.
  - o However, arteritic ischemic optic neuropathy might also present without disc edema (posterior ischemic optic neuropathy).
- Etiology
  - o GCA is a small- to medium-sized vessel vasculitis with a predilection for the ocular circulation.
  - o The cause of A-AION is believed to be vasculitis and secondary occlusion of the posterior ciliary circulation with ischemic infarction of the optic nerve.
- Symptoms
  - o Acute visual loss in the involved eye(s) of an elderly patient
  - o The visual loss may be unilateral or bilateral, and if bilateral might be simultaneous or rapidly sequential.
  - o As opposed to NAION, which is typically unilateral, bilateral simultaneous ischemic optic neuropathy (ION) should be considered to be GCA until proven otherwise.
  - o In arteritic ION, there may be a variable loss of visual acuity and/or visual field, but more severe loss (eg, no light perception or light perception vision) is a "red flag" for arteritic ION.
  - o Patients with GCA may have associated constitutional symptoms including headache, neck or ear pain, scalp tenderness, pain in the jaw while chewing (ie, jaw claudication), polymyalgia rheumatica, fever, weight loss, and malaise.
  - o Involvement of other vessels is uncommon but has been reported in GCA (eg, cranial arteritis, aortitis, and other branches of the aorta).
- Signs
  - o Visual acuity and/or visual field loss
  - o An RAPD will be present in unilateral or in bilateral but asymmetric cases.
  - o In the acute setting, the optic disc may be swollen in a sector or diffuse fashion.
  - o Pallid edema (ie, pale and swollen optic nerve), retrobulbar optic neuropathy (posterior ischemic optic neuropathy), and simultaneous involvement of multiple ocular circulations (eg, AION and choroidal or retinal circulation ischemia) are suggestive of GCA.
  - o Although most visual loss in GCA is due to AION, nonembolic central retinal artery occlusion can also be a presenting sign (Figure 11-18).
  - o Another "red flag" for GCA in patients with AION is the absence of the structural "disc at risk" in the fellow eye. Patients with AION and a large rather than small cup in the fellow eye should be considered for GCA (Figure 11-19).
  - o Fluorescein angiography might demonstrate the choroidal perfusion deficit in GCA (Figure 11-20).
  - o Optic atrophy develops over time in the affected eye(s).
  - o There may be temporal artery or scalp tenderness or nodularity.
- Differential diagnosis
  - o The differential diagnosis of an acute optic neuropathy is extensive and includes ischemic, inflammatory, infiltrative, demyelinating, toxic, and hereditary optic neuropathies and papilledema. In most cases, the acute onset of unilateral optic disc edema with visual loss in a vasculopathic patient can be diagnosed clinically as AION

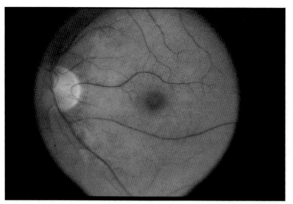

Figure 11-18. Nonembolic central retinal artery occlusion with "cherry red spot" in macula.

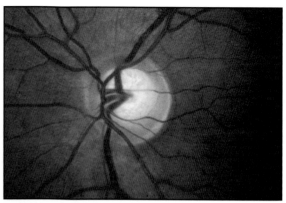

Figure 11-19. Large cup-to-disc ratio (not the "disc at risk" as seen in NAION) in the fellow eye of a patient with GCA.

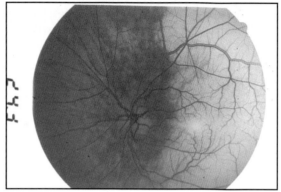

Figure 11-20. Choroidal perfusion deficit seen on fluorescein angiography.

- ○ The presence of anterior or posterior segment inflammation (eg, iritis, vitreitis, retinitis) generally suggests an inflammatory optic neuropathy but rarely may occur in GCA.
- ○ The major diagnostic consideration in anterior ischemic optic neuropathy is distinguishing arteritic from NAION. An elderly patient with visual loss should be considered to have GCA until proven otherwise.
- Evaluation
  - ○ The diagnosis of A-AION is a clinical one, supported by laboratory testing and confirmed by temporal artery biopsy (TAB).
  - ○ A stat serum ESR and/or C-reactive protein should be performed in every case of suspected GCA.
  - ○ A TAB should be performed as soon as possible (ie, within a few weeks of clinical diagnosis).
    - ■ If the clinical suspicion of GCA is low (eg, NAION in a vasculopathic patient with a borderline ESR) then a unilateral TAB might be sufficient to exclude the diagnosis of GCA.
    - ■ On the other hand, in a patient with high clinical suspicion of GCA (eg, elderly patient with pallid edema, no light perception vision, headache, jaw claudication, and scalp tenderness), a normal ESR or CRP or even a negative unilateral TAB may not be sufficient to exclude the diagnosis of GCA. Multiple studies have shown that the concordance rate for a unilateral versus bilateral TAB is about 96%. A bilateral sequential or simultaneous TAB may be performed depending upon the individual clinician's preferences. A TAB is useful for pathologic confirmation of the diagnosis, in order to deter the inappropriate or too rapid tapering of corticosteroid therapy and to provide justification for continued therapy when steroid side effects develop. The pathologic diagnosis does not require giant cells to be present in the TAB specimen, and some patients (especially those who have biopsies performed after steroid therapy has been initiated) have evidence for "healed arteritis" without active inflammatory infiltrate.

o Neuroimaging is not necessary for typical GCA but patients with a negative TAB but persistent clinical findings (eg, headache, optic neuropathy) may benefit from cranial and orbital imaging to exclude alternative etiologies.

o Patients with retrobulbar optic neuropathy (ie, posterior ischemic optic neuropathy) should also be considered for neuroimaging.

o The pretest likelihood of disease determined by clinical suspicion and the laboratory testing (eg, ESR, CRP) should drive the decision making for further management.

- Management
  o Corticosteroids should be initiated immediately in every case of suspected GCA.
  o Although no prospective controlled evidence exists, some authors recommend IV over oral steroids for GCA especially for those who are monocular, who have visual loss, or who have premonitory transient visual loss.
  o Most patients require long-term (months to years) steroid therapy. Tapering of treatment should be dictated by the activity of symptoms and the laboratory testing (eg, ESR, CRP).
  o Many elderly patients develop significant side effects on corticosteroids. Close follow up with an internist or rheumatologist is advisable for patients on long-term steroid treatment including calcium and vitamin D supplementation, monitoring for osteoporosis, blood pressure, and blood sugar.
  o Methotrexate and other immunosuppressives have been used as steroid-sparing agents in patients who are intolerant of corticosteroid therapy, but the evidence for their efficacy is conflicting.
- Prognosis
  o The goal of corticosteroid therapy is to prevent visual loss in the unaffected eye(s).
  o Improvement is unlikely once visual loss occurs, but patients on adequate steroid therapy do not often lose vision in an unaffected eye or progress after the first week in the affected eye.
  o Although corticosteroids do not cure GCA, many patients achieve a remission with adequate long-term therapy.
  o Although the visual manifestations of GCA are the most feared, aortic, intracranial, and other vessel involvement can be life-threatening.

Papilledema/Increased Intracranial Pressure

- Definition
  o *Papilledema* is a term that should be reserved for optic disc edema due to increased intracranial pressure.
  o All other forms of optic disc edema should be referred to as simply *optic disc edema* if the cause is unknown or by etiologic classification if the cause is known (eg, optic neuritis, anterior ischemic optic neuropathy).
  o It is important to use the term *papilledema* specifically in order to provide accurate documentation in the medical record and to avoid miscommunication with other specialists (eg, neurology, neurosurgery).
  o Papilledema should be considered an ophthalmic emergency that requires evaluation.
- Etiology
  o Any cause of increased intracranial pressure can produce papilledema including the following:
    ▪ Intracranial mass lesions (eg, mass effect, obstructive hydrocephalus)
    ▪ Overproduction of cerebrospinal fluid (CSF) (eg, choroid plexus papilloma)
    ▪ Underabsorption of CSF (eg, meningitis, subarachnoid hemorrhage)
    ▪ Decreased venous outflow (eg, cerebral venous sinus thrombosis, jugular venous obstruction, or cardiac overload)
    ▪ Idiopathic intracranial hypertension (IIH) (ie, pseudotumor cerebri)
- Symptoms
  o Headache
  o Pulse-synchronous tinnitus
  o Diplopia (due to nonlocalizing sixth nerve palsy)
  o Nausea/vomiting
  o Transient visual obscurations lasting seconds at a time (due to papilledema)

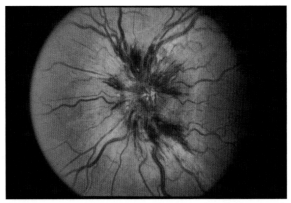

Figure 11-21. Fundus photograph shows papilledema with peripapillary.

- ○ Blurred vision (due to papilledema or macular fluid, exudate, or hemorrhage)
- Signs
  - ○ The optic disc edema in papilledema is typically bilateral but markedly asymmetric, or rarely frankly unilateral cases may occur (Figure 11-21).
  - ○ Patients with papilledema typically have normal visual acuity but can have visual field loss (ie, enlarged blind spots, nasal step, arcuate defects, or other glaucomatous-like field loss).
  - ○ Visual acuity loss can occur, however, in chronic or severe papilledema or due to macular hemorrhage, exudate, fluid, or subretinal neovascular membrane formation.
  - ○ Although optic disc edema with a macular star figure of exudate may be due to infectious neuroretinitis (eg, cat scratch neuroretinitis), a bilateral presentation (especially in the absence of compelling history or anterior or posterior uveitis) should prompt evaluation for papilledema.
  - ○ The sixth nerve palsy is a nonlocalizing finding of increased intracranial pressure and is presumably due to stretching along the course of the sixth nerve within the subarachnoid space.
  - ○ An RAPD may occur in patients with either unilateral or bilateral but asymmetric visual loss.
  - ○ Patients may have other localizing neurological findings as the result of the underlying process producing the increased intracranial pressure (eg, mass effect, meningeal signs).
  - ○ There should not be any signs of anterior or posterior inflammation (eg, uveitis) in routine papilledema unless the cause is inflammatory (eg, sarcoid).
- Differential diagnosis
  - ○ Optic disc edema can be due to infectious, infiltrative, demyelinating (ie, optic neuritis), ischemic (ie, AION), toxic, or hereditary optic neuropathies (eg, Leber's hereditary optic neuropathy).
  - ○ Malignant hypertension-related optic neuropathy can mimic papilledema, and the blood pressure should probably be measured in all patients with bilateral optic disc edema.
  - ○ Papilledema can usually be differentiated clinically from other causes of optic disc edema by the bilateral and simultaneous onset and the relative preservation of central acuity (see Table 11-7)
- Evaluation
  - ○ Patients with papilledema should undergo a semiemergent neuroimaging study, preferably a contrast cranial MR scan.
  - ○ MR venography should also be considered to rule out cerebral venous sinus thrombosis.
  - ○ Patients presenting in the emergency room setting may be screened with a computed tomography (CT) scan but may still require a follow-up MR scan
  - ○ If the imaging study is negative for an intracranial mass lesion or other etiology for the increased intracranial pressure, then a lumbar puncture should be performed to measure the opening pressure and to rule out meningeal etiologies for increased intracranial pressure (eg, infectious, inflammatory, or carcinomatous meningitis).
  - ○ If both the neuroimaging study and the lumbar puncture are normal except for an elevated opening pressure, then the diagnosis of IIH is established. Most patients with IIH are young, overweight females, and the diagnosis should be suspect in thin, elderly, or male patients.
  - ○ The blood pressure should be measured in patients with papilledema.

TABLE 11-7. DIFFERENTIATING FEATURES OF OPTIC DISC EDEMA

	PAPILLEDEMA	OPTIC NEURITIS (ON)	ANTERIOR ISCHEMIC OPTIC NEUROPATHY
Age	Any age	Young adults or children	Older aged individuals
Associated features	Other signs or symptoms of increased intracranial pressure	May have history of prior neurologic events in demyelinating disease or systemic symptoms (eg, fever, prodromal illness) if not demyelinating ON	Vasculopathic risk factors (eg, hypertension or diabetes) or arteritic symptoms and signs in A-AION
Laterality	Usually bilateral but may be asymmetric or rarely frankly unilateral	Usually unilateral in demyelinating ON but can be bilateral in children or in systemic (eg, infectious, inflammatory, or infiltrative) causes of ON	Usually unilateral but can be bilateral in temporal arteritis (ie, A-AION) or postsurgical AION (eg, lumbar spine or cardiac surgery)
Visual acuity	Usually preserved until late, unless concomitant macular pathology present	Usually decreased visual acuity	Often decreased visual acuity
Visual field loss	Typically enlarged blind spot with nerve fiber bundle defects	Often central depression or central scotoma but may have any optic nerve-related visual field defect	Often altitudinal or arcuate field loss but may have any optic nerve-related visual field defect
Associated retinal findings	May have dilated vasculature, peripapillary hemorrhages and exudate	Usually only mild hyperemia if optic disc edema is present without secondary vascular changes, hemorrhage, or exudates	May have secondary hemorrhages and uncommonly exudate

- Management
  - Patients with an underlying etiology for the increased intracranial pressure (eg, intracranial tumor or meningitis) should undergo therapy directed at the primary etiology (eg, surgical resection of tumor, steroid therapy, antibiotic therapy for meningitis). Treatment of the underlying etiology typically leads to resolution of the papilledema.
  - Because the spinal fluid reforms rapidly within 24 hours after a spinal tap, it is unlikely that there would be significant persistent treatment effect from serial spinal taps.
  - Patients with IIH should undergo serial eye exams (including formal visual field examinations) until the optic disc edema resolves. Medial treatment of IIH includes acetazolamide (or other diuretics) and weight loss.
  - Patients who fail, are intolerant to, or are noncompliant with medical therapy who have progressive visual loss might benefit from surgical decompression of the optic nerve sheath (ie, sheath fenestration) or a shunting procedure (eg, lumboperitoneal or venticuloperitoneal shunting).
- Prognosis
  - Most patients with papilledema retain good visual acuity and visual field.
  - Some patients may present with an aggressive and rapid visual loss due to papilledema, and in these cases urgent surgical treatment may be necessary.

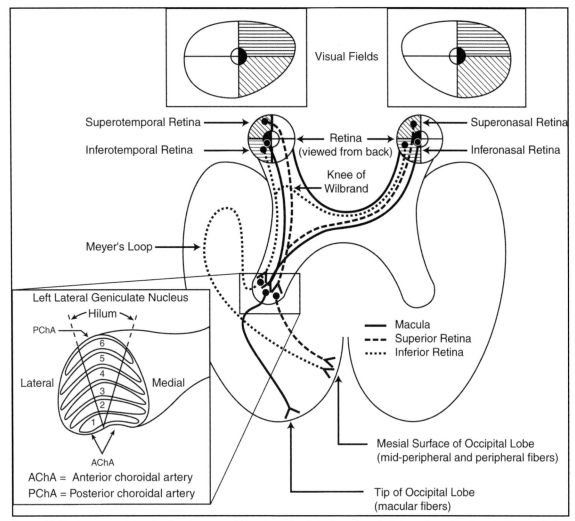

Figure 11-22. Anatomy of the visual pathways and blood supply of the lateral geniculate nucleus. (Reprinted with permission from Kline LB, Bajandas FJ. *Neuro-Ophthalmology.* 5th ed. Thorofare, NJ: SLACK Incorporated; 2004.)

- Loss of central acuity is a late finding in papilledema but can occur due to superimposed macular disease (subretinal fluid, macular exudates, or hemorrhage) or AION.
- Most patients with IIH respond to medical treatment, but some patients have persistent or recurrent visual loss.

Visual Field Defects

- Definition/anatomy
  - The visual fibers begin in the retina and travel in the ipsilateral optic nerve. At the junction of the optic nerve and optic chiasm, the nasal fibers cross, and the temporal fibers remain uncrossed.
  - After the chiasm, crossed nasal fibers and uncrossed temporal fibers form the optic tract.
  - The fibers then travel to the lateral geniculate body (LGB) and continue as the optic radiations in the temporal (Meyer's loop) and parietal lobe
  - The radiations terminate in the occipital cortex (Figure 11-22). The anterior portion of the calcarine cortex is subserved by monocular temporal crescent of vision in the contralateral eye.
  - Lesions affecting each of the parts of the visual pathway produce specific and localizing visual field loss. The normal visual field is 50 degrees nasally, 60 degrees superiorly, 70 degrees inferiorly, and 80 to 90 degrees temporally.

- o Monocular visual field defects are due to lesions of the ipsilateral retina or optic nerve. The one exception is the monocular temporal crescent, which results from occipital cortex involvement. Binocular visual field defects may be due to bilateral retinal or optic nerve disease or if bitemporal may be chiasmal or if homonymous may be retrochiasmal lesions.
- Evaluation
  - o There are a number of methods for testing the visual field.
    - ▪ One easy method at the bedside or in the clinic is the confrontation visual field testing. The examiner uses his or her own hand or fingers presented in 4 quadrants. The examiner's own visual field serves as the control. Colored test objects (eg, red) may enhance the sensitivity of the testing. Confrontation testing is a reasonable routine peripherally screening test for new patients. Testing of the central field can also be performed quickly using the examiner's face as the central test object (eg, "Looking at my face, are any parts missing?").
    - ▪ One useful test of the central 10 to 20 degrees is the Amsler grid. The grid is held at 30 cm by the patient, and the test is especially helpful in macular disease or small central or paracentral scotomas. The patient can draw directly on the grid the size, shape, and density of the scotoma and outline the presence and location of any metamorphopsia.
    - ▪ The tangent screen tests the central 20 to 40 degrees. This test is particularly helpful in patients who are unable to be tested by formal perimetry (eg, Goldmann, automated). Testing is typically performed at various distances (eg, 1 and 2 meters) using test objects of various colors (eg, white or red) and sizes on a black-tipped wand against a black felt background. The tangent screen is a good test for detecting nonorganic "tunnel" fields. Nonorganic tunnel visual fields fail to expand appropriately with doubling of the test distance and test object size.
    - ▪ The Goldmann perimeter can be used for static or kinetic testing of the visual field. The advantages of the Goldmann technique include its utility in patients with unreliable computerized static testing; its helpfulness for patients with very poor visual acuity (<20/200); its ability to detect peripheral islands of intact visual field outside the central visual field (eg, residual temporal island); testing for visual field defects in the extreme periphery (eg, monocular temporal crescent); and its value in the evaluation of the shape of visual field defects (eg, homonymous or bitemporal hemianopsias). The disadvantages of the technique include that the quality of results are highly technician dependent; the results are not as reliably reproducible as computerized perimetry; the test is time intensive; and Goldmann perimetry is not universally available.
    - ▪ Automated computerized perimetry has several advantages including standardized data with a reproducible method of documenting, quantifying, and following visual field defects. The disadvantages include that it requires a cooperative and alert patient; it may be difficult for very young or very old patients; it requires good central and steady vision; it is subject to artifacts (overly sensitive); and it is subject to some intratest and intertest variability.
- Signs/symptoms
  - o Specific visual field defects are topographically localizing.
    - ▪ Arcuate or nerve fiber bundle defects (eg, scotoma extends to blind spot) are usually due to lesions of the ipsilateral optic nerve or retina.
      - □ The nerve fiber bundle visual field defect may be monocular or binocular (depending on bilateral or unilateral disease process) (Figure 11-23)
      - □ The temporal nerve fibers traverse an arcuate course around the fovea to the optic nerve, and thus lesions in this area create arcuate-shaped field loss that inserts into the blind spot (representing the optic nerve).
      - □ The nasal fibers traverse a straight line to the optic nerve nasally.
      - □ Glaucoma is the most common cause of nerve fiber layer defects, but other optic neuropathies (eg, optic disc drusen, papilledema) and retinal disease of any type may produce similar visual field loss.
      - □ The visual field defects should correlate with the ophthalmoscopically visible pathologic changes in the retina or optic disc (eg, glaucomatous cupping or atrophy, nerve fiber layer loss).

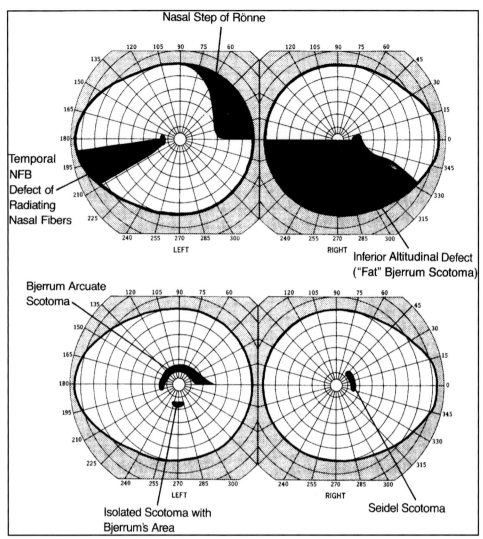

Figure 11-23. Composite diagram depicting different optic nerve-type field defects. (Reprinted with permission from Kline LB, Bajandas FJ. *Neuro-Ophthalmology.* 5th ed. Thorofare, NJ: SLACK Incorporated; 2004.)

- Involvement of the nerve fibers from the macula (ie, the papillomacular bundle) may be due to any optic neuropathy (eg, optic neuritis) or macular disease (eg, macular hole).
  - The central scotoma may be unilateral or bilateral (depending on laterality of the process).
  - A related scotoma, the cecocentral scotoma or Siedel scotoma (see Figure 11-23), is a central scotoma extending to the blind spot.
  - Bilateral central or cecocentral scotomas suggest toxic/nutritional or hereditary optic neuropathy, but other optic neuropathies or maculopathies may also cause similar field loss.
  - Likewise, either macular disease or an optic neuropathy can produce a central scotoma from papillomacular bundle involvement.
- An arcuate defect that progresses and becomes more confluent may produce an altitudinal defect that respects the horizontal midline (see Figure 11-23).
  - The altitudinal loss may be superior or inferior, unilateral or bilateral, and may occur after any optic neuropathy or retinal disease (eg, artery occlusion).

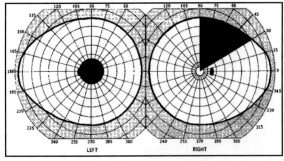

Figure 11-24. Junctional scotoma: A central scotoma in one eye with a superior-temporal defect in the fellow eye; indicates a lesion at the junction of the optic nerve (left eye in this case) and the chiasm. (Reprinted with permission from Kline LB, Bajandas FJ. *Neuro-Ophthalmology.* 5th ed. Thorofare, NJ: SLACK Incorporated; 2004.)

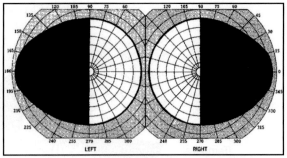

Figure 11-25. Bitemporal hemianopia due to interruption of decussating nasal fibers in the chiasm. (Reprinted with permission from Kline LB, Bajandas FJ. *Neuro-Ophthalmology.* 5th ed. Thorofare, NJ: SLACK Incorporated; 2004.)

Figure 11-26. A chiasmatic lesion may affect only the decussating nasal-macular fibers, resulting in a central bitemporal hemianopia. Therefore, a complete visual field evaluation of a patient suspected of a chiasmatic lesion must include a search of the central field. (Reprinted with permission from Kline LB, Bajandas FJ. *Neuro-Ophthalmology.* 5th ed. Thorofare, NJ: SLACK Incorporated; 2004.)

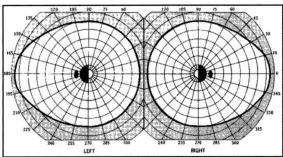

- □ Altitudinal defects are common after ION, perhaps due to preferential involvement of the blood supply to the upper or lower pole of the optic nerve, but altitudinal visual field defect is not pathognomonic for ION.
- □ Bilateral and adjacent homonymous quadrantanopsias (inferior or superior) can mimic altitudinal loss.
- Historically, inferonasal fibers crossing in the anterior chiasm loop were postulated to travel for a short course into the medial portion of the opposite optic nerve (the so called "Wilbrand's knee").
  - □ Clinically, a lesion at the junction of the optic nerve and chiasm may cause an ipsilateral optic neuropathy with a central scotoma and a contralateral superior temporal defect (the junctional scotoma) (Figure 11-24)
  - □ The Wilbrand's knee may be an artifact of enucleation, however, rather than a distinct anatomic entity; nevertheless, the clinical localizing value of the junctional scotoma (ipsilateral optic neuropathy with contralateral superotemporal field loss) remains valid.
  - □ A monocular hemianopia, also referred to as hemianopsia, (nasal or temporal unilateral hemianopic field loss) may occur at junction and is referred to as junctional scotoma of Traquair (differs from superotemporal junctional scotoma).
  - □ In either case of junctional visual loss (junctional scotoma or junctional scotoma of Traquair), the clinician should suspect a compressive lesion at the junction of the optic nerve and chiasm.
- A bitemporal hemianopia (Figure 11-25) respects the vertical midline and produces temporal field loss bilaterally.
  - □ The bitemporal loss may be paracentral (Figure 11-26) or peripheral and indicates a lesion at the level of the optic chiasm until proven otherwise.
  - □ Neuroimaging is generally required for any unexplained bitemporal hemianopic visual loss.

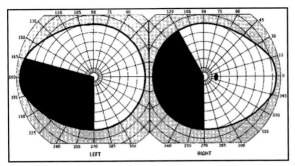

Figure 11-27. Incongruous left homonymous hemianopia due to a right optic tract lesion. (Reprinted with permission from Kline LB, Bajandas FJ. *Neuro-Ophthalmology*. 5th ed. Thorofare, NJ: SLACK Incorporated; 2004.)

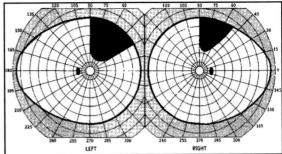

Figure 11-28. Anterior temporal lobe lesion of Meyer's loop produces incongruous, midperipheral and peripheral-contralateral, homonymous, superior ("pie in the sky") quadrantanopia. This is an example of a patient with a left temporal lobe lesion. (Reprinted with permission from Kline LB, Bajandas FJ. *Neuro-Ophthalmology*. 5th ed. Thorofare, NJ: SLACK Incorporated; 2004.)

- □ Patients may have a concomitant optic neuropathy in one or both eyes.
- □ Drift across the vertical meridian may occur, and any bitemporal "flavor" to the visual field loss should be considered seriously.
- ■ Homonymous hemianopsias are due to retrochiasmal lesions on the contralateral side to hemianopic field loss.
  - □ The homonymous hemianopia may be complete or incomplete (Figure 11-27).
  - □ A complete homonymous hemianopia is lateralizing to the contralateral side, but is otherwise nonlocalizing (the lesion could exist anywhere within the retrochiasmal pathway).
  - □ The more congruous (or similar in appearance) the defect, the more posterior (eg, occipital) in the retrochiasmal pathway is the lesion location, and conversely the more incongruous the lesion, the more anterior (eg, optic tract) the lesion is in the retrochiasmal pathway. The term *congruity*, however, should not be used in a complete homonymous hemianopsia.
  - □ The clinician should look for specific clinical signs to help localize homonymous defects.
    - • In optic tract lesions, for example, there may be a contralateral RAPD and a specific form of optic atrophy (band atrophy) due to the involvement of nasal fibers (temporal field) in the contralateral eye. The optic tract lesion generally produces an incongruous homonymous hemianopsia.
    - • LGB lesions may produce an incongruous wedge defect ("spears to fixation") due to the unusual blood supply to the LGB. For example, involvement of the lateral choroidal branch may spare this horizontal strip of field, whereas involvement of the anterior choroidal branch of the internal carotid artery may involve only a horizontal wedge of visual field.
  - □ Temporal lobe lesions produce a contralateral homonymous hemianopia that is typically denser superiorly (Meyer's loop).
    - • The homonymous hemianopia resembles a "pie in the sky" visual field defect and is often incongruous (Figure 11-28).
  - □ Parietal lobe lesions on the other hand produce homonymous hemianopic defects that are denser inferiorly resembling a "pie on the floor" (Figure 11-29).
  - □ Lesions in the parietal or temporal lobe tend to produce other associated neurological signs and symptoms (eg, hemiplegia, hemisensory loss, visual or other neglect).
  - □ Occipital lobe lesions produce homonymous hemianopsias that may occur in isolation without other neurological deficit.

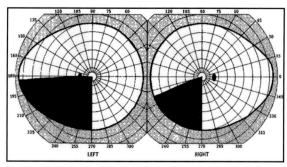

Figure 11-29. Parietal lobe lesions tend to affect the inferior, contralateral visual field quadrants first. This is an example of a patient with a right parietal lobe lesion. (Reprinted with permission from Kline LB, Bajandas FJ. *Neuro-Ophthalmology*. 5th ed. Thorofare, NJ: SLACK Incorporated; 2004.)

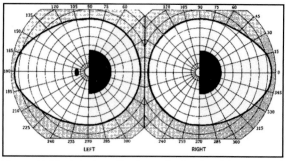

Figure 11-30. A lesion affecting only the tip of the occipital lobe produces a defect of only the central homonymous hemifields. This is an example of a patient with a left occipital tip lesion. (Reprinted with permission from Kline LB, Bajandas FJ. *Neuro-Ophthalmology*. 5th ed. Thorofare, NJ: SLACK Incorporated; 2004.)

TABLE 11-8. DIFFERENTIAL DIAGNOSIS OF VISUAL FIELD DEFECTS

Optic neuropathy	Glaucoma Demyelinating Ischemic Inflammatory Traumatic Toxic/nutritional Infectious Hereditary
Junctional visual field loss and bitemporal hemianopsia	Pituitary adenoma Craniopharyngioma Meningioma Internal carotid artery aneurysm Demyelinating Traumatic
Homonymous hemianopsia	Ischemic Neoplastic Vascular Demyelinating Traumatic

- The homonymous defects tend to be very congruous (Figure 11-30); may be paracentral or peripheral; may be complete or incomplete; and may demonstrate macular sparing of the central 5 degrees.
- The anterior calcarine cortex of the occipital lobe represents monocular temporal visual field (ie, the monocular temporal crescent). Thus, sparing or involvement of temporal crescent localizes to occipital lobe.
- Differential diagnosis
  - Table 11-8 lists the differential diagnosis of visual field defects.

Suggested Readings

Arnold AC. Ischemic optic neuropathies. *Ophthalmol Clin North Am.* 2001;14:83–98.

Balcer LJ. Anatomic review and topographic diagnosis. *Ophthalmol Clin North Am.* 2001;14:1–21, vii.

Bennett JL, Pelak VS. Palsies of the third, fourth, and sixth cranial nerves. *Ophthalmol Clin North Am.* 2001;14:169–185, ix.

Bremner FD. Pupil assessment in optic nerve disorders. *Eye.* 2004;18:1175–1181.

Corbett JJ. The bedside and office neuro-ophthalmology examination. *Semin Neurol.* 2003;23:63–76.

Donahue SP. Perimetry techniques in neuro-ophthalmology. *Curr Opin Ophthalmol.* 1999;10:420–428.

Gottlob I. Nystagmus. *Curr Opin Ophthalmol.* 1998;9:32–38.

Mathews MK, Sergott RC, Savino PJ. Pseudotumor cerebri. *Curr Opin Ophthalmol.* 2003;14:364–370.

Optic Neuritis Study Group. Long-term brain magnetic resonance imaging changes after optic neuritis in patients without clinically definite multiple sclerosis. *Arch Neurol.* 2004;61:1538–1541.

Su GW, Foroozan R. Update on giant cell arteritis. *Curr Opin Ophthalmol.* 2003;14:332–338.

Questions

1. Which of the following is least likely to be true regarding the RAPD?
    a. The RAPD correlates roughly with the size and density of the visual field defect but is less tightly correlated with visual acuity.
    b. A RAPD can occur in patients with retinal, optic nerve, or optic tract disease.
    c. **There can be a large RAPD from media disease (eg, cataract, corneal disease, refractive error) alone.**
    d. There may not be a RAPD if there is bilateral and symmetric anterior visual pathway involvement (eg, bilateral optic neuropathy).

2. Which of the following regarding an isolated incomplete external dysfunction third nerve palsy with no pupil involvement is true?
    a. Patients with an incomplete external (ie, extraocular) muscle involvement but no pupil involvement (eg, divisional palsy) still require MR scan to rule out a mass lesion and an MRA or CTA to consider aneurysm.
    b. If the MRI and MRA (or CTA) are normal, an aneurysm has been completely excluded.
    c. **Cerebral angiography remains the "gold standard" to exclude cerebral aneurysm.**
    d. The combination of an adequately performed and interpreted MRI and MR angiography or CTA may be up to 98% sensitive in the detection of an aneurysm that will bleed.

3. Which of the following is true in the evaluation of a non-neurologically isolated fourth nerve palsy?
    a. Observation for improvement in a vasculopathic patient is a reasonable option for nonisolated palsies.
    b. A CT scan is superior to the MR scan in the evaluation of the fourth nerve.
    c. A cerebral angiogram should be performed.
    d. **The neuroimaging study should be directed toward the topographical localization of the lesion.**

4. Which of the following regarding sixth nerve palsy is least true?
    a. Patients with a nonisolated palsy should have neuroimaging.
    b. **Patients with a sixth nerve palsy should have a lumbar puncture prior to neuroimaging.**
    c. Vasculopathic patients with a neurologically isolated sixth nerve palsy may be observed for improvement.
    d. Patients with presumed vasculopathic palsies should undergo diagnosis and treatment of the underlying risk factors (eg, diabetes, hypertension).

5. Which of the following regarding nystagmus is not true?
    a. Patients not taking any medications or not exposed to any toxins that can produce nystagmus should probably undergo neuroimaging.
    b. Neuroimaging should be directed to the topographical localization of the clinical findings.
    c. MRI with contrast is the imaging of choice.
    d. **Neuroimaging is unnecessary in the evaluation of nystagmus.**

6. Which of the following regarding the treatment of optic neuritis (according to the ONTT) is false?
   a. There were 3 treatment arms in the ONTT: IV steroids followed by an oral taper; oral steroids; or oral placebo.
   b. All 3 treatment groups recovered visual function equally, but IV treatment sped the rate of visual recovery.
   c. Oral steroids did not improve final visual outcome and increased the rate of new attacks.
   d. Oral steroids in conventional doses should be prescribed for typical optic neuritis.

7. Which of the following is true regarding NAION?
   a. Steroids have been proven effective for NAION.
   b. Surgical decompression is effective in NAION.
   c. Patients with NAION should be evaluated and treated for any underlying vasculopathic risk factors.
   d. One aspirin per day improves final visual outcome in NAION.

8. Which of the following regarding GCA is true?
   a. Few elderly patients develop significant side effects on corticosteroids.
   b. Close follow up with an internist or rheumatologist is advisable for patients on long-term steroid.
   c. Methotrexate can be substituted for steroid therapy in the acute therapy of visual loss in GCA.
   d. The Medrol dose pack can be used to provide a short-term treatment of GCA with tapering over a few days.

9. Which of the following is not part of the evaluation of papilledema?
   a. Neuroimaging study, preferably a contrast cranial MR scan
   b. MR venography to rule out cerebral venous sinus thrombosis
   c. Lumbar puncture
   d. Measurement of blood pressure
   e. Temporal artery biopsy

10. Which of the following is incorrect about a homonymous hemianopsia?
    a. Homonymous hemianopsias are due to retrochiasmal lesions on the contralateral side to hemianopic field loss.
    b. The homonymous hemianopia may be complete or incomplete.
    c. A complete homonymous hemianopia is lateralizing to the contralateral side, but is otherwise nonlocalizing (the lesion could exist anywhere within the retrochiasmal pathway).
    d. The more incongruous (or similar in appearance) the defect, the more posterior (eg, occipital) in the retrochiasmal pathway is the lesion location, and conversely the more congruous the lesion, the more anterior (eg, optic tract) the lesion is in the retrochiasmal pathway.

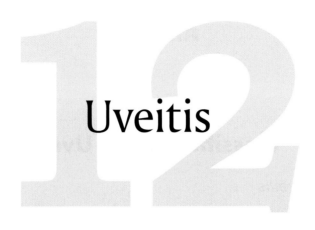

Uveitis

Thomas J. Federici, MD, and Julie H. Tsai, MD

Outline

1. Anatomy
2. Classification of Uveitis
   a. Granulomatous Uveitis
   b. Nongranulomatous Uveitis
3. Grading of Inflammation
   a. Anterior Uveitis
   b. Intermediate Uveitis
   c. Posterior Uveitis
   d. Panuveitis
4. Infectious Uveitis
   a. Syphilis
   b. Lyme
   c. Bartonella
   d. Tuberculosis
   e. Leptospirosis
   f. Herpes Viruses
      i. Herpes Simplex Virus/Varicella Zoster Virus
   g. Cytomegalovirus
   h. Presumed Ocular Histoplasmosis Syndrome
   i. Candidiasis
   j. Toxoplasmosis
      i. Ocular Toxoplasmosis
   k. Toxocariasis
   l. Cryptococcus
5. Immune-Mediated Uveitic Conditions
   a. Seronegative Spondyloarthropathies
      i. HLA B27 Related Uveitis
         1. Psoriatic Arthritis
         2. Ankylosing Spondylitis
         3. Inflammatory Bowel Disease
         4. Reiter Syndrome
   b. Behçet's Disease
   c. Fuchs' Heterochromic Iridocyclitis
   d. Posner-Schlossman Syndrome (Glaucomatous Cyclitic Crisis)
   e. Uveitis-Glaucoma-Hyphema Syndrome
   f. Multiple Sclerosis
   g. Sarcoidosis
   h. Sympathetic Ophthalmia
   i. Vogt-Koyanagi Harada Syndrome (Uveomeningitic Syndrome)
   j. White Dot Syndromes
      i. Multiple Evanescent White Dot Syndrome
      ii. Acute Posterior Multifocal Placoid Pigment Epitheliopathy
      iii. Multifocal Choroiditis and Panuveitis Syndrome
      iv. Birdshot Retinochoroidopathy
      v. Punctate Inner Choroidopathy
      vi. Serpiginous Choroiditis
   k. Phacogenic Uveitis
   l. Idiopathic Intermediate Uveitis

Probst LE, Tsai JH.
Ophthalmology: Clinical and Surgical Principles (pp. 453–478).
© 2012 SLACK Incorporated

Anatomy

- The uvea
  - Iris
  - Ciliary body
  - Choroid

Classification of Uveitis

Granulomatous Uveitis

- Inflammation of the uvea associated with nodular collections of epithelioid and giant cells surrounded by lymphocytes

Nongranulomatous Uveitis

- Typically, iris and ciliary body inflammation without associated granuloma formation
- Differential diagnosis of uveitis based on anatomical location (Figure 12-1)

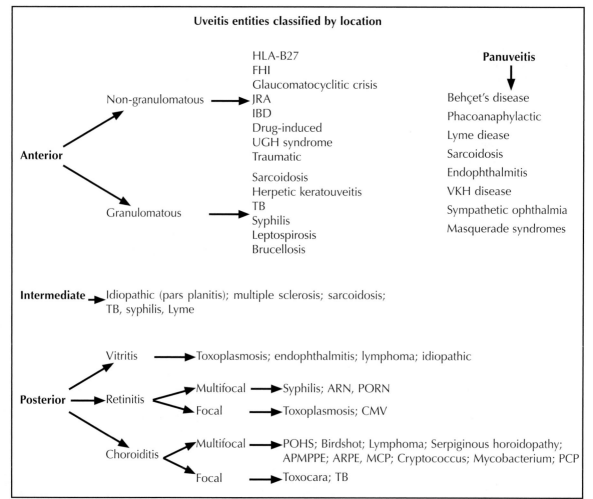

Figure 12-1. Differential diagnosis of uveitis based on anatomical location.

TABLE 12-1. GRADING OF ANTERIOR CHAMBER CELL AND FLARE

ANTERIOR CHAMBER	GRADE	DESCRIPTION (CELLS/HPF)
Cells	0	No inflammatory cells
	Trace	<5
	1+	5 to 10
	2+	10 to 20
	3+	20 to 30
	4+	Too numerous to count
Flare	0	None noted
	1+	Barely detectable
	2+	Moderate (iris details still visible
	3+	Marked (iris details hazy)
	4+	Intense (coagulated aqueous and fibrin)

Adapted from Hogan MJ, Kimura SJ, Thygeson P. Signs and symptoms of uveitis, I. Anterior uveitis. *Am J Ophthalmol.* 1959;47(5, Part 2):155–170.

TABLE 12-2. GRADING OF VITREOUS INFLAMMATION (CELLS/OPACITIES)

GRADE	DEFINITION
0	No cells/opacities
1+	Few fine cells/coarse opacities (fundus details still clear)
2+	Moderate cells/opacities (slight obscuration of fundus details)
3+	Many cells/opacities (marked obscuration of fundus details)
4+	Dense opacities (no fundus details visible)

Adapted from Kimura SJ, Hogan MJ, Thygeson P. Signs and symptoms of uveitis, II. Classification of the posterior manifestations of uveitis. *Am J Ophthalmol.* 1959;47(5 Part 2):171–176.

Grading of Inflammation

Anterior Uveitis

- Inflammation involving the anterior uveal structures, the iris and ciliary body, producing conjunctival injection and anterior chamber cell and flare (Table 12-1)
- Photophobia and blurry vision are frequent symptoms.
- Longstanding and/or recurrent bouts may produce keratic precipitates (KPs), iris nodules, and synechiae, cataract, glaucoma, and cystoid macular edema (CME).

Intermediate Uveitis

- Inflammation involving primarily the anterior vitreous; may be associated with inflammatory infiltrate along the pars plana ("snowbanks") (Table 12-2)
- Can often be seen in association with other infectious and immunologically mediated causes of uveitis
- Idiopathic cases are referred to as pars planitis.

Posterior Uveitis

- Inflammation involving primarily the vitreous, ciliary body, and choroid
- Retinal vasculitis and optic nerve edema and hyperemia may also be seen.
- Chronic complications include cataract, retinal neovascularization, glaucoma, and CME.
- Conditions that disrupt Bruch's membrane, such as serpiginious choroiditis, may be complicated by the development of choroidal neovascularization.

Panuveitis

- Inflammation that involves the anterior and posterior segments of the eye simultaneously
- A panophthalmitis refers to a panuveitis due to an infectious etiology.

Infectious Uveitis

Syphilis

- Etiology
  - Infection caused by the spirochete *Treponema pallidum* (*T. pallidum*) through maternal-fetal or sexual transmission
- Signs/symptoms
  - Ocular syphilis is uncommon, but uveitis is the most common ocular presentation.
  - Clinically, there are 4 stages of infection
    - Primary
      - Painless chancre appears 3 weeks following inoculation at site of infection. May be seen on genitalia, mouth, conjunctiva, and eyelids.
    - Secondary
      - Spirochetemia. Maculopapular rash may be found on soles of feet and palms of hands.
    - Latent
      - Follows secondary stage in which clinical disease is not detectable and the patient is not contagious
    - Tertiary
      - Obliterative endarteritis. Three subtypes are tertiary syphilis, cardiovascular syphilis, or neurosyphilis.
- Common signs of syphilitic uveitis
  - Anterior
    - May occur 6 weeks to 6 months following infection. Often bilateral, granulomatous inflammation with iris nodules. May also have dilated iris vessels (roseolae). Corneal involvement may be seen (interstitial keratitis).
  - Posterior
    - Chorioretinitis
      - May be focal or disseminated; most common presentation of posterior disease. Multiple yellow lesions located in the posterior pole and equatorially, but can be seen in periphery (Figure 12-2). Vitreous cell is also noted on exam. Retinitis, optic nerve edema, and serous retinal detachment may accompany chorioretinitis.
    - Vasculitis
      - May involve large and small arteries and veins of the retinal circulation. May occur in isolation from other ocular manifestations.
    - Intermediate uveitis
      - May appear like idiopathic intermediate uveitis (formerly pars planitis) if the posterior vitreal cell is more prominent than the anterior reaction; however, true pars plana exudates are absent.
    - Panuveitis
      - The entire uveal tract can be involved. As many as 27% to 50% of patients presented with panuveitis.

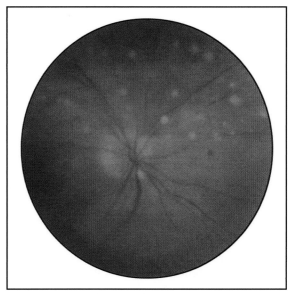

Figure 12-2. Multiple yellow chorioretinal lesions can be seen with overlying vitritis. (This figure was published in *The Retina Atlas*. Yannuzzi LA, Guyer DR, Green WR. Copyright Elsevier [1995].)

- Diagnosis
  - Nonspecific tests
    - Rapid plasma reagin (RPR) and the Venereal Disease Research Laboratory (VDRL) tests show high activity in active disease and revert to normal following treatment, whereas specific tests (ie, fluorescent treponemal antibody absorption [FTA-ABS] and treponemal micro-hemagglutinin [MHA-TP] tests) quantify the amount of serum antibody against treponemal antigens. Both will remain positive once a patient is infected even following treatment.
- Treatment
  - Center for Disease Control recommendations include penicillin intramuscular every week for 3 weeks. Some consider ocular syphilis akin to neurosyphilis and treat accordingly with intravenous penicillin G 18 to 20 million units daily for 10 to 14 days. If the patient is penicillin allergic, one may try desensitization or tetracycline 500 mg by mouth 4 times daily for 30 days *or* doxycycline 100 mg orally twice daily for 14 days.
- Prognosis
  - If diagnosed early and treated appropriately, cure is possible.

Lyme

- Etiology
  - Caused by the spirochete *Borrelia burgdorferi* (*B. burgdorferi*) carried by the Ixodes ticks
- Incidence
  - Affects men more than women without age predilection
- Signs/symptoms
  - Systemic disease
    - Early stage
      - Erythema migrans (bull's eye rash) is diagnostic of disease but may not occur in 20% to 40% of patients. Patients may exhibit fever, malaise, and fatigue.
    - Disseminated stage
      - Erythema chronicum migrans, large joint arthritis, and central and peripheral nervous system manifestations can occur. Atrioventricular block is the most common manifestation of cardiac involvement.

- Persistent stage
  - □ Patients may develop acrodermatitis chronica atrophicans, a blue-red lesion on the ex-tremities, most often seen in women. Encephalopathy may occur, and joint disease may persist.
- Ocular disease
  - ○ Early stage
    - Photophobia, conjunctivitis, episcleritis
  - ○ Disseminated stage
    - Bells' palsy and optic nerve involvement common
  - ○ Uveitis
    - Most commonly intermediate uveitis with a severe vitritis. A granulomatous anterior reac-tion, retinitis, and optic nerve involvement may accompany the vitritis. Anterior, posterior, intermediate, and panuveitis can be seen with Lyme disease.
  - ○ Persistent stage
    - Episcleritis, keratitis
- Diagnosis
  - ○ Erythema chronicum migrans is confirmatory as is a late manifestation (musculoskeletal, ner-vous, or cardiovascular system findings) plus laboratory confirmation (isolation of *B. burgdorferi*, IgM/ Immunoglobulin G [IgG] in serum/cerebrospinal fluid [CSF])
- Treatment
  - ○ Adults
    - Doxycycline 100 mg orally twice daily
    - Amoxicillin 500 mg by mouth 4 times daily (or cefuroxime 500 mg by mouth twice a day for 2 to 3 weeks)
  - ○ Jarisch-Herxheimer reaction following treatment may occur.
- Prognosis
  - ○ With early diagnosis and treatment, cure is possible; however, if left untreated, involvement of the cardiac and nervous systems can be devastating.

Bartonella

- Etiology
  - ○ Infection with *Bartonella henselae*, a gram-negative bacillus
- Signs/symptoms
  - ○ Parinaud's oculoglandular syndrome
    - Primary inoculation occurs from a cat scratch or bite on the hands, arms, or neck. A small erythematous papule develops at the inoculation site, followed by a follicular unilateral con-junctivitis with associated lymphadenopathy.
  - ○ Neuroretinitis
    - Patients complain of decreased vision. Usually unilateral, a relative afferent pupillary defect is seen on exam. Optic disc edema with macular star is seen on ophthalmoscopy.
  - ○ Uveitis
    - Anterior and intermediate uveitis have been reported.
- Diagnosis
  - ○ Relies on clinical findings and indirect fluorescent antibody test, with titers more than 1:64 as positive.
- Treatment
  - ○ There are no guidelines to treatment.
  - ○ May consider doxycycline or trimethoprim-sulfamethoxazole (Bactrim) for a 10- to 14-day course
- Prognosis
  - ○ Those with neuroretinitis have a good prognosis, as most recover excellent visual acuity.

Tuberculosis

- Etiology
  - Infection with *Mycobacterium tuberculosis* (or *M. bovis*, *M. africanum*, *M. microti*). Disease risk factors include HIV infection and close contact with someone with tuberculosis (TB).
- Signs/symptoms
  - Disseminated choroiditis
    - Most common presentation of TB uveitis. Well circumscribed, yellow, gray, or white lesions deep in the choroid, typically in the posterior pole. Anterior uveitis may be absent, mild, or severe. Optic disc edema may accompany the choroiditis.
  - Anterior uveitis
    - Granulomatous with mutton-fat KPs. A vitritis may be present.
  - Panuveitis
    - Inflammation can start acutely, be severe, and result in loss of the eye within several days. Enucleation or evisceration may be required if the eye becomes blind and painful.
    - Uveitis may result in posterior synechiae, retinal detachment, and neovascular glaucoma. In patients with HIV, choroidal lesions may be observed on routine ophthalmoscopy.
- Diagnosis
  - Fluorescein angiography
    - A lesion will show early fluorescence with diffuse hyperfluoresence in the late stages.
  - Tuberculin skin test
    - Indicates mycobacterium infection, not TB
  - Acid-fast staining
    - Sputum, urine, or gastric aspirate samples can be used as well as cervical lymph node biopsy.
  - Nucleic acid amplification
    - Anterior chamber tap can be sent for transcription-mediated amplification (TMA) and polymerase chain reaction (PCR).
- Treatment
  - Recommend a physician knowledgeable of TB be consulted to aid in treatment.
  - Regimens often include isoniazid, rifampin, and pyrazinamide (all bactericidal). Direct observed therapy is also implemented to help ensure compliance.
- Prognosis
  - If treated quickly, cure is possible.
  - The most common reason for treatment failure is noncompliance.
  - With respect to ocular complications, the presentation of disease, aggressiveness of treatment, and underlying immune status plays a role in determining final visual outcomes.

Leptospirosis

- Etiology
  - Infection with the spirochete *Leptospira interrogans*
  - Often seen in tropical and subtropical climate zones
  - Natural hosts are rodents, dogs, pigs, and cattle.
  - Transmission to humans occurs through contact with contaminated soil or surface water.
- Signs/symptoms
  - Nonocular disease
    - Subclinical to fatal infections; may produce hemorrhage and end-organ failure (kidneys, liver, heart). Acute phase marked by fever, headache, and fatigue. The spirochetemic phase results in organisms in the blood, CSF, kidneys, and other organs. The disease may be considered anicteric (90%) or icteric (10%), depending upon how much liver involvement occurs.
  - Ocular disease
    - Earliest and most common sign is conjunctival injection or hemorrhage. Uveitis is the most serious ocular complication and may occur months after initial infection.
  - Anterior uveitis
    - Benign; red eye, blurry vision, pain, and photophobia. Most common form of uveitis.
  - Posterior uveitis
    - Vitritis, choroiditis, optic nerve edema, or panuveitis

- Diagnosis
  - Microscopic agglutination test (MAT) detects antibodies but is complex, requiring special laboratories and personnel.
  - Isolation of organisms or DNA in body fluids is more commonly done, but requires near daily sampling in order to ensure finding organisms/DNA.
- Treatment
  - Controversial
  - Standard treatment is doxycycline 100 mg twice daily for 10 to 14 days.
- Prognosis
  - Favorable
  - Good care of uveitis can result in reasonable outcomes.

Herpes Viruses

- All herpes viruses have a core of linear double-stranded DNA surrounded by an icosahedral capsid.
- Herpes simplex virus (HSV), varicella zoster virus (VZV), Epstein-Barr virus (EBV), and cytomegalovirus (CMV) are in the herpes family.
- All herpes viruses produce infectious virus particles within the cytoplasm of the host cell, eventually leading to host cell death.
- Also, all viruses in this family have a latent period.

Herpes Simplex Virus/Varicella Zoster Virus

- Signs/symptoms
  - Keratitis
    - May involve epithelium, stroma, and/or endothelium. Therapy may include topical and/or antivirals and topical and/or oral steroids.
  - Anterior uveitis
    - In HSV, iritis and trabeculitis may be seen with or without corneal lesions. Patients complain of redness, photophobia, pain, and blurry vision. Cell, flare, and mutton-fat KPs may be seen. Hypopyon, fibrin deposition, post synechiae, and glaucoma can occur. Iritis is often seen in association with stromal keratitis or endotheliitis. Trabeculitis, or inflammation of the trabecular endothelium, may result in increased intraocular pressure (IOP).
  - Acute retinal necrosis (ARN)
    - Begins with anterior uveitis. White or yellow exudative lesions deep in the retina and retinal pigment epithelium (RPE) develop in the mid- and far periphery. Over the next several days, retina necrosis spreads posteriorly and peripherally, and the retina appears white. The macula may be spared. A dense vitritis may develop along with retinal nonperfusion and neovascularization (Figure 12-3). May lead to retinal detachment. Typically, the disease is unilateral, but if left untreated, may affect the fellow eye.
  - Progressive outer retinal necrosis (PORN) syndrome
    - Similar to ARN, except it occurs in the immunocompromised population, typically those with HIV/AIDS. Multiple deep retinal lesions, often involving the macula, begin to coalesce and leave large areas of necrosis. The inner retina and retinal vasculature is relatively spared. There is a "cracked-mud" appearance. Minimal inflammatory signs are seen due to the altered immune status of the patient. May lead to retinal detachment.
- Diagnosis
  - HSV/VZV iridocyclitis/trabeculitis is made clinically and is aided by a history of or active keratitis
  - ARN: Fluorescein angiogram (FA) demonstrates leakage from the retinal vasculature. Retinal neovascularization may be seen.
- Treatment
  - Iridocyclitis/trabeculitis
    - Topical antiviral therapy has little or no effect. Oral acyclovir may be helpful. The inflammation usually responds to topical steroids. IOP may be managed with antiglaucomatous medications.

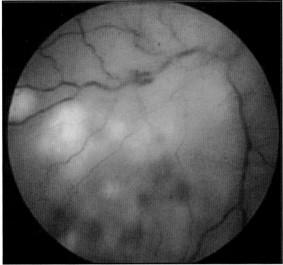

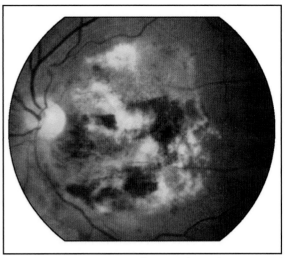

Figure 12-3. Typical presentation for ARN, with intraretinal hemorrhages, peripheral retinal necrosis, and overlying vitritis. (This figure was published in *Retina*. Ryan SJ, Ed. Copyright Elsevier [2006].)

Figure 12-4. CMV retinitis with areas of retinal necrosis and intraretinal hemorrhage. (This figure was published in *The Retina Atlas*. Yannuzzi LA, Guyer DR, Green WR. Copyright Elsevier [1995].)

- o ARN
  - ▪ Acyclovir may produce lesion regression as early as 2 days after treatment is initiated. The vitritis may worsen as this is a secondary reaction to the retinal necrosis, not the viral infection. In patients with HIV/AIDS, acyclovir may not be useful, and other agents such as foscarnet may be more beneficial. Acyclovir has been shown to reduce fellow eye involvement.
- Prognosis
  - o Patients with iridocyclitis/trabeculitis may do well if IOP is controlled; however, in chronic cases, band keratopathy and phthisis may occur.
  - o In patients with ARN, retinal detachment, vaso-occlusive disease, and optic nerve involvement may produce visual devastation.

Cytomegalovirus

- Most common ocular manifestation is retinitis
- Is a frequent cause of blindness in AIDS patients
- Signs/symptoms
  - o CMV retinitis
    - ▪ Patients with CD4+ counts <50 cells/mm^3 are at risk. Patients complain of blurry vision and/or floaters. Begins in peripheral retina with small white infiltrate. The retinitis may appear as a white, fluffy, confluent retinal opacification with multiple retinal hemorrhages (Figure 12-4). Disease may appear more granular with central atrophy. A low-grade vitritis can be seen. The retinitis can progress 0.2 mm per week.
  - o Immune recovery uveitis
    - ▪ Occurs following introduction of highly-active antiretroviral therapy (HAART) in patients with CMV retinitis. Inflammatory response is seen in a previously quiet eye with CMV retinitis.
- Diagnosis
  - o Based on clinical criteria, history of immunocompromised status (AIDS)
- Treatment
  - o CMV retinitis
    - ▪ HAART has been beneficial in preserving immune status. Usually given intravenously, gancyclovir, foscarnet, and cidofovir can be used systemically to treat ocular disease. If the patient cannot tolerate intravenous dosing or is failing therapy, intravitreous gancyclovir can be given 2 to 3 times a week during induction and then weekly thereafter for

maintenance. Gancyclovir implants can also be surgically placed. Treatment with ocular antivirals, although effective, does not protect the fellow eye from disease.
- o Immune-recovery uveitis
  - Oral or sub-Tenon's injections may be considered.
- Prognosis
  - o With the advent of new medications, disease can be held at bay; however, retinal detachment due to areas of necrosis can be visually devastating despite pars plana vitrectomy with silicone oil.

Presumed Ocular Histoplasmosis Syndrome

- Etiology
  - o Possible infection/exposure to the dimorphic yeast *Histoplasma capsulatum* (*H. capsulatum*)
  - o Increased prevalence in the population of the Ohio River valley
- Signs/symptoms
  - o Sudden blurring of vision, metamorphopsia, and micropsia. A central scotoma in one eye may also be present. Patients often report having lived in the east and southeastern part of the United States. Clinically, there is an absence of vitreous inflammation.
  - o Clinical triad
    - Peripapillary scarring, peripheral retinal pigment epithelial atrophic spots ("histo spots"), and disciform macular scars
  - o Classically describes the ocular findings of the disease
  - o Choroidal neovascularization (CNV) is a vision-threatening complication of disease.
- Diagnosis
  - o Clinical
    - The absence of vitreous cell helps distinguish disease from other conditions such as multifocal choroiditis and panuveitis (MFC-PU) syndrome or punctate inner choroidopathy (PIC).
    - Approximately 90% of patients with presumed ocular histoplasmosis syndrome (POHS) will have a positive skin test for histoplasmin.
    - Higher frequency of HLA-B7 positivity.
    - Postmortem studies in an infected patient with AIDS uncovered histoplasma spores in the visual tract and optic nerve.
    - FA
      - □ Window defects showing underlying choroidal vessels expose the peripheral atrophic spots; peripapillary atrophy of the RPE is demonstrated by choroidal fluorescence in the early stages of the angiogram. CNV will demonstrate early hyperfluoresence with late leakage.
- Treatment
  - o Limited to the management of the CNV
  - o Macular Photocoagulation Study (MPS)
    - Indicated laser ablation of the juxtafoveal CNV prevents loss of vision in the affected eye. To date, laser photocoagulation of extrafoveal and juxtafoveal CNV in OHS is the treatment of choice. Photodynamic therapy (PDT) with verteporfin for subfoveal lesions may be beneficial.
- Prognosis
  - o Visual outcomes related to macular involvement
  - o If CNV develops and is diagnosed early, vision-saving therapy such as laser photocoagulation and PDT with verteporfin may be applied.

Candidiasis

- Etiology
  - o Infection due to *Candida albicans*
- Signs/symptoms
  - o Endophthalmitis/chorioretinitis

- ○ Endogenous
  - ▪ Typically, patients are asymptomatic due to either the peripheral location of the disease or the mental status of the patient. Discomfort, red eye, floaters, and vision loss have been reported. The lesion begins as a fluffy white choroidal infiltrate that will involve the retina and eventually break through to the vitreous. When involving the vitreous, the fungus, inflammatory cells, and debris can form a mass. A "string-of-pearls" can sometimes be seen. Anteriorly, cells, flare, hypopyon, and conjunctival hyperemia may be noted.
  - ○ Exogenous
    - ▪ May be post-traumatic due to contaminated foreign material or rarely postsurgical
- Diagnosis
  - ○ High suspicion in those with risk factors, including immunocompromised state, total parenteral nutrition (TPN), and newborns
  - ○ Cultures from blood, urine, catheters, and any other site of potential source are helpful.
  - ○ Repeated fundus examinations are required in the presence of candidemia without ocular findings.
- Treatment
  - ○ Infectious disease consultation is warranted.
  - ○ A combination of system and intraocular antifungals may be required. Amphotericin B IV 0.5 to 1.0 mg/kg/day (average dose 40–50 mg/day) is given until retinal lesions become small, fibrose, or resolve completely. Intravitreal amphotericin (10 mcg or 2.5 mcg/mL) given through the pars plana is effective. Pars plana vitrectomy may be required; it allows for biopsy, reduction of infectious/inflammatory load, and easy access for administration of intravitreal antifungal agents.
- Prognosis
  - ○ Candidal endophthalmitis can be devastating.
  - ○ Outcomes are dependent upon organism virulence, degree of inflammatory response, and the rapidity of detection and appropriate treatment.

Toxoplasmosis

- Etiology
  - ○ Infection with *Toxoplasma gondii* (*T. gondii*), an obligate intracellular parasite. Felines are the only definitive host; humans are an intermediate host group that support asexual reproduction of the organism.
- Life cycle
  - ○ Asexual cycle
    - ▪ Begins with a host ingesting mature oocysts, tissue cysts, or tachyzoites in raw meat. Tachyzoites are destroyed by gastric acid, but mature oocysts and tissue cysts are broken down and release sporozoites and bradyzoites, which then enter the cells of the intestinal tract and transform into tachyzoites. These tachyzoites then are carried via the lymphatics and bloodstream to various parts of the body.
  - ○ Sexual cycle
    - ▪ Occurs only in the feline intestine. Cats will ingest contaminated meat containing oocysts or tissue cysts. In the cat's intestines, tachyzoites enter intestinal cells and multiply. Gametocytes are formed and are fertilized to produce oocysts, which are excreted for up to 20 days; occurring approximately 3 to 24 days after ingestion.
- Signs/symptoms
  - ○ Congenital toxoplasmosis
    - ▪ Severity of disease is inversely related to trimester in which infection occurs; first-trimester infection may lead to abortion/severe disease.
  - ○ Retinochoroiditis
    - ▪ 70% to 90% of cases
  - ○ Intracranial calcifications
  - ○ Acquired toxoplasmosis
    - ▪ Initially thought to be rare. The majority of immunocompetent patients are symptom-free. Some develop a flu-like illness. Ocular involvement may present simultaneously with systemic signs/symptoms. Lymphadenopathy may be present.

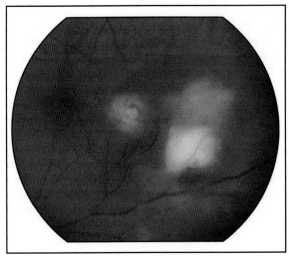

Figure 12-5. Toxoplasmosis. There is an area of acute retinal hemorrhage, retinitis adjacent to an old chorioretinal scar, and overlying vitritis. Perivasculitis can be seen adjacent to the site of infection. (This figure was published in *The Retina Atlas*. Yannuzzi LA, Guyer DR, Green WR. Copyright Elsevier [1995].)

- o Immunocompromised patients
  - ▪ May develop acute toxoplasmosis from reactivation of congenital disease or newly acquired infection. The prognosis is particularly poor. Multiple organ involvement can be seen.

Ocular Toxoplasmosis

- Congenital infection accounts for 80% to 98% of disease.
- Peripheral retinochoroidal scars are most common finding.
- Two-thirds of patients suffer from recurrences; recurrent lesions often occur adjacent to old lesions. Initially, lesions begin in the superficial retina and appear yellow-white with ill-defined margins. The lesion will become more defined and the borders pigmented. A dense vitritis is usually present ("fog in the headlight"). Phlebitis can also be seen. Kyrieleis arteriolitis, the presence of exudates or periarterial plaques without associated leakage or vascular obstruction, is of unknown etiology and can occasionally be seen in toxoplasmosis (Figure 12-5).
- Lesions affecting the macula can be devastating
- Atypical forms
  - o Punctate outer retinal toxoplasmosis (PORT)
    - ▪ Gray-white outer retinal and RPE lesions with little or no vitritis. Significant optic nerve involvement.
  - o Neuroretinitis
    - ▪ Severe optic nerve edema with disc hemorrhages, venous dilation, and vitritis
  - o Neuritis
    - ▪ Optic nerve involvement along with a distant retinal lesion
- Diagnosis
  - o Clinical findings are key, whereas serologic testing is only supportive as IgG and/or IgM titers may be low or negative initially.
  - o FA: Lesions demonstrate central hypofluorescence with late leakage
- Treatment
  - o Should be considered when the lesion is vision-threatening either due to vitreous haze or proximity to the macula or optic nerve. Some believe all lesions should be treated. Total treatment time has not been established.
  - o Standard regimen
    - ▪ Includes pyrimethamine, sulfadiazine, clindamycin, folinic acid, and prednisone. Pyrimethamine and sulfadiazine impair DNA synthesis by inhibiting folic acid synthesis; therefore, patients require folinic acid rescue therapy to prevent bone marrow suppression.

- o Pregnancy
  - ▪ Pyrimethamine should be avoided as it is teratogenic. Sulfadiazine should be avoided in the third trimester. Spiramycin can be used in combination with sulfadiazine, but is not available in the United States. Treatment during pregnancy is associated with decreased percentage of children developing chorioretinal scars in first 2 years of life.
- Prognosis
  - o Lesions not involving the macula or optic nerve have a good prognosis.

Toxocariasis

- Etiology
  - o Human infection usually due to *T. canis*
- Life cycle
  - o Dogs acquire intestinal infection by ingestion of eggs or larvae. The eggs/larvae mature and enter the systemic circulation where they eventually reach the lungs. They are coughed up, swallowed, and mature in the intestines and are excreted.
  - o Humans are infected by eating contaminated soil or contaminated meat. In the intestine, the larvae migrate into the blood stream by which they find their target organs. As the organism cannot pass into the tracheal system of humans, they encyst in focal granulomata.
- Signs/symptoms
  - o Visceral larva migrans (VLM) syndrome
    - ▪ Affects children 1 to 4 years of age; demonstrate fever, cough, malaise, and nodules on the trunk and legs
  - o Ocular toxocariasis
    - ▪ Presents as either a central or peripheral granuloma
- Diagnosis
  - o Clinical findings are important.
  - o Enzyme-linked immunosorbent assay (ELISA)
    - ▪ 90% sensitivity and specificity
- Treatment
  - o If inflammatory response is present, topical steroids can be used.
  - o Pars plana vitrectomy, cryotherapy, and photocoagulation can be used on patients who fail medical therapy, have dense vitreous haze, and/or retinal detachment.
- Prognosis
  - o Depends on lesion location and sequelae of inflammation

Cryptococcus

- Etiology
  - o Infection with *Cryptococcus neoformans* (fungus), which is found in pigeon feces and contaminated soil. Usually affects immunocompromised patients.
- Signs/symptoms
  - o May produce meningitis, pneumonia, endocarditis, and ocular infection
  - o Ocular manifestations are thought to arise from optic nerve extension and are often seen in concert with meningitis.
  - o Most common intraocular manifestation is chorioretinitis. A yellow-white focal choroiditis is seen first and will progress to retinal and vitreous inflammation. An anterior reaction may be seen if left untreated.
  - o Endogenous endophthalmitis
    - ▪ Blurred vision, redness, pain, and photophobia. Anterior reaction consists of cell, flare, and mutton-fat KPs.
- Diagnosis
  - o May be presumptive
  - o CSF analysis in immunocompetent patients often reveals increased opening pressure, elevated protein, and leukocytosis. Immunocompromised patients may not have any abnormalities.
  - o Absence of growth from cultures does exclude infection.

TABLE 12-3. COMPARISON OF HLA-B27-ASSOCIATED UVEITIDES

	PSORIATIC ARTHRITIS	ANKYLOSING SPONDYLITIS	INFLAMMATORY BOWEL DISEASE	REITER SYNDROME
Systemic associations	Psoriasis; spondyloarthropathy (with sacroiliitis in up to 20%); pitting of nail beds; inflammatory bowel disease	Inflammation of vertebrae/hip joints; sacroiliac spine involvement common (sacroiliitis)	Ulcerative colitis (5% to 12% develop uveitis) Crohn's disease (2.4% develop uveitis)	Seronegative arthritis; keratoderma blennorhagicum; aphthous stomatitis; balanitis; urethritis; onycholysis; plantar fasciitis; sacroiliitis (up to 80%)
Diagnostic testing		HLA-B27–positive in 90%; sacroiliac x-rays	Colonoscopy	HLA-B27–positive in 85% to 95%
Disposition		Co-management with rheumatology	Co-management with gastroenterology	

- Treatment
  - Meningitis is fatal without treatment
  - 50% relapse rate in AIDS patients
  - Combination therapy with flucytosine 25 to 35 mg orally every 6 hours and amphotericin B 0.4 to 0.6 mg/day IV
  - Endophthalmitis may require systemic antifungals, intravitreal therapy, and pars plana vitrectomy.
- Prognosis
  - Mortality rate in patients
    - Immunocompromised without AIDS—25%
    - Lymphoreticular malignancy or steroid use—55%
    - 25% relapse
    - 40% suffer permanent sequelae

Immune-Mediated Uveitic Conditions

Seronegative Spondyloarthropathies

HLA-B27–Related Uveitis

- Etiology
  - Nonsystemic disease affects young men
- Systemic conditions (PAIR mnemonic) (Table 12-3 and Figure 12-6)

Psoriatic Arthritis

- Skin scales and arthropathy affecting sacroiliac joints and distal joints of the hands and feet
- About 20% develop uveitis
- Topical steroids and cycloplegics

Ankylosing Spondylitis

- Men > women
- 25% uveitis, 80% bilaterally affected—not necessarily simultaneously
- Uveitis does not correlate to joint disease.
- Sacroiliac joints: sclerosis and eventual obliteration of joint space
- Aortic insufficiency, cardiomegaly, and conduction defects may be present.

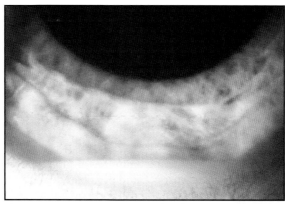

Figure 12-6. Hypopyon associated with anterior uveitis in an HLA-B27–positive patient. (Reprinted from *Cornea Atlas*. 2nd ed. Krachmer JH, Palay DA. Copyright [2006], with permission from Elsevier.)

Inflammatory Bowel Disease

- Uveitis in ulcerative colitis and Crohn's disease
- About 5% develop uveitis with ulcerative colitis.
- Conjunctivitis, episcleritis, and posterior uveitis may occasionally be seen.

Reiter Syndrome

- May develop following dysentery by gram-negative bacteria or after nongonococcal urethras (*Chlamydia trachomatis* and *Ureaplasma urealyticum*)
- Polyarthritis, conjunctivitis, and urethritis
- Other major signs: keratoderma blennorrhagica, circinate balanitis
- Conjunctivitis more frequently seen than iritis
- Ocular disease is mild; systemic disease may require immunosuppression.

Behçet's Disease

- Etiology
  - Chronic relapsing inflammatory condition, etiology unknown
- Signs/symptoms
  - Classic triad of recurrent oral and genital aphthous ulcers, ocular inflammation, and skin lesions (eg, erythema nodosum). A slight preponderance of those who live along the Silk Trade Route may be affected.
- Ocular manifestations
  - Anterior
    - Classically nongranulomatous iridocyclitis with shifting hypopyon. Conjunctival injection, ciliary flush, cell, and flare are present. Patients complain of blurry vision, redness, photophobia, and pain.
  - Posterior
    - Vitreous cell, posterior vitreous detachment, and an obliterative, necrotizing vasculitis (arterioles and venules). Retinal edema and retinal ischemia may be present. Ischemia may lead to neovascularization and possibly neovascular glaucoma. Disc edema and optic atrophy may occur.
- Systemic manifestations
  - Oral and genital aphthous ulcers
  - Skin lesions
    - Erythema nodosum (usually on tibia), superficial thrombophlebitis, and acne vulgaris
  - Vascular
    - Vasculitis (any vessel size), arterial occlusion, aneurysms, venous occlusion, and varices. Cardiac involvement is possible.

- o Central nervous system (CNS)
  - ▪ 3% to 10%, but most serious manifestations. Palsies of cranial nerves 6 and 7, central scotoma from optic nerve edema, and papilledema from idiopathic intracranial hypertension.
  - o Gastrointestinal (GI)/Genitourinary (GU)
    - ▪ Ulcers anywhere along GI tract. Epididymitis and acute glomerulonephritis.
  - o Pulmonary
    - ▪ Pulmonary arteritis
  - o Musculoskelatal
    - ▪ Arthritis (50% of cases involve the knee)
- Diagnosis
  - o Serum HLA-B51. According to Research Committee of Japan, Behçet's disease is broken down into 4 types (complete, incomplete, suspect, and possible) depending upon major/minor criteria and eye involvement. Major criteria include recurrent oral aphthae, skin lesion, recurrent genital ulcers, and ocular inflammation. Minor criteria include bowel ulcers, arthritis, vasculitis, and neuropsychiatric symptoms.
  - o Complete
    - ▪ 4 major
  - o Incomplete
    - ▪ 3 major, or 1 major + ocular
  - o Suspect
    - ▪ 2 major, no eye
  - o Possible
    - ▪ 1 major
- Treatment
  - o Systemic and local steroids may be used but disease becomes resistant.
  - o Immunomodulating agents such as azathioprine, chlorambucil, cyclophosphamide, cyclosporine, and tacrolimus may be required.
- Prognosis
  - o Cataract, CME, glaucoma, and neovascularization may all limit visual acuity.
  - o Due to the vitreal and retinal manifestations, retinal detachment and vitreous hemorrhage may occur, and the obliterative vasculitis may be devastating.

Fuchs' Heterochromic Iridocyclitis

- Etiology
  - o Unknown
- Signs/symptoms
  - o Iris heterochromia, mild anterior chamber reaction, and stellate-appearing KPs not limited to Arlt's triangle
    - ▪ Heterochromia
      - □ An affected blue eye will appear more blue, a brown eye will be less brown, and a gray eye may appear green.
  - o Other findings
    - ▪ Cataract; fine iris vessels may be seen on gonioscopy but rarely lead to neovascular glaucoma
  - o Patients are frequently asymptomatic.
- Diagnosis
  - o Purely based on clinical examination
- Treatment
  - o The anterior chamber reaction is typically mild, and long-term steroid use further potentiates the development of cataract.
  - o Cataract extraction can be done safely.
- Prognosis
  - o Complications from uveitis manifest mainly as cataract and glaucoma.
  - o Cataract surgery is typically uneventful if inflammation is controlled.
  - o Although glaucoma is often linked to the degree of inflammation initially and will respond to topical steroids, later in the disease, antiglaucoma medications will be needed, and 20% require glaucoma surgery.

Posner-Schlossman Syndrome (Glaucomatous Cyclitic Crisis)

- Etiology
  - Unknown
- Signs/symptoms
  - Mild anterior chamber reaction, fine KPs, mydriasis, and an elevated IOP
- Diagnosis
  - Based upon clinical examination
- Treatment
  - The inflammation is treated with topical steroids; the IOP is managed with aqueous suppressants.
- Prognosis
  - Glaucoma may be controlled with topical medications; however, surgical therapy may be warranted. Both eyes may be susceptible to open-angle glaucoma and its sequelae.

Uveitis-Glaucoma-Hyphema Syndrome

- Etiology
  - Uncommon disorder, may be due to iris irritation from a malpositioned intraocular lens, particularly closed-loop anterior chamber lens
- Signs/symptoms
  - Anterior chamber cell and flare, hyphema, and increased IOP
- Treatment
  - Treat inflammation with topical steroids and cycloplegics; treat increased IOP with aqueous suppressants.

Multiple Sclerosis

- Etiology
  - Chronic inflammatory demyelinating disease that affects the central nervous system, typically in young adults
  - Manifestations of disease are dependent upon the location of the demyelination in the brainstem and/or brain.
  - Patients are between the ages of 20 and 40 years at the time of first episode.
  - Women develop multiple sclerosis (MS) more frequently than men (approximately 2:1).
- Signs/symptoms
  - Systemic
    - Patients may experience fatigue, clumsiness, paresthesias, and neuralgias. Bladder and bowel dysfunction can also occur. Memory impairment and depression are seen.
  - Ocular
    - Diplopia/nystagmus: The third and sixth cranial nerves can be affected leading to extraocular motility disturbances and diplopia. Internuclear ophthalmoplegia (INO) is due to a lesion in the medial longitudinal fasciculus (MLF) that produces an ipsilateral adduction deficit and a jerk nystagmus in the contralateral abducting eye.
  - Optic neuritis
    - Considered a forme fruste of MS and can be the initial presentation of disease. Patients complain of an acute-onset loss of vision and pain behind the eye that is present at rest and may be exacerbated during eye movement. On examination, a relative afferent papillary defect can be seen. Occasionally, optic nerve edema can be seen, but most cases are retrobulbar in location; therefore, the nerve head appears unremarkable. Left untreated, visual acuity will recover; however, color vision and visual field defects may be noted. L'hermitte's sign (flashes of light with eye movement), Pulfrich's phenomenon (disturbed depth perception, particularly with a moving target), and Uhthoff's phenomenon (worsening of neurologic symptoms with heat) can occur. Resolution will produce optic atrophy and pallor.
  - Uveitis
    - The most common presentation of uveitis is intermediate disease and is indistinguishable from idiopathic intermediate uveitis (pars planitis). Anterior uveitis is uncommon, but may appear granulomatous.

- Diagnosis
  - MS
    - The diagnosis of MS requires a lesion affecting different areas of the CNS separated by both space and time. MRI should show white matter plaques, preferably at least 3 lesions with 1 in a periventricular location. CSF will show elevated protein, increased white blood cells, and increased IgG.
  - Optic neuritis
    - Diminished color vision, scotomata on visual field testing, and leakage of dye from arterioles/venules (vasculitis) on FA
- Treatment
  - MS
    - Glucocorticoids and interferon-beta can be employed, but, to date, no medications completely halt progression of disease
  - Optic neuritis
    - The Optic Neuritis Treatment Trial discovered that optic neuritis associated with white matter lesions/plaques on magnetic resonance imaging (MRI) should be treated with intravenous methylprednisolone 250 mg IV every 6 hours for 3 days followed by an 11-day course of prednisone 1 mg/kg/day and a rapid taper 20 mg/day and 10 mg/day on days 12 and 13 to 15, respectively, produced faster visual recovery (but not finial vision) and delayed the onset of MS over 2 years but not at 3 years. Do not use oral steroids alone, as this was associated with an increased risk of recurrent optic neuritis.
  - Uveitis
    - Should be treated as intermediate uveitis. Topical steroids and injectable steroids are therapeutic options.
- Prognosis
  - Overall, the prognosis of ocular disease is good; however, recurrent optic neuritis produces significant color vision, visual field, and visual acuity decline.

Sarcoidosis

- Etiology
  - Granulomatous inflammation that affects multiple organ systems, particularly the lungs, skin, and eye
  - The presentation and course of sarcoidosis is variable.
  - In the United States, the majority of patients are African American, whereas in Europe, mostly whites are affected
- Signs/symptoms
  - Systemic
    - The lung is the most frequently affected organ. Lesions involve the peribronchial and perivascular lymphatics. Hilar and mediastinal lymphadenopathy is common. Splenomegaly can be seen in as many as 18% of patients. As many as 37% of patients develop integumentary involvement, lupus pernio, plaques, subcutaneous nodules, and erythema nodosum.
    - Heerfordt's syndrome
      - □ Uveoparotid fever consists of uveitis, parotitis, fever, and cranial nerve palsies (often facial nerve).
    - Lofgren's syndrome
      - □ Consists of erythema nodosum, fever, arthropathy, and bilateral hilar adenopathy
  - Ocular
    - The most common ocular manifestation (85%) of all patients with ocular sarcoidosis is anterior segment involvement. Conjunctival granulomas, uveitis, and iris nodules can be seen.
    - Anterior uveitis
      - □ Typically chronic in nature and granulomatous; cell, flare, and mutton-fat KPs are seen.
    - Posterior uveitis
      - □ Vitritis, intermediate uveitis, posterior uveitis, and retinal vasculitis can occur. Vitritis is the most common posterior segment manifestation. Choroidal nodules may be visible, and inflammation may produce CME and serous/exudative retinal detachment.

Periphlebitis may be associated with yellow perivenous exudates ("taches de bougie" or candle wax drippings).
- ■ Neurosarcoidosis
  - □ Patients with posterior segment disease may have associated CNS involvement leading to Babinski reflexes, spinal cord compression, and cranial nerve paresis.
- ■ Orbit/adnexae
  - □ Lacrimal gland involvement, the most frequently affected area of the orbit, can lead to dry eye disease. The lacrimal gland may be visibly enlarged. Extraocular muscles may show involvement leading to diplopia or painful external ophthalmoplegia.
- ● Diagnosis
  - ○ Chest x-ray
    - ■ Shows bilateral hilar lymphadenopathy, lung infiltration, and lung fibrosis
  - ○ Gallium scan
    - ■ Abnormal uptake in parotid and/or submandibular glands ("panda sign") and in the para-hilar and infrahilar lymph nodes along with the mediastinal lymph nodes ("lambda sign")
  - ○ Serology
    - ■ Angiotensin converting enzyme (ACE)
      - □ Elevated in 60% to 90% of patients with active sarcoidosis. ACE levels may be normal in subclinical disease.
    - ■ Hypercalcemia
      - □ Elevated in 10% to 15% of patients with sarcoidosis
    - ■ Lysozyme
      - □ Age-dependent increase over age 60 years. Will elevate as ACE elevates, but levels may be high in association with other conditions.
    - ■ Tissue
      - □ Transbronchial lung biopsy
        - • Mucosal and/or lung biopsy via fiberoptic bronchoscope. Four biopsies increase diagnostic yield to 90%.
      - □ Conjunctival biopsy
        - • Topical antibiotic and anesthetic is applied, and a tissue sample is removed using Westcott scissors. Suture closure is not required.
      - □ Lacrimal gland biopsy
        - • More fruitful if lacrimal glands are enlarged and in patients with positive gallium scan. Avoid palpebral lobe as it may lead to dry eye syndrome.
- ● Treatment
  - ○ Mild anterior uveitis may be treated with topical steroids and cycloplegics. If not responsive to topical therapy, sub-Tenon's and intravitreal steroids may be used, but systemic therapy may be required.
  - ○ Posterior uveitis is typically unresponsive to topical therapy and may require more immediate aggressive therapy.
- ● Prognosis
  - ○ Sarcoid-related uveitis can be visually debilitating, particularly those with chronic posterior disease.
  - ○ Complications such as glaucoma, CME, and epiretinal membrane can lead to vision loss.

Sympathetic Ophthalmia

- ● Etiology
  - ○ May be due to disruption of immune privilege and activity to S-antigen
- ● Signs/symptoms
  - ○ A bilateral panuveitis that develops following penetrating ocular trauma or surgery
  - ○ The onset of inflammation in the sympathizing eye (atraumatic) is usually 2 weeks to several months.
  - ○ The inflammatory process is usually granulomatous, producing cell, flare, and mutton-fat KPs in the anterior chamber (Figure 12-7).
  - ○ Posteriorly, vitritis, optic nerve edema, and vasculitis may be seen. Yellow choroidal lesions (the histopathologic Dalen-Fuchs nodules) can be present. Serous/exudative retinal detachment may occur.

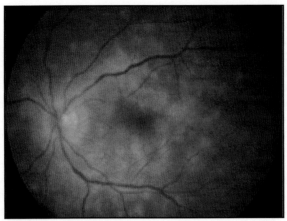

Figure 12-7. Multiple choroidal granulomas seen in sympathetic ophthalmia. (This figure was published in *Retina*. Ryan SJ, Ed. Copyright Elsevier [2006].)

- Diagnosis
  - Clinical and historical information is required.
  - High suspicion of sympathetic ophthalmia (SO) is required, particularly in the setting of penetrating ocular trauma or recent eye surgery with inflammation in the fellow eye.
- Treatment
  - Enucleation is the only known prevention of SO.
  - Must be done before autoimmunity begins
  - Steroids may be given topically or by sub-Tenon's or intravitreal injection for control of inflammation.
  - Systemic administration should also be considered.
  - If patients are steroid-resistant, cyclosporine and other cytotoxic agents may be considered.
- Prognosis
  - Rare condition, but can cause blindness if not treated appropriately and with vigilance.

Vogt-Koyanagi Harada Syndrome (Uveomeningitic Syndrome)

- Etiology
  - Experimental models show similarities between SO and Vogt-Koyanagi Harada (VKH); at the molecular level, susceptibility to melanocytic proteins may play a role. Affects Asians, Mestizos, and Hispanics. There may be a genetic susceptibility.
- Signs/symptoms
  - Ocular manifestations
    - Prodromal phase
      - Fever, headache, vertigo, and tinnitus; lasts several days
    - Acute uveitic phase
      - Bilateral granulomatous uveitis; thickened posterior choroid and disc hyperemia early on, with eventual development of disc edema. Harada syndrome is the combination of posterior uveitis, serous retinal detachment, and CSF pleocytosis. VKH syndrome is the bilateral iridocyclitis associated with vitiligo, poliosis, and auditory disturbance. The acute uveitic phase may last several weeks.
    - Convalescent phase
      - Depigmentation begins to occur, often within 1 month following onset of disease. Suigiura's sign is perilimbal vitiligo, seen mostly in Japanese patients. Yellow-white choroidal lesions, similar to Dalen-Fuchs nodules, can be seen in the midperiphery.
    - Chronic recurrent phase
      - Manifests commonly as anterior uveitis. Focal iris pigment atrophy and nodules may be seen. Chronic uveitis may result in cataract, glaucoma, retinal and optic disc neovascularization, and choroidal neovascularization.

- Systemic manifestations
  - Integumentary system
    - Alopecia, poliosis, and vitiligo
  - Nervous system
    - Headache, confusion, and meningismus; CSF pleocytosis with a predominance of lympho-cytes and monocytes
  - Auditory system
    - Hearing loss, often high frequencies, and vestibular dysfunction
- Diagnosis
  - There is no confirmatory test for VKH.
  - To aid diagnosis, the American Uveitis Society Criterion for diagnosis of VKH requires the ab-sence of previous ocular trauma or surgery and at least 3 or 4 of the following:
    - Bilateral chronic iridocyclitis
    - Posterior uveitis (exudative retinal detachment, disc hyperemia or edema, and sunset glow fundus)
    - Neurologic signs of tinnitus, meningismus, headache, cranial/CNS problem, or CSF pleo-cytosis, and/or
    - Alopecia, poliosis, or vitiligo
  - FA
    - Multiple pinpoint hyperfluoresence at the level of the RPE, which pool in areas of subretinal fluid
  - B-scan
    - Diffuse thickening of the posterior choroid, serous retinal detachment, and/or posterior thickening of the sclera
  - Lumbar puncture
    - CSF pleocytosis with a predominance of lymphocytes
- Treatment
  - Aggressive treatment with systemic steroids and possibly immunomodulatory agents is usually nec-essary to effectively control inflammation and prevent the sequelae of chronic ocular inflammation.
- Prognosis
  - Early therapy with the use of systemic steroids and immunosuppressive treatment yields a fair prognosis.
  - Poor predictors of outcome include increased age at disease onset, chronic inflammation requir-ing prolonged treatment with steroids, and choroidal neovascularization.

White Dot Syndromes

- Consist of several entities that present with varying degrees of inflammation, but all produce white lesions at the level of the choroid, RPE, or retina
- ICG for the lesions below all show hypofluoresence
- Treatment has not been standardized, but, for chronic cases, may require systemic immunosuppres-sion including, but not limited to, prednisone, azathioprine, or cyclophosphamide.
- A brief summary of each is provided.

Multiple Evanescent White Dot Syndrome

- Etiology
  - Multiple Evanescent White Dot syndrome (MEWDS) affects those aged 20 to 40 years, is seen in women more than men, and is associated with a viral prodrome.
- Signs/symptoms
  - Multiple white dots at the level of RPE/choroids (Figure 12-8)
  - Usually unilateral, may be asymmetrically bilateral
- Diagnosis
  - The FA reveals lesions that hyperfluoresce early and late; wreath-like pattern
- Prognosis
  - Vision returns to baseline

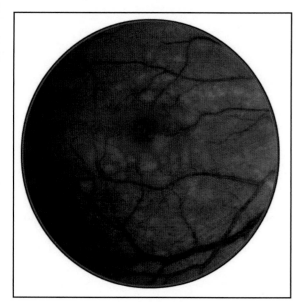

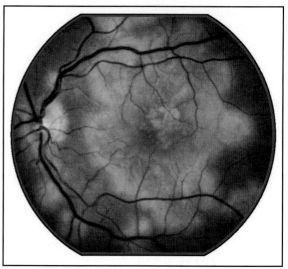

Figure 12-9. Multiple acute and resolving lesions associated with APMPPE. (This figure was published in *The Retina Atlas*. Yannuzzi LA, Guyer DR, Green WR. Copyright Elsevier [1995].)

Figure 12-8. Characteristic findings associated with MEWDS: granularity of the macula with whitish spots at the level of the RPE/choroid. (This figure was published in *The Retina Atlas*. Yannuzzi LA, Guyer DR, Green WR. Copyright Elsevier [1995].)

Acute Posterior Multifocal Placoid Pigment Epitheliopathy

- Etiology
  - Acute posterior multifocal placoid pigment epitheliopathy (APMPPE) affects patients aged 20 to 30, no sexual predilection, associated with severe viral prodrome
- Signs/symptoms
  - Bilateral, with yellow, placoid lesions (Figure 12-9)
- Diagnosis
  - FA demonstrates early hypofluoresence followed by late hyperfluoresence.
- Prognosis
  - Vision returns to baseline

Multifocal Choroiditis and Panuveitis Syndrome

- Etiology
  - Unknown; affects those from age 20 to 60 with greater preponderance among women
- Signs/symptoms
  - Bilateral, with iritis/vitritis, multiple punched-out lesions in midperiphery, CME
- Diagnosis
  - The FA demonstrates early hypofluoresence (blockage) with late staining; petalloid pooling in macula may be due to CME.
- Prognosis
  - Can be progressive and vision-threatening, particularly with CME or choroidal neovascularization

Birdshot Retinochoroidopathy

- Etiology
  - Unknown; affects patients aged 30 to 60, women much more than men; associated with HLA-A29 locus
- Signs/symptoms
  - Bilateral, with vitritis, and creamy white lesions that follow choroidal circulation; appear like "birdshot," often in midperiphery (Figure 12-10)

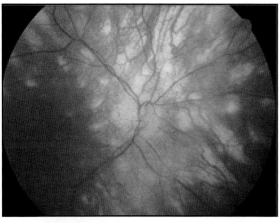

Figure 12-10. Characteristic findings of birdshot retinochoroidopathy showing the depigmented spots surrounding the optic disc. (This figure was published in *Retina*. Ryan SJ, Ed. Copyright Elsevier [2006].)

- Diagnosis
  - FA shows late staining of the lesions; disc hyperfluoresence
- Prognosis
  - Often diminished final vision; may be recurrent/progressive

Punctate Inner Choroidopathy

- Etiology
  - Unknown, affects individuals aged 20 to 40, with greater preponderance among women as compared to men
- Signs/symptoms
  - May be unilateral or bilateral, with multiple punctate chorioretinal lesions in the posterior pole
- Diagnosis
  - The FA shows early hyperfluoresence of the lesions.
- Prognosis
  - Diminished vision; CNV may occur

Serpiginous Choroiditis

- Etiology
  - Unknown, affects those aged 20 to 60 without sexual predilection
- Signs/symptoms
  - Bilateral, with yellow peripapillary lesions that are serpentine in appearance
- Diagnosis
  - FA demonstrates late hyperfluoresence of the lesions.
- Prognosis
  - Generally poor; disease is often chronic, progressive. CNV may occur. Vision may be stable if lesions do not involve the macula.

Phacogenic Uveitis

- Previously termed *phacolytic*, *phacoantigenic*, *phacotoxic*, and *phacoanaphylactic uveitis*
- Etiology
  - Lens-induced uveitis is a spectrum of disease.
  - May occur after trauma with exposure of lens proteins or in cases of hypermature cataract with leakage of lens protein through the lens capsule
- Signs/symptoms
  - Uveitis may be granulomatous or nongranulomatous.
  - Cell, flare, and KPs can be seen in the anterior chamber.
  - Hypopyon can be seen. The anterior lens capsule can be wrinkled or lacerated. The lens is typically opaque. Vitreous cell will develop if left untreated.

Figure 12-11. Snowbank seen in pars planitis. (This figure was published in *The Retina Atlas*. Yannuzzi LA, Guyer DR, Green WR. Copyright Elsevier [1995].)

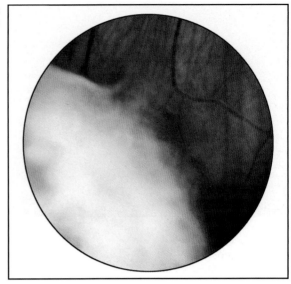

- Diagnosis
  - A clinical history of trauma or previous ocular surgery is often elicited. Additionally, an anterior chamber tap can be performed.
  - Histopathologic examination will reveal giant macrophages engorged with lens material.
- Treatment
  - Requires removal of lens material
  - Topical/systemic steroids and cycloplegia may be required.
- Prognosis
  - If the lens material is not removed, chronic inflammation may lead to glaucoma, neovascularization, macular edema, band keratopathy, and loss of the eye.

Idiopathic Intermediate Uveitis

- Etiology
  - Idiopathic inflammation without an associated underlying etiology (infectious, autoimmune, or medication-related) that primarily affects the ciliary body with some involvement of the anterior vitreous and peripheral retina
- Signs/symptoms
  - Patients may complain of floaters, occasionally mildly blurry vision.
  - Clinical examination may reveal a mild vitritis, snowballs, and snowbanking (collections of inflammatory cells in the inferior vitreous and on the pars plana, respectively) (Figure 12-11).
  - Peripheral vasculitis may be evident.
- Diagnosis
  - This is a diagnosis of exclusion, with emphasis placed on clinical findings. A chest x-ray may be helpful in evaluating for TB or syphilis.
  - Serologies include ACE, RPR, and FTA-ABS.
  - FA may reveal CME and peripheral vasculitis.
  - Differential diagnosis includes the following:
    - Bartonella
    - Syphilis
    - TB
    - Sarcoidosis
    - MS
- Treatment
  - Varies depending upon the degree of inflammation
  - Treatment options include topical steroid therapy (usually less effective), but IU usually requires periocular or intravitreal corticosteroids.

- o Systemic steroids and immune-modulating agents are also an option in refractory cases.
- o Pars plana vitrectomy can also be used to debulk the vitreous inflammation.
- o Retinal laser photocoagulation can be used to treat retinal neovascularization.
- Prognosis
  - o The typical course of pars planitis involves 3 major categories: a benign course, a chronic smoldering course, and a chronic progressive course involving the formation of cyclitic membranes and retinal detachment.
  - o Several studies indicate that the majority of patients suffer a waxing and waning course of disease.
  - o Good control of inflammation and management of complications such as CME and cataract can optimize visual potential.
  - o When considered as a separate group, children generally have a worse visual prognosis than adults.

Suggested Readings

Bodaghi B, LeHoang P. Ocular tuberculosis. *Curr Opin Ophthalmol.* 2000;11(6):443–448.

Bonfioli AA, Orefice F. Toxoplasmosis. *Semin Ophthalmol.* 2005;20(3):129–141.

Damico FM, Kiss S, Young LH. Sympathetic ophthalmia. *Semin Ophthalmol.* 2005;20(3):191–197.

Gaynor BD, Margolis TP, Cunningham ET. Advances in diagnosis and management of herpetic uveitis. *Int Ophthalmol Clin.* 2000;40(2):85–109.

Jones NP. Sarcoidosis and uveitis. *Ophthalmol Clin North Am.* 2002;15(3):319–326, vi.

La Hey E, de Jong PT, Kijlstra A. Fuchs' heterochromic cyclitis: review of the literature on the pathogenetic mechanisms. *Br J Ophthalmol.* 1994;78(4):307–312.

Prasad AG, Van Gelder RN. Presumed ocular histoplasmosis syndrome. *Curr Opin Ophthalmol.* 2005;16(6): 364–368.

Raja SC, Jabs DA, Dunn JP, et al. Pars planitis: clinical features and class II HLA associations. *Ophthalmology.* 1999;106(3):594–599.

Suhler EB, Martin TM, Rosenbaum JT. HLA-B27-associated uveitis: overview and current perspectives. *Curr Opin Ophthalmol* 2003;14(6):378–83.

Zaidman GW. The ocular manifestations of Lyme disease. *Int Ophthalmol Clin.* 1997;37(2):13–28.

Questions

1. The most common ocular manifestation of sarcoidosis is which of the following?
   a. Vitritis
   b. Periphlebitis with "candle wax drippings" seen on clinical examination
   c. CME with chronic posterior uveitis
   d. Anterior uveitis

2. A 25-year-old woman presents for her yearly examination. She has a history of contact lens wear but notes that her vision has not changed. On clinical examination, you find that she has one hazel-colored iris and one dark brown iris. There is mild anterior inflammation associated with stellate KPs on the corneal endothelium. Gonioscopic findings reveal the following:
   a. Pigmented trabecular meshwork
   b. Peripheral anterior synechiae
   c. Irregular iris insertion
   d. Fine vessels bridging the angle

3. ARN is most often associated with which of the following?
   a. *Borrelia burgdorferi*
   b. *Candida albicans*
   c. *Herpes zoster*
   d. *Treponema pallidum*

4. A patient presents with genital ulcers and an anterior uveitis with shifting hypopyon. She notes a history of an unusual rash on her legs. You decide to get a laboratory test in order to confirm your diagnosis. Which test would you order?
   a. HLA-A29
   b. HLA-B27
   c. HLA-B51
   a. HLA-DR5

5. Anterior uveitis is seen most commonly in which of the seronegative spondyloarthropathies?
   a. Ankylosing spondylitis
   a. Psoriatic arthritis
   b. Reiter syndrome
   c. Inflammatory bowel disease

6. The following are clinical features seen in ocular histoplasmosis *except*
   a. Peripapillary atrophy
   b. Peripheral granuloma
   a. Peripheral chorioretinal scars
   b. Macular chorioretinal scars

7. A patient presents with decreased vision in his left eye. He denies trauma or previous injury. Past medical history includes a history of oral candidiasis treated with fluconazole. A review of systems is positive for a recurrent cough, for which he takes Bactrim (sulfamethoxazole and trimethoprim). Clinical examination reveals multiple areas of retinal hemorrhage with minimal vitritis. What medication should be initiated promptly?
   a. Intravenous acyclovir
   b. Intravenous gancyclovir
   a. Oral acyclovir
   b. Oral valgancyclovir

8. The most common presentation of posterior disease in syphilitic uveitis is which of the following?
   a. Chorioretinitis
   a. Vitritis
   b. Phlebitis
   c. Optic neuritis

9. A young woman presents with decreased visual acuity and light sensitivity. Clinical examination reveals a dense vitritis with an ill-defined lesion in the peripheral retina adjacent to a chorioretinal scar. Which of the following is the likely etiologic agent?
   a. *T. pallidum*
   b. *T. gondii*
   c. *T. canis*
   d. *T. cati*

10. A middle-aged man recently returned from his summer home in Connecticut after a week of camping and fishing. He notes that since his return, he has had a fever and developed aches and pains all over his body. Moreover, he noticed a large red bump on the side of his arm, which appears to be surrounded by redness in a ring-like fashion. He states that he has never had arthritis, but his knees have also been bothering him. When questioned about his eyes and his vision, he states that the vision in his left eye is slightly blurry, but he is more concerned about the fever. What treatment would be indicated for this condition?
    a. Penicillin G
    b. Levofloxacin
    c. Gatifloxacin
    d. Doxycycline

Retina and Vitreous

13

T. Mark Johnson, MD, FRCS(C)

Outline

Probst LE, Tsai JH.
Ophthalmology: Clinical and Surgical Principles (pp. 479–522).
© 2012 SLACK Incorporated

Clinical Examination of the Retina

It is impossible to approach the patient with retinal disease without a complete and thorough mastery of the examination of the retina. Complete retinal examination includes both the clinical exam as well as adjuvant investigations that provide information regarding the anatomy and physiology of the retina, its vascular supply, and the choroid.

Symptomatology of the Patient With Retinal Disease

In its simplest form, the retina contains cells with 2 primary functions: rods that provide for peripheral and dim light vision and cones that provide central and color vision. The vitreous, while important in the development of the eye, undergoes progressive syneresis throughout life, leading to potential secondary complications resulting from vitreoretinal traction.

Floaters

- Opacities in the optical media of the vitreous
- Typically described as webs or spots in the visual field that track eye movements with a slight lag
- Floaters can result from a variety of processes.
    - Age-related vitreous syneresis/posterior vitreous detachment (PVD)
    - Hemorrhage in the vitreous
    - Inflammatory process involving the vitreous

Photopsia

- Photopsia are pinpoint flashing lights that may appear anywhere in the visual field.
- They are more often noticeable in dim light situations due to enhanced contrast.
- Photopsia may result from the following:
    - Vitreous traction on the retina
    - Retinal edema
    - Outer retinal inflammation

Distortion and Micropsia

- Distortion of lines is easily observed with the use of an Amsler grid.
- Any process that produces structural alteration of the macular anatomy will result in distortion.
- Distortion is usually nonspecific; however, central tapering of lines is usually indicative of a macular hole.
- Micropsia, or the perception of objects appearing smaller, results from elevation of the macula with relative preservation of the retinal architecture.
- In general, distortion results from the following:
    - Accumulation of material (blood, fluid, drusen) in the subretinal space
    - Edema of the retina secondary to vascular leakage
    - Structural distortion of the macula due to vitreoretinal traction (ie, epiretinal membrane [ERM], macular hole)

Visual Field Deficits and Nyctalopia

- Interruption of function of the peripheral rod systems will result in the perception of loss of peripheral visual field.
- Symptoms are typically more apparent under dim light conditions where rod function predominates.
- In general, peripheral visual field defects and nyctalopia can result from the following:
    - Peripheral retinal degenerations
    - Posterior uveitis with predominant peripheral retinal involvement
    - Progressive peripheral retinal ischemia
    - Peripheral retinal detachment

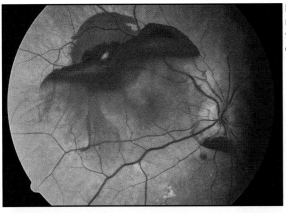

Figure 13-1. Patient with a ruptured retinal arterial macroaneurysm. Hemorrhage is present both above and below the retinal vessels, indicating the presence of both pre- and subretinal hemorrhage. This finding is typical of patients with macroaneurysms.

Clinicopathologic Correlations of Ophthalmoscopy

Clinical examination allows localization of pathology, development of a differential diagnosis, and selection of appropriate investigations. Examination typically involves examination at the slit lamp with a contact lens or handheld biomicroscopy lens (78 D or 90 D lens), binocular indirect ophthalmoscopy, and dynamic examination of the peripheral retina with scleral depression.

Localization of pathology relative to the retina is crucial in developing a differential diagnosis. The retinal blood vessels are located in the inner retina. They serve as a useful guide for the localization of pathology. Pathology located in the vitreous or preretinal or subinternal limiting membrane space will obscure the view of the retinal vessels. Pathology located in the outer retina, subretinal space, and choroids will allow the retinal vessels to pass over without obstruction.

While a vast number of disorders can result from retinal pathology, there are a limited number of appearances of pathology in the fundus. Recognition of characteristic pathologic processes allows the examiner to narrow the differential diagnosis.

The color of the pathology observed in the fundus often provides helpful clues to the underlying pathologic process.

- Red
  - Red lesions in the fundus typically result from vascular processes. These include proliferation of abnormal vessels, pathologic dilation of normal retinal blood vessels, and hemorrhages associated with either of these processes. Localization of hemorrhages relative to the retina is important in characterizing the pathology (Figure 13-1).
- White
  - White lesions in the fundus can indicate the formation of scar tissue (fibrosis), the presence of myelin, retinal edema of the inner retina (cotton wool spot), or retinal inflammation and necrosis (retinitis).
- Gray
  - Gray lesions are typically the result of significant edema of the outer retina, accumulation of subretinal fluid, or accumulation of abnormal metabolic materials in the retina.
- Yellow
  - Yellow lesions in the fundus include accumulation of lipid deposits (hard exudates and lipofuscin drusen).
- Black
  - Black lesions in the fundus are the result of retinal pigment epithelial hypertrophy that may be associated with scarring or degenerative processes or from the proliferation of melanocytic cells (nevi and melanoma).

Fluorescein Angiography

Interpretation of fluorescein angiography is central to the diagnosis and management of many retinal vascular problems. Understanding of the basic physiology of the test allows for simple interpretation and utilization in the development of differential diagnosis and management.

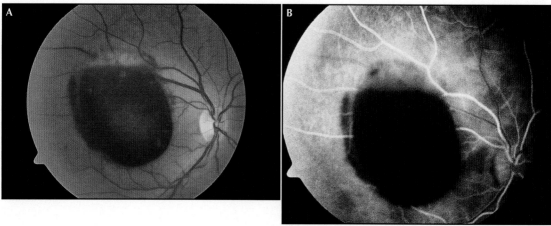

Figure 13-2. (A) Color photo of a patient with a preretinal hemorrhage. The blood obscures the view of the underlying retinal vessels, confirming the location of the hemorrhage relative to the retina. (B) Frame from fluorescein angiogram from the same patient. The hemorrhage blocks the view of the underlying retina. The blood vessel clearly lies beneath the hemorrhage.

Fluorescein Dye

- Sodium fluorescein
- Excites at 465 nm (blue), and emits at 525 nm (yellow green)

Phases of the Angiogram

- Choroidal filling occurs in 8 to 10 seconds with irregular patchy filling of the choroid that becomes more confluent with leakage from the choriocapillaris.
- Arterial filling occurs within 1 second of the choroidal filling.
- Venous filling begins with laminar flow.

Angiographic Terms

- Autofluorescence
  - Fluorescence that occurs with blue light illumination. Observed with optic disc drusen and lipofuscin accumulations over melanoma, Best's Disease
- Hyperfluorescence
  - An area characterized by increasing amounts of brightness during the study. Typical causes include leaking, dilated vascular structures, or an absence of pigment that normally blocks fluorescence.
- Hypofluorescence
  - An area characterized by an absence of normal fluorescence, also referred to as blocked fluorescence. Typical causes include accumulations of blood (Figure 13-2), subretinal fluid, or pigment.
- Leaking
  - An area characterized by increasing amounts of hyperfluorescence that increase both in intensity and size during the course of the study. Typical causes include neovascularization.
- Staining
  - An area that increases in intensity of fluorescence during the study but remains the same size. Typical causes include areas of retinal pigment epithelium (RPE) atrophy.
- Classic choroidal neovascularization
  - A well-defined area of early subretinal hyperfluorescence that leaks in the late frames of the angiogram
- Occult choroidal neovascularization
  - A poorly defined area of early hyperfluorescence that leaks late or an area of late leakage without a defined early source

Indocyanine Green Angiography

Indocyanine Green Dye

- Excites at 790 to 805 nm and emits at 835 nm
- High degree of protein binding prevents indocyanine green (ICG) from leaking from choriocapillaris, thus improving visualization of the choroidal vasculature.
- Longer wavelength allows penetration and emission through pigment and blood.'

Indocyanine Green Angiography

- Early phase occurs within 1 minute of dye injection.
  - o Medium and large choroidal vessels are visualized.
- Middle phase occurs 6 to 15 minutes after injection.
  - o Diffuse choroidal fluorescence appears.
- Late phase occurs 18 minutes after injection.
  - o Choroidal fluorescence fades, leaving vessels as hypofluorescent.
  - o Maximal contrast demonstrates abnormal hyperfluorescence.

High-Speed Indocyanine Green Angiography

- ICG is administered as a small bolus dose followed by flush.
- Scanning laser ophthalmoscope records images immediately following injection.
- Phi motion playback provides perception of continuous motion angiogram that concentrates on the early filling of the choroids.
- Allows for identification of "feeder vessels" that represent channels in the Sattler's layer of the choroids that preferentially fill choroidal neovascular membranes.

Optical Coherence Tomography

- Based on principles of low coherence interferometry
- Partially coherent, continuous 810-nm diode light serves as the optical beam that is divided into a beam directed into the eye and a reference beam.
- The time for reflection of the beam from the eye is compared to that of the reference beam by interference detected by a photosensor.
  - o The time for reflection determines the distance of the reflecting tissue.
  - o Analogous to an A-scan ultrasound using light rather than sound

Electrophysiology

Electroretinography

- Components of electroretinography (ERG)
  - o A wave
    - Initial negative deflection due to hyperpolarization of the photoreceptor cell
  - o B wave
    - Positive deflection due to Müller's cell depolarization
    - B wave is dependent upon the presence of the A wave.
    - Disorders of the inner retina will affect only the B wave but the not A wave.
  - o C wave
    - Prolonged negative deflection due to hyperpolarization of the RPE
    - Oscillatory potentials
      - High-frequency oscillations of the ascending B wave due to activity of the amacrine and interplexiform cells
      - May reflect inner retinal function

- Measuring the ERG
  - Photopic
    - Light adaptation bleaches the rods and isolates the cone responses.
  - Scotopic
    - Dark adaptation tests rods and cones; however, the rod response dominates.
    - Low-intensity (blue) stimulus isolates the rod response.
  - Flicker
    - Increasing stimulus frequency isolates cone responses.

Electrooculogram

- Measuring the electrooculogram (EOG)
  - Measures the electrical potential between the positive cornea and negative posterior pole
  - Eyes are swept between 2 lights located 30 degrees eccentric to a fixation light.
  - Electrodes are placed at medial and lateral canthi with a ground on the forehead.
  - Recorded with lights off for 15 minutes and on for 15 minutes.
  - Amplitude of response decreases in the dark to a trough at 8 to 12 minutes and increases in light to a peak at 6 to 9 minutes.
  - Arden ratio is the ratio of the light peak to the dark trough.
    - Normally more than 1.80

Hereditary Retinal Disease

Rod Cone Degenerations (Retinitis Pigmentosa)

- Epidemiology
  - Prevalence
    - In the United States, 1 in 3400
    - Highest prevalence in Navajo Indians (1 in 1800)
- Etiology
  - Autosomal dominant (10%)
  - Autosomal recessive (84%)
    - Family history may be difficult to document
  - X-linked (6%)
  - Multiple genetic defects have been described in rhodopsin, retinal degeneration slow gene/peripherin, retinal outer segment membrane protein 1 gene (ROM1), and other genes to produce the retinitis pigmentosa (RP) phenotype.
- Clinical features
  - Symptoms
    - Progressive nyctalopia
    - Later central vision loss
  - Signs
    - Posterior subcapsular cataract
    - Retinal vascular attenuation
    - Intraretinal pigment migration
    - Waxy optic nerve pallor
    - Cystoid macular edema (CME)
- Investigations
  - Visual field
    - Progressive visual field constriction
  - ERG
    - Initial depression of scotopic ERG with loss of rods
    - Later decline in photopic ERG
- Management
  - Vitamin A supplementation may slow progression.

Cone Rod Degenerations

Stationary Cone Rod Degenerations

- Complete rod monochromatism (achromatopsia)
  - Epidemiology
    - 1 in 30,000
  - Etiology
    - Autosomal recessive
    - Three identified genes
      - CNGA3 (25%)
      - CNGB3 (50%)
      - CNAT2 (2%)
  - Clinical features
    - Symptoms
      - Stable poor visual acuity (VA) (20/200)
      - Hemeralopia: Poorer vision in bright light
    - Signs
      - Pendular nystagmus
      - Absent foveal reflex

Progressive Cone Rod Degenerations

- Etiology
  - Autosomal recessive is most common form.
- Clinical features
  - Symptoms
    - Progressive visual and color vision loss
  - Signs
    - Progressive macular atrophy with development of bull's eye atrophy
- Investigations
  - Visual fields
    - Central scotoma
  - Color vision
    - Severe deutan–tritan defect
  - ERG
    - Progressive decline in photopic ERG with preserved scotopic ERG

Stargardt's Disease

- Etiology
  - Autosomal recessive defect in the ATP-binding transporter (ABCR) gene
  - Gene codes for an ABCR gene in the retina
- Clinical features
  - Symptoms
    - Progressive decreased VA
  - Signs
    - Initially, macula may appear normal.
    - Early atrophy produces "beaten metal" appearance (Figure 13-3A).
    - Progressive RPE atrophy may produce bull's eye appearance or progressive central geographic atrophy (Figure 13-3B).
    - Midperipheral pisciform yellow flecks
- Investigations
  - Fluorescein angiography
    - About 85% have early blocked choroidal fluorescence referred to as the "dark choroid phenomenon."
    - Later hyperfluorescence of atrophic areas

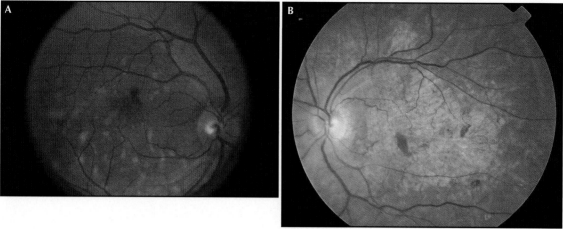

Figure 13-3. (A) Patient with early Stargardt's disease. Note yellow "pisciform" lesions in the macular region. VA is 20/30. (B) Same patient re-evaluated 20 years later demonstrates extensive macular atrophy. VA is now 20/400.

Best's Disease

- Etiology
  - Autosomal dominant
- Clinical features
  - Symptoms
    - Variable degree of visual impairment (20/30 to 20/200)
  - Signs
    - Various stages of maculopathy
      - Stage 0: Normal fundus with abnormal EOG
      - Stage 1: Fine speckled pigmentary changes in macula
      - Stage 2: Egg yolk lesion
      - Stage 3: Yellow fluid forms a level (pseudohypopyon) with later degenerative phase with lesion breaking up (scrambled egg)
      - Stage 4: Degenerative phase with atrophy, fibrosis, or secondary choroidal neovascular membrane (CNVM)
- Investigations
  - EOG
    - Marked depression
    - Carriers have abnormal EOG.

Diseases of the Macula

Age-Related Macular Degeneration

Dry Age-Related Macular Degeneration

- Epidemiology
  - Prevalence
    - Represents 80% of cases of age-related macular degeneration (AMD)
    - Increases with age
      - Patients older than 52 years—6%
      - Patients older than 75 years—20%
  - Incidence of CNVM
    - The 5-year incidence of development of CNV in patients with bilateral drusen is approximately 13%.

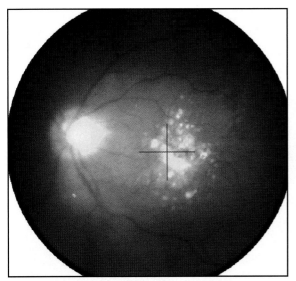

Figure 13-4. Patient with dry age-related macular degeneration. Extensive drusen are noted with areas of macular atrophy.

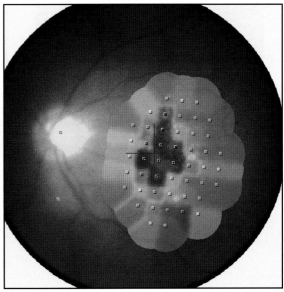

Figure 13-5A. Macular perimetry (MP1) of patient in Figure 13-4 shows focal central scotoma related to atrophic changes in the macula.

- o Risk factors
  - ▪ Family history
  - ▪ Light racial pigmentation
  - ▪ Smoking
  - ▪ Hypertension
  - ▪ Cardiovascular disease
- ● Clinical features
  - o Symptoms
    - ▪ Asymptomatic
    - ▪ Decreased vision
    - ▪ Distortion
  - o Signs
    - ▪ Drusen
      - □ Yellow subretinal deposits
    - ▪ Hard drusen: Well-defined yellow deposits (Figure 13-4)
    - ▪ Soft drusen: Ill-defined deposits (Figure 13-5A)
      - □ Coalescence produces drusenoid RPE detachment
    - ▪ Pigmentary hypertrophy
    - ▪ Geographic atrophy
      - □ Well-defined RPE and choriocapillaris leaving areas of visible deep choroids and sclera
- ● Investigations
  - o Fluorescein angiography (Figure 13-5B and 13-5C)
    - ▪ Indications
      - □ Rule out evidence of CNVM
    - ▪ Results
      - □ Soft drusen have pooling of dye under the drusen, resulting in late hyperfluorescence without leakage.
      - □ Areas of atrophy show well-defined choroidal staining.
- ● Management
  - o Antioxidant therapy
    - ▪ Indications
      - □ Extensive intermediate (63 to 124 μm) drusen
      - □ At least one large drusen (>124 μm)

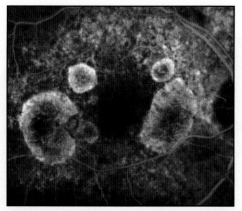

Figure 13-5B. Fluorescein angiogram of patient with dry AMD shows window defects in areas of atrophy.

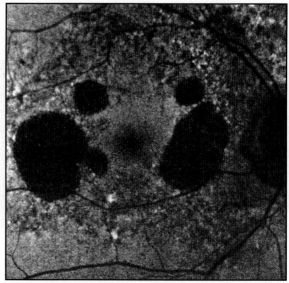

Figure 13-5C. Scanning laser autofluorescence demonstrated decreased autofluorescence in the areas of geographic atrophy.

- □ Noncentral geographic atrophy
- □ CVNM in fellow eye
- ■ Methods
  - □ Supplementation with high-dose beta carotene, vitamin C, vitamin E, and zinc
  - □ Smokers should receive zinc supplementation alone due to concerns about related lung cancers.
- ■ Results
  - □ Age Related Eye Disease Study (AREDS) demonstrated a significant reduction in the risk of development of advanced macular degeneration.
  - □ AREDS II study will examine the role of additional supplementation with lutein and omega-3 fatty acids.
    - • In addition, a lower-dose zinc arm will be included in the study.
- ○ Laser
  - ■ Macular laser has been observed to reduce the number of drusen evident in the macula.
  - ■ Initial clinical trials observed a reduction in drusen with a marginal visual benefit but possible increased risk of developing CNVM.
  - ■ Currently considered investigational
- ○ Future investigations
  - ■ Phase 2 clinical trials are ongoing with several pharmacologic agents.
    - □ Fenretinide
      - • Promotes renal clearance of retinol
      - • Hypothesis that reduction in retinol entering the RPE reduces the accumulation of toxic metabolites including apolipoprotein 2E (A2E)
      - • Phase 2 data suggest that a 300-mg dose may reduce progression of geographic atrophy.
    - □ Othera
      - • Downregulates expression of nuclear factor kappa B and thus may regulate inflammatory mediators in AMD
    - □ Manipulation of complement
      - • Phase 1 and 2 trials are examining the role of monoclonal antibodies and aptamers targeting complement component 3,5 and D.
    - □ Ciliary neurotrophic factor
      - • Encapsulated cell technology that may protect photoreceptors

Exudative (Wet) Age-Related Macular Degeneration

- Epidemiology
  - Prevalence
    - Accounts for 10% of macular degeneration
      - Accounts for the majority of legal blindness secondary to AMD
    - About 80% of legal blindness secondary to AMD is due to exudative AMD.
      - Prevalence of legal blindness in Caucasian population secondary to exudative AMD is 2.7/1000 people.
  - Incidence
    - The 5-year incidence of CNVM in patients with bilateral drusen is about 13%.
    - The 3-year incidence of CNVM in patients with unilateral CNVM is about 30%.
  - Risk factors
    - Family history
    - Smoking
    - Cardiovascular disease
    - Hypertension
- Clinical features
  - Symptoms
    - Decreased VA
    - Distortion
  - Signs
    - Subretinal fluid: Appears as turbid, gray elevation of retina
    - Subretinal hemorrhage
    - Lipid exudation: Typically at margins of exudation
    - Serous pigment epithelial detachment (PED): Dome-shaped elevation of RPE, may have a notch at the margin of the choroidal neovascular membrane
    - Fibrovascular PED: Irregular elevation of RPE, may have associated fibrosis
    - Subretinal fibrosis: Fibrotic tissue indicative of regressed choroidal neovascularization
- Investigations
  - Fluorescein angiography: Describes the pattern of the choroidal neovascularization
    - Location
      - Subfoveal
        - Located under the center of the fovea
      - Juxtafoveal
        - 1 to 199 μm from fovea
      - Extrafoveal
        - Greater than 200 μm from fovea
- Pattern of CNVM
  - Classic
    - Well-defined early hyperfluorescence with late leakage (Figure 13-6A and 13-6B)
  - Occult
    - Ill-defined early hyperfluorescence with late leakage or ill-defined late leakage with an obvious early source
- ICG angiography
  - Allows visualization of CNV through areas of blood, subretinal fluid, or PED
    - Plaque
      - More than 1 disc area of hyperfluorescence that is less intense than a hot spot
    - Hot spot
      - Bright hyperfluorescent lesion less than 1 disc area, typically indicative of retinal angiomatous proliferation (RAP) lesion or polypoidal CNV
  - High-speed ICG angiography
    - Uses rapid capture of the early perfusion of the retina; phi motion produces a continuous motion of early vascular flow, allowing visualization of arterial and venous flow of the CNVM
- Optical coherence tomography (OCT)
  - Visualize intraretinal edema, subretinal fluid, and PED

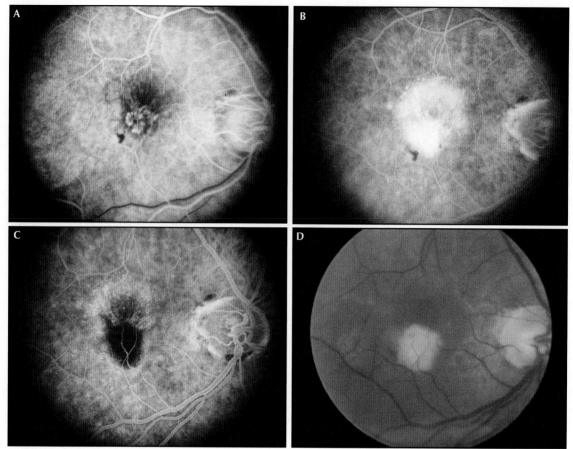

Figure 13-6. (A, B) Early and late fluorescein angiogram of patient with a well-defined CNVM with late leakage. (C) Color photo of patient immediately postlaser photocoagulation. (D) Postoperative fluorescein angiogram shows blockage of fluorescence with ablation of CNVM.

- Management
  - Focal laser (Figure 13-6)
    - Indications
      - Extrafoveal CNVM
      - Juxtafoveal
        - The scotoma generated by focal laser has led most practitioners to use alternative treatments.
      - Subfoveal CNVM
    - Methods
      - Confluent ablation of the entire CNV complex with treatment border of 100 µm beyond the CNV margin
    - Results
      - Treatment reduces the risk of severe visual loss (<20/200).
      - Treatment is associated with permanent scotoma.
      - While subfoveal macular photocoagulation study (MPS) trial showed better stabilization of vision with treatment, the scotoma and immediate visual decline has led to alternative therapies.
      - Recurrence rates are high.
        - Extrafoveal MPS had a 54% 5-year recurrence rate with the majority of recurrences extending into the fovea.
        - Recurrence is associated with a greater risk of visual loss.

- The overall utilization of laser has decreased significantly with advances in pharmaco-therapy.
- Focal laser ablation may still play some role in the management of select cases of CNVM.
  o Photodynamic therapy (PDT)
  - Indications
    - Subfoveal choroidal neovascularization
    - Juxtafoveal choroidal neovascularization
  - Methods
    - Intravenous infusion of verteporfin dye
      - Administer 6 mg/m^2
    - Application of 689-nm laser to lesion at 50 J/cm^2
    - Treatment is extended 300 to 500 μm beyond the border of the lesion.
  - Results
    - PDT slows the rate of visual loss with exudative AMD.
    - CNVM with more than 50% classic component may experience a greater benefit from treatment with PDT.
  o Transpupillary thermotherapy (TTT)
  - Indications
    - Subfoveal choroidal neovascularization
  - Methods
    - A 810-nm diode laser is applied to the entire CNVM to obtain light gray burn to the entire neovascular complex.
  - Results
    - Initial case series demonstrated promising results.
    - Randomized controlled trial (RCT) failed to show significant benefit for TTT in patients with AMD, and thus this treatment modality is largely obsolete.
  o Intravitreal antivascular endothelial growth factor (anti-VEGF) therapy
  - Indications
    - Monotherapy for choroidal neovascularization
    - Role in combination therapy
  - Methods
    - Available agents
      - Macugen (pegaptanib)
      - Lucentis (ranibizumab)
      - Avastin (bevacizumab)
    - Method of administration
      - Intravitreal injection
      - Frequency of dosing is generally every 4 to 6 weeks
    - Long-term dosing schedule is being studied.
  - Complications
    - Endophthalmitis
    - Cataract
    - Retinal detachment
    - Uveitis
  - Results
    - Macugen Trial (VISION Trial)
      - Clinical trials have demonstrated pegaptanib to be better than placebo at stabilizing visual loss.
        - About 70% of treated patients lost less than 15 letters of acuity over 2 years.
      - Repeated injections are required every 6 weeks.
      - Limited subset of patients regains VA.
    - Lucentis (ranibizumab) trials
      - Several RCTs of ranibizumab have been completed (MARINA, ANCHOR)
      - RCTs demonstrate that ranibizumab is superior to the natural history of CNVM and is superior to monotherapy with PDT.

- Patients with occult subfoveal CNVM treated with monthly intravitreal ranibizumab injections had a more than 90% rate of stabilization of vision.
  - Average visual improvement of 6 to 7 ETDRS letters
  - About 30% achieve better than 20/40 VA
- Controversy exists as to the optimal dosing schedule for anti-VEGF therapy.
  - ANCHOR and MARINA trials used monthly fixed dosing for 2 years.
  - PIER study used 3 monthly doses followed by quarterly injections.
    - Mean VA change of -0.2 letters at 12 months.
    - Suggests fixed, low-frequency dosing is inferior to monthly dosing
  - EXCITE study compared PIER dosing to fixed monthly dosing
  - At month 12, 4 to 5 letters were gained in low-frequency fixed dosing versus 8.3 letters in monthly dosing.
  - Individualized anti-VEGF studies (PrONTO, SUSTAIN, SAILOR) suggest that as needed dosing (PRN) treatment according to strict criteria-based retreatment may allow for adequate control of neovascularization with a reduction in number of overall treatments.
  - Optimal dosing regimen is not yet known.
  - □ Avastin (bevacizumab)
    - Case series of patients treated with Avastin intravenously and intravitreally have been reported.
    - Efficacy and safety approximating that observed in the ranibizumab trials coupled with a lower cost has led to widespread usage of bevacizumab.
    - A direct head-to-head trial of bevacizumab versus ranibizumab is being conducted (comparison of age-related macular degeneration treatment trial [CATT] study).
- o Intravitreal steroid
  - ■ Indications
    - □ Monotherapy for occult CNVM
    - □ Combination therapy with PDT, feeder vessel treatment
  - ■ Methods
    - □ Intravitreal injection
  - ■ Results
    - □ Case series describing combined use of triamcinolone with PDT suggest a prolonged treatment effect and possibly improved visual outcomes.
    - □ Use of triamcinolone as monotherapy is not well-supported by published studies.
- o Submacular surgery
  - ■ Indications
    - □ Unclear at present time
    - □ Subfoveal CNVM in elderly patient without significant drusen
  - ■ Methods
    - □ Vitrectomy with removal of the subfoveal CNVM
  - ■ Results
    - □ Submacular Surgery Trial did not show significant benefit to surgery compared with observation at 2-year follow up.
- o Macular translocation
  - ■ Indications
  - ■ Unclear at this time
- o Methods
  - ■ 360-degree translocation
    - □ Vitrectomy followed by cutting the retina 360 degrees, allowing a large degree of macular translocation
    - □ Secondary extraocular muscle surgery is required due to torsional diplopia.
  - ■ Limited translocation
    - □ Vitrectomy with creation of localized macular detachment
    - □ Scleral imbrication allows small degree of macular translocation.
  - ■ Results
    - □ Case series described benefit in selected patients; however, no RCT has been conducted to date.

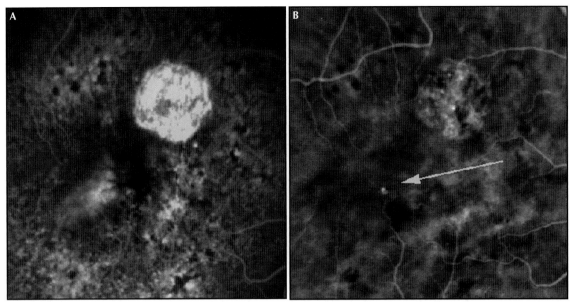

Figure 13-7. (A) Fluorescein angiogram demonstrating occult leakage inferonasally with cystoid macular edema. Small flecks of intraretinal hemorrhage block fluorescence. Clinical features are typical for a RAP lesion. Geographic atrophy is noted superiorly. (B) Single frame from high-speed ICG angiogram demonstrates small focus of intraretinal neovascularization (RAP).

Age-Related Macular Degeneration Variants

- RAP
  - o Variant of AMD believed to originate with intraretinal neovascularization rather than subretinal
  - o Epidemiology
    - Female > Male
    - Elderly
  - o Clinical features
    - Signs of AMD
    - Intraretinal hemorrhage (versus subretinal hemorrhage)
    - Cystic intraretinal edema
    - PED
    - Later development of subretinal neovascularization with retinal-choroidal anastamoses
  - o Classification
    - Stage I: Neovascularization confined to the neurosensory retina
    - Stage II: Neovascularization extending from the retina into the subretinal space
    - Stage III: Neovascularization extending from the retina into the choroid
  - o Investigations (Figure 13-7)
    - Fluorescein angiography
      - □ Majority have occult CNVM
    - ICG angiography
      - □ Focal hot spot
        - Intraretinal neovascularization
      - □ Plaque
        - Associated subretinal neovascularization
    - High-speed ICG
      - □ Demonstrates the intraretinal and subretinal components of neovascularization
    - OCT
      - □ Intraretinal cystic edema
      - □ Intraretinal neovascularization may be demonstrated in some cases.

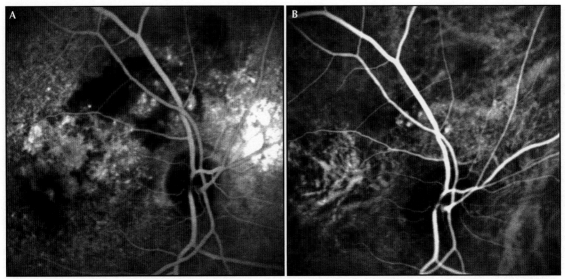

Figure 13-8. (A) Fluorescein angiogram shows subretinal hemorrhage and ill-defined leakage of dye superior to the optic nerve. Window defects consistent with macular drusen are present centrally. (B) ICG angiogram shows multiple focal hot spots typical of polypoidal neovascularization.

    o Management
        ■ Focal laser
        ■ PDT
        ■ Anti-VEGF therapy
    o Results
        ■ To date, no large trials have been conducted comparing treatment modalities.

Polypoidal Choroidal Vasculopathy

- Epidemiology
  - o Middle-aged woman
  - o More common in pigmented racial groups
  - o Association with hypertension
- Clinical features
  - o Large subretinal or sub-RPE hemorrhages
  - o Lesions center on optic nerve rather than fovea.
- Investigations (Figure 13-8)
  - o Fluorescein angiography
    - ■ Mainly occult CNV
  - o ICG angiography
    - ■ Focal hot spots in grape-like clusters
  - o High-speed ICG
    - ■ Central feeder vessel supplying dilated vascular clusters
- Management
  - o Focal laser
  - o Feeder vessel laser
  - o PDT
  - o Anti-VEGF therapy
- Results
  - o No comparative trials of therapy for polypoidal CNVM exist.

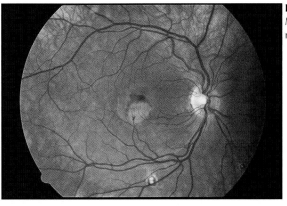

Figure 13-9. Subretinal hemorrhage secondary to CNV. Midperipheral circumscribed chorioretinal scars are evident inferiorly, typical of POHS.

Presumed Ocular Histoplasmosis Syndrome

- Epidemiology
  - ○ Predominates in watershed areas of major river systems (ie, Mississippi, Ohio)
  - ○ Approximately 2000/year in the United States lose central vision secondary to CVNM in presumed ocular histoplasmosis (POHS)
- Clinical features
  - ○ Symptoms
    - ▪ Asymptomatic
    - ▪ Symptomatic CNVM
  - ○ Signs
    - ▪ Signs of CNVM
      - □ Subretinal hemorrhage (Figure 13-9)
      - □ Fluid
    - ▪ Bilateral, punched-out midperipheral chorioretinal scars
    - ▪ Peripapillary atrophy
    - ▪ Linear areas of choroidal atrophy
    - ▪ No vitreous cells
- Investigations
  - ○ Fluorescein angiography
    - ▪ Peripheral chorioretinal scars show late staining
    - ▪ CNVM evident in macula
  - ○ High-speed ICG
    - ▪ Feeder vessel typically originates in the macular chorioretinal scar.
- Management
  - ○ Focal laser ablation
    - ▪ Indications
      - □ Extrafoveal CNVM
      - □ Juxtafoveal CNVM
    - ▪ Methods
      - □ Complete ablation of CNVM complex
    - ▪ Results
      - □ Laser ablation of CNVM prevents significant visual loss compared with observation.
        - • Has a 30% recurrence rate
      - □ Recurrences occur under fovea associated with more significant vision loss.
  - ○ PDT
    - ▪ Indications
      - □ Subfoveal CNVM
    - ▪ Results
      - □ No large trials exist.
      - □ Median VA and leakage seems to improve 2 years after PDT therapy with approximately 4 treatments.

- o Anti-VEGF therapy
  - ▪ Indications
    - □ Subfoveal CNVM
  - ▪ Results
    - □ Case series suggest that anti-VEGF therapy is efficacious in the treatment of CNVM in POHS.
- o Submacular surgery
  - ▪ Indications
    - □ Subfoveal CNVM
  - ▪ Methods
    - □ Small-gauge retinotomy with complete removal of CNVM complex
  - ▪ Results
    - □ Multiple case series suggest benefit to removal.
    - □ Recurrent neovascularization occurs.
    - □ RCT suggested possible benefit to surgery in patients with subfoveal CNVM and VA less than 20/100.

Central Serous Retinopathy

- • Epidemiology
  - o Risk factors
    - ▪ Type A personality
    - ▪ Male > Female (9:1)
    - ▪ Young to middle age
    - ▪ Corticosteroids
    - ▪ Mild hyperopia
- • Clinical features
  - o Symptoms
    - ▪ Decreased vision
      - □ Usually mild (50% better than 20/30)
    - ▪ Decreased color perception
    - ▪ Micropsia
    - ▪ Distortion
  - o Signs
    - ▪ Localized round or oval area of subretinal fluid
    - ▪ Subretinal yellow precipitates
    - ▪ PED
    - ▪ Pigmentary atrophy with previous episodes
- • Investigations
  - o Fluorescein angiography (Figure 13-10)
    - ▪ Focal hyperfluorescence with expanding late leakage
    - ▪ "Smokestack" leak is classic finding in central serous retinopathy (CSR) and is present in 15% of cases.
- • Management
  - o Observation
    - ▪ Majority of cases will resolve spontaneously in 12 to 16 weeks.
    - ▪ Recurrence occurs in 30% to 50% of cases.
  - o Focal laser
    - ▪ Indications
      - □ Prolonged CSR (greater than 16 weeks) with well-defined leakage point
      - □ Professional incapacity
    - ▪ Methods
      - □ Focal laser over the area of leakage
        - • 100- to 200-µm spot, long duration, low-intensity application
        - • Mild gray burn over the leak site

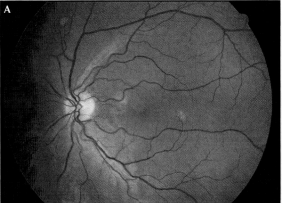

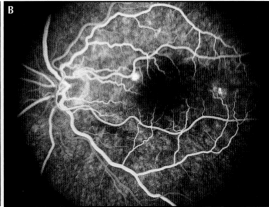

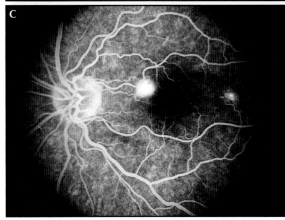

Figure 13-10. (A) Color photo of patient with CSR. Blister of subretinal fluid is present in the macula. Temporal RPE depigmentation suggestive of previous episodes of CSR. (B) Early fluorescein angiogram frame shows hyperfluorescence superonasally. Window defects are present temporally at prior site of CSR leakage. (C) Late fluorescein angiogram frame shows progressive leakage superonasally.

Epiretinal Membranes

- Etiology
  - Idiopathic
  - Branch/central retinal vein occlusion
  - Uveitis
  - Trauma
  - Proliferative vitreoretinopathy
- Clinical features
  - Symptoms
    - Decreased vision
    - Metamorphopsia
  - Signs (Figure 13-11)
    - Glistening sheen over macula with associated retinal vascular distortion
    - Retinal edema
    - Cystoid retinal changes
    - Pseudohole
- Investigations
  - Fluorescein angiography
    - Retinal vascular distortion
    - Late intraretinal leakage
  - OCT
    - ERM is demonstrated on retinal surface.
    - Associated intraretinal edema and distortion
    - Pseudohole appears as abrupt break in ERM.

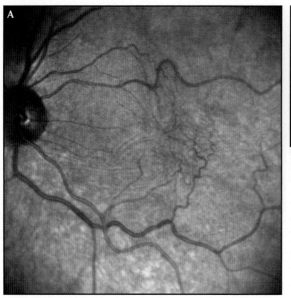
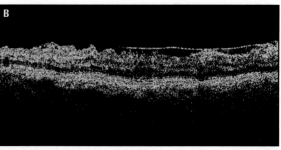

Figure 13-11. (A) Infrared photo of patient with ERM demonstrates retinal striae secondary to contracture of membrane. (B) Horizontal OCT of same patient shows distortion of retina with visible ERM.

- Management
  - Vitrectomy
    - Indications
      - Symptomatic decreased vision with ERM
    - Methods
      - Pars plana vitrectomy with stripping of ERM complex
    - Results
      - About 87% have improved VA
      - Better visual outcome with
        - Preoperative VA > 20/100
        - Thin ERM
        - Absence of traction retinal detachment
        - Shorter symptom duration

Vitreomacular Traction Syndromes

- Etiology
  - Idiopathic
  - Uveitis
  - Diabetic retinopathy
- Clinical features
  - Symptoms
    - Decreased vision
    - Distortion
  - Signs
    - Incomplete PVD
    - ERM in 50% of cases
    - Tractional detachment of fovea
- Investigations
  - OCT
    - Demonstrates persistent vitreous adhesion to macula with associated traction on fovea (Figure 13-12)
    - May have associated retinal detachment

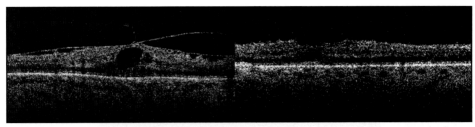

Figure 13-12. Pre- and postvitrectomy OCT of patient with ERM and vitreomacular traction syndrome. Note preoperative cystoid macular edema and insertion of posterior hyaloid into the ERM complex.

- Management
  - Vitrectomy
    - Indications
      - Symptomatic VMT
    - Methods
      - Pars plana vitrectomy with complete removal of posterior hyaloid and ERM

Macular Hole

- Epidemiology
  - Prevalence
    - Less than 1% of the population
  - Risk factors
    - Female > Male
    - About 10% of cases are bilateral.
- Etiology
  - Idiopathic
    - May represent an advanced form of vitreomacular traction
      - Trauma
      - High myopia
- Clinical features
  - Symptoms
    - Decreased vision
      - Correlates with the size of the hole
    - Distortion
  - Signs
    - Full-thickness defect in the macula with central yellow deposits in the base of the hole
    - Watzke Allen sign
      - A thin slit-lamp beam placed across the hole is perceived as having a gap.
      - Commonly, patients perceive a narrowing of the beam rather than a complete gap.
    - Cuff of retinal edema or subretinal fluid
    - Associated ERM
- Classification
  - Stage 1: Central yellow spot or ring with flattening of the foveal depression
  - Stage 2: Eccentric, oval full-thickness hole
  - Stage 3: Complete, round full-thickness hole without PVD
  - Stage 4: Full-thickness hole with PVD
- Investigations
  - Autofluorescence imaging
    - Increased autofluorescence due to absence of macular xanthophyll
  - Fluorescein angiography
    - Window defect at base of hole
  - OCT
    - Complete gap in retina with associated intraretinal edema and subretinal fluid at margin (Figure 13-13)

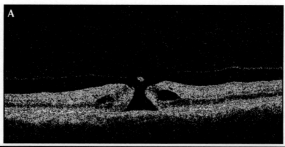

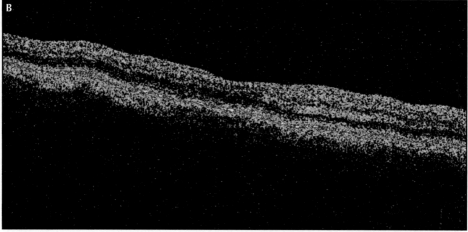

Figure 13-13. (A) Horizontal OCT shows full-thickness macular hole with perifoveal vitreous separation. Centrally, there is vitreous condensation consistent with clinically observed pseudo-operculum. (B) Postvitrectomy OCT shows complete closure of macular hole.

- Management
  - Vitrectomy
    - Indications
      - Stage 2, 3, or 4 hole
    - Methods
      - Pars plana vitrectomy with removal of posterior hyaloid and ERM
      - Removal of internal limiting membrane appears to increase success rate but may delay visual recovery.
      - Gas tamponade with facedown positioning
    - Results
      - A 80% to 90% single-procedure macular hole closure rate reported
      - Predictors of anatomic success and visual improvement
        - Shorter duration hole (<6 months)
        - Smaller diameter hole (<400 μm)

Cystoid Macular Edema

- Epidemiology
  - Prevalence
    - Varies with the underlying cause and definition
      - Intermediate uveitis: 30%
      - Postcataract angiographic CME: 50%
      - Postcataract CME with VA <20/40: 8%
- Etiology
  - Congenital
    - RP
    - Autosomal dominant CME
    - Familial exudative vitreoretinopathy

- o Acquired
    - Central/branch retinal vein occlusion (BRVO)
    - Diabetic retinopathy
    - Perfoveal telangiectasias
    - Uveitis
    - Postsurgical
    - ERM/vitreomacular traction
    - Drugs
        - □ Nicotinic acid
        - □ Prostaglandin analogues
        - □ Topical epinephrine
- Clinical features
    - o Symptoms
        - Decreased vision
        - Micropsia
    - o Signs
        - Visible cystic changes in macula
- Investigations
    - o Fluorescein angiography
        - Late fluorescein leakage into cystic intraretinal spaces
    - o OCT
        - Demonstrates intraretinal cystoid spaces
        - Able to demonstrate vitreomacular traction
- Management
    - o Observation
        - Many cases of postcataract CME will resolve without treatment.
        - Treatment is indicated with prolonged CME with visual impairment.
    - o Topical nonsteroidal anti-inflammatory drug (NSAID)
        - Demonstrated to be beneficial in prolonged postoperative CME
        - Typically given as 3- to 6-week course of treatment
        - Longer courses may be required in chronic cases of CME
    - o Topical steroids
        - Often combined with topical NSAID
        - Traditional experience suggests benefit; however, no comparative trials have been conducted
    - o Injectable steroids
        - Used in cases of prolonged CME
        - Can be administered as sub-Tenon's or intravitreal injection
    - o Laser
        - Nd:YAG vitreolysis can be performed to divide vitreous strands in the anterior chamber
    - o Surgery
        - Vitrectomy with meticulous removal of vitreous incarceration in anterior segment
        - Multicentered prospective trial demonstrated benefit in aphakic patients with chronic CME (>6 months) and vitreous incarceration.
        - Case series demonstrate benefit in pseudophakic CME with anterior prolapsed vitreous.

Retinal Vascular Disease

Diabetic Retinopathy

- Epidemiology
    - o Prevalence
        - Prevalence of diabetes is increasing
        - Estimated prevalence of diabetes in the United States is approximately 8% of the total population.
            - □ About 30% of patients are undiagnosed.

- All diabetics will develop some retinopathy.
- The prevalence of retinopathy varies with the following:
  - Type of diabetes
  - Duration of diabetes
    - Type I diabetes
      - >10 years duration: 70% have retinopathy
      - >30 years: 95% have retinopathy
    - Type II diabetes
      - >16 years: 60% have retinopathy
- Incidence
  - 10-year incidence of retinopathy
    - Type I diabetes without retinopathy at baseline
      - 89% will develop some retinopathy
    - Type II diabetes without retinopathy at baseline
      - 79% will develop some retinopathy
- Clinical features
  - Symptoms
    - Asymptomatic
    - Decreased VA
    - Floaters
  - Signs

Nonproliferative Diabetic Retinopathy

- Retinal microaneurysms: Outpouchings of the capillary walls
- Dot and blot-shaped hemorrhages
- Venous caliber changes: Venous "beading" and tortuosity
  - Indicative of increasing retinal edema
- Intraretinal microvascular abnormalities (IRMA): Composed of early neovascularization within the retina or shunting vessels in of poor capillary perfusion
- Cotton-wool spots: Infarctions in the nerve fiber layer of the retina
- Higher risk of progression to proliferative retinopathy with the following:
  - Severe retinal hemorrhages in 4 quadrants
  - Venous beading in 2 quadrants
  - IRMA in 2 quadrants

Proliferative Diabetic Retinopathy

- Neovascularization: On or near the optic disc (NVD) or elsewhere (NVE), often located at the watershed zone between perfused and nonperfused retina (Figure 13-14)
- High-risk proliferative retinopathy
  - Any neovascularization with vitreous hemorrhage
  - Neovascularization greater than half the disc area
- Fibrovascular proliferation: Often beginning at the optic disc and vascular arcades
- Preretinal hemorrhage: Adjacent to or within areas of neovascularization
- Vitreous hemorrhage
- Tractional retinal detachment
- Rhegmatogenous retinal detachment: From retinal tears and holes secondary to traction

Diabetic Macular Edema

- CME: Leakage of capillaries into cystoid spaces within the outer plexiform layer of the retina (Figures 13-15A to 13-15C)
- Retinal thickening: Within or adjacent to the center of the macula
- Hard exudates: Lipid that precipitated as intraretinal fluid was absorbed
- Clinically significant macular edema
  - Retinal thickening within 500 μm of center of foveal avascular zone (FAZ)
  - Hard exudates within 500 μm from center of FAZ associated with retinal thickening
  - Retinal thickening more than 1 disc diameter within 1 disc diameter of the center of the FAZ

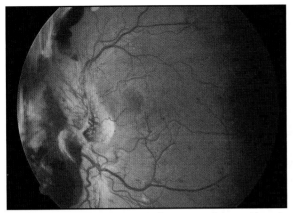

Figure 13-14. Extensive neovascularization of disc with early fibrosis and preretinal hemorrhage.

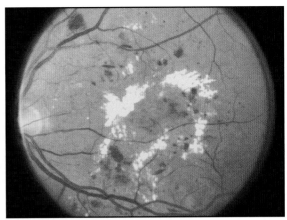

Figure 13-15A. Color photo demonstrates retinal edema with hard exudates and microaneurysms.

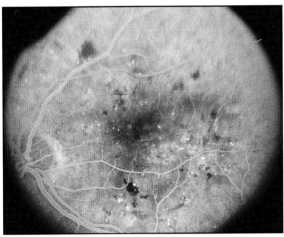

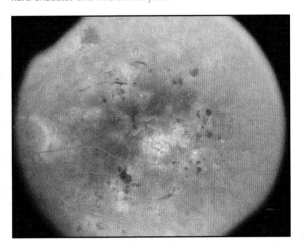

Figures 13-15B and 13-15C. Fluorescein angiogram demonstrates microaneurysms in early frame with extensive leakage in late frame. Early cystoid macular edema is present.

- Investigations
  - Fluorescein angiography
    - Diabetic macular edema (DME)
      - Hyperfluorescent microaneurysms with late leakage
      - Diffuse late leakage
        - Generalized vascular leakage
        - Associated with midperipheral capillary nonperfusion
      - Capillary nonperfusion
    - Proliferative retinopathy
      - Early, preretinal vascular complexes that leak diffusely late
      - Occur at margin of perfused and nonperfused retina
  - OCT
    - Can localize and determine the extent of macular edema
      - Volumetric maps may be useful in monitoring therapy
    - Can determine the extent of tractional forces on the retina from fibrovascular proliferation
  - Ultrasonography
    - Indicated if posterior segment cannot be visualized due to vitreous hemorrhage or other media opacification
- Management
  - Prevention
    - Indications
      - Primary and secondary prevention of retinopathy

- Methods
  - Intensive therapy to maintain glucose control
  - Hemoglobin A1C should be maintained less than 7%.
- Results
  - Large trials demonstrate beneficial effects of excellent glycemic control in type I and type II diabetes.
- Ophthalmic screening eye examination
  - Baseline exam
    - Type I: 5 years after onset or in puberty
    - Type II: At time of diagnosis
  - Follow up is determined by the severity of retinopathy
    - One-year incidence of progression to proliferative diabetic retinopathy (PDR)
      - Mild nonproliferative diabetic retinopathy (NPDR): 0.8%
      - Moderate NPDR: 3%
      - Severe NPDR: 40%
- Laser photocoagulation
  - Focal laser treatment indications
    - Indications
      - Clinically significant macular edema
    - Methods
      - Focal application of laser to microaneurysms to achieve light blanching
      - Grid laser may be applied to areas of diffuse retinal thickening.
    - Results
      - Randomized trial of laser has demonstrated a significantly reduced risk of visual loss with laser therapy.
        - Fewer patients regained significant amounts of vision.
      - Focal laser may be less effective in cases of extensive diffuse macular edema.
  - Panretinal photocoagulation (PRP)
    - Indications
      - High-risk PDR
      - Non–high-risk PDR in patients with poor compliance
      - Severe NPDR in select patients
    - Methods
      - 1600 to 2000 200-μm burns in retinal periphery
      - Multiple sessions reduce risk of choroidal effusion.
    - Results
      - PRP reduces the risk of severe visual loss in patients with high-risk PDR.
      - PRP reduces risk of severe visual loss in non–high-risk PDR and severe NPDR; however, the risk of severe visual loss is lower in these patient groups.
- Corticosteroids
  - Indications
    - Nonresponsive macular edema
  - Methods
    - Intravitreal or sub-Tenon's triamcinolone
  - Results
    - Numerous case series demonstrate clear reduction in retinal edema.
      - No large randomized trials published to date
    - May be associated with significant visual improvement in some cases
    - Effects of treatment may be transient with edema recurring in 4 to 6 months.
    - Comparative trial of steroids versus focal laser demonstrated that laser at the 2-year endpoint yielded better visual results.
      - Thus, steroids may play a role of adjunct therapy but are not likely to be effective as monotherapy.

- o Anti-VEGF therapy
  - ▪ Indications
    - □ Neovascular glaucoma
    - □ Macular edema
    - □ Retinal neovascularization
  - ▪ Methods
    - □ Intravitreal injection
  - ▪ Results
    - □ Case series indicate that anti-VEGF therapy may be useful in controlling anterior segment neovascularization and macular edema.
    - □ Anti-VEGF therapy may offer possibility of visual improvement as monotherapy or as adjunct therapy to patients with DME
      - • READ2 study suggests that ranibizumab therapy in patients with chronic macular edema may be superior to laser therapy.
      - • RESTORE study showed an average visual improvement of 6 letters in ranibizumab monotherapy, 5.9 letters in ranibizumab plus laser therapy, and 0.8 letters in laser monotherapy.
- o Surgical
  - ▪ Indications
    - □ Nonclearing vitreous hemorrhage
    - □ Vitreomacular traction with visual loss
    - □ Tractional retinal detachment
  - ▪ Methods
    - □ Pars plana vitrectomy
    - □ Complete removal of posterior hyaloid and associated ERM
    - □ Complete photocoagulation

Branch Retinal Vein Occlusion

- • Epidemiology
  - o Prevalence
    - ▪ Second most common retinal vascular disorder after diabetic retinopathy
    - ▪ Over 90% of retinal vein occlusions occur in patients over the age of 50.
  - o Risk factors
    - ▪ Hypertension
    - ▪ Cardiovascular disease
    - ▪ Glaucoma
- • Clinical features
  - o Symptoms
    - ▪ Painless, unilateral sudden decrease in VA
    - ▪ Partial loss of visual field
    - ▪ Asymptomatic especially if located nasally
  - o Signs
    - ▪ Flame-shaped intraretinal hemorrhages and venous tortuosity in the distribution of the obstructed vein
      - □ Obstruction occurs at site of arteriovenous crossing
      - □ Distribution of hemorrhages is typically triangular with the apex pointing to the site of obstruction
    - ▪ Macular edema
    - ▪ Cotton wool spots
    - ▪ Collateral vessels
      - □ Extend across the horizontal raphe
    - ▪ Retinal neovascularization, at the borders of perfused and nonperfused retina
    - ▪ Vitreous hemorrhage
    - ▪ Tractional retinal detachment, rarely
    - ▪ Iris neovascularization, rarely

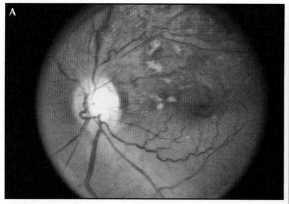

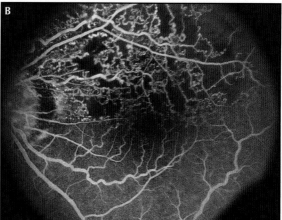

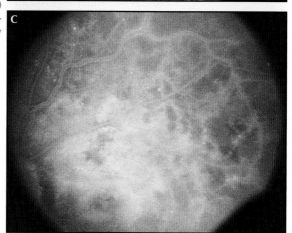

Figure 13-16. (A) Intraretinal hemorrhage, cotton wool spots, and retinal edema secondary to superotemporal BRVO. (B) Early FA shows extensive capillary nonperfusion. (C) Late intraretinal leakage with cystoid macular edema centrally secondary to BRVO.

- Investigations (Figure 13-16)
  - Fluorescein angiography
    - Blockage from intraretinal hemorrhages
    - Macular edema with diffuse leakage
    - Capillary nonperfusion
  - OCT
    - Can localize and determine the extent of macular edema
    - Can determine the extent of tractional forces on the retina from fibrovascular proliferation
  - Ultrasonography
    - Indicated if posterior segment cannot be visualized due to vitreous hemorrhage or other media opacification
  - Gonioscopy
    - To identify angle neovascularization
- Management
  - Laser photocoagulation
    - Indications
      - Perfused macular edema with VA <20/40 for greater than 3 months duration
      - Retinal neovascularization
      - Extensive nonperfusion in noncompliant patients
    - Methods
      - Macular grid for edema
        - 50- to 100-μm low-intensity burns in the area of edema
      - PRP for neovascularization
        - 200- to 500-μm burns in the sectors of retinal nonperfusion

- Results
  - Grid laser significantly improves the chances of gaining 2 or more lines of VA compared to observation.
    - Average VA is better with treatment.
  - PRP reduces the risk of neovascularization; however, given that neovascularization responds well to PRP, treatment is usually reserved for cases with neovascularization.
- Corticosteroids
  - Indications
    - Nonresponsive macular edema
  - Methods
    - Intravitreal triamcinolone
  - Results
    - Case series report benefit with reduction of CME and improved visual function.
    - SCORE study examined the role of preservative-free triamcinolone versus grid laser for macular edema in BRVO.
      - No difference in visual outcome with 26% to 29% of patients gaining 15 letters of VA.
      - Higher rate of elevation of intraocular pressure (IOP) and cataract in the 4-mg triamcinolone group
    - Limited duration of effect
- Anti-VEGF therapy
  - Indications
    - Retinal neovascular
    - Macular edema
  - Methods
    - Intravitreal injection with bevacizumab
  - Results
    - Case series indicate that anti-VEGF therapy may be useful in controlling neovascularization and macular edema.
    - BRAVO Trial was a 12-month trial consisting of an initial 6-month treatment phase and a 6-month observation phase with PRN treatment.
      - Patients receiving 6 months of intravitreal ranibizumab have significantly better visual improvement and greater reductions in OCT central retinal thickness compared with sham treatment arm.
      - Patients in sham group receiving treatment during the observation phase of the study do gain vision but do not appear to match gains achieved with early therapy.
- Surgical
  - Indications
    - Nonresponsive macular edema
    - Nonclearing vitreous hemorrhage
  - Methods
    - Pars plana vitrectomy with induction of PVD
    - Decompression of arteriovenous crossing
  - Results
    - Case series show possible benefit to arteriovenous crossing
    - Induction of PVD alone may be beneficial

Central Retinal Vein Occlusion

- Epidemiology
  - Prevalence
    - Occurrence in patients older than 50 years—90%
  - Risk factors
    - Glaucoma
    - Hypertension
    - Diabetes mellitus

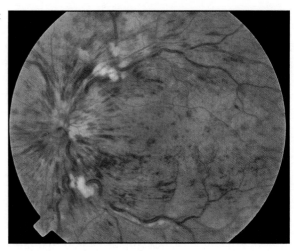

Figure 13-17. Intraretinal hemorrhage with venous engorgement in all 4 quadrants of fundus typical of CRVO.

- Clinical features
  - Symptoms
    - Sudden onset of painless, unilateral decrease in VA
    - Worse VA in ischemic form of central retinal vein occlusion (CRVO), better VA in the non-ischemic form
  - Signs
    - Pupil
      - Afferent pupillary defect more consistent with ischemic retina
    - Iris
      - Neovascularization with ischemic retinopathy
      - Occurs in 50% to 80% of nonperfused CRVO
    - Retina
      - Flame-shaped and blot-shaped intraretinal hemorrhages and venous tortuosity in all quadrants of the retina (Figure 13-17)
      - Macular edema with CME
      - Cotton wool spots
      - Optic disc swelling
      - Later collateral vessels form at optic disc
- Investigations
  - Fluorescein angiography
    - Blockage secondary to intraretinal hemorrhage
    - Capillary nonperfusion
      - Greater than 10 disc areas increases risk of neovascularization
    - Late intraretinal leakage
  - Systemic workup
    - In patients less than 50 years
      - Complete blood count (CBC)
      - Protein C and S deficiency
      - Antithrombin III deficiency
      - Activated protein C resistance (Factor V Leiden mutation)
      - Anticardiolipin antibodies
      - Lupus anticoagulant
- Management
  - Laser photocoagulation
    - Indications
      - Secondary iris or retinal neovascularization
      - Macular edema in younger patients

- Methods
  - Macular grid laser for macular edema
  - PRP for neovascularization
- Results
  - Macular grid reduces retinal edema
    - Visual benefit is limited.
    - Visual recovery may be more likely in patients less than 60 years.
  - PRP is indicated in patients with neovascularization and regresses iris neovascularization
  - PRP may be considered in cases of extensive nonperfusion with poor follow up.
- Corticosteroids
  - Indications
    - Extensive macular edema
  - Methods
    - Intravitreal corticosteroids
  - Results
    - Case series indicate benefit in selected patients.
    - SCORE study compared treatment with preservative-free triamcinolone to observation in the treatment of macular edema secondary to CRVO.
      - At 12 months, treated patients were significantly more likely to gain 15 letters of VA compared to sham (27% versus 7%).
      - Treatment with 4-mg dose was associated with a higher rate of elevated IOP and cataract.
- Anti-VEGF therapy
  - Indications
    - Neovascular glaucoma
    - Macular edema
  - Methods
    - Intravitreal injection with bevacizumab
  - Results
    - Case series indicate that anti-VEGF therapy may be useful in controlling anterior segment neovascularization and macular edema.
    - CRUISE study was a 12-month study of macular edema secondary to CRVO.
      - Patients underwent a 6-month treatment phase and a 6-month observation phase with PRN treatment.
      - Patients treated with monthly ranibizumab were significantly more likely to gain 15 letters of acuity and were more likely to have significant reductions in OCT retinal thickness compared to sham treatment.
      - Patients receiving delayed treatment gained vision but did not appear to match the gains of patients undergoing early therapy.
- Creation of chorioretinal anastamoses
  - Indications
    - Perfused CRVO with retinal edema
    - Possibly nonperfused CRVO
  - Methods
    - Laser
      - High-intensity small spot size laser burn breaking Bruch's membrane and inducing anastamoses
    - Surgical
      - Radial incision at the margin of the optic nerve triggering anastamoses between choroid and retina
  - Results
    - Multiple techniques for creation of anastamoses exist.
      - No clearly reproducible technique for all cases
    - Creation of anastamoses improves vascular flow.
    - Visual improvement depends upon macular perfusion.
    - May be associated with complications

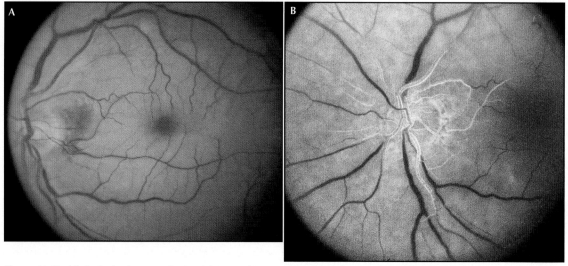

Figure 13-18. (A) Retinal edema producing "cherry red spot" in patient with central retinal artery occlusion. (B) Fluorescein angiogram shows delayed perfusion in patient with CRAO.

Retinal Arterial Occlusion

- Epidemiology
  - Risk factors
    - Cardiac risk factors: hypertension, smoking, elevated cholesterol
- Clinical features
  - Symptoms
    - Sudden painless visual loss
  - Signs (Figure 13-18)
    - Afferent pupillary defect
    - Pale retinal edema
      - Central artery occlusion is associated with "cherry red spot" due to visible choroidal flow.
    - Arterial narrowing with sluggish venous flow producing "boxcarring"
    - Retinal embolus
- Investigations
  - Fluorescein angiography
    - Delayed arterial filling with sluggish venous flow
  - ERG
    - Reduced B wave with normal A wave due to ischemia in inner retina
  - Ultrasound
    - Investigation of potential carotid artery disease
  - Management
    - Lower IOP
      - Glaucoma drops
      - Anterior chamber paracentesis
    - Fibrinolytic agents
      - No large trials exist
      - Potential for secondary hemorrhagic complications
    - Laser clot lysis
      - YAG laser disruption of intra-arterial clot

Radiation Retinopathy

- Epidemiology
  - Prevalence
    - Prevalence varies with the total dose of radiation and duration of follow up.
    - Onset average of 18 months postexposure
  - Risk factors
    - Higher radiation dose (usually >3000 rads)
    - Diabetes
    - Adjuvant chemotherapy may reduce tolerable dose of radiation
- Clinical features
  - Symptoms
    - Asymptomatic
    - Decreased vision
  - Signs (see Figure 13-18A)
    - Retinal vascular telangiectasia
    - Retinal edema with CME and hard exudates
    - Secondary neovascularization
- Investigations
  - Fluorescein angiography (see Figure 13-18B)
    - Capillary nonperfusion
      - Nonperfusion may be more common with external beam radiation
    - Late intraretinal leakage
- Management
  - Intravitreal steroids
  - Focal laser

Parafoveal Telangiectasias

- Epidemiology
  - Risk factors
    - Radiation exposure
    - Diabetes
- Clinical features
  - Symptoms
    - Decreased vision
    - Distortion
  - Signs
    - Perifoveal telangiectatic capillaries
    - Drained by right angled veins
    - Secondary exudation, pigmentary changes or CNVM
    - Classification
      - Group 1
        - Unilateral temporal telangiectasia with secondary exudation
        - Occurs mainly in young males
      - Group 2
        - Bilateral temporal telangiectasia with secondary exudation
        - Occurs in middle aged men and women
      - Group 3
        - Rare form with progressive capillary closure and enlargement of FAZ
- Investigations
  - Fluorescein angiography
    - Telangiectasia in the temporal macula with secondary leakage
- Management
  - Observation
  - Laser photocoagulation
  - Intravitreal steroids

Figure 13-19. Horseshoe peripheral retinal tear.

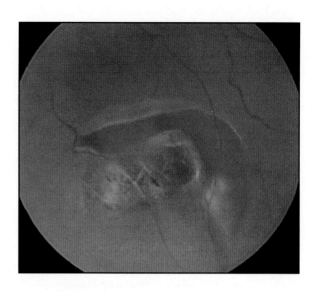

Peripheral Retinal Disorders

Posterior Vitreous Detachment and Retinal Tears

- Epidemiology
  - Prevalence
    - Increases with age
- Clinical features
  - Symptoms
    - Floaters
    - Flashes
  - Signs
    - Weiss ring: Round condensation of cortical vitreous anterior to the optic nerve
    - Vitreous pigment
      - Highly predictive of patients with retinal tear associated with PVD
    - Retinal tear (Figure 13-19)
- Management
  - Observation
    - Between 10% and 15% of patients have a retinal tear associated with acute PVD.
    - Within 6 weeks of follow up, 2% will develop a retinal tear.
  - Retinopexy
    - Indications
      - Untreated symptomatic retinal tears have a high risk of progression to retinal detachment.
    - Methods
      - Laser retinopexy
      - Cryopexy in cases with vitreous hemorrhage

Lattice Degeneration

- Epidemiology
  - Prevalence
    - Approximately 10% of general population
  - Risk factors
    - Myopia
    - Family history

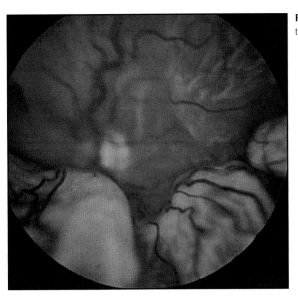

Figure 13-20. Total retinal detachment. Retina is elevated and translucent due to edema.

- Clinical features
  - Signs
    - Oval lesions located between the equator and ora serrata
    - Overlying vitreous liquefaction with adherent vitreous at margins
    - White "lattice" lines
    - Secondary atrophic retinal holes
- Management
  - Observation
    - While lattice is present in about 20% of retinal detachments, the risk of lattice to an individual patient is low (about 1% lifetime).
  - Laser retinopexy
    - Indications
      - Symptomatic tear in lattice
      - Atrophic hole with increasing subretinal fluid
      - Prophylaxis of fellow eye with retinal detachment
        - May be considered in patients with extensive areas of lattice
        - Frequently, retinal breaks occur in areas outside of clinically evident lattice

Retinal Detachment

- Epidemiology
  - Incidence
    - 1/10,000 population/year
  - Risk factors
    - Myopia
      - Lifetime risk increases with increasing degrees of axial myopia
    - Aphakia
    - Pseudophakia
      - Higher rate in patients with vitreous loss
    - Lattice degeneration
- Clinical features (Figure 13-20)
  - Symptoms
    - Flashes
    - Floaters
    - Progressive visual field defect

- Signs
  - IOP
    - May be lower than normal
    - Some cases have elevated IOP due to obstruction of trabecular meshwork by photore-ceptor outer segments
  - Vitreous
    - Vitreous pigment
  - Retinal break
    - Atrophic hole
      - More prevalent in myopic retinal detachment in young patients
    - Horse shoe tear
      - More common in middle-aged patients with PVD
  - Retinal detachment (RD)
    - Translucent, mobile, elevated retina
- Management
  - Pneumatic retinopexy
    - Indications
      - Retinal break in the superior 8 clock hours
      - Retinal breaks within 1 clock hour of each other
      - No significant PVR
    - Methods
      - Intravitreal injection of gas
      - Sulfur hexafluoride (SF6): Volume doubles, lasts 10 to 14 days
      - Perfluoropropane (C3F8): Volume quadruples, lasts about 30 days
    - Results
      - Pneumatic Retinopexy Trial
      - Similar success rate to scleral buckle
        - Single procedure success rate 80% to 85%
      - Possible higher rate of VA >20/50
  - Scleral buckle
    - Indications
      - Retinal detachment
      - Proliferative vitreoretinopathy
    - Methods
      - Silicone rubber or silicone sponge exoplant
      - Buckle may be segmental in the area of retinal pathology or encircle the entire globe
    - Results
      - Single procedure success rate of 85%
    - Complications
      - Infection
      - Diplopia
      - Increased myopia
  - Vitrectomy
    - Indications
      - Recurrent retinal detachment with proliferative vitreoretinopathy
      - Primary vitrectomy for pseudophakic RD
      - Primary vitrectomy for phakic RD with large or posterior breaks
    - Methods
      - May be combined with scleral buckle procedure
    - Results
      - Single procedure success rate is more than 85%.
    - Complications
      - Cataract progression in phakic patients

TABLE 13-1 DIFFERENTIATING FEATURES OF RETINAL DETACHMENT VERSUS RETINOSCHISIS

	RETINAL DETACHMENT	*RETINOSCHISIS*
Transparency	Little	Very
Mobility	Yes	No
Surface	Undulations	Smooth
Visual field	Relative	Absolute
Laser spot test	Negative	Positive

Retinoschisis

- Epidemiology
  - Prevalence
    - Affects 5% to 10% of population
- Clinical features
  - Symptoms
    - Typically asymptomatic
    - Visual field testing may show absolute scotoma.
  - Signs
    - 70% located inferotemporal
    - Smooth, nonmobile, transparent inner layer elevation of retina
    - Yellow dots believed to be Müller cell footplates
    - Outer layer has beaten metal appearance and may demonstrate white with pressure during scleral depression.
    - Breaks
      - Outer layer breaks tend to be large oval breaks.
      - Inner layer breaks are small and more numerous.
- Differentiation from retinal detachment (Table 13-1)
  - Most cases are differentiated on clinical examination.
  - In difficult cases, application of laser to the area in question can be helpful.
    - In retinoschisis, the outer retinal layer is attached to the RPE, and, therefore, laser produces a visible spot unlike detached retina, which cannot be lasered.
- Management
  - Observation
  - Surgery
    - Required in cases of secondary retinal detachment

Tumors of the Posterior Pole

Choroidal Nevus

- Epidemiology
  - Prevalence
    - Approximately 10% of the population
- Clinical features
  - Symptoms
    - Asymptomatic
    - Distortion with subretinal fluid

Figure 13-21. Elevated pigmented choroidal mass due to choroidal melanoma.

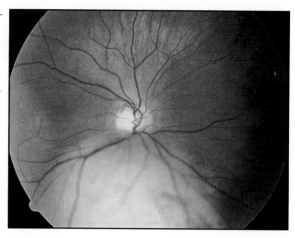

- o Signs
  - ▪ Flat slate gray pigmentation
  - ▪ Thickness less than 2 mm
  - ▪ Overlying changes
    - □ Subretinal fluid
    - □ Orange pigment
    - □ Drusen
- • Management
  - o Observation
    - ▪ Factors suggestive of progression to melanoma
      - □ Thickness >2 mm
      - □ Orange pigment
      - □ Subretinal fluid
      - □ Adjacent to optic nerve

Choroidal Melanoma

- • Epidemiology
  - o Incidence
    - ▪ 6/million per year
- • Clinical features
  - o Symptoms
    - ▪ Asymptomatic
    - ▪ Decreased vision secondary to retinal detachment, unilateral cataract, glaucoma
    - ▪ Blind painful eye
  - o Signs
    - ▪ Subretinal pigmented mass (Figure 13-21)
      - □ Dome-shaped elevation
      - □ Mushroom-shaped with penetration of Bruch's membrane
    - ▪ Subretinal fluid
- • Management
  - o Observation
    - ▪ Indications
      - □ Small melanoma
    - ▪ Prognosis
      - □ By 7 years, 33% have been treated with enucleation or plaque therapy.
      - □ Has a 5-year melanoma specific mortality rate of 1%

- o Plaque therapy
  - Indications
    - □ Medium-sized melanoma
  - Treatment methods
    - □ External iodine 125 plaque therapy
  - Prognosis
    - □ Collaborative Ocular Melanoma Study compared plaque therapy to enucleation.
    - □ No difference in 5-year melanoma-specific mortality (approximately 10%)
    - □ VA declines secondary to radiation effects.
      - Median enrollment VA 20/30
      - In 3-year follow up median acuity 20/125
- o Enucleation
  - Indications
    - □ Large melanoma
    - □ Total retinal detachment
    - □ Secondary glaucoma

Choroidal Hemangioma

- Etiology
  - o Circumscribed hemangiomas appear as isolated lesions.
  - o Diffuse hemangiomas are typically associated with Sturge Weber syndrome.
- Clinical features
  - o Symptoms
    - Asymptomatic
    - Decrease vision due to tumor exudation
  - o Signs
    - Circumscribed
      - □ Discrete, smooth tumor that is reddish orange in color
      - □ Located typically posterior to the equator
      - □ Secondary exudation with serous retinal detachment, CME, and lipid exudation
    - Diffuse
      - □ Large, flat lesions extending to large areas of fundus
      - □ Produces "tomato ketchup fundus"
- Investigations
  - o Fluorescein angiography
    - Large vascular spaces fill with choroids producing a mottled appearance with late leakage
  - o Ultrasound
    - Choroidal mass with high internal reflectivity
- Management
  - o Indications
    - Exudative complications
  - o Methods
    - Laser photocoagulation
    - PDT

Endophthalmitis

- Epidemiology
  - o Incidence
    - 0.11% penetrating keratoplasty
    - 0.072% cataract extraction
    - 0.062% glaucoma surgery
    - 0.051% pars plana vitrectomy
    - 0.05% intravitreal injection

- o Time of onset
  - ▪ Average 6 days post operatively
- o Risk factors
  - ▪ Posterior capsule rupture
    - ▫ Vitreous provides media for bacterial proliferation
- Etiology
  - o In the Endophthalmitis Vitrectomy Study (EVS)
    - ▪ 70% staphylococcus epidermidis
    - ▪ 10% staphylococcus aureus
    - ▪ 9% streptococcus
    - ▪ 2% enterococcus
    - ▪ 6% gram negative
  - o Bleb associated endophthalmitis
    - ▪ Delayed onset from surgery
    - ▪ Streptococcus is the classic pathogen
  - o Post intravitreal injection
    - ▪ Appears to have higher rate of streptococcal infections
- Clinical features
  - o Symptoms
    - ▪ Blurred vision (95% of EVS patients)
    - ▪ Red eye (82% of EVS patients)
    - ▪ Pain (75% of EVS patients)
    - ▪ Swollen upper lid (35% of EVS patients)
  - o Signs
    - ▪ Vision
      - ▫ Vision is decreased
      - ▫ EVS presentation
        - • 26% light perception
        - • 44% hand motion
        - • 16% <5/200
        - • 14% >5/200
    - ▪ Pupils
      - ▫ Afferent pupillary defect is predictor of poorer outcome and infection more likely to be non staph epidermidis
    - ▪ Lid
      - ▫ Upper lid swelling
    - ▪ Cornea
      - ▫ May have corneal infiltrate or ring ulcer in severe cases
    - ▪ Anterior chamber
      - ▫ Hypopyon
    - ▪ Vitreous
      - ▫ Vitreous haze
      - ▫ 80% of EVS patients had no view of the posterior pole
      - ▫ 23% had red reflex in EVS
    - ▪ Retina
      - ▫ Vasculitis
      - ▫ Intraretinal hemorrhages
- Management
  - o Prevention
    - ▪ Povidone iodine
    - ▪ Meticulous sterile surgical technique
    - ▪ Routine use of prophylactic antibiotics has not been shown to clearly reduce the risk of endopthalmitis
  - o Treatment
    - ▪ Intravitreal antibiotics
      - ▫ The EVS demonstrated that post cataract surgery endophthalmitis could be managed with intravitreal antibiotics

- Most commonly used antibiotics are:
  - Vancomycin 1.0 mg in 0.1 ml saline
  - Ceftazidime 2.25 mg in 0.1 ml saline
- Vitrectomy
  - Vitrectomy is utilized to clear vitreous debris.
  - The EVS demonstrated no benefit to vitrectomy/intravitreal antibiotics over vitreous tap/intravitreal antibiotics
  - A subgroup of patients presenting with light perception or worse visual acuity had improved visual outcome with vitrectomy.
- Systemic antibiotics
  - EVS did not demonstrate visual benefit to the routine use of intravenous antibiotics (ceftazidime and amikacin).
  - There may be some role of the use of oral fourth generation fluoroquinolones due to better vitreous penetration.
- Adjuvant corticosteroids
  - Controversial
  - No clear evidence that corticosteroids improve visual outcomes and some evidence that they may be harmful

Laser Techniques

Laser Theory

- Majority of retinal laser treatment is performed by photocoagulation.
- Laser energy raises tissue temperature.
- Absorption properties of tissues determine which wavelength may be optimal.
  - Pigment and hemoglobin absorb green and yellow light best.
  - Red light is less absorbed by blood and therefore may be preferable in cases of extensive vitreous or subretinal hemorrhage.

Practical Applications of Laser Treatment

- Delivery system
  - Slit lamp
    - Contact lens allows visualization of retina.
    - Macular contact lens
      - A –60 D lens that produces a virtual upright image of macula
      - High detailed view but limited field
    - High plus lens
      - Produce real inverted fundus image
        - Low magnification lenses allow peripheral view.
          - Minified view results in spot size magnification.
        - Higher magnification lenses are used for macular treatment.
          - Wider field of view than traditional contact lens
  - Indirect laser
    - Spot size is variable with the power of the condensing lens, the patient's refractive status, and the distance from the patient to the physician.
      - Spot size
        - Macular treatment: 50 to 100 µm
        - Peripheral treatment: 100 to 500 µm
      - Burn intensity
        - Lower-intensity burns are typically used for focal macular laser.
        - Moderate-intensity burns are used for PRP or peripheral retinopexy.
        - Heavy burns are used for ablative treatments for CNVM.

Suggested Readings

BRVO Study Group. Argon laser scatter photocoagulation for prevention of neovascularization and vitreous hemorrhage in branch vein occlusion. *Arch Ophthalmol.* 1986;104:34–41.

COMS. The COMS randomized trial of I125 brachytherapy for choroidal melanoma I: visual acuity after 3 years. COMS Report No. 16. *Ophthalmology.* 2001;108:348–366.

CRVO Study Group. A randomized trial of early photocoagulation for ischemic CRVO. *Ophthalmology.* 1995;102:1434–1444.

de Bustros S, Thompson JT, Michels RG, Rice TA, Glaser BM. Vitrectomy for idiopathic epiretinal membranes causing macular pucker. *Br J Ophthalmol.* 1988;72(9):692–695.

Diabetic Retinopathy Study Group. Indications for photocoagulation. Report #14. *Int Ophthalmol Clin.* 1987;27(4):239–253.

Freeman WR, Azen SP, Kim JW, el-Haig W, Mishell DR 3rd, Bailey I. Vitrectomy for the treatment of full thickness stage 3 or 4 macular holes. *Arch Ophth.* 1997;115:11–21.

Hawkins BS, Bressler NM, Bressler SB, et al, Submacular Surgery Trials Research Group. Surgical removal vs. observation for subfoveal choroidal neovascularization, either associated with the ocular histoplasmosis syndrome or idiopathic: I. Ophthalmic findings from a randomized clinical trial: Submacular Surgery Trials (SST) Group H Trial: SST Report No. 9. *Arch Ophthalmol.* 2004;122:1597–1611.

Klein R, Klein B, Moss SE, et al. The Wisconsin Epidemiologic Study of Diabetic Retinopathy XIV: 10 year incidence and progression of diabetic retinopathy. *Arch Ophthalmol.* 1994;112:1217–1228.

Macular Photocoagulation Study. Laser photocoagulation of subfoveal neovascular lesions in age related macular degeneration. *Arch Ophthalmol.* 1991;109:1220–1231.

The Choroidal Neovascularization Prevention Trial Research Group. Laser treatment in eyes with large drusen. Short term effects seen in a pilot randomized clinical trial. *Ophthalmology.* 1998;105:11–23.

Questions

1. Which of the following statements about indocyanine green dye is *false*?
   a. ICG is highly protein bound.
   b. Classic choroidal neovascular membranes leak significantly in the late frames of the angiogram.
   c. Long wavelength emission of ICG allows penetration through blood and PED.
   d. Scanning laser imaging allows creation of a real-time ICG angiogram.

2. The B wave of the ERG
   a. Is a negative deflection
   b. Can indicate outer retinal dysfunction
   c. Is dependent upon an intact A wave
   d. Results from the photoreceptors

3. RP is associated with all *except*
   a. Anterior subcapsular cataract
   b. Waxy pallor of the optic nerve
   c. Intraretinal pigment migration
   d. CME

4. Which of the following statements regarding dry macular degeneration is *true*?
   a. The 5-year incidence of progression to wet AMD in patients with bilateral drusen is greater than 50%.
   b. Beta carotene supplementation is an important component of therapy in smokers with dry AMD.
   c. Laser treatments reduce the number of observed drusen, but long-term safety remains a concern.
   d. Lutein is a well-demonstrated beneficial supplement in the treatment of dry AMD.

5. Current treatment for choroidal neovascularization in patients with macular degeneration includes which of the following:
   a. Focal laser ablation of CNVM
   b. PDT
   c. Intravitreal anti-VEGF therapy
   d. Combination therapy
   e. All of the above

6. An 80-year-old woman presenting with 20/100 VA and intraretinal hemorrhage, CME with extensive drusen is most likely to also have
   a. A focal hot spot on ICG
   b. A classic CNVM on fluorescein angiogram
   c. A primary subretinal focus of neovascularization
   d. A low 3-year risk of occurrence in the fellow eye

7. The following statements about macular holes are correct *except*
   a. Trauma is the most common cause of macular holes.
   b. Large macular holes have the best visual prognosis.
   c. Stage 3 macular holes are associated with a PVD.
   d. Vitreomacular traction typically precedes hole formation.

8. Clinically significant macular edema in diabetic retinopathy is defined as
   a. Retinal thickening within 500 μm of center of FAZ
   b. Hard exudates within 500 μm from center of FAZ associated with retinal thickening
   c. Retinal thickening more than 1 disc diameter within 1 disc diameter of the center of the FAZ
   d. All of the above

9. High-risk proliferative diabetic retinopathy is characterized by all *except*
   a. Neovascularization more than 2 disc diameters located at the superotemporal arcade
   b. Neovascularization 1.5 disc diameters located at the inferotemporal arcade with vitreous hemorrhage
   c. Neovascularization more than 0.5 disc diameter on the optic nerve
   d. Neovascularization less than 0.25 disc diameter on the optic nerve with vitreous hemorrhage

10. The indications for pneumatic retinopexy include the following:

    (1) Retinal break in the superior 8 clock hours

    (2) Retinal breaks within 1 clock hour of each other

    (3) No significant PVR

    a. (1) and (2)
    b. (2) and (3)
    c. (3) only
    d. (1), (2), and (3)

Common Abbreviations in Ophthalmology

A/C or AC	Anterior chamber
ACG	Angle closure glaucoma
ALT	Argon laser trabeculoplasty (for glaucoma)
AMD	Age-related macular degeneration
ANA	Antinuclear antibody
APD	Afferent pupillary defect
AVM	Arteriovenous malformation
BCa, BCC	Basal cell cancer (carcinoma)
BCVA	Best corrected visual acuity
BCDA	Best corrected distance acuity
BRVO	Branch retinal vein occlusion
c or cc	With refractive correction
C:D	Cup-to-disc ratio of the optic nerve
CF	Count fingers visual acuity
CTL	Contact lenses
CME	Cystoid macular edema
CRAO	Central retinal artery occlusion
CRVO	Central retinal vein occlusion
CSR or CSCR	Central serous chorioretinopathy
CSF	Cerebrospinal fluid
CVF	Confrontation visual field
cyl	Cylinder (in refraction)
D	Diopter
DCR	Dacryocystorhinostomy
DVD	Dissociated vertical deviation (a form of strabismus)
ECCE c IOL	Extracapsular cataract extraction with intraocular lens implantation
EOG	Electrooculogram
ERG	Electroretinogram
EOM	Extraocular muscle
ERM	Epiretinal membrane
ET, E(T), E, E'	Esotropia, intermittent esotropia, esophoria, and esophoria at near
FA	Fluorescein angiogram
HAART	Highly active antiretroviral therapy
HLA	Human leukocyte antigen
HM	Hand motion vision
HRT	Heidelberg retinal tomograph
I/A	Irrigation/aspiration
ICCE	Intracapsular cataract extraction
ICG	Indocyanine green
Ig	Immunoglobulin
IK	Interstitial keratitis
IM	Intramuscular
INH	Isoniazid
IO	Inferior oblique
IOL	Intraocular lens
IOOA	Inferior oblique overaction
IOP	Intraocular pressure
IR	Inferior rectus
IV	Intravenous
K	Keratometer reading (measures the curvature of the cornea), or abbreviation for cornea
KCS	Keratoconjunctivitis sicca
KP	Keratic precipitate
LHT, RHT	Left hypertropia and right hypertropia
LPI	Laser peripheral iridectomy
LP	Light perception
LR	Lateral rectus
MR	Manifest (noncyclopleged) refraction
NLP	No light perception
NPDR	Nonproliferative diabetic retinopathy
NS or NSC	Nuclear sclerotic cataract
NTG	Normotension glaucoma
NVA	Neovascularization of the angle
NVD	Neovascularization of the disc
NVE	Neovascularization of the retina elsewhere (outside the disc)
NVI	Neovascularization of iris
OD, OS, OU	Right eye, left eye, both eyes
OHT	Ocular hypertension
PAS	Peripheral anterior synechiae

Probst LE, Tsai JH.
Ophthalmology: Clinical and Surgical Principles (pp. 523–524).
© 2012 SLACK Incorporated

PC	Posterior chamber or posterior capsule	RPE	Retinal pigment epithelium
PD	Prism diopters	s or sc	Without refractive correction
PE, PHACO	Phacoemulsification	SCTL, EWSCTL	Soft and extended wear
PEE	Punctate epithelial erosions	SLE	Slit lamp exam
PEK	Punctate epithelial keratitis or keratopathy	SPK	Superficial punctate keratitis
PERL	Pupils equal and reactive to light	SR	Superior rectus
		SRN, SRNVM	Subretinal neovascular membrane
PF, PA 1%	Pred Forte eye drops, prednisolone acetate	Ta	Applanation tonometry
		T ½, T ¼	Timoptic (with concentrations)
PH	Pinhole	UCVA	Uncorrected visual acuity
PKP or PK	Penetrating keratoplasty (cornea transplant)	UCDA	Uncorrected distance acuity
		Va	Visual acuity
POAG	Primary open angle glaucoma	VDRL	Venereal Disease Research Laboratory
POHS	Presumed ocular histoplasmosis syndrome	VF	Visual field
		vit	Vitreous
PRP	Panretinal photocoagulation	VTX	Vitrectomy
PSC	Posterior subcapsular cataract	W4D	Worth 4 dot test (in strabismus)
PVD	Posterior vitreous detachment	XT, X(T)	Exotropia, intermittent exotropia
RD	Retinal detachment	X, X′	Exophoria, exophoria at near
RF	Rheumatoid factor	YAG	Neodymium-yttrium aluminum garnet laser
ROP	Retinopathy of prematurity		
RP	Retinitis pigmentosa	Δ	Prism diopter

Financial Disclosures

Dr. *Peter Bergenske* is an employee of Alcon Laboratories, Inc., a division of Novartis AG.

Dr. *Catherine M. Birt* has acted as a consultant and/or speaker for Alcon, Allergan, Merck Frosst, and Pfizer.

Dr. *Louis C. Blumenfeld* is a consultant/equity owner for Pediavision.

Dr. *Paul Ernest* has no financial or proprietary interest in the materials presented herein.

Dr. *Thomas J. Federici* has no financial or proprietary interest in the materials presented herein.

Dr. *Robert S. Gold* receives lecture fees from Alcon Laboratories and Bausch and Lomb, Inc.; is a consultant for Bausch and Lomb, Inc., Pediavision, and Quest Medical; and is an equity owner in Pediavision.

Dr. *George Goodman* has no financial or proprietary interest in the materials presented herein.

Dr. *Khalid Hasanee* has no financial or proprietary interest in the materials presented herein.

Dr. *Edward J. Holland* receives grant support from Abbott Medical Optics, Alcon Laboratories, Inc., QLT Phototherapeutics, Inc., and Wavetec Vision Systems, Inc. Dr. Holland also receives lecture fees from Alcon Laboratories, Inc., Allergan, and Bausch & Lomb. In addition, Dr. Holland is a consultant for Abbott Medical Optics, Advanced Vision Research, Inc., Alcon Laboratories, Inc., Allergan, Bausch & Lomb, QLT Phototherapeutics, Inc., Senju Pharmaceutical Co., LTD., and Wavetec Vision Systems, Inc.

Dr. *T. Mark Johnson* has no financial or proprietary interest in the materials presented herein.

Dr. *Jemshed A. Khan* has no financial or proprietary interest in the materials presented herein.

Dr. *Andrew G. Lee* has no financial or proprietary interest in the materials presented herein.

Dr. *Irmingard Neuhann* has no financial or proprietary interest in the materials presented herein.

Dr. *Thomas Neuhann* has no financial or proprietary interest in the materials presented herein.

Dr. *Louis E. Probst* is a consultant for Abbott Medical Optics and TLCVision.

Dr. *Paul Rafuse* is a speaker for Merck and Alcon and is a consultant and speaker for Pfizer and Allergan.

Dr. *Naval Sondhi* has not disclosed any relevant financial relationships.

Dr. *Jeff Steeves* has no financial or proprietary interest in the materials presented herein.

Dr. *Julie H. Tsai* has no financial or proprietary interest in the materials presented herein.

Financial Disclosures

Index

Wait...There's More!

SLACK Incorporated's Health Care Books and Journals offers a wide selection of books in the field of Ophthalmology. We are dedicated to providing important works that educate, inform and improve the knowledge of our customers. Don't miss out on our other informative titles that will enhance your collection.

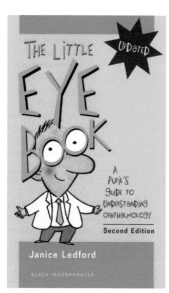

The Little Eye Book: A Pupil's Guide to Understanding Ophthalmology, Second Edition
Janice K. Ledford, COMT

192 pp., Soft Cover, 2008
ISBN 13 978-1-55642-884-5
Order# 68845, **$25.95**

The Little Eye Book: A Pupil's Guide to Understanding Ophthalmology is an easy-to-understand introduction to the field of eye care that has been updated into a new Second Edition. This book is written with the non-physician in mind, so you won't be bogged down with heavy details, yet every basic fact that you need is right here. With photographs as well as drawings and helpful tables and charts, this conversational-style text packs a big punch.

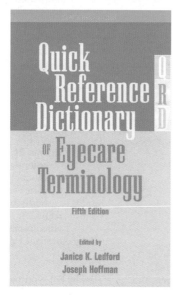

Quick Reference Dictionary of Eyecare Terminology, Fifth Edition
Janice K. Ledford, COMT; Joseph Hoffman

504 pp., Soft Cover, 2008
ISBN 13 978-1-55642-805-0
Order# 68057, **$41.95**

Compact, concise, and informative, *Quick Reference Dictionary of Eyecare Terminology, Fifth Edition,* provides quick access to over 3,700 terms and their definitions, including over 400 new words. This pocket-sized companion also contains 25 appendices. Additionally, pronunciations have been added—an attribute users are sure to appreciate.

Please visit **www.slackbooks.com** to order any of the above titles!

24 Hours a Day...7 Days a Week!

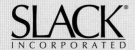